QUALITY IN HEALTHCARE

Corinne M. Karuppan, PhD, CPIM, is professor emerita of operations management at Missouri State University. She continues to teach quality measurement and management in healthcare in the MHA program. For over 25 years, she taught business process management and management science. Her work has been published in the *Journal of Operations Management*, *Production and Operations Management*, *International Journal of Operations and Production Management*, *European Journal of Information Systems*, *Journal of Healthcare Management*, *Journal of Emergency Nursing*, and *Disability and Rehabilitation*. Dr. Karuppan is currently one of the area editors of *Operations Management Research*. She co-authored *Operations Management in Healthcare: Strategy and Practice*, Second Edition (Springer Publishing, 2022).

Corinne holds a BA in Langues Étrangères Appliquées from the University of Lille III (France), an MBA from Creighton University, and a PhD in business administration from the University of Nebraska–Lincoln. She is certified in production and inventory management by the Association for Operations Management (APICS).

Nancy E. Dunlap, MD, PhD, MBA, is professor emerita of medicine at the University of Alabama at Birmingham (UAB). She practiced medicine in the field of pulmonary critical care for over 25 years and held executive positions in two academic medical centers, most recently as dean of the School of Medicine at the University of Virginia. She served as vice president for ambulatory services of the UAB Health System and chief operating officer of the Kirklin Clinic, the faculty practice site for UAB. Nancy participated in the Robert Wood Johnson Foundation Health Fellowship Program and served as physician-in-residence at the Center for Best Practices at the National Governor's Association in Washington, D.C. Throughout her career, she has worked to improve healthcare quality and outcomes through more efficient patient care delivery processes and information technology. Nancy holds an MD from Duke University School of Medicine, a PhD in microbiology from the University of Alabama at Birmingham, and an MBA from the University of Michigan.

Robert Cavagnol, MD, MHA, FACS, currently serves as the president of the North region for Froedtert-Thedacare Health (FTCH). In this capacity, he is the accountable executive for the overall strategic direction and operational execution of all elements of the nine-hospital health system in Northeastern Wisconsin. Prior to joining FTCH, Dr. Cavagnol served as the president of St. Luke's Clinic based in Boise, Idaho, leading the physician enterprise composed of 1,600 providers across the health system.

Dr. Cavagnol received his bachelor's degree in health sciences from Kalamazoo College and his medical degree from Wayne State University, School of Medicine. He completed his surgical training at the University of Cincinnati. Following his general surgery residency, Dr. Cavagnol spent 3 years on active duty with the U.S. Navy, stationed at Camp Lejeune, North Carolina. During his naval career, Dr. Cavagnol deployed twice, first on the hospital ship *USNS Comfort* in support of the humanitarian relief after Hurricane Katrina, and then as a trauma surgeon to Fallujah, Iraq, in support of Operation Iraqi Freedom.

After completing his commitment to the Navy, Dr. Cavagnol joined Mercy Health System in Springfield, Missouri, as a practicing general surgeon. He attended Missouri State University during his time with Mercy and earned a master's in healthcare administration. While at Mercy, he was recognized with the Young Physician of the Year award in his third year with the health system. He also held numerous leadership positions with Mercy including medical director of patient safety and quality, section chair for general surgery, vice president of surgery, chief physician officer, and president for the Mercy Springfield clinic.

QUALITY IN HEALTHCARE

A Lean Six Sigma Project Approach

Corinne M. Karuppan, PhD, CPIM

Nancy E. Dunlap, MD, PhD, MBA

Robert Cavagnol, MD, MHA, FACS

SPRINGER PUBLISHING

Springer Publishing Company, LLC
902 Carnegie Center/Suite 140, Princeton, NJ 08540
www.springerpub.com
connect.springerpub.com

Acquisitions Editor: David D'Addona
Production Editor: Joe Stubenrauch
Compositor: S4Carlisle Publishing Services

ISBN: 978-0-8261-7975-3
e-book ISBN: 978-0-8261-7976-0
DOI: 10.1891/9780826179760

SUPPLEMENTS:

SPRINGER PUBLISHING CONNECT™ | A robust set of instructor resources designed to supplement this text is located at **http://connect.springerpub.com/content/book/978-0-8261-7976-0.** Qualifying instructors may request access by emailing **textbook@springerpub.com**.

Instructor Materials:
LMS Common Cartridge—With All Instructor Resources ISBN: 978-0-8261-8343-9
Instructor Manual ISBN: 978-0-8261-7977-7
Instructor Test Bank ISBN: 978-0-8261-7982-1
Instructor PowerPoints ISBN: 978-0-8261-7979-1
Instructor Sample Syllabus ISBN: 978-0-8261-7978-4
Instructor Data Files ISBN: 978-0-8261-8858-8

Student Materials:
Student Resources ISBN: 978-0-8261-7981-4
Interview Video Transcripts ISBN: 978-0-8261-5182-7
Excel Tutorial Video Transcripts ISBN: 978-0-8261-7983-8

25 26 27 28/ 5 4 3 2 1

Library of Congress Control Number: 2024061499

To all the healthcare workers who commit their lives in service to others in the spirit of promoting health and wellness

CONTENTS

Preface *xix*
Tutorial Video List *xxiii*
On The Job! Interview Video List *xxv*
Resources *xxvii*

PART I. INTRODUCTION

1. Quality First *3*

Learning Objectives ***3***
Introduction ***3***
The Long Pursuit of Value-Based Care ***4***
Current Threats to Value-Based Care ***4***
High Costs *4*
Inadequate Quality *7*
Errors *7*
Variation *7*
Approaches to Increasing Value ***8***
The Six Aims *8*
Care Delivery Models *9*
New Opportunities *10*
Systems Thinking *12*
The Strategic Importance of Quality ***12***
What to Do *12*
SWOT Analysis *13*
How to Do It *14*
The Cumulative Model: Quality First *17*
What Is a Process? ***18***
Processes Are Everywhere *19*
Total Quality Management ***19***
Deming Wheel *20*
Deming's 14 Points *20*
Point #1: Create Constancy of Purpose Toward Improvement *21*
Point #2: Adopt the New Philosophy *21*
Point #3: Cease Dependence on Inspection to Achieve Quality *21*
Point #4: End the Practice of Awarding Business on the Basis of Price Tag Alone *21*
Point #5: Improve Constantly and Forever the System of Production and Service *21*
Point #6: Institute Training *21*
Point #7: Institute Leadership *21*
Point #8: Drive Out Fear *21*
Point #9: Break Down Barriers Between Departments *21*
Point #10: Eliminate Slogans Asking for Zero Defects and Unattainable Productivity *22*
Point #11: Eliminate the Emphasis on Numerical Quotas *22*
Point #12: Remove Barriers That Rob People of Pride of Workmanship *22*
Point #13: Institute a Vigorous Program of Education and Self-Improvement *22*
Point #14: Put Everybody in the Company to Work to Accomplish the Transformation *22*
Purpose and Focus of This Book ***22***
Summary ***26***
Key Terms ***26***
Review Questions ***26***
Learning Activities ***27***
References ***28***

2. Introduction to Lean Six Sigma: Doing It Right the First Time 32
Learning Objectives *32*
Introduction *33*
Lean *34*
Lean Culture *35*
Importance of Leadership and Training for Lean *35*
Waste Elimination *36*
Lean Principles *37*
Identify Value *37*
Map the Value Stream *38*
Create Flow *39*
Establish Pull *39*
Seek Perfection *41*
Shortcomings of Lean Implementations in Healthcare *42*
Six Sigma *43*
History of Six Sigma *44*
Principles of Six Sigma *44*
Define—What Is the Process? *45*
Measure—Where Is the Waste and How Bad Is It? *46*
Analyze—Why Is There Waste in the Process? *46*
Improve—How to Eliminate Waste? *47*
Control—How to Keep Waste at Bay? *49*
The A3 Report *50*
The Learning Culture in Six Sigma and Key Players *50*
Benefits of Lean and Six Sigma *52*
Summary *53*
Certification Tips *53*
Key Terms *54*
Review Questions *54*
Learning Activities *55*
References *55*

PART II. DEFINE—WHAT IS THE PROCESS?

3. Process Selection and Description 61
Learning Objectives *62*
Introduction *62*
Selecting a Project for Improvement *62*
Business Case for Action *63*
Benefits/Effort Matrix *64*
Describing the Process *65*
High-Level View *65*
Customers *67*
Patients' Perspectives *67*
Providers' Perspectives *67*
Third-Party Payers' Perspectives *68*
Accrediting Agencies *68*
Process Steps *68*
Process Modeling *69*
Flowchart *70*
Swimlane Diagram *72*
The 5W2H Framework *72*
Summary *76*
Certification Tips *76*
Key Terms *76*
Review Questions *77*
Solve Bright Angel Medical Center's Problems *77*
Learning Activities *79*
References *79*

4. The Voice of the Customer and the Voice of the Process *81*

Learning Objectives *81*
Introduction *82*
What Is Quality? *82*
The House of Quality **82**
The Kano Model *85*
The Critical-to-Quality Tree *87*
The Voice of the Customer *90*
Data Collection Methods *91*
Affinity Diagram *92*
Consumer Assessment of Healthcare Providers and Systems Survey Instrument *93*
SERVQUAL Survey Instrument *95*
The Voice of the Process *97*
Structure *97*
Process *98*
Outcomes *99*
The Vital Few *99*
Use of Quality Measures *100*
The Overall Hospital Quality Star Rating *100*
Hospital Value-Based Purchasing Program *101*
Leapfrog *101*
Benchmarking *102*
Balanced Scorecard *103*
Dashboards *104*
Building the A3 Report *108*
Summary *109*
Certification Tips *109*
Key Terms *110*
Review Questions *110*
Solve Bright Angel Medical Center Problems *111*
Learning Activities *113*
References *113*

Appendix 4.1 Basic Concepts of Questionnaire Design *116*
Introduction *116*
Questionnaire Development *116*
Translate the Data Requirements Into a Set of Questions *117*
Check the Questionnaire for Form, Relevance, Wording, Sequencing, Layout, and Appearance *117*
Form *117*
Relevance *117*
Wording *117*
Sequencing *118*
Appearance and Layout *118*
Pretest *119*
Reliability and Validity *119*
Reliability *119*
Construct Validity *120*
Key Terms *121*
Review Questions *121*
Problems *121*
Learning Activities *122*
References *122*

For More Advanced Content on Measurement System Analysis, see eChapter 15: Gage Repeatability and Reproducibility

5. Project Management 123
Learning Objectives 123
Introduction 123
What Is Project Management? 124
Project Charter and Roles 125
The Project Charter 125
The Project Manager 127
The Project Team 128
Characteristics of a Good Project Team 128
Employees in Functional Areas 128
Executives 128
Project Champions 128
Importance of Leadership in Project Management 129
Phases of a Project 131
Initiation 132
Planning 132
Execution 136
Control 136
Closure 137
The Critical Path Method 137
The Network Diagram 137
The Critical Path 139
The Activity Schedule 140
Computing Slack 143
Evaluating the Critical Path Method 145
Advantages 145
Disadvantages 145
Why Projects Fail 145
Team Dynamics and Communication 146
Summary 148
Certification Tips 148
Key Terms 148
Review Questions 148
Solve Bright Angel Medical Center's Problems 149
Learning Activities 152
References 153

PART III. MEASURE—WHERE IS THE WASTE AND HOW BAD IS IT?

6. Process Measurement 157
Learning Objectives 157
Introduction 157
Collecting Data 158
A Closer Look at Value-Added Activities and Waste 158
Value Stream Map 159
Process Activity Chart 164
Flow Process Chart 166
Yield 166
Check Sheet 170
Spaghetti Diagram 170
Building the A3 Report 171
Summary 174
Certification Tips 174
Key Terms 174
Review Questions 174
Solve Bright Angel Medical Center's Problems 174

Learning Activities *177*
References *178*

7. Data Visualization and Description *179*

Learning Objectives *179*
Introduction *179*
Types of Data Analytics *180*
Data Sets *181*
Measurement Levels *182*
Data Visualization Examples for Different Measurement Levels *183*
Nominal and Ordinal Data *183*
Bar Chart *183*
Pie and Doughnut Charts *184*
Interval and Ratio Data *186*
Histogram *186*
Line Chart *187*
Dashboard *189*
Population and Sample *190*
Probabilities *191*
Theoretical and Empirical Distributions *191*
Some Important Theoretical Distributions *193*
Discrete Distributions *193*
Continuous Distributions *195*
Measures of Central Tendency *198*
The Mode *198*
The Median *198*
The Mean *200*
Measures of Dispersion *200*
The Range *200*
The Variance *201*
The Standard Deviation *202*
The Standard Error *202*
Summary *203*
Certification Tips *203*
Key Terms *204*
Review Questions *204*
Solve Bright Angel Medical Center's Problems *205*
Learning Activities *208*
References *208*

For More Advanced Content on Probabilities and Distributions see eChapter 14: Expanded Coverage of Probabilities and Distributions

Appendix 7.1 Probability and Nonprobability Sampling *209*
Learning Objectives *209*
Introduction *209*
Probability Sampling *210*
Simple Random Sampling *210*
Simple Random Sampling Using Excel *213*
Proportionate Stratified Random Sampling *216*
Systematic Sampling *216*
Cluster Sampling *218*
Nonprobability Sampling *219*
Convenience Sampling *219*
Judgment Sampling *220*
Summary *221*
Certification Tips *221*
Key Terms *222*
Review Questions *222*

Solve Bright Angel Medical Center's Problems *222*
Learning Activity *223*

8. Process Stability and Capability *224*

Learning Objectives *224*
Introduction *224*
Variation *225*
Assignable Causes of Variation *225*
Common or Random Causes of Variation *226*
Fundamentals of Statistical Process Control *227*
The Centerline *228*
The Control Limits *228*
Process Control Charts *229*
Attribute or Variable *230*
Control Charts for Attributes *230*
p-*Charts* *230*
np-*Charts* *235*
c-*Charts* *236*
u-*Charts* *240*
Control Charts for Variables *243*
IX *and* MR *Charts* *243*
$\bar{X}$ *and* R *Charts* *249*
$\bar{X}$ *and* s-*Charts* *253*
Control Chart Patterns *255*
Pattern Tests *257*
Cumulative Sum Control Charts *257*
Process Capability *262*
Is the Process Distribution Too Wide? *263*
Is the Process Well Centered? *265*
Summary *267*
Certification Tips *267*
Key Terms *267*
Review Questions *268*
Solve Bright Angel Medical Center's Problems *268*
Learning Activities *274*
References *275*

Appendix 8.1 Factors for Control Charts *276*

For More Advanced Content on Measurement System Analysis, see eChapter 15: Gage Repeatability and Reproducibility

PART IV. ANALYZE—WHY IS THERE WASTE IN THE PROCESS?

9. Problem-Solving *279*

Learning Objectives *279*
Introduction *280*
Basic Tools *280*
Organizing the Team's Thoughts *280*
Cause-and-Effect Diagram *280*
Interrelationship Diagram *284*
Failure Mode and Effects Analysis *285*
Verifying Association Between Potential Cause and Effect *289*
Scatter Diagram *289*
Correlation Analysis *290*
Predicting the Effect of the Cause on the Problem *291*
Regression Analysis *291*

Simple Linear Regression *292*
Multiple Regression *295*
Prioritizing Causes ***297***
Pareto Chart *297*
Building the A3 Report ***298***
Summary ***300***
Certification Tips ***300***
Key Terms ***301***
Review Questions ***301***
Solve Bright Angel Medical Center's Problems ***301***
Learning Activities ***304***
References ***304***

For More Advanced Content on Confidence Intervals and Hypothesis Tests, see eChapter 16: Estimation and Hypothesis Testing

PART V. IMPROVE—HOW TO ELIMINATE WASTE?

10. Process Redesign (I): The Toolbox for Higher Value ***309***
Learning Objectives ***309***
Introduction ***309***
Secondary Sources of Information ***310***
Process Design ***311***
Design Principles ***312***
Principle #1: Reduce Fragmentation *312*
Flexible System *312*
Principle #2: Avoid Excessive Delegation *314*
Jidoka *314*
Total Productive Maintenance *314*
Principle #3: Capture the Information Once, at the Source *314*
Quality at the Source *314*
Principle #4: Perform Activities in Parallel Whenever Possible *315*
Principle #5: Link Parallel Activities Instead of Merely Integrating Their Output *315*
Principle #6: Design for the Mainstream, Not the Exceptions *316*
Standardization *316*
6S *316*
Workload Leveling (heijunka) *318*
Principle #7: Mistake-Proof the Process *319*
Checklists *319*
Principle #8: Optimize the Whole System and Stop Focusing on Local Optimization *320*
Principle #9: Eliminate Buffers *321*
Just-In-Time *321*
Undercapacity Scheduling *322*
Principle #10: Link Layout and Process *322*
The Relationship Between Process and Layout ***322***
Designing Product Layouts for Repetitive Processes *323*
Designing Functional Layouts for Nonrepetitive Processes *324*
Relationship Diagramming *325*
Cellular Layouts *325*
Theory of Constraints ***328***
Summary ***332***
Certification Tips ***332***
Key Terms ***332***
Review Questions ***332***
Solve Bright Angel Medical Center's Problems ***333***
Learning Activities ***335***
References ***335***

11. Process Redesign (II): Ensuring Success 337

Learning Objectives *337*
Introduction *337*
The Future State *338*
Value Stream Map *338*
Process Activity Chart *339*
General Process Chart *342*
Spaghetti Diagram *342*
Simulation *344*
Cost–Benefit Analysis *346*
Documenting the Improvement *351*
Process Activity Chart *351*
Statistical Process Control Charts *351*
Six Sigma Metrics *353*
Yield and Throughput Yield *353*
Sigma Level *356*
Dashboards *358*
Building the A3 Report *361*
Summary *363*
Certification Tips *363*
Key Terms *363*
Review Questions *363*
Solve Bright Angel Medical Center's Problems *364*
Learning Activities *366*
References *366*

PART VI. CONTROL—HOW TO KEEP WASTE AT BAY?

12. Sustaining the Improvement 371

Learning Objectives *371*
Introduction *372*
Documenting the New Process *372*
Control Plan *372*
Standard Operating Procedures *373*
Document Control *375*
Auditing *376*
Systematizing the Improvement *377*
Statistical Process Control (Revisited) *377*
6S (Revisited) *379*
Total Productive Maintenance *379*
Types of Maintenance *380*
Benefits of Total Productive Maintenance *380*
Visual Workplace *381*
Benefits of Visual Management *381*
Huddles *382*
Benefits of Huddles *383*
Institutionalizing the Improvement *383*
Quality Circles *383*
Rapid Process Improvement Workshops *384*
Benefits *384*
Closure: Lessons From the Project and Moving On *384*
Summary *387*
Certification Tips *387*
Key Terms *388*
Review Questions *388*
Learning Activities *388*
References *389*

PART VII. REAPING THE REWARDS AND BUILDING RESILIENCE

13. Accreditation, Awards, and the Highly Reliable Organization 393

Learning Objectives 394
Introduction 394
Accreditation 394
The Joint Commission 395
How Is Accreditation Achieved? 395
Priorities 396
Performance Measurement 396
Benefits of Accreditation 397
Det Norske Veritas 397
National Committee for Quality Assurance 398
Certification 399
The International Organization for Standardization 399
Malcolm Baldrige National Quality Award 400
Leadership 402
The Governing Body 404
The CEO and Other Senior Leaders 404
Strategy 404
Customers 405
Measurement, Analysis, and Knowledge Management 405
Workforce 405
Operations 405
Business/Organizational Performance Results 406
New Baldrige Award Criteria for 2024 407
The Highly Reliable Organization 407
Common Principles of Highly Reliable Organizations 408
The Importance of Mindfulness in Highly Reliable Organizations 411
Summary 413
Key Terms 413
Review Questions 413
Solve Bright Angel Medical Center's Problems 413
Learning Activities 414
References 414

eChapter Part VIII: Advanced Quality Management and Lean Six Sigma Project Tools (eChapters 14, 15, and 16) 415

Appendix A: Cumulative Standard Normal Distribution Table 417
Appendix B: Tool Kit 419
Index 425

Glossary The Glossary for this title may be accessed by visiting www.springerpub.com/courseconnect. See inside front cover and tear-out card for CourseConnect details.

PART VIII. ADVANCED QUALITY MANAGEMENT AND LEAN SIX SIGMA PROJECT TOOLS

eChapters 14, 15, and 16 are designed for students seeking more advanced Lean Six Sigma tools and content. To access Part VIII, visit www.springerpub.com/courseconnect. See inside front cover and tear-out card for CourseConnect details.

14. Expanded Coverage of Probabilities and Distributions

Learning Objectives
Introduction
Basic Probability Rules
- Mutually Exclusive Events
- Conditional Probability
- Independent Events

Other Continuous Distributions
- Student's *t*-Distribution
- Chi-Square Distribution
- *F*-Distribution

Summary
Certification Tips
Key Terms
Review Questions
Solve Bright Angel Medical Center's Problems
References

15. Gage Repeatability and Reproducibility

Learning Objectives
Introduction
Measurement Analysis
Gage Repeatability and Reproducibility
- Attribute Gage Repeatability and Reproducibility
- Variable Gage Repeatability and Reproducibility

Summary
Certification Tips
Key Terms
Review Questions
Solve Bright Angel Medical Center's Problems
Learning Activities
References

16. Estimation and Hypothesis Testing

Learning Objectives
Introduction
Estimation: Confidence Intervals
- Means
  - *Confidence Interval for the Mean (Sample Size Is Large)*
  - *Confidence Interval for the Mean (Sample Size Is Small)*
- Proportions

Hypothesis Testing
- One- or Two-Tailed Tests
- Type I and Type II Errors
- Tests of Means
  - *One-Sample Mean Test (Sample Size Is Large)*
  - *One-Sample Mean Test (Sample Size Is Small)*
  - *Two-Independent-Samples Mean Test*

Test of Means for More Than Two Independent Samples
Test of Means for Two Paired Samples
Tests of Proportions
One-Sample Test
Two-Independent-Samples Test
Nonparametric Tests
One Variable: Chi-Square Goodness-of-Fit Test
Multiple Variables: Chi-Square Test of Independence
Summary
Certification Tips
Key Terms
Review Questions
Solve Bright Angel Medical Center's Problems
Learning Activities
References

PREFACE

"We are what we repeatedly do. Excellence, then, is not an act, but a habit" (Aristotle).

It's all about the patient! In healthcare, excellence is thus the habit of exceeding patients' expectations. This requires an organizational culture that nurtures everyone's commitment to continuous improvement. It does take a village to produce outstanding care. A systems approach is therefore the only way to create and manage the conditions that make it hard, or nearly impossible, to fail and disappoint. More than ever, healthcare professionals must develop the skills to produce value for the patient, adapt to new demands, and navigate nimbly in a rapidly evolving environment. With its focus on Lean Six Sigma (LSS), this book is written for anyone dedicated to the relentless pursuit of value-based healthcare. As a result, it addresses the learning needs of a very diverse market: business students enrolled in curricula emphasizing healthcare (undergraduate and graduate), healthcare administration/public health students (undergraduate and graduate), nursing students (undergraduate and graduate), medical students and clinicians, allied health professionals, and administrators.

WHAT IS THE APPROACH OF THIS BOOK?

Facing pressures to improve quality while reining in costs, healthcare organizations must continuously rethink their way of delivering care. Over the past decades, they have increasingly turned to LSS to create better *value* along the care continuum. Some have boasted success, whereas others have failed miserably. To optimize the chances of success and avoid common pitfalls, this book steers learners through an LSS project from start to finish. Our team combines educators', clinicians', and administrators' viewpoints and uses a hands-on approach so that students can go from lecture to next-day execution at work.

From the start, the book emphasizes the strategic importance of quality in healthcare operations. It then integrates the concepts, tools, and techniques necessary to optimize flow and eliminate defects. To create a robust mental model of process improvements, we repeatedly illustrate how the tools work together to visualize, understand, analyze, and improve deficient productive systems. This synergy also demonstrates that progress does not have to be slow and linear, but rather can be accelerated through clear and cohesive communication.

To increase the relevance of the material in the real world, the book provides a solid foundation for the LSS Green Belt certification. Our focus is on the American Society for Quality's (ASQ) standards, but the material is applicable to the examination requirements of other certification bodies. Yet, we recognize that certification is not the primary objective of the course. Therefore, the book lends itself to three teaching styles:

- a qualitative approach emphasizing leadership, culture, and organizational and team dynamics;
- a quantitative approach focusing on tools and statistical techniques; or
- a mixed approach seeking a balance between qualitative and quantitative notions.

Finally, in order to bring the project and cultural context to life, we take you through an LSS project composed of a continuous series of short stories featuring the struggles and successes of a fictitious healthcare organization, *Bright Angel Medical Center*.

HOW IS THIS BOOK ORGANIZED?

The book follows the Six Sigma Define-Measure-Analyze-Improve-Control (DMAIC) framework.

1. **Introduction**

   This part defines value-based care. It identifies the obstacles to its implementation, but it also highlights avenues to make it a universal reality. The critical role of quality in a healthcare organization's operations strategy is demonstrated, and Deming's teachings provide the foundation for building quality into processes. Lean and Six Sigma principles are also presented, and the logic of their fusion is explained.

2. **Define—What Is the Process?**

   In this section, we identify which process is the best candidate for improvement and make a compelling argument for redesign. The process is described and depicted. Because customers decide what quality means to them, their voice is captured and then translated into process characteristics. These measures will be used for quality reporting, benchmarking, tracking progress, and mapping activities to strategic objectives. A project charter will be the roadmap for the approved improvement project, and a team will ensure that each phase of the project is well executed while meeting time and cost requirements.

3. **Measure—Where Is the Waste and How Bad Is It?**

   In this part, process data tell the story. Process measurements are incorporated into a depiction of the process from a Lean perspective. Value-added and non–value-added steps are identified, throughput yield is determined, and the layout is scrutinized for effectiveness and efficiency. Visualization of the data in graphical format promotes understanding and sets the stage for assessing the stability of the process and its capability to meet specifications. Several sampling techniques are discussed as well. Additional material on probabilities, distributions, and measurement system analysis for students or professionals seeking Six Sigma Green Belt certification can be found in the final part, Advanced Quality Management and Lean Six Sigma Project Tools. See list number eight for details on how to access this material.

4. **Analyze—Why Is There Waste in the Process?**

   Now that we know the locations and quantities of waste in the process, it is time to eliminate it or, at least, reduce it. However, to proceed, the root causes of defects, delays, and other types of waste must be uncovered. Several tools help accomplish this task. To make sure that the identified causes are indeed the factors creating waste, it is critical to verify the associations between causes and problems. Causes are then prioritized for elimination based on the magnitude of their impact. For any readers seeking Six Sigma Green Belt certification, additional material on data analysis (CIs and hypothesis testing) can also be found in the final part, Advanced Quality Management and Lean Six Sigma Project Tools.

5. **Improve—How to Eliminate Waste?**

   This is the most exciting phase of the project as the root causes of waste are removed and the process is redesigned. Simplification, standardization, mistake-proofing, and other LSS tools and techniques facilitate this endeavor. The layout is also rearranged to support the workflow and maximize safety. A visualization of the future state of the process provides a blueprint for the planned changes and may signal the need for adjustments or reconfigurations. Once the improvement is implemented, its benefits will be assessed and documented.

6. **Control—How to Keep Waste at Bay?**

   After improvement, it is easy to go back to the old ways of doing things. In order to sustain the improvement, the new process and procedures must be documented. Visual management, daily huddles, standard organization of the workplace, and maintenance responsibilities will help systematize the improvement. Because the pursuit of excellence never ends, employees will be continuously engaged in perfecting the system. The lessons learned during the project will shape the planning and implementation of future projects.

7. **Reaping the Rewards and Building Resilience**

   The concluding part covers the completion of a successful journey to excellence. It mentions the merits of accreditation but urges organizations to go beyond meeting the standards and become *highly reliable organizations*. The Malcolm Baldrige National Quality Award Framework is described, and the concepts covered in this book are mapped onto the framework. To conclude, we show how dedication to excellent quality engenders resilience.

8. **Advanced Quality Management and Lean Six Sigma Project Tools**

   This additional part provides advanced guidance on using LSS tools including an expanded coverage of probabilities and distributions, Gage repeatability and reproducibility, and estimation and hypothesis testing. These topic areas may not be covered in a traditional quality management course but are essential for anyone preparing for Six Sigma Green Belt certification and are found on the exam. The chapters in this part can be used in a course with advanced cohorts; if you are an instructor, you can find a sample course schedule for how to implement these additional chapters in your semester. If you are using the print book and want to dive into these tools, you can access these chapters by visiting www.springerpub.com/courseconnect. See inside front cover and tear-out card for CourseConnect details.

WHAT ARE THE PRIMARY FEATURES OF THIS BOOK?

The approach taken in this book is very practical and experiential. Not only should you learn the concepts and tools, but you should also be able to apply them in a variety of contexts. As a result, the tools are presented using step-by-step instructions and are fully integrated with the chapter materials. Most of our students have felt they were able to use these decision aids on the job right away.

To promote learning and reflection on important topics, the book includes the following features:

- **Complete process improvement project with A3 report** is weaved into the chapter materials through an interactive running case involving *Bright Angel Medical Center*. Each chapter starts with a project challenge that the protagonists overcome using the chapter material. The concepts, techniques, and story are intermixed, and you are asked to reflect on the issues confronting the characters.
- **Focus on careers and jobs** with interviews of healthcare professionals demonstrating their use of the chapter materials in a hospital. Discussion questions on the projects they oversaw foster engagement.
- **Ethical scenarios** are used to promote discussions about challenging decisions in a constantly changing healthcare environment.
- **FAQs** and their answers appear in boxed features within several chapters.
- **Extensive tool kit** is summarized in a table format in Appendix B.
- **Tutorial videos** demonstrating the use of selected tools and/or techniques and providing guided practice are offered.
- **Boxed features** (Quality in Practice!) are presented with real-world implementations of the various concepts and tools covered in the book.
- **Comprehensive and flexible coverage** of leadership, culture, organizational dynamics, tools, and statistical techniques is provided to accommodate a variety of learning emphases.
- **Certification tips** are offered for students seeking Six Sigma Green Belt certification.
- **Engaging end-of-chapter questions, problems, and learning activities**:
    - ***Review Questions:*** This section includes basic questions about the material covered in the chapter.
    - ***Solve Bright Angel Medical Center's Problems:*** Readers discuss/solve various problems faced by *Bright Angel Medical Center*. Numerous problems involving quantitative decision-making are provided in this section. Several data sets similar to those found in an actual hospital are provided.
    - ***Learning Activities:*** These include experiential activities involving ChatGPT, mock interviews, role-playing, Pecha Kuchas, field work, and team collaboration.

WHAT SUPPLEMENTAL MATERIALS ARE INCLUDED?

Instructor Resources:

- Instructor's manual (This features a project; teaching tips; YouTube video links; answers to end-of-chapter questions and problems; suggested answers to Bright Angel Medical Center, ethical scenario, and On the Job! video questions; and supplemental essay questions and problems.)
- Sample syllabi for qualitative, quantitative, or balanced teaching approaches

- Test bank
- PowerPoint slides
- Excel solutions for all chapter examples and end-of-chapter problems

Student Resources:

- Data for each end-of-chapter problem (Excel files)
- Data sets for analysis and decision-making
- Links to Excel, Word, and online templates
- Excel solutions for all chapter examples
- Three e-only chapters on advanced concepts

Videos:

- Eighteen chapter-specific tutorial videos cover the techniques used to solve chapter problems presented in select tables, figures, exhibits, and appendices.
- Sixteen "On the Job!" videos feature interviews with healthcare professionals who describe how they use the chapter materials in their jobs.

All chapter-specific Excel tutorial and "On the Job!" videos may be viewed by accessing the book through CourseConnect and visiting www.springerpub.com/courseconnect. See inside front cover and tear-out card for CourseConnect details.

Your concerns and opinions matter to us! Please contact Corinne Karuppan (ckaruppan@missouristate.edu) to let us know how we can serve you better.

TUTORIAL VIDEO LIST

Throughout chapters of *Quality in Healthcare: A Lean Six Sigma Project Approach*, the authors have included 18 tutorial videos connected to various tables, figures, exhibits, and appendices that present the techniques used to solve several chapter examples. Students can follow these step-by-step solution methods in Excel and practice along with the videos. In most cases, the videos end with a section, *Your Turn!*, asking students to put in practice their newly acquired knowledge and skills. To access the videos and transcripts, visit www.springerpub.com/courseconnect. See inside front cover and tear-out card for CourseConnect details.

Chapter 6

Excel Video 6.1: Yield (Exhibit 6.1)

Chapter 7

Excel Video 7.1: Bar Chart (Figure 7.3)
Excel Video 7.2: Pie Chart (Figure 7.4)
Excel Video 7.3: Line Chart (Figure 7.9)

Appendix 7.1

Excel Video A.7.1: Simple Random Sampling (Figures A.7.1.1–A.7.1.5)

Chapter 8

Excel Video 8.1: *p*-Chart (Exhibit 8.1)
Excel Video 8.2: *np*-Chart (Table 8.1)
Excel Video 8.3: *c*-Chart (Exhibit 8.2)
Excel Video 8.4: *u*-Chart (Table 8.2)
Excel Video 8.5: *IX-MR* Charts (Exhibit 8.4)
Excel Video 8.6: $\bar{X}$ and *R* Charts (Exhibit 8.5)
Excel Video 8.7: $\bar{X}$ and *s* Charts (Exhibit 8.6)
Excel Video 8.8: CUSUM Chart (Table 8.3)

Chapter 9

Excel Video 9.1: Scatter Diagram (Figure 9.3)
Excel Video 9.2: Correlation Coefficient (Figure 9.4)
Excel Video 9.3: Simple Linear Regression (Figure 9.5)
Excel Video 9.4: Multiple Regression (Figure 9.8)
Excel Video 9.5: Pareto Chart (Table 9.2)

ON THE JOB! INTERVIEW VIDEO LIST

Chapters in the textbook include video-recorded interviews with healthcare professionals. These individuals discuss their roles and responsibilities within a healthcare organization, address the strategic importance of quality, and demonstrate their own use of specific Lean Six Sigma tools in quality improvement projects and everyday activities. Students can see for themselves what quality at work really is. To access the videos and transcripts, visit www.springerpub.com/courseconnect. See inside front cover and tear-out card for CourseConnect details.

Chapter 1

Interview Video 1.1 It's All About Patient Care!
Alicia Young, MSN, RN, MBA

Chapter 2

Interview Video 2.1 Making Change a Gift, Not a Threat!
Bethany Rogers, MSML, BSN, RN, LSSMBB, CPHQ, CPHRM

Chapter 3

Interview Video 3.1 Creating Action Based on Data
Sharon Erickson, RN, BSN, LSSBB

Chapter 4

Interview Video 4.1 Humanizing Healthcare
Jami Momberger, JD, MPA

Chapter 5

Interview Video 5.1 Creating Sustainable Change
Liliana Mathis, MBA, BSN, RN, PMP, LSSGB

Chapter 6

Interview Video 6.1 Meeting Federal and State Quality Reporting Requirements
Hongmey Zhen Castillo, MBA, MHA, LSSGB

Chapter 7

Interview Video 7.1 Using Data to Optimize Learning
Paula Lewis, MBA, BSN, RN-C

Chapter 8

Interview Video 8.1 Visualizing Progress Toward Standardization
John Barnes, MBA
Interview Video 8.2 Making the Right Thing to Do the Easy Thing to Do
Mandy Studebaker, PA-C, LSSBB, CPHQ

Chapter 9

Interview Video 9.1 Prioritizing Areas Needing Improvement
Stuart Carson, MBA, MHA, LSSBBP, MLS(ASCP)^CM

Chapter 10

Interview Video 10.1 Every Vital Every Time Initiative
Summer Johnson, MBA

Chapter 11

Interview Video 11.1 Cross-Functional Collaboration to Ensure Success
Brian Dotter, PharmD, MBA
Interview Video 11.2 Human Subjects Versus Process Improvement Research
Laura J. Tivis, CCRP, LSSGB

Chapter 12

Interview Video 12.1 Daily Huddles to Drive and Sustain Change
Jennifer Gartner

Chapter 13

Interview Video 13.1 Continual Readiness
Danika Severe, MSN, RN, CPPS

eChapter 16

Interview Video 16.1 Leveraging Technology to Improve Patient and Clinician Experience
Shelby Darland, MSN, RN, NI-BC

RESOURCES

STUDENT RESOURCES

- **Interview Videos and Transcripts**
- **Excel Tutorial Videos and Transcripts**
- **Online Glossary**
- **Excel Chapter Example Solutions/Data Sets for the End-of-Chapter Problems**
- **Tool Templates**

SPRINGER PUBLISHING CONNECT™ | A robust set of instructor resources designed to supplement this text is located at **http://connect.springerpub.com/content/book/978-0-8261-7976-0**. Qualifying instructors may request access by emailing **textbook@springerpub.com**.

INSTRUCTOR RESOURCES

- **LMS Common Cartridge With All Instructor Resources and Instructions for Use**
- **Instructor Manual**:
  - Learning Objectives
  - Teaching Tips
  - YouTube video links
  - Answers to End-of-Chapter Questions
  - Learning Activities
  - Answers to Ethical Scenario Questions
  - Answers to On the Job! Video Questions
  - Additional essay questions and problems
- **Sample Syllabi** featuring course description, course objectives, course schedules, and more for three different teaching perspectives: Qualitative, Quantitative, and Balanced
- **Test Bank** with more than 150 multiple-choice questions (including full rationales)
- **Instructor Chapter PowerPoints** summarizing chapter content
- **Instructor Excel Solutions** for all chapter examples and end-of-chapter problems.

SPRINGER PUBLISHING

Instructor resources are available online by http://connect.springerpub.com /content/book/978-0-8261-7976-0

PART I

Introduction

CHAPTER 1

QUALITY FIRST

LEARNING OBJECTIVES

After reading this chapter, you will be able to:

- Appreciate the long journey to value-based care.
- Identify the challenges value-based healthcare still faces today.
- Describe multiple options to increase value in healthcare.
- Recognize the importance of systems thinking and organizational culture.
- Explain the business strategy development process.
- Underscore the strategic significance of quality and its impact on competitiveness.
- Describe processes and the need to build quality into each one.
- Define total quality management and the ongoing pursuit of perfection.
- Understand how this textbook is organized.

INTRODUCTION

What does quality healthcare mean to you? You may say good health outcomes, ease of getting appointments, short wait at the doctor's office, compassion, safety, and so forth. All these answers are right! Quality means many different things to different people. It is a complex concept that must be assessed and managed formally by knowledgeable professionals. It plays an important part in producing value-based healthcare, a top priority for decades. We associate "**value**" with good quality for the money. Essentially, it is quality divided by cost. In healthcare, it means the health outcomes relative to the costs spent to achieve them (Porter & Lee, 2015). Contrary to long-held beliefs, lower-cost hospitals treat the same patients—same acuity levels, same socioeconomic strata—at a lower cost and achieve the same outcomes. Basically, there is no trade-off between cost and quality (Bailey, 2022). In the United States, healthcare expenditures are the highest among industrial nations, and yet, the quality of care leaves a lot to be desired. In other words, value remains elusive. Although the link between healthcare quality and health outcomes is well understood, the contribution of quality to cost reduction is less evident to many. This first chapter explains the central role of quality in policy, strategy, and practice to promote value-based healthcare. It also shows how putting "quality first" positions an organization to excel in multiple dimensions of competitiveness. At its core is a holistic, systems-oriented approach designed to engrain quality into the organizational culture and to create value-added clinical and administrative processes. Finally, this first chapter introduces you to a fictional health system, Bright Angel Medical Center (BAMC), whose journey from predicament to success will highlight the lessons of failure, the dynamics of decision-making, and the rewards of teamwork.

WHY IS THIS MATERIAL USEFUL?

The ultimate purpose of this textbook is to help healthcare professionals deliver superior value to patients while building highly reliable organizations. The challenges are significant, but so are the rewards for a job well done. This chapter provides an overview of how policy, strategy, and practice shape value-based healthcare. It also introduces the mindset that you, as a clinician or administrator, will have to adopt in order to achieve excellence in patient-centered care.

ON THE JOB! INTERVIEW VIDEO 1.1

Alicia Young
Ambulatory Chief Nursing Officer

It's All About Patient Care!

Setting standards for clinical practice
Aligning programs and resources with strategic priorities
Medication safety at point-of-care

1. Alicia discusses the triage nurse project and the work they do to help patients avoid unnecessary ED visits. What are the benefits to the patients who avoid an unnecessary ED encounter?
2. The in-basket resource nurses respond to patient messages in real time either through phone calls or email messages. How does this program improve access to care for all patients?
3. Alicia discussed using barcode identification to ensure that the right patient receives the right medication. Discuss other methods that the healthcare team could employ to ensure the correct patient gets the intended medication at the appropriate dose.

The interview is available online by visiting www.springerpub.com/courseconnect. See inside front cover and tear-out card for CourseConnect details.

THE LONG PURSUIT OF VALUE-BASED CARE

Much has been written about the ills of healthcare organizations, but before we embark on our journey to treat them, we need to understand the events that shaped the environment in which providers operate today. Until the beginning of the 20th century, healthcare was essentially primitive, and medical remedies were quite eccentric. Fortunately, this type of care was cheap. In 1900, the cost of healthcare for the average resident in the United States was $5.00 a year, which is equivalent to about $160 today. Medical colleges did exist, but clinical instruction was provided in underequipped facilities, was limited in scope, and largely ignored scientific research. By the end of the century, science had taken over, modern medicine was born, and organization for a better healthcare system began. A brief history of the U.S. healthcare system is presented in Table 1.1.

CURRENT THREATS TO VALUE-BASED CARE

HIGH COSTS

At approximately $13,000 per capita, the United States spends more of its national income on healthcare than any other industrialized country (Peterson-KFF, 2024; Figure 1.1). Several factors, including increased trauma and injuries in young people, high obesity rates and their complications, and an aging population, do contribute to high expenditures. But interestingly, although the

TABLE 1.1 BRIEF HISTORY OF THE U.S. HEALTHCARE SYSTEM

Milestone	Time	Events
Founding of the AMA	1847	• Pushed for medical scientific research and improvement of medical education (AMA, 1847)
Birth of modern medicine	Early 1900s	• Standards for medical licensure • Standards for hospitals (Silverman & Danner, 2000) • Government regulation of pharmaceuticals (Swann, 2001)
Birth of health insurance	1920–1939	• The Baylor Plan: prepaid program similar to health insurance • Farmers' Union Cooperative Health Association is the first **health maintenance organization** • No national health insurance program, but private plans gain popularity (Goodridge & Arnquist, 2009)
Growth and progress	1940–1969	• Numerous medical and technological breakthroughs: widespread use of penicillin, polio vaccine, pacemakers, first heart transplant, EMRs (Chapman, 2016; Grossman, 2008; Quinn, 2013) • Expansion of private insurance (Goodridge & Arnquist, 2009) • Creation of the **JCAH** to provide voluntary accreditation • Social Security Amendments of 1965 and creation of Medicare and Medicaid programs providing healthcare coverage for the older adults and for the poor, blind, and disabled (Centers for Medicare & Medicaid Services [CMS], 2009). Use of **"fee-for-service."** Only hospitals accredited by the JCAH could participate in the Medicare and Medicaid programs
Looming crisis and rise of HMOs	1970–1989	• New diseases emerge • Fragmented, inefficient system of hospitals, pharmaceutical companies, insurers, and government programs • Medicare adoption of the **diagnosis-related group (DRG)** system to control costs (Goodridge & Arnquist, 2009; Rosenthal et al., 2002; Silverman & Danner, 2000) • Despite early success in lowering costs, HMOs lose popularity because of quality issues and denial of some procedures
Toward universal healthcare	1990s–to date	• Pharmaceutical companies' direct-to-consumer advertising, greater use of expensive technologies, and higher demand for drugs and medical services contribute to unsustainable cost increases • Significant proportion of U.S. population cannot afford health insurance (U.S. Census Bureau, 2010) • Sustainability of Medicare program is questioned • The IOM's report, *To Err Is Human*, places the number of preventable deaths from medical errors between 44,000 and 98,000 (Institute of Medicine [IOM], 1999) • Enactment of the **ACA**: Everyone must be insured or pay a penalty; measures to control costs and improve quality are enforced • MACRA: Medicare rewards clinicians for value and streamlines multiple quality programs (CMS, 2019) • Despite several efforts to repeal or weaken the ACA such as the removal of the individual mandate penalty (Norris, 2023), most of it remains in effect

Abbreviations: ACA, Affordable Care Act; AMA, American Medical Association; EMRs, electronic medical records; HMOs, health maintenance organization; IOM, Institute of Medicine; JCAH, Joint Commission on Accreditation of Hospitals; MACRA, Medicare Access and CHIP Reauthorization Act.

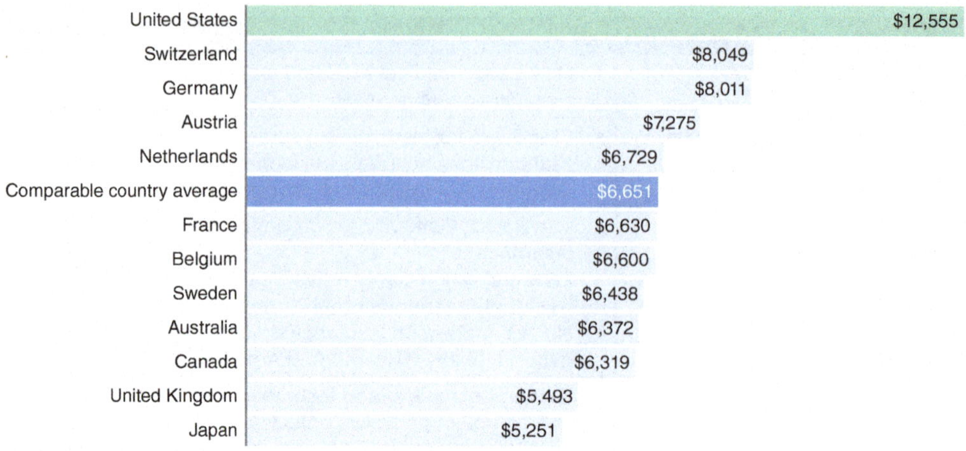

Notes: Data from Australia, Belgium, France, Japan, Switzerland, and the United States are estimated.
Data from Austria, Canada, Germany, the Netherlands, Sweden, and the United Kingdom are provisional.

FIGURE 1.1 National health spending for Organisation for Economic Co-operation and Development (OECD) countries for the year 2022.

Source: **KFF analysis of OECD data. Copyright by Peter G. Peterson Foundation. Used with permission.**

United States spends more than twice as much as other high-income countries on medical care, healthcare utilization per capita in the United States is not substantially different from the others' (Papanicolas et al., 2018). The cost of labor and goods, including drugs and devices, and administrative overhead appear to be the major drivers of the high U.S. costs. Excessive administrative costs mostly stem from the U.S. system's complexity (Gee & Spiro, 2019):

- Each provider has a mix of multiple payers and quasi-customized insurance products with different coverage structures, deductibles, and copayments. Providers must negotiate contracts with insurers or plan sponsors. A single physician negotiation might consume several hours, but for large groups of providers with numerous contracts, the time spent on negotiation is significant.
- A plurality of payment mechanisms makes it difficult for the provider to standardize its claim-filing procedures. This requires more staff to file claims and understand the nuances of each payment mechanism.
- The multiple standards for coding, prescribing medicine, credentialing, reporting of quality metrics, and so forth, create hours of work for administrative personnel and frequently result in errors and duplication of work.
- Complying with federal and state regulations requires additional staff and adds millions of dollars to the cost of care annually. Staff must understand and comply with each regulation or penalties to the providers are incurred.

This complex administrative structure paves the way for unscrupulous people to engage in both fraud and abuse. **Fraud** involves deceit and misrepresentation to obtain something of value without being entitled to it. Examples include *knowingly* billing for services or supplies not provided, altering claims, upcoding, and kickbacks. **Abuse** occurs when providers or suppliers follow improper practices that result in unnecessary costs or payments, such as overcharging for services or supplies and billing for medically unnecessary treatments or procedures. Unnecessary treatments and tests—**overuse**—is considered wasteful, but may also be considered a type of kickback, if the provider intends to benefit from the revenue generated. The Office of Inspector General and the CMS enforce the fraud and abuse laws (Office of the Inspector General, 2023), and the penalties for violation are severe.

A tightening labor market with heavy reliance on contract labor and the need to staff new technical positions have also contributed to major increases in healthcare labor costs over the past few years (KaufmanHall, 2022).

We often say that we get what we pay for, implying that there is a positive correlation between costs and quality. As the United States ranks on top as far as healthcare costs are concerned, you would therefore expect the same for quality. Unfortunately, the facts paint a different picture, as explained in the next section.

INADEQUATE QUALITY

Errors

It is difficult to assess how much progress has been made since the 1999 IOM report (see Table 1.1), but despite the large expenditures for healthcare, the "quality crisis" endures. Sadly, preventable **medical errors**—using the wrong plan or failing to implement the right plan when providing care—have remained a major concern since estimates have placed them as the third-leading cause of death (Makary & Daniel, 2016). These errors can be diagnostic, treatment, preventive, or system-related (IOM, 1999). Data from the United States and other high-income peer countries were compared in terms of medication and treatment errors, and the United States ranked poorly (Wager et al., 2024; Figure 1.2). The United States even ranks last in life expectancy at birth, but it has started to rebound (Rakshit et al., 2024; Figure 1.3). Although this does not give a complete picture of the quality of U.S. healthcare, it does provide a glimpse of where we stand relative to other countries in providing all our citizens with quality care.

It can be argued that comparing the U.S. healthcare system to other countries' healthcare systems is inappropriate because the metrics used to measure the quality dimensions vary greatly. However, in 2019, a Global Burden of Disease (GBD) study assessed that most of the 369 causes of death could be positively impacted by effective healthcare treatment (GBD, 2020). Especially disconcerting was the finding that improvements in health had been reversed in the United States over the past 10 years.

Variation

A 2022 study by the Commonwealth Fund examined 56 metrics of health system performance that represented measurable aspects of care in each of the U.S. states (Radley et al., 2022). The authors found that health system performance varied significantly among states and regions

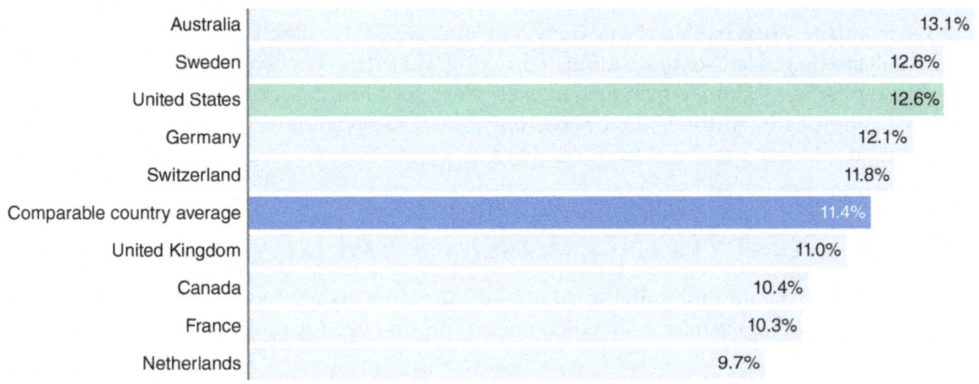

Note: Share responding that in the past 2 years, they had been given the wrong medication or wrong dose by a doctor, nurse, hospital, or pharmacist, or if there was a time they thought a medical mistake was made in their treatment.

FIGURE 1.2 Prevalence of healthcare-related errors in selected OECD countries.

Abbreviation: OECD, Organisation for Economic Co-operation and Development.

Source: Wager, E., Telesford, I., Rakshit, S., Kurani, N., & Cox, C. (2024). How does the quality of the U.S. health system compare to other countries? https://www.healthsystemtracker.org/chart-collection/quality-u-s-healthcare-system-compare-countries. Used with permission.

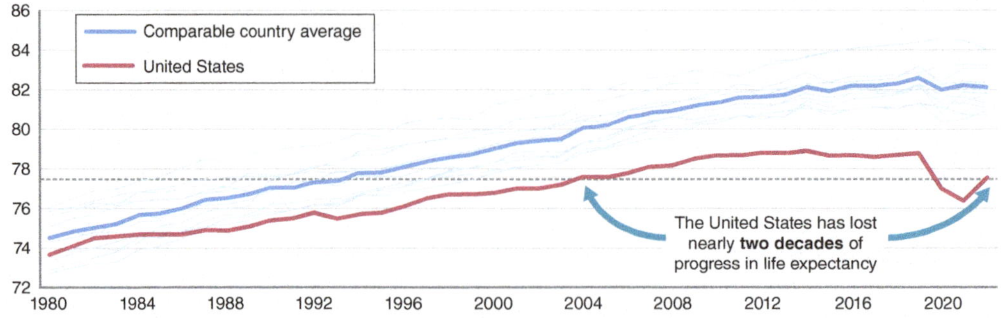

Notes: Comparable countries include Australia, Austria, Belgium, Canada, France, Germany, Japan, the Netherlands, Sweden, Switzerland, and the United Kingdom. See methods section of "How Does U.S. Life Expectancy Compare to Other Countries?"

FIGURE 1.3 Life expectancy at birth in selected OECD countries.

Abbreviation: OECD, Organisation for Economic Co-operation and Development.

Source: Rakshit, S., McGough, M., & Amin, K. (2024, January 30). How does U.S. life expectancy compare to other countries? https://www.healthsystemtracker.org/chart-collection/u-s-life-expectancy-compare-countries. Used with permission.

of the country. In addition to deaths from COVID-19, U.S. deaths from preventable or treatable causes increased significantly from 2020 to 2022. Mortality due to drug overdose reached a record high in most states in 2020. Encouragingly, states with already high-performing health systems fared relatively well during the pandemic and registered lower mortality rates and better health outcomes. If every state adopted the practices of the top-ranked state for each measure, the gains in healthcare quality for the country would improve dramatically.

Differences in care quality exist not only among the states, but also within them. **Health disparities** are differences in health status that are closely linked to social, economic, and/or environmental disadvantage (Centers for Disease Control and Prevention [CDC], 2023). They adversely affect groups of people who have barriers to care due to race or ethnicity, religious beliefs, disability, sexual orientation, or geographic location. In a study of all census tracts in the United States, socioeconomic disadvantage was the primary factor of disparity in health outcomes, and social and neighborhood environment characteristics combined accounted for almost as much variation. Besides their economic disadvantage, areas of extreme poverty may indicate deinvestment in healthcare facilities and structural collapse (e.g., lead contamination of drinking water, lead exposure, and parasitic worm outbreaks due to poor sanitation), which further exacerbate poor health outcomes. The study confirmed that 60% of early deaths in the United States are related to nonclinical factors (Kolak et al., 2019). Urgent solutions to these problems are needed before we can truly improve the health of the nation.

APPROACHES TO INCREASING VALUE

Addressing inadequate and inequitable quality of care is hardly a new concern. It has been a staple on the agendas of U.S. health policy, academia, and practice for more than two decades.

THE SIX AIMS

Following up on the alarming number of deaths due to preventable medical errors (IOM, 1999), the IOM set new directives to improve the quality of care. It released another report, *Crossing the Quality Chasm*, which specified six aims for quality improvement (IOM, 2001). Their acronym, STEEEP, has helped guide providers on their quality journey (Ballard, 2015):

- **Safety** refers to the prevention of harm. Keeping patients safe has long been a priority in healthcare, but the incidence of medical errors remains high, and continued efforts are needed to decrease these rates.

BOX 1.1 QUALITY IN PRACTICE!

Time Is Money

The earliest appointment is 26 days out in 15 of the largest cities in the United States. In Portland, Oregon, the average time to see a physician (cardiologist, dermatologist, orthopedic surgeon, OB/GYN, or primary care provider) is 45.6 days (Merritt Hawkins, 2022). Americans also spend an average of 34 minutes traveling to doctors' appointments and another 18 minutes in the waiting room once they get there (First Stop Health, 2022). Besides taking their tolls on people's mental and physical health, treatment delays may result in further complications and thus excess costs. For example, during the pandemic, a delay of 6 days almost doubled the cost of treatment compared to no delay (Haque, 2021). Deeper understanding of demand and capacity patterns and streamlined processes are useful approaches providers may use to decrease waits and treatment delays.

- **Timeliness** refers to minimal waits and absence of harmful delays for patients seeking access, treatment, and information (Box 1.1)
- **Effectiveness** means to provide care based on scientific knowledge and deliver this care to all those who can benefit. Medicine has made progress in the treatment of many chronic conditions, such as blood pressure control and treatment of heart disease and diabetes, but many patients do not have access to the treatments that could benefit them.
- **Efficiency** involves producing the desired outcome with minimal waste of human resources, equipment, supplies, ideas, and energy. Improving efficiency can decrease healthcare costs without affecting health outcomes.
- **Equitable treatment** means giving *all* patients the care they need when they need it. The IOM defines health equity as providing care that does not vary in quality because of an individual's gender, sexual preference or identity, race, ethnicity, socioeconomic status, or geographic region.
- **Patient-centeredness** encompasses the characteristics of compassion and empathy to respond to the patient's needs, values, and personal preferences. A major component of patient-centeredness is clear communication. It is vital that the provider understands and addresses the patient's needs and that the patient understands the provider's diagnosis and recommendations for treatment. The Patient-Centered Outcomes Research Institute (PCORI) sponsors clinical effectiveness research that focuses on outcomes aligned with patients' circumstances and preferences.

To this day, the six aims, or STEEEP, have provided a framework for developing value-based care delivery models.

CARE DELIVERY MODELS

Value-based healthcare is a healthcare delivery model where providers are paid based on the health outcomes and not the volume of services delivered. In value-based practices, providers are rewarded for improving patients' health and reducing the effects of chronic disease.

There are different care delivery models that translate into value-based healthcare. These are noted in the following list:

1. **Medical homes.** A medical home is an approach to care where primary, specialty, and acute care are all integrated. A primary care physician directs the team to address patient access and care for all of the patient's medical issues.
2. **Accountable care organizations (ACOs).** ACOs are organizations where the patient and providers are partners in care decisions. In an ACO, hospitals, doctors, and other healthcare professionals work as a team to deliver coordinated and high-quality care at the lowest cost.

BOX 1.2 QUALITY IN PRACTICE!

The Hospital VBP Program

According to CMS, "The Hospital VBP Program encourages hospitals to improve the quality, efficiency, patient experience andtsafety of care that Medicare beneficiaries receive during acute care inpatient stays by:

- Eliminating or reducing adverse events (healthcare errors resulting in patient harm). — Safety
- Adopting evidence-based care standards and protocols in order to obtain the best outcomes for Medicare patients. — Effectiveness and equitability
- Incentivizing hospitals to improve patient experience. — Patient-centeredness and timeliness
- Increasing the transparency of care quality for consumers, clinicians, and others. — Effectiveness
- Recognizing hospitals that provide high-quality care at a lower cost to Medicare" (CMS, 2024). — Efficiency

Notice how the objectives mirror five of the six aims of quality proposed by the IOM (2001).

3. **Hospital value-based purchasing (VBP).** Acute care hospitals receive adjusted payments based on the efficiency and quality of care that their patients receive. This program is administered by the CMS and encourages hospitals to continuously improve the quality and safety of care within the institution. The premises of VBP are closely aligned with STEEEP (Box 1.2).
4. **Merit-based incentive payment system (MIPS).** Under the Quality Payment Program, Medicare rewards clinicians providing high-quality, high-value care with higher payments; the opposite is true if performance is unsatisfactory. Clinicians can participate in the program via the MIPS or participation in alternative payment models. With MIPS, performance is evaluated in terms of quality and cost of patient care, process improvements and increased patient engagement, and use of certified electronic health record technology (CMS, 2023).

As providers are shifting to value over volume, coordination of services and competition among stakeholders are creating new and exciting opportunities.

NEW OPPORTUNITIES

- **Mergers and acquisitions**. The trend of mergers and acquisitions between health systems continues. These transactions are being driven by complementary capabilities or robust revenue streams that help the parties build competitive strength. New entrants are driving industry disruption to the healthcare market. For example, Walmart has opened locations that serve as "health super-centers" where patients can have access to primary care, dental services, behavioral health, and more (Carmouche, 2023). CVS Health also provides services such as primary care, condition and disease management, mental health, and home infusion and tube feeding therapy in addition to its pharmacies (CVS Health, 2023). In the past, healthcare organizations focused on aggregation to leverage economies of scale. Although cost reduction has not materialized yet, organizations continue to expand in the hopes of transforming the process of care and changing industry dynamics.
- **Insurers' roles in care delivery**. Insurers' primary role is to enable people to stay healthy. There are several opportunities for them to do so: (a) protecting people in the case of

catastrophic health events, (b) providing broad access to free or low-cost services, (c) obtaining price concessions from providers and screening out high-cost providers from their networks, (d) measuring and tracking providers' performance on quality and holding them accountable, (e) encouraging healthy behaviors through reductions in premium or out-of-pocket expenses, and (f) improving equitability through wealth transfers from older to younger individuals and from healthier to sicker patients (Dey & Bach, 2019).

- **Direct-to-employer arrangements**. Hoping to cut costs and improve quality, some innovative, typically self-funded employers bypass traditional health insurance companies and contract directly with hospitals and other providers. Although Walmart's contracts with centers of excellence like the Cleveland Clinic are well-known, small- and medium-sized businesses also have the opportunity to enter into such arrangements. The design of tailored plans, the negotiation of rates and reference-based pricing plans, increased price transparency, and requirements for performance on quality and financial indicators are some of the benefits that make these arrangements attractive to businesses. For providers, these partnerships provide the opportunity to eliminate middlemen, fend off competition from provider-insurer mergers, and diversify revenue streams (Livingston, 2018).
- **Population health. Population health** is an approach that connects social determinants of health and health outcomes. The **social determinants of health** are nonmedical factors that include "the conditions in which people are born, grow, work, live, and age." They affect a wide range of health and quality-of-life risks and outcomes (CDC, 2022). Population health brings these factors into consideration to develop interventions that improve health outcomes and incentivize partnerships, collaboration, and integration.
- **Health co-creation**. Co-creation requires that the stakeholders of a process partner to achieve better value. At its core is the recognition that the expertise and perspective of the target customer (here, the patient) complement those of the service providers. Together, they participate in creating and implementing processes that benefit both (Chapter 4). This collaboration promotes a patient-centric model that can improve satisfaction, efficiency, and outcomes (Peng et al., 2022).
- **Innovation centers.** A growing number of health systems have created innovation centers to develop a variety of health solutions: processes, procedures, digital platforms, medical devices, and so forth. The centers promote their own staff's creative ideas and/or partner with startups to improve patient care. For example, the Innovation Studio at Children's Hospital Los Angeles assembled internal and external communities to design, test, and implement new processes and technologies that can transform care delivery in pediatrics. Design thinking (Chapter 10) and an innovative culture drive these incubators of new ideas (AHA Center for Health Innovation, 2023; Children's Hospital Los Angeles, 2022).
- **Green healthcare**. Green healthcare refers to the incorporation of environmentally responsible practices into care delivery. The healthcare sector generates millions of tons of waste and hazardous materials. In the United States alone, hospitals produce about 6 million tons of garbage each year (Jain & LaBeaud, 2022). This has prompted the advocacy of more responsible waste management with an emphasis on the pillars of sustainability: reduce (e.g., packaging, paper, and mercury-containing equipment); reuse (e.g., binders, water pitchers, sterilization trays, thermometer probes); and recycle (e.g., newspapers, plastics, glass bottles; Thomas, 2022; World Medical Association, 2023). Besides saving money and protecting the environment, these eco-friendly practices give healthcare institutions the opportunity to lead their communities by example.
- **Information technology**. Health systems are listening to patients' demands for better care as well as increased access and convenience. Electronic health records, clinical decision support systems, and telehealth have transformed care delivery by improving care coordination, facilitating diagnosis and treatment, and increasing patient access to care and their health information. Artificial intelligence improves diagnosis accuracy (Lenharo, 2024), enables the identification of hidden conditions at an early stage (Johnson, 2024), and identifies

trends in health data that otherwise would be missed (National Institutes of Health, 2024). Analysis of data at the population level has targeted interventions to improve the health of communities as a whole. The use of data analytics, especially on big data sets, is central to uncovering patterns and relationships and setting directions for the future.

SYSTEMS THINKING

A value-based healthcare system will require significant efforts from all of its major stakeholders if we are to improve the health of the nation. Patients must be more actively involved in their health and well-being. Policy makers must create an environment favorable to the pursuit of uniform quality and cost control. Providers must reevaluate their ways of delivering care and strive for both effectiveness (doing it right the first time) and efficiency (doing it with minimum waste of time and resources). Insurers must acknowledge and support providers' performance, and the reimbursement system must be modified. Change is happening in healthcare and the tools to manage change are more important than ever. Professionals who understand how to build quality in all facets of their productive systems are in the best position to steer their operations on the path to excellence. What does it take to get there? Adopting a "systems approach" is crucial.

Systems thinking is a way of viewing interconnections and patterns of change—as opposed to discrete and static elements—in the structures and processes of a whole entity. This way of thinking improves one's ability to work with others, identify the root causes of problems, and produce creative solutions benefitting the whole system. It forms the foundation on which strategies are formulated and implemented. Systems thinkers are known to:

- Study the big picture and observe how elements within a system interact and change over time.
- Recognize patterns and trends as well as useful connections within and across systems.
- Identify cause-and-effect relationships and factors that alter these relationships.
- Acknowledge the consequences of time delays.
- Resist drawing quick conclusions and consider the unintended consequences of actions.
- Test assumptions, check results, and be willing to change course of action, if needed.

Overall, systems thinking provides better patient-centered care, improves problem-solving, and fosters collaboration (Henry, 2023).

THE STRATEGIC IMPORTANCE OF QUALITY

The competitiveness of any organization heavily rests on its ability to deliver quality to its customers. In fact, the pursuit of quality paves the way for success on multiple fronts. Following our discussion on systems thinking, we want to briefly review the strategy formulation process at the organizational level before delving into the central position of quality in achieving world class status.

WHAT TO DO

A **business strategy** focuses on *WHAT* business units need to do to compete in the marketplace (Vadarajan & Clark, 1994). It specifies the game plan the business has selected to maximize its long-term value to customers, and it outlines the resource deployments necessary to "win the game." Executives do not select the courses of action articulated in the strategy in a vacuum. They are derived from a rigorous process; a full discussion of strategy development is beyond the scope of this text. However, it is important to understand the basic framework used to develop strategies. It usually starts with a deep understanding of the organization and the environment in which it conducts business. This process is known as a "SWOT analysis" (Schooley, 2023).

SWOT Analysis

A **SWOT analysis** identifies the business's internal strengths (**S**) and weaknesses (**W**) and evaluates the environmental opportunities (**O**) and threats (**T**; Figure 1.4 offers some examples). Its objective is to leverage the business's internal capabilities and to benefit from market opportunities while mitigating external threats. This matching procedure helps the firm evaluate the viability of various strategies and position itself favorably in the marketplace, but risks remain (Box 1.3).

After conducting a SWOT analysis, the organization must formulate alternative, feasible strategic options that improve the chances of gaining and/or sustaining market dominance and assuring financial success. All strategic choices determine the position of the business unit relative to its competitors. Porter's (1985) typology of generic business strategies focuses on the actions an organization takes to produce greater value: (a) minimizing costs through greater efficiency (cost leadership), (b) developing and offering different and more attractive products or services (differentiation), (c) minimizing costs in a niche market (cost focus), and (d) increasing differentiation in a particular market segment (differentiation focus). It is important to note that few organizations adopt a strictly pure strategy. Many times, there will be "spillovers" from one to the other. For instance, some of the services offered by an organization pursuing differentiation may be of low cost and high quality. As the focus strategies imply, there can be different strategies for different markets.

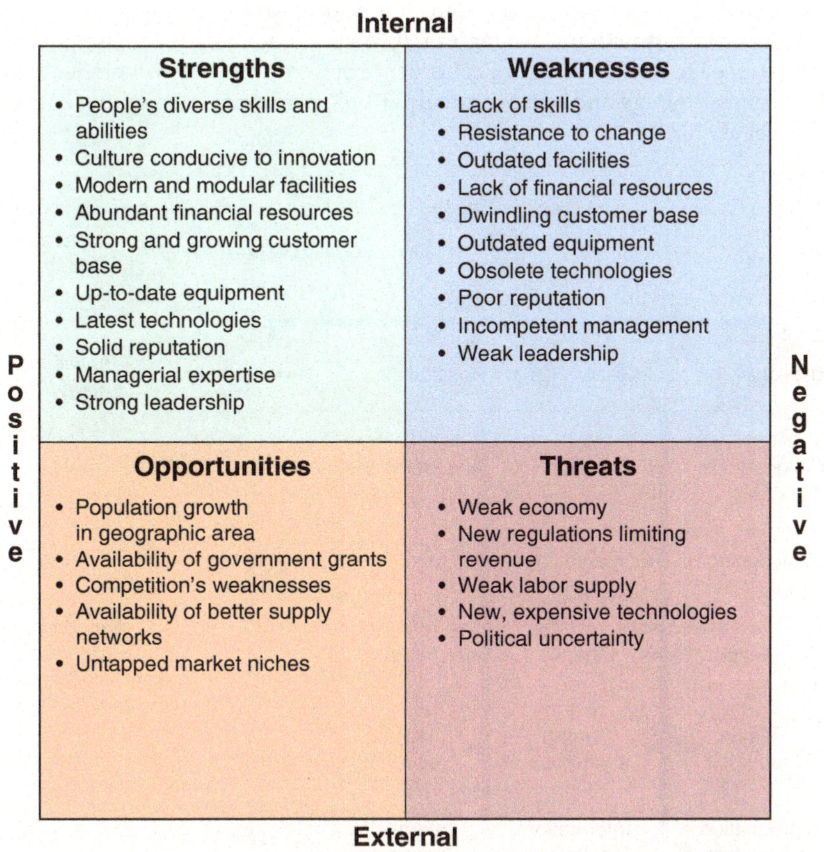

FIGURE 1.4 Examples of strengths, weaknesses, opportunities, and threats.

BOX 1.3 QUALITY IN PRACTICE!

Haven Healthcare: A Missed Opportunity

In 2018, Amazon, Berkshire Hathaway, and JP Morgan Chase joined forces to launch a health-care system intended to "provide high-quality and transparent care at a reasonable cost" for their employees and families. They attracted top talent: Atul Gawande, the renowned surgeon, for the CEO position, and Jack Stoddard, the former general manager for digital health at Comcast, for the COO job. Despite their founders' clout in the United States, the new venture was extinct after only 3 years. What happened?

First, the three companies' large workforce was still too small to generate the market power necessary to persuade providers to lower their prices. Second, U.S. health systems had no financial incentive to focus on prevention rather than treatment tied to the lucrative fee-for-service reimbursement system unless they were insurers themselves. Third, the COVID-19 pandemic undermined Haven's efforts to gain overwhelmed, cash-strapped providers' support for any new, potentially risky venture. With mounting challenges, both Stoddard and Gawande promptly left their positions, and Haven disbanded less than 3 years after its launch (Toussaint, 2021).

HOW TO DO IT

The question now is, "HOW do you execute the business strategy?" Again, systems thinking guides the process. All functional areas of the organization (operations, finance, marketing, and information technology [IT]) must be engaged in the successful implementation of the business strategy. In other words, **functional strategies** (HOW) must be designed to support the business strategy (WHAT; see Figure 1.5). A lack of congruence between the two will hinder the implementation of the business strategy and will potentially cripple performance, resulting in organizational failure (Dohale et al., 2022).

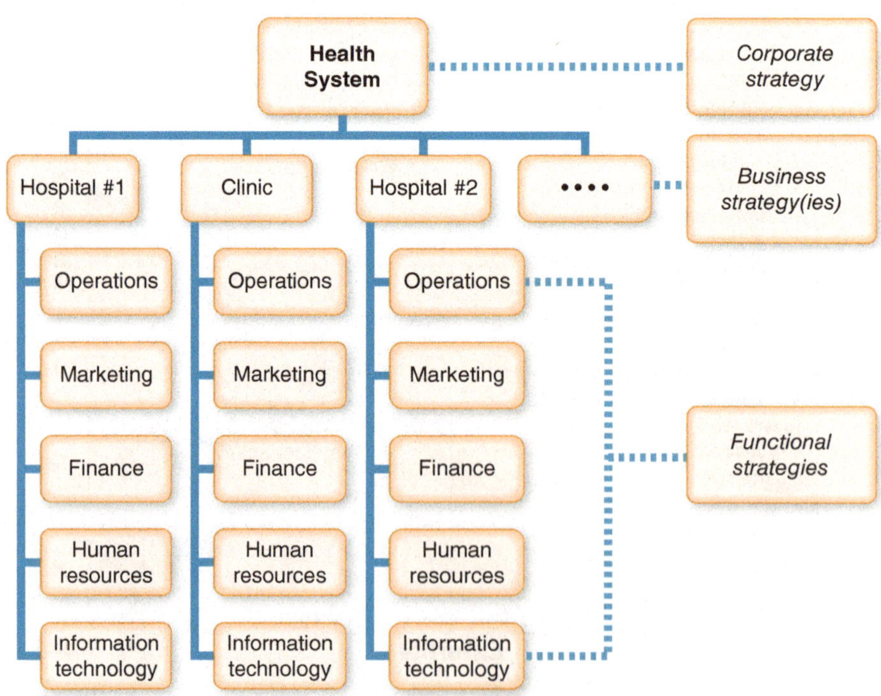

FIGURE 1.5 Strategy levels.

Where does quality fit in all this? Quality is one of the pillars of an operations strategy. **Operations**, in general, represent the core activities of an organization. They are what the business is essentially about. What is the first thing that comes to your mind when you hear "General Motors"? They make cars. The post office? It delivers mail and packages. A hospital? It provides healthcare to patients. Of course, these different organizations provide a variety of other services that complement the core activities. For example, a health system may offer health plans, provide education, and fund research and development projects in order to enrich the core of healthcare delivery.

An **operations strategy** specifies HOW the operations function plans to align its resources (facilities, people, equipment, technology, and supply networks) with the demands of the business strategy (Waters, 2006). In short, it is the blueprint for achieving competitiveness through superior operations.

In order to be effective, an operations strategy must also produce a distinctive competitive advantage. Using A. Hill and T. Hill's (2018) conceptualization of operations strategy, we can view it as a set of operations-oriented strategic priorities (competitive priorities) that help increase market share by "winning orders." In a healthcare environment, "winning orders" means attracting patients and health insurers to consume your services instead of your competitors'. The **competitive priorities** are quality, cost, timeliness, and flexibility (Figure 1.6).

- **Quality:** Competing on quality means accomplishing better patient outcomes (clinical and experiential) than those produced by your competition.
- **Cost:** Competing on cost refers to the ability to offer services at lower prices than those charged by the competition.
- **Timeliness:** Competing on timeliness refers to the ability to provide services on time (on-time delivery) or to deliver the services faster (fast delivery) than the competition.
- **Flexibility:** Competing on flexibility refers to the ability to respond to changes with minimal cost and time penalties and uniform outcomes for services.

Patient safety and effective care are definitely within the scope of operations strategy. To improve patient safety, the IOM (1999, p. 2) suggests the design of a health system that "makes it harder . . . to do something wrong and easier . . . to do something right." This statement suggests that process redesign or reengineering might be the key to ensuring a care delivery process that minimizes medical errors and optimizes clinical outcomes. Such a process often includes a minimum number of steps to minimize **handoffs**, that is, passing the responsibility for an activity onto another person, unit, or department. Why? At each step of a process, there is an opportunity to make an error. The lower the number of steps, the fewer the opportunities for error.

Excellent performance in clinical care, in general, and patient safety, in particular, boost a healthcare organization's reputation and improves its standing relative to its competitors. Other quality attributes, such as well-designed and maintained facilities, prompt service, responsive staff, and effective communication, shape the patient's experience. A first-class experience drives patient loyalty, which in turn improves competitiveness through repeat business. Finally, the ability of a healthcare provider to produce excellent patient outcomes—clinical and experiential—will increase reimbursement.

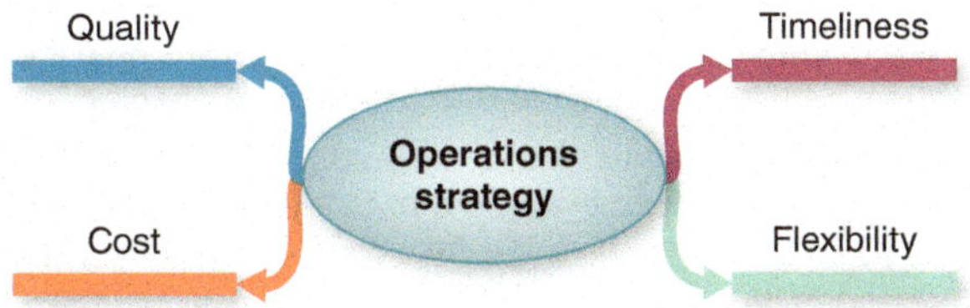

FIGURE 1.6 Competitive priorities in operations strategy.

BOX 1.4 FAQs

Is healthcare quality expensive?

Well, let's try to answer this question with another. What attributes do you consider when you shop?

I try to balance the quality of the product with its cost.

Exactly! You search for VALUE. Customer value captures the relationship between cost and quality:

$$\text{Value} = \frac{\text{Quality}}{\text{Cost}}$$

In healthcare, it is health outcome per $ spent (Porter's definition)

To improve value, you can increase quality, decrease cost, or do both. Porter recommends doing both. He argues that the best way to decrease costs is to drive quality up!

Porter's perspective on value (Box 1.4) is strongly anchored in the operations management tradition, which views quality as a means to decrease the costs associated with poor performance, such as rework, retesting, inefficient utilization, scrapped supplies, litigation, and lower reimbursements from Medicare (see Table 1.2). Ultimately, superior value wins orders and leads to greater competitiveness. How else does quality contribute to competitiveness? The answer is in the next section.

TABLE 1.2 THE COSTS OF QUALITY

Cost Category	Description
Prevention costs	Costs associated with decreasing the likelihood of making errors in the first place. They include training programs, process improvement efforts (e.g., collecting patient information, process analysis, process redesign), and maintenance of records and quality data.
Appraisal costs	Costs involved in evaluating the quality of products or services. They include the costs of conducting inspections or audits. Appraisal does not prevent errors from occurring, but it is hoped that it will help identify them and correct them before the customer of the process is affected.
Internal failure costs	Costs of fixing errors before the customer is affected. They include the costs of rework to correct the errors, of outdated supplies that must be discarded, and of downtime caused by failures in the process (e.g., malfunctioning equipment).
External failure costs	Costs of errors that are detected too late and affect the customer. They include customer complaints, readmissions, litigation, and loss of customers.

THE CUMULATIVE MODEL: QUALITY FIRST

In operations, there was a long-held belief of trade-offs among the competitive priorities (Skinner, 1966). This is especially true in healthcare. Cost cutting is often seen as a threat to the quality of clinical outcomes. In fact, many healthcare professionals claim that the U.S. healthcare system is costly because it is "the best in the world." There is a sound logic behind the high-cost, high-quality paradigm. Employing surgeons with outstanding track records, using the latest and most sophisticated equipment and technologies, acquiring premium supplies, continuously developing the skills of the nursing and support staff, and so on, should, in theory, yield the best possible outcomes. By the same token, cost savings that threaten the quality of these inputs would likely jeopardize the quality of the outputs.

Now, let us reflect for a while. In the previous section, we said that improving quality could actually lower the costs of rework, inventory, litigation, poor resource utilization, and so on. The IOM's (2012) report, *Best Care at Lower Cost: The Path to Continuously Learning Health Care in America,* further supports this relationship. It explores the potential to attack the higher costs associated with increasingly complex medical care. Opportunities resulting from increased computational power, connectivity allowing for improved dissemination of information, progress in organizational capabilities, and patient empowerment are now present to help improve the quality of care while reining in the costs.

We also said that improving quality through a simplification of processes with fewer handoffs improved patient flow and rapid response to evolving needs (timeliness). Logically, businesses with excellent performance on cost, quality, and timeliness should be best positioned to adapt to the rapid changes required by a dynamic environment with negligible performance decrements (flexibility). There appears to be a synergistic effect among all the competitive priorities. This was first noticed by Nakane (1986), who realized that world-class manufacturers excelled in all competitive priorities. He also established a sequence. World-class companies should first devote their efforts to achieving excellence in quality, then to timeliness, cost, and flexibility. Others (Ferdows & De Meyer, 1990; Noble, 1995; Sum et al., 2012) came up with a different sequence, but there was a consensus that *quality* was the building block of outstanding performance in all dimensions. Therefore, improving quality in order to decrease costs made sense, but not vice versa. This practice of accumulating capabilities, starting with quality, is known as the **cumulative model** (Figure 1.7).

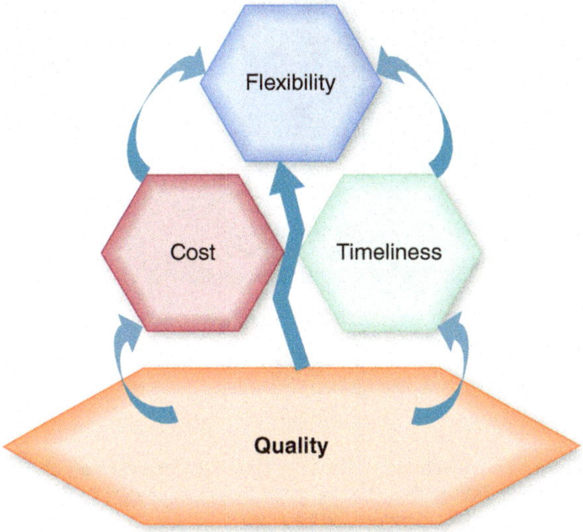

FIGURE 1.7 Cumulative model.

Nevertheless, the companies that excelled at everything also distinguished themselves by "beating the competition" or differentiating themselves on one or several dimensions. T. Hill (2000) captured this phenomenon in his distinction between "order winners" and "order qualifiers." **Order winners** are literally the competencies that enable the business to *win* orders or customers, that is, the competencies on which a particular business's performance outclasses that of the competition. However, **order qualifiers** merely *qualify* the business to be competitive in the marketplace, that is, performance on these competencies is on par with that of the competition. Let us take timeliness, for example. If the ED's average wait is 3 hours at Hospital X, and this wait is comparable to the wait in the other EDs in town, timeliness is a qualifier for Hospital X. If its average wait time is only 2 hours compared to the competition's 3 hours, then it is an order winner. Now, let's say that Hospital X averages wait times of 4 hours or more. It no longer meets the threshold for competitiveness and risks losing as opposed to winning some market share to its competitors. For this reason, you should never underestimate the significance of order qualifiers.

Designing a healthcare system that makes it easier to do something right starts with ensuring that quality is built into every step of every process, be it clinical or administrative.

WHAT IS A PROCESS?

At its most basic level, a process is a **productive system** that involves the transformation of inputs into outputs of greater value (Figure 1.8) to the customer. An efficient transformation is achieved when the desired output is produced with the least resources and waste. To ensure that the transformation processes are carried out to produce the desired outputs, data collection at various stages of the healthcare delivery process should take place. These measurements (feedback) should be gauged against preestablished standards to determine whether corrective action is needed at the input and/or transformation process levels. For example, patients' complaints about long wait times in the ED may lead to changes in triage procedures and reallocation of resources. Similarly, poor utilization of hospitalists' time during their rounds may result in floor redesign to minimize steps between patient rooms.

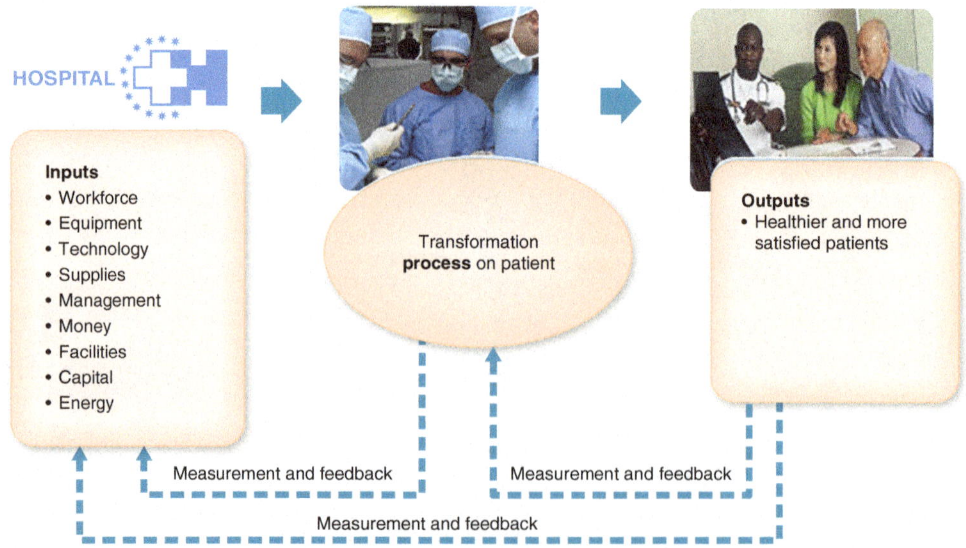

FIGURE 1.8 Clinical productive system.

PROCESSES ARE EVERYWHERE

The transformation process involving the care of a sick patient is supported by a myriad of other transformation processes throughout the healthcare organization: registering patients, ordering medical supplies and storing them, billing, filing insurance claims, training employees, preparing financial statements, archiving medical records, housekeeping, and so on (Figure 1.9). Every activity in a business organization is part of a process, which should be designed and managed to deliver value to its customers. In healthcare, the ultimate customer is the patient. However, the direct customer of any given process is the recipient of its output. Therefore, the doctor who ordered a lab test is the customer of the lab doing the test, the vice president who requested a financial report on a new project is the customer of the team preparing the report, and so forth.

Whether or not you plan to work in the field of quality management, there is a compelling reason to learn more about it. Striving for excellence permeates all areas and processes of an organization; it can thus be the key to reducing fragmentation among the various parts of a business and offering a unified "way of doing things" that is both customer-focused and efficiency-driven. For example, rifts between physicians and administrators are quite common as physicians often view administrators' cost-cutting initiatives as threats to the quality of care. Lean Six Sigma has been a catalyst as it positions error reduction (better quality) and smarter process design as major drivers of cost reduction. This approach brings both groups together. Physicians subscribe to it when they see that it provides opportunities for better patient care; administrators appreciate its emphasis on waste elimination.

TOTAL QUALITY MANAGEMENT

The ubiquity of processes requires that companies delivering value to their customers engrain quality in their culture. This managerial philosophy is commonly known as **total quality management (TQM)**. The three major principles of TQM underscore what is meant by "total." The first principle is a commitment to provide customers with total satisfaction by exceeding their expectations. The second principle requires that all members of the value chain share this commitment. In other words, quality is the responsibility of suppliers, schedulers, physicians, vice presidents, chief

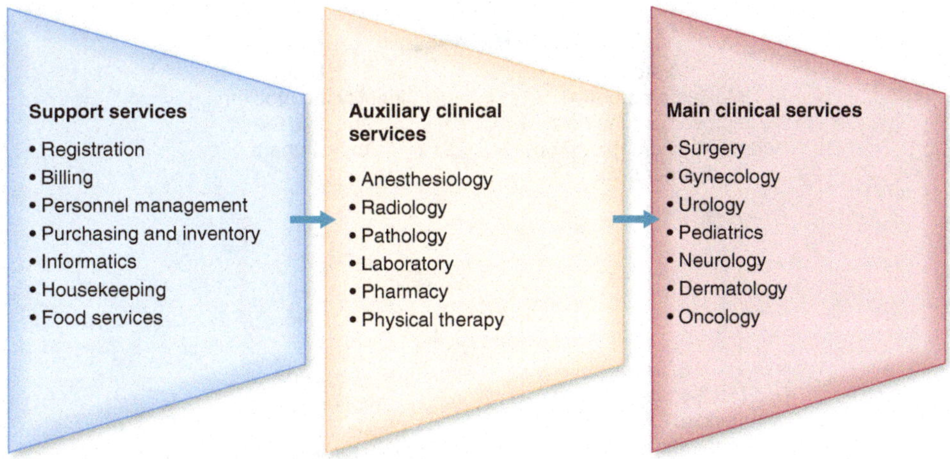

FIGURE 1.9 Processes in a hospital.

Source: Adapted from Amberg, M., & Graber, S. (1996). Specifying information systems using business process modeling. In J. Brender, J. P. Christensen, J.-R. Scherrer, & P. McNair (Eds.), *Medical informatics Europe '96* (pp. 1037–1041). IOS Press.

executive officers, nurses, cooks, janitors, and so on. The third principle advocates a never-ending journey focused on continuous improvement. The relentless pursuit of perfect quality—getting it right the first time—becomes an integral part of the organizational culture.

DEMING WHEEL

TQM's orientation is definitely long term as incremental improvements are sought continuously. This approach is best illustrated by the **plan-do-study-act (PDSA) cycle**, also known as the *Deming Wheel*. As shown in Figure 1.10, four stages make up the PDSA cycle:

1. **Plan:** Carefully select the process that needs improvement. Then develop a deeper understanding of the process by collecting data. Based on the data analysis, formulate a plan for improvement that includes performance measures.
2. **Do:** Implement the improvement on a limited scale. During this phase, do not forget to collect data on the performance of the process.
3. **Study:** Analyze the data collected during the Do phase and check whether the improvement has yielded the results anticipated in the Plan phase. If the results are negative, go back to the Plan phase and modify the improvement. If they are positive, proceed to the next phase.
4. **Act:** Make the improved process the new standard and deploy it on a larger scale. During this phase, make sure that everyone involved in the process understands its new dynamics, and provide training on the new methods if necessary.

Is the process perfect? Certainly not! It is, therefore, time to plan the next improvement and repeat the cycle.

DEMING'S 14 POINTS

In 1984, the Navy was one of the first adopters of TQM principles in the United States. It had asked researchers to evaluate some of its operations and make recommendations for improved performance. The researchers proposed TQM and Deming's works. Deming's (1982) 14 points embody his ideas about quality. They emphasize the importance of the three TQM principles and of human capital development to its success.

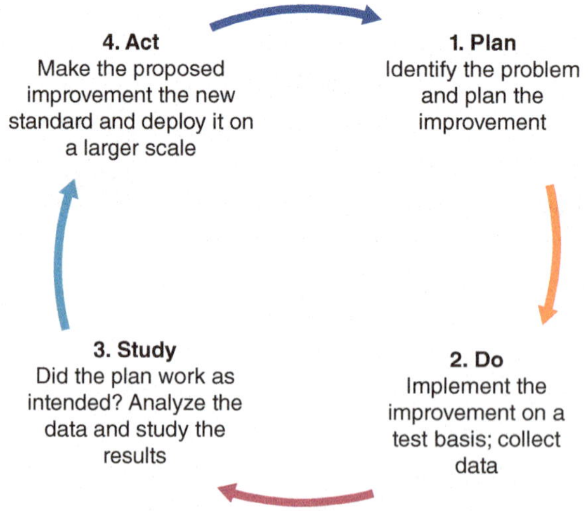

FIGURE 1.10 Deming wheel.

Point #1: Create Constancy of Purpose Toward Improvement

This point underscores the importance of instituting a culture of continuous improvement to become or remain competitive.

Point #2: Adopt the New Philosophy

Leadership must rise to the challenge of letting go of the old ways and embrace change for improvement.

Point #3: Cease Dependence on Inspection to Achieve Quality

This point highlights the need for productive systems that focus on prevention rather than correction of defects or errors (see IOM's recommendation in the introductory section of this chapter). Inspections are basically needed because errors are made. If one could develop a system that makes it difficult for the most serious errors to occur, patient safety would improve greatly, and the scarce resources now consumed with error detection and correction would be utilized more efficiently (Table 1.2).

Point #4: End the Practice of Awarding Business on the Basis of Price Tag Alone

This point emphasizes abandoning the practice of switching from one vendor to another while pursuing the lowest possible price. Instead, Deming advocated the selection of few suppliers based on their ability to deliver quality products and supplies consistently.

Point #5: Improve Constantly and Forever the System of Production and Service

As perfection does not exist, the pursuit of perfect quality is a never-ending journey. Seeking this perfection throughout the organization results in an overall decrease in costs associated with poor quality (e.g., rework, scrap, lost productivity; see Table 1.2).

Point #6: Institute Training

All employees must be trained to use the methods, tools, and techniques that help them achieve a higher quality output in their jobs.

Point #7: Institute Leadership

Because lives are at stake, good leadership is especially critical to a healthcare organization's success. **The Joint Commission**, a major healthcare accreditor, likens a healthcare organization to a watch (Schyve, 2009). A watchmaker could gather the best components in the world and put them together, but the resulting watch would be unlikely to run. The individual components, although necessary, are not enough. It is how the components work together that creates a quality watch. In other words, healthcare organizations must be appreciated as a system, the components of which work together to provide high-quality care. Thus, when we talk of leadership in healthcare, it implies that the many leaders within the organization (the governing body, the CEO and other senior leaders, and the leaders of the licensed independent practitioners) work well together to formulate and implement their shared vision of success.

Point #8: Drive Out Fear

Perfecting quality requires some experimentation with new concepts and processes. As a result, mistakes will be made. Penalizing workers for these mistakes is essentially guaranteeing that they will never try again. They will avoid improvement rather than seek it.

Point #9: Break Down Barriers Between Departments

As discussed earlier, a major problem of the U.S. healthcare system is fragmentation. This fragmentation is the result of an organizational structure that emphasizes silos rather than team collaboration. Collaboration across departments and units reduces the errors and inefficiencies resulting from a lack of communication and overall system perspective.

Point #10: Eliminate Slogans Asking for Zero Defects and Unattainable Productivity

Lean Six Sigma aims for zero defects but provides the training and tools to get close over time.

Setting lofty goals that seem out of reach for the employees will only contribute to poor morale and adversarial relationships. Rather, it is important to set reasonable goals that make employees take pride in achieving the goals. Over time, these goals or targets will be revised to set higher standards, but again, meeting the new expectations must be perceived as achievable.

Point #11: Eliminate the Emphasis on Numerical Quotas

The piece rate system of yesteryear often sacrificed quality for quantity. Point #11 does not call for the elimination of reasonable quotas. Rather, it urges supervisors and leaders to stop relying heavily on those for performance evaluations. Physicians could see a very large number of patients if they spent very little time with them. This might lead the physicians to overlook important symptoms and misdiagnose. The poor quality of care and deficient physician–patient interaction would threaten not only patient safety but also patient satisfaction. At the other extreme, a physician could extend the exam time beyond what is necessary, which would then hurt the bottom line because of low volume and make it difficult for patients to schedule timely appointments. Therefore, Point #11 implies balance. A certain numerical target may be set, but it should never jeopardize quality.

Point #12: Remove Barriers That Rob People of Pride of Workmanship

This point is related to the previous one. Numerical goals that prevent employees from doing their jobs well and enjoying the pride of fully exercising their skills must be eradicated. These goals should be replaced with a system that emphasizes problem-solving and the delivery of a superior product or service.

Point #13: Institute a Vigorous Program of Education and Self-Improvement

Deming recognized the importance of training and professional development. He viewed self-improvement as a driver of quality improvements throughout the organization.

Point #14: Put Everybody in the Company to Work to Accomplish the Transformation

Point #14 stresses that quality becomes everyone's purpose and part of everyone's job. In other words, quality is engrained in the organizational culture. **Culture**, or the basic set of values, assumptions, and beliefs in an organization, is what guides people when no one is looking. A healthcare organization's culture reflects the beliefs, attitudes, and priorities of the staff, including physicians and leadership. When quality is approached as a set of values, as a general orientation, and as an organizational ideology, there evolves a sense of engagement and a desire to strive to do better (Eva, 2023).

Deming's 14 points have passed the test of time across industries. A consistent approach to meaningful measurement and continuous improvement contribute to increased quality of care and patient safety. Two dominant methodologies have built on the concepts of leadership, measurement, analysis, and continuous improvement. They are called Lean and Six Sigma and are the focus of this textbook. An overview is presented in the next chapter.

PURPOSE AND FOCUS OF THIS BOOK

It is hoped that you now have a better glimpse of the threats to a value-based healthcare system: spiraling costs, disappointing overall quality performance, complex regulatory environment, and unfavorable population demographics. If you are in the healthcare field, you must deal with these seemingly insurmountable problems and contribute to the solution. The rest of this book is devoted to equipping you with the knowledge and tools necessary to use quality as a strategic competitive weapon. This is accomplished through the completion of a process improvement project using an integrated Lean Six Sigma (LSS) framework.

First, we *Define* the process improvement project and model the process (Chapter 3). It is critical at that stage to identify the customer(s) of the process, identify their needs and expectations (the Voice of the Customer), and translate those into process requirements (the Voice of the Process; Chapter 4). We are then ready to formulate a plan for the execution of the project and specify the deliverables (Chapter 5).

Second, we *Measure* the current process by mapping it and identifying the steps that do not contribute value (Chapter 6). We also collect process performance data, describe them graphically for better understanding (Chapter 7), and assess the process stability and capability (Chapter 8).

Third, we *Analyze* the process. We identify the root causes of the process inefficiencies that will spearhead improvement. To do so, we use a battery of tools and techniques (Chapter 9).

Fourth, we *Improve* the process by implementing process design principles, reconfiguring the layout, and eliminating bottlenecks (Chapter 10). We then assess whether the plan for improvement worked as intended (Chapter 11).

Finally, we *Control* the improved process by establishing standard operating procedures and sticking to a control plan. The improvement is standardized and becomes the norm. Lessons learned from the project are documented for future reference (Chapter 12).

Because the pursuit of excellence is a continuous journey, we seek further improvements and transition toward achieving high reliability and resiliency (Chapter 13).

Throughout the book, we adopt a very "hands-on" approach with multiple examples, tutorial videos with practice, vignettes that showcase real-world implementations, FAQ sections based on actual student questions, a focus on jobs with interviews of healthcare professionals involved in quality improvement projects, and tips for **Lean Six Sigma certification**. Students seeking certification will also have access to additional online resources. Furthermore, we thought it best to present the concepts in a work context. Meet the employees of Bright Angel Medical Center (BAMC)! Because successful process improvements require systems thinking and teamwork, the personal and cultural challenges that you will face must be anticipated. The story about the trials and successes of a fictional health system *puts the patient first* while narrating situations that you will probably encounter. You will see how the employees use chapter materials to solve problems day after day to achieve world class quality.

BRIGHT ANGEL MEDICAL CENTER 1.1

Bright Angel Medical Center (BAMC) has served its community well for the past 45 years. Over that time, the health system has grown with the population and now consists of two acute care hospitals, two critical access hospitals, an ambulatory surgery center, a long-term care facility, and several physician offices. The long-time CEO, Richard Cline, had been in his role for 22 years and had recently announced his plans to retire. He had been working with the board of directors for the past 12 months to find a successor. The chairman of the board, Stewart Baldrige, spearheaded the search committee, and they eventually brought in an external candidate, Kimberly Mitchell, to succeed Mr. Cline. The board was split on hiring an outside candidate versus promoting from within, and there had been some fierce discussions over the past few months. When the final vote tallied in favor of Kimberly Mitchell, two long-standing board members resigned in protest.

Kimberly officially assumed her duties as president and CEO 2 weeks ago and she has uncovered some troubling news. Bright Angel has a long history of success in this community, but over the past several years, complacency has set in, and the financial performance of the organization has deteriorated. Recently, a private equity firm opened a brand-new imaging center in town, and that was cutting into their market share. In addition, many of the departments had been stuck in their traditional methods of delivering care and had not improved their processes or safety protocols to keep pace with current regulations.

One week after stepping into the role, a prominent board member asked to meet with Kimberly to share an awful experience he had had while waiting to be seen in the ED for

(*continued*)

BRIGHT ANGEL MEDICAL CENTER 1.1 (*CONTINUED*)

a finger laceration. Kimberly was also notified of two sentinel events related to wrong site surgery in the ambulatory surgery center.

She was wondering if taking on the CEO role for a system with so many problems was a mistake. Kimberly had also learned that the system chief operating officer, Mira Martinez, was one of the finalists for the job, and she worried that Mira would have a bruised ego from not being selected for the role. Kimberly thought about the challenging landscape and pondered where she should begin. Does the ED need attention first? Or the surgery center? What about the concerning financial numbers? She was convinced that some of these areas would benefit from her Lean Six Sigma training and started to prioritize her first meetings. After completing a SWOT analysis (Exhibit 1.1) with her executive team, they came to an agreement that due to the importance of the ED as the front door to the hospital and the overall poor performance, that should be their first area of focus.

EXHIBIT 1.1 BAMC'S SWOT ANALYSIS

Internal

	Positive	**Negative**
Internal	**Strengths** • Strong brand in the market • Long, well-established history of providing care in the market • Hub and spoke model with outlying clinics that refer to the larger hospital • Ambulatory surgery center that allows for outpatient operations • Well-established orthopedic and neurosurgery service lines • New CEO willing to challenge the status quo	**Weaknesses** • Poor reputation in the ED for long wait times and low patient satisfaction • Aging operating rooms, ED, and patient care areas • Significant staffing shortages in some departments leading to a dependence on traveling nurses, especially in the ED • Recent deterioration in financial performance due to shift in payer mix and increased expense • Challenging primary care access • Lack of agility and slow decision-making leading to an inability to respond to competitor threats • Poor case turnover in the surgery center and quality concerns in the care delivery
External	**Opportunities** • Recent dissolution of large cardiology group creates an opening for new business • Higher cost of labor forcing a redesign of care teams • Other critical access hospitals looking to partner for more complex referrals	**Threats** • Lower payer reimbursements in ED • Shifting competitor landscape with new entrants looking to capture high-end imaging and urgent care business • Wage pressure • Looming physician shortage • Aging population (higher portion on Medicare, more costly care) • Increased supply costs

External

Abbreviations: BAMC, Bright Angel Medical Center; SWOT, strengths, weaknesses, opportunities, and threats.

(*continued*)

BRIGHT ANGEL MEDICAL CENTER 1.1 (*CONTINUED*)

Bright Angel Medical Center Characters and Their Roles

Board Members

- Richard Cline — Retiring CEO
- Stewart Baldrige — Board chair
- Jamal Nelson — New board member
- Emily Bates — New board member

Executive Leadership Team

- Kimberly Mitchell — New CEO
- Joe García — CFO
- Mira Martinez — Chief operating officer (COO)
- Michael Chen — Chief nursing officer (CNO)
- Dr. Paul Tibbets — Chief medical officer (CMO)
- Samantha Enapay — Chief human resources officer (CHRO)

Project Team

- Dr. Paul Tibbets — Executive sponsor
- Adeleke Mensah — ED improvement project manager
- Barbara Waters — ED director
- Ali Hussein — Patient experience manager
- Dr. Hana Aoki — ED medical director
- Olina Petrenko — Director of quality and Six Sigma Master Black Belt
- Loretta Romero — ED nurse manager

Other People at BAMC

- Philip Robinson — Chief pharmacy officer
- Dr. C. P. Rao — Surgery center director

The healthcare industry is full of challenging questions which sometimes do not have a clear answer. The end of each chapter will present an ethical scenario to reflect and discuss the pros and cons of various options.

ETHICAL SCENARIO 1.1

Selecting Patients Based on Insurance Status

Physicians in private practice across the United States are running their own small businesses. They are responsible for every element of the business including managing HR issues, recruitment, business development, marketing, and fiscal management, among other responsibilities. In markets where patient demand exceeds physician supply, doctors can be motivated to fill as many slots as possible with commercially insured patients. Patients with government insurance, such as Medicare and Medicaid, reimburse at a lower rate than commercial insurance. Uninsured or "self-pay" patients, many of whom are unable to afford to pay for their care, are responsible for the entire balance for the services they receive. The disparity between payments for identical services often leads private offices to limit the number of patients seen with government insurance and may require payment upfront for the uninsured.

What does this mean for access to care for the uninsured and underinsured?

What are the possible outcomes for patients who cannot find outpatient appointments due to their insurance status?

What would you recommend to improve the situation?

ETHICAL SCENARIO 1.2

Moving From Volume to Value

Most of the reimbursement models across the United States are based on a fee-for-service model. This payment method pays physicians for an activity—office visit, procedure, or encounter. Likewise, hospitals are reimbursed for every lab order and imaging test completed for ambulatory patients. The financial incentives of fee-for-service reimbursement encourage healthcare utilization. CMS has begun shifting from volume to value and paying more based on outcomes than on the number of visits. As healthcare spending continues to rise, CMS has set a target that, by 2030, all payments will be in some type of value-based arrangement. Some physicians and hospitals have resisted the transition from volume to value with the argument that patients are not held accountable for complying with medical regimens.

What are the downsides of maintaining a fee-for-service reimbursement model?

What is needed for physicians and hospitals to effectively move from volume to value?

SUMMARY

This chapter reviewed the history of healthcare and healthcare reform in the United States. This reform was driven primarily by quality, costs, and access concerns. Unfortunately, serious challenges to value-based healthcare remain. Building quality into a health system will help you tackle these challenges effectively and increase value for the patient. Gaining expertise in the field of quality will enable you to design processes that are mistake-proof, robust, and devoid of waste. Total quality management and Lean Six Sigma principles provide a treasure trove of tools and best practices that will help you achieve quality excellence. As you work along BAMC's team in this book, you will prepare yourself for Lean Six Sigma certification and the careers it opens up.

KEY TERMS

Value
Health maintenance organization (HMO)
Diagnosis-related group (DRG)
Affordable Care Act (ACA)
Fraud
Abuse
Overuse
Medical error
Health disparity
Safety
Timeliness (aim for quality)
Effectiveness
Efficiency
Equitable treatment
Patient-centeredness
Medical home
Accountable care organization (ACO)
Hospital value-based purchasing (VBP)
Value-based purchasing (VBP)
Merit-based incentive payment system (MIPS)
Population health
Social determinants of health
Systems thinking
Business strategy
SWOT analysis
Functional strategy
Operations
Operations strategy
Competitive priorities
Quality
Cost
Flexibility
Handoff
Prevention costs
Appraisal costs
Internal failure costs
External failure costs
Cumulative model
Order winners
Order qualifiers
Productive system
Total quality management (TQM)
Plan-do-study-act (PDSA) cycle
The Joint Commission (TJC)
Culture
Lean Six Sigma certification
Fee-for-service (FFS)

REVIEW QUESTIONS

1. What is value in general? What is value in healthcare?
2. Select five major events that shaped healthcare in the 20th century and describe them.

3. What are the current threats to value-based care? Describe each one.
4. What are the roots of the administrative complexity of the U.S. healthcare system?
5. What are the six aims for healthcare quality?
6. What is patient-centeredness? Give examples.
7. What is health disparity? Give examples.
8. List and explain the care delivery models that contribute to value-based healthcare.
9. List and briefly explain five of the new healthcare opportunities that may contribute to improving value.
10. Why is "systems thinking" necessary to improve the value of healthcare?
11. What is a business strategy?
12. An operations strategy is based on four competitive priorities. What are they?
13. What is the cumulative model? Illustrate it with a healthcare example.
14. What is a process?
15. Give examples of inputs and outputs in healthcare.
16. What is TQM? What are its principles?
17. What is the PDSA cycle? What are its elements?
18. What are the costs of quality?
19. Deming's third point is consistent with a recommendation from the IOM. What is it?
20. Look at the issues that have contributed to the increase in healthcare costs in the United States, list the one(s) that is (are) under the influence of operations management.

LEARNING ACTIVITIES

1. Select a piece of healthcare legislation that was passed in the last 10 years. What are its benefits to society? What are its unintended drawbacks?
2. Think about a memorable experience that you had as a patient. Describe all the positive and negative aspects of the experience. If you encountered some problems, how do you think they could be fixed?
3. In the video *Why US Health Care Is Getting More Expensive*, by CNBC, February 28, 2022 (https://www.youtube.com/watch?v=QRihG16iSug)
   a. What are the reasons why costs continue to go up?
   b. What are some of the approaches that can control them?
4. Research the term *value* in healthcare. What does this term really mean? Are models designed to provide value for the patient, physician, or insurer? Explain your answer.
5. The video *Systems Thinking Is Not Optional: Lessons From a Pandemic | Steve Woodsmall | TEDxLake-Junaluska*, by TEDx Talks, April 1, 2021 (https://www.youtube.com/watch?v=yuvHvi84TFw), applies the principles of systems thinking to the pandemic. How does it help you think about different issues? Give an example in your organization.
6. Ask ChatGPT or any other chatbot to formulate a plan to decrease the fall rate at a nursing facility. Explain why implementation of the plan will require systems thinking.

REFERENCES

AHA Center for Health Innovation. (2023). *The AHA Center for Health Innovation: Where disruption, collaboration and innovation-at-scale converge to reimagine health care*. American Hospital Association. https://www.aha.org/center

American Medical Association. (1847). *Code of medical ethics*. AMA Press. https://code-medical-ethics.ama-assn.org/

Bailey, V. (2022, March 2). *High hospital prices do not always lead to better health outcomes*. RevCycle Intelligence. https://revcycleintelligence.com/news/high-hospital-prices-do-not-always-lead-to-better-health-outcomes

Ballard, D. J. (2015). *The guide to achieving STEEP health care: Baylor Scott & White health's quality improvement journey*. CRC Press.

Carmouche, D. (2023, March 2). *Walmart health nearly doubles in size with launch into two new states in 2024*. https://corporate.walmart.com/newsroom/2023/03/02/walmart-health-nearly-doubles-in-size-with-launch-into-two-new-states-in-2024

Centers for Disease Control and Prevention. (2024). *Social determinants of health at CDC*. U.S. Department of Health & Human Services. https://www.cdc.gov/about/priorities/social-determinants-of-health-at-cdc.html

Centers for Disease Control and Prevention. (2023). *Health disparities*. U.S. Department of Health & Human Services. https://www.cdc.gov/healthyyouth/disparities/index.htm

Centers for Medicare & Medicaid Services. (2009, November 13). *Key milestones in CMS programs*. Author. http://www.cms.hhs.gov/History

Centers for Medicare & Medicaid Services. (2019). *MACRA*. https://www.cms.gov/medicare/quality/value-based-programs/chip-reauthorization-act

Centers for Medicare & Medicaid Services. (2023). *Reporting options overview*. Author. https://qpp.cms.gov/mips/reporting-options-overview

Centers for Medicare & Medicaid Services (2024). *The Hospital Value-Based Purchasing (VBP) Program*. https://www.cms.gov/medicare/quality/value-based-programs/hospital-purchasing

Chapman, S. (2016). A solution inside a problem. *For The Record*, *28*(5), 24. https://www.fortherecordmag.com/archives/0516p24.shtml

Children's Hospital Los Angeles. (2022). *CHLA innovation studio*. https://www.chla.org/chla-innovation-studio

CMS.gov. (2023). *The hospital value-based purchasing (VBP) program*. Centers for Medicare & Medicaid Services. https://www.cms.gov/Medicare/Quality-Initiatives-Patient-Assessment-Instruments/Value-Based-Programs/HVBP/Hospital-Value-Based-Purchasing

CVS Health. (2023). *Other health care services*. https://www.cvshealth.com/services/health-care-and-wellness/other-health-care-services.html

Deming, W. E. (1982). *Out of the crisis*. The MIT Press.

Dey, P., & Bach, P. B. (2019). The 6 functions of health insurance. *JAMA*, *321*(13), 1242–1243. https://jamanetwork.com/journals/jama/fullarticle/2729357

Dohale, V., Gunasekaran, A., Akarte, M. M., & Verma, P. (2022). 52 Years of manufacturing strategy: An evolutionary review of literature (1969–2021). *International Journal of Production Research*, *60*(2), 569–594. https://doi.org/10.1080/00207543.2021.1971788

Eva, K. W. (2023). Quality improvement as a statement of values. *Medical Education*, *57*(1), 2–3. https://doi.org/10.1111/medu.14972

Ferdows, K., & De Meyer, A. (1990). Lasting improvements in manufacturing performance. *Journal of Operations Management*, *9*(2), 168–184. https://doi.org/10.1016/0272-6963(90)90094-T

First Stop Health. (2022, July 4). *How much time does a doctor visit really take?* Author.

Gee, E., & Spiro, T. (2019). *Excess administrative costs burden the U.S. health care system*. https://www.americanprogress.org/issues/healthcare/reports/2019/04/08/468302/excess-administrative-costs-burden-u-s-health-care-system

Global Burden of Disease. (2020). Global burden of 369 diseases and injuries in 204 countries and territories, 1990–2019: A systematic analysis for the Global Burden of Disease Study 2019. *The Lancet, 396*, 1204–1222. https://www.thelancet.com/pdfs/journals/lancet/PIIS0140-6736(20)30925-9.pdf

Goodridge, E., & Arnquist, S. (2009). A history of overhauling health care. *The New York Times*. http://www.nytimes.com/interactive/2009/07/19/us/politics/20090717_HEALTH_TIMELINE.html?_r=0

Grossman, C. M. (2008). The first use of penicillin in the United States. *Annals of Internal Medicine, 149*(2), 135–136. https://doi.org/10.7326/0003-4819-149-2-200807150-00009

Haque, L. A. (2021). The effect of delays in acute medical treatment on total cost and potential ramifications due to the coronavirus pandemic. *Harvard Public Health Review, 26*. https://doi.org/10.54111/0001/Z7

Henry, T. A. (2023, May 18). *Why you need a systems thinker in health care*. American Medical Association. https://www.ama-assn.org/education/changemeded-initiative/why-you-need-be-systems-thinker-health-care

Hill, A., & Hill, T. (2018). *Operations strategy: Design, implementation, and delivery*. Palgrave.

Hill, T. (2000). *Manufacturing strategy: Text and cases* (3rd ed.). McGraw-Hill.

Institute of Medicine. (1999). *To err is human*. National Academies Press. https://nap.nationalacademies.org/resource/9728/To-Err-is-Human-1999--report-brief.pdf

Institute of Medicine. (2001). *Crossing the quality chasm: A new health system for the 21st century*. National Academies Press. https://www.ncbi.nlm.nih.gov/books/NBK222271/

Institute of Medicine. (2012). *Best care at lower cost: The path to continuously learning health care in America*. National Academies Press. https://nap.nationalacademies.org/catalog/13444/best-care-at-lower-cost-the-path-to-continuously-learning

Jain, N., & LaBeaud, D. (2022). How should US health care lead global change in plastic waste disposal? *AMA Journal of Ethics, 24*(10), E986–E993. https://doi.org/10.1001/amajethics.2022.986

Johnson, M. (2024, January 16). How doctors are using AI to diagnose a hidden heart condition in kids. *The Washington Post*. https://www.washingtonpost.com/science/2024/01/16/ai-diagnose-rheumatic-heart-disease

KaufmanHall. (2022). *The financial effects of hospital workforce dislocation: A special workforce edition of the National Hospital Flash Report*. https://www.kaufmanhall.com/sites/default/files/2022-05/KH-NHFR-Special-Report-2.pdf

Kolak, M., Bhatt, J., Park, Y. H., Padrón, N. A., & Molefe, A. (2019). Quantification of neighborhood-level social determinants of health in the continental United States. *JAMA Network Open, 3*(1), e1919928. https://doi.org/10.1001/jamanetworkopen.2019.19928

Lenharo, M. (2024). *Google AI has better bedside manner than human doctors—and makes better diagnoses*. Nature. https://www.nature.com/articles/d41586-024-00099-4

Livingston, S. (2018, January 27). *Left out of the game: Health systems offer direct-to-employer contracting to eliminate insurers*. Modern Healthcare. https://www.modernhealthcare.com/article/20180127/NEWS/180129919/left-out-of-the-game-health-systems-offer-direct-to-employer-contracting-to-eliminate-insurers

Makary, M. A., & Daniel, M. (2016). Medical error—the third leading cause of death in the US. *The British Medical Journal, 353*, i2139. https://doi.org/10.1136/bmj.i2139

Merritt Hawkins. (2022). *2022 Survey of physician appointment wait times and Medicare and Medicaid acceptance rates*. https://www.merritthawkins.com/uploadedFiles/MerrittHawkins/Content/News_and_Insights/Articles/mha-2022-wait-time-survey.pdf

Nakane, J. (1986). *Manufacturing futures survey in Japan, a comparative survey 1983–1986*. Waseda University, System Science Institute.

National Institutes of Health. (2024, January). *Artificial intelligence and your health: How computers are helping medicine*. NIH News in Health. https://newsinhealth.nih.gov/2024/01/artificial-intelligence-your-health

Noble, M. A. (1995). Manufacturing strategy: Testing the cumulative model in a multiple country context. *Decision Sciences, 26*(5), 693–721. https://doi.org/10.1111/j.1540-5915.1995.tb01446.x

Norris, L. (2023, April 16). *Is there a penalty for being uninsured in 2023?* Verywell Health. https://www.verywellhealth.com/obamacare-penalty-for-being-uninsured-4132434

Office of the Inspector General. (2023). *Fraud and abuse laws*. HHS Office of Inspector General. https://oig.hhs.gov/compliance/physician-education/fraud-abuse-laws

Papanicolas, I., Woskie, L. R., & Jha, A. K. (2018). Health care spending in the United States and other high-income countries. *JAMA, 319*(10), 1024–1039. https://doi.org/10.1001/jama.2018.1150

Peng, Y., Wu, T., Chen, Z., & Deng, Z. (2022). Value cocreation in health care: Systematic review. *Journal of Medical Internet Research, 24*(3), e33061. https://doi.org/10.2196%2F33061

Peterson-KFF. (2024, January 23). *How does health spending in the U.S. compare to other countries?* https://www.healthsystemtracker.org/chart-collection/health-spending-u-s-compare-countries

Porter, M. E. (1985). *The competitive advantage: Creating and sustaining superior performance*. Free Press.

Porter, M. E., & Lee, T. H. (2015). Why strategy matters now. *The New England Journal of Medicine, 372*(18), 1681–1684. https://doi.org/10.1056/NEJMp1502419

Quinn, R. (2013). Rethinking antibiotic research and development: World War II and the penicillin collaborative. *American Journal of Public Health, 103*(3), 426–434. https://doi.org/10.2105/AJPH.2012.300693

Radley, D. C., Baumgartner, J. C., & Collins, S. R. (2022). *2022 Scorecard on state health system performance: How did states do during the COVID-19 pandemic?* https://www.commonwealthfund.org/publications/scorecard/2022/jun/2022-scorecard-state-health-system-performance

Rakshit, S., McGough, M., & Amin, K. (2024, January 30). *How does U.S. life expectancy compare to other countries?* https://www.healthsystemtracker.org/chart-collection/u-s-life-expectancy-compare-countries

Rosenthal, M. B., Berndt, E. R., Donohue, J. M., Frank, R. G., & Epstein, A. M. (2002). Promotion of prescription drugs to consumers. *New England Journal of Medicine, 346*(7), 498–505. https://doi.org/10.1056/NEJMsa012075

Schooley, S. (2023). What is a SWOT analysis? (And when to use it). *Business News Daily*. https://www.businessnewsdaily.com/4245-swot-analysis.html

Schyve, P. M. (2009). *Leadership in healthcare organizations: A guide to Joint Commission leadership standards*. https://psnet.ahrq.gov/issue/leadership-healthcare-organizations-guide-joint-commission-leadership-standards

Silverman, F., & Danner, B. (2000, November 3). *Healthcare timeline (classroom materials). Healthcare crisis: Who's at risk?* Public Broadcasting Service. https://www.pbs.org/healthcarecrisis/classroom_timeline.html

Skinner, W. (1966). Production under pressure. *Harvard Business Review, 44*(6), 139–146.

Sum, C. C., Singh, P. H., & Heng, H. Y. (2012). An examination of the cumulative capabilities model in selected Asia-Pacific countries. *Production Planning and Control, 23*(10–11), 735–753. https://doi.org/10.1080/09537287.2011.642135

Swann, J. P. (2001). Pharmaceutical industry. In P. S. Boyer (Ed.), *The Oxford companion to United States history (pp. xx-xx)*. Oxford University Press.

Thomas, L. (2022, July 7). *The sustainable management of healthcare waste*. News Medical Life Sciences. https://www.news-medical.net/health/The-Sustainable-Management-of-Healthcare-Waste.aspx

Toussaint, J. S. (2021, January 6). *Why Haven healthcare failed*. Harvard Business Review. https://hbr.org/2021/01/why-haven-healthcare-failed

U.S. Census Bureau. (2010). *Income, poverty, and health insurance coverage in the United States: 2009.* https://www.census.gov/library/publications/2010/demo/p60-238.html

Vadarajan, P. R., & Clark, T. (1994). Delineating the scope of corporate, business, and marketing strategy. *Journal of Business Research, 31*(2–3), 93–105. https://doi.org/10.1016/0148-2963(94)90074-4

Wager, E., Telesford, I., Rakshit, S., Kurani, N., & Cox, C. (2024). How does the quality of the U.S. health system compare to other countries? https://www.healthsystemtracker.org/chart-collection/quality-u-s-healthcare-system-compare-countries/

Waters, D. (2006). *Operations strategy*. Cengage Learning.

World Medical Association. (2023). *Green health: Reducing the environmental impact of healthcare.* https://www.wma.net/what-we-do/public-health/green-health

CHAPTER 2

INTRODUCTION TO LEAN SIX SIGMA: DOING IT RIGHT THE FIRST TIME

BRIGHT ANGEL MEDICAL CENTER 2.1

The restaurant opened at 6:00 a.m. for breakfast, and Kimberly Mitchell was grateful that the board chair, Stewart Baldrige, was willing to meet her so early to discuss her plans. Kimberly shared with him that she had two initial priorities—first was to ask the nominating committee of the board to find some new business leaders to fill the two vacant board positions.

"We need some fresh blood on our board, Stewart," Kimberly stated in a matter-of-fact tone. Stewart agreed. The two board members who had resigned had each served for over 20 years and were frequently barriers to innovative ways of thinking.

Stewart added, "I will call the chair of the nominating committee today. We have several influential leaders in this community, and we should not have trouble finding a few of them interested in helping us get Bright Angel back on track."

Kimberly was glad to hear they were on the same page. "If you agree, I would also like to tell the board about transforming Bright Angel Medical Center (BAMC)'s culture. We had success in my last organization with utilizing Lean Six Sigma principles to drive quality improvement. It's not just about tools, it's about changing the way we all think about reaching excellence," Kimberly shared. "Change is hard, and I will need your support as we move forward." Stewart nodded, but he wondered where this was going.

Which is better: A board member with experience in the organization or one with an outside perspective?

Should Lean Six Sigma be discussed at a board meeting?

LEARNING OBJECTIVES

After reading this chapter, you will be able to:

- Recognize the importance of leadership and culture in organizations that adopt Lean Six Sigma (LSS) methodologies.
- Describe the eight types of waste found in healthcare processes.
- List the five Lean principles and explain briefly how each one is used to examine a process.
- Understand the importance of flow in Lean.
- List some of the barriers to a successful Lean implementation.

- Explain the basis for Six Sigma.
- Describe the steps in DMAIC (define, measure, analyze, improve, control).
- Describe the various roles in Six Sigma projects.
- List the major benefits of LSS.
- Determine if LSS certification is valuable to you now.

INTRODUCTION

In Chapter 1, we made a strong argument for building quality into processes. In this chapter, we present a general overview of Lean Six Sigma (LSS). These complementary methodologies are powerful drivers of process improvements and mistake prevention. They were both derived from manufacturing, but they are increasingly used to improve healthcare. Each brings to the improvement process something the other does not.

In practice, Lean is often used first, when the process needing improvement has not previously been refined. Think of Lean as a house painter, using broad strokes and a wide brush. It looks at steps in the process fairly quickly, identifies areas for improvement, and allows you to check whether the change creates an improved process flow. After using Lean methods, if specific steps need refinement and a high level of reliability, the more technical Six Sigma tools help decrease variation and improve process outcomes. Think of Six Sigma as an artist, using precise strokes to refine the picture.

We describe the methodologies of Lean and Six Sigma, illustrate how each methodology can be used, and show how their fusion, LSS, can steer improvement in healthcare.

WHY IS THIS MATERIAL USEFUL?

LSS helps improve both efficiency and effectiveness by eliminating waste and reducing defects which, in healthcare, can be deadly. Together, the two methodologies aim at increasing the value of care provided. However, their careful implementation is the key to success. The tools and principles presented in this book will guide you in the successful delivery of patient-centered care and will facilitate your journey toward LSS certification.

ON THE JOB! INTERVIEW VIDEO 2.1

Bethany Rogers
Director of Performance Improvement, Master Black Belt

Making Change a Gift, Not a Threat!

Strategy deployment
Mini Kaizen: N95 mask fit-testing in high volume
Advantages of LSS training

1. What is the value of LSS training for those who are working on process performance improvements?
2. Bethany discusses the use of Lean principles in speeding up the N95 mask fit-testing process. What are some of the key elements that helped to optimize this process?
3. Change management is a core competency for anyone in a leadership role. Discuss some strategies leaders can implement to help team members better embrace organizational change.

The interview is available online by visiting www.springerpub.com/courseconnect. See inside front cover and tear-out card for CourseConnect details.

LEAN

Although some trace the idea of rigorous process analysis back to the 1450s' shipbuilding industry in Venice, most attribute Henry Ford with seizing the idea of streamlining the process of building automobiles (H. Ford & Crowther, 1922). He set up the moving assembly line and lined up fabrication processes in sequence to produce cheaper automobiles. However, a limitation of the assembly line was that it did not allow for variety. Henry Ford's famous quote, "Any customer can have a car painted any color that he wants so long as it is black" (H. Ford & Crowther, 1922, p. 112), sums up this problem!

In the 1930s, Kiichiro Toyoda founded Toyota Motor Corp. After initial failures in the American market, the company built on the basic assembly line concept and invented what is now called the "Toyota Production System (TPS)." Toyota shifted the focus of the automobile assembly process to the flow of the automobile throughout the total process. The TPS began to right-size machines for the volume needed, introduce self-monitoring machines that ensured quality, line up the machines in process sequence, and develop quick setups so that each machine could make small volumes of many part numbers. The TPS was much more than an improved assembly line. It focused on the customer, and the push was to give the customer *value*. A major component of the TPS was treating employees with respect and allowing employees to think about and improve processes when they saw the need. W. Edwards Deming's teachings had greatly influenced the company's quality transformation and worldwide success, prompting Toyota's honorary chairman to say: "There is not a day I don't think about what Dr. Deming meant to us. Deming is the core of our management" (Hunter, 2013).

Lean is a system. It "is a way of thinking about creating needed value with fewer resources and less waste. And Lean is a practice consisting of continuous experimentation to achieve perfect value with zero waste. Lean thinking and practice occur together" (Lean Enterprise Institute, 2023b). The core idea of Lean involves distinguishing what adds value to a process from what does not. The non–value-added steps are called "**waste**" (or *muda* in Japanese). In fact, the term *Lean* means with little or no fat. The goal is to ensure each process is as streamlined as possible, and designed to provide the customer with the most value. In its comprehensive form, Lean is a complete management system in which the values that permeate the organization are aligned with the guiding principles of Lean.

Healthcare organizations have shown that when Lean practices are rigorously applied throughout the organization, efficiency, cost, timeliness, quality, and flexibility are dramatically improved (Antony et al., 2019; Virginia Mason Institute, 2021). The reason that Lean is so useful in healthcare is that care processes in large organizations have generally evolved over time and have rarely been the result of thoughtful analysis. The focus tends to be on optimal time utilization for doctors and nurses, and not on patients. Care is usually segmented into departments, and often the only people who experience the entire patient care process are the patients themselves. In these systems, a patient can spend hours going from area to area, waiting at each step, for only a few minutes of value-added effort. Lean has the potential to break down the silos between departments and provide care that will add value from the patient's viewpoint (Graban, 2019; Box 2.1).

BOX 2.1 QUALITY IN PRACTICE!

Harnessing the Power of Lean at Virginia Mason Medical Center

Virginia Mason Medical Center began using Lean management principles in 2002. It developed the Virginia Mason Production System based on the TPS and deployed it throughout its system. For example, in its pursuit of improved patient safety, it focused on sepsis, a major cause of mortality in the United States. Through a series of improvement events designed to identify sepsis early, a protocol called the "Power Hour" was developed. With systematic use of the protocol, recognition time at the hospital dropped from 8 hours to 30 minutes, and time to antibiotic administration was reduced from 140 minutes to 66 minutes for inpatients. Because of its success, the Power Hour was expanded to outpatient services where time to treatment declined from 9 hours to less than an hour (Virginia Mason Franciscan Health, 2023).

LEAN CULTURE

A Lean culture is the backdrop for the use of Lean principles. Culture is a learned process that is cultivated within an organization in response to the working environment established by the leadership and management team. A Lean culture requires a framework with guiding principles and behavioral expectations for the whole organization. But more than that, Lean links the behavioral expectations with policies and procedures to achieve the vision. If you are a leader who wants to develop a culture in which Lean practices are pervasive, you cannot do it by edict. Your employees must learn the actions expected of them, and they will have to build these actions into their daily work. Not only do the frontline people need to learn what actions are expected, but leaders must also model the desired behaviors. Because respect is a necessary component of a Lean culture, everyone within the organization needs to be trained in the Lean methodology. Cultural change can take years to take root, so the leadership team must be committed to the practices as the new way of doing business.

Importance of Leadership and Training for Lean

To be a leader in a Lean organization, you must work differently. You must understand that when making decisions, you need to know the reality of what is happening in the field. You need to go where the problem is occurring, personally observe how the product or service is delivered, and gather facts for yourself. This process is called a "**Gemba walk.**" You ask the frontline employees questions and understand that they are the experts when it comes to the activity under investigation. Because respect is a fundamental value in a Lean organization, leaders and frontline staff work together and listen to each other as problems are solved. There are four types of conversations that, when *used at the right time*, can contribute to a more productive and considerate work environment (J. Ford & Ford, 2009). The "**Four Conversations**" framework includes:

- **Initiative conversations** are meant to share new ideas, objectives, and anticipated benefits with all stakeholders who can make them happen.
- **Understanding conversations** are true dialogs designed to foster a complete understanding of an idea, a barrier, a method, or an anticipated benefit. Constructive feedback is a vital part of those conversations; the intent is to eliminate as much ambiguity as possible about what needs to be done, by whom, and how.
- **Performance conversations** include specific requirements for the deliverables of a project. As such, their purpose is to foster commitment and accountability.
- **Closure conversations** take place when a deliverable, or part of it, has been completed. They involve praise for a job well done or a candid discussion of the failures or missed opportunities experienced along the way.

Lean leaders do not only model desired behaviors, they inspire others to also become leaders. All people must be challenged by their work and understand how what they do fits into the whole system. Their mindset should be to solve problems, not just follow instructions. A Lean leader involves the entire team in every step of the improvement process. Lean leaders need to foster cross-functional teamwork, be willing to have their decisions challenged, and be open to contrary opinions. Ultimately, the Lean leader must successfully guide teams to a common goal.

Training is essential in creating a Lean culture. Because Lean uses data, measurements, and statistics to identify process inefficiencies and because it has a vocabulary to describe different types of waste and process improvement activities, it is important that everyone involved be well-versed in the methodology. Investing in Lean training for employees at all levels within an organization can be a catalyst to increase efficiencies. When the number of employees who have obtained Lean training reaches a critical mass, productivity and profitability can rise dramatically (McKinsey & Company, 2017).

BRIGHT ANGEL MEDICAL CENTER 2.2

Kimberly gathered her executive team to share what had happened at the last board meeting. "We are getting fresh blood on the board, and everyone seems ready for a change. They seemed very intrigued by transforming our culture and asked me how I planned to do so. I mentioned training and more teamwork. What do you think?"

Samantha Enapay, the chief human resources officer, replied that the first thing to do to make the staff receptive to any change was to fill the staffing holes and help improve morale in the ED.

Barbara Waters, the ED director, agreed. "We have so many traveling nurses down there right now. It is hard to build a culture when half of the staff are temporary. If we can replace them with permanent staff, it will help us develop comprehensive Lean training programs, build a Lean culture, and reduce our wasteful expenses. Moreover, we will be able to develop sets of best practices to encourage sustained participation and better communication in improvement projects."

That was music to the ears of Mira Martinez, the hospital chief operating officer (COO). She had noted a steady rise in traveling nurses over the past 18 months and was racking her brain on how to tackle that one. Barbara and Mira also agreed to dedicate time to look at the ED workflows and find opportunities to improve efficiencies. "It is going to take all hands on deck to get that unit functioning like it needs to be. Our teams are counting on us as is the board of directors. We have targeted the ED for improvement—now we need to execute on it." encouraged Kimberly.

How do high turnover and numerous temporary nurses impact the culture of a patient care unit?

Do healthcare teams function better when the members know each other?

WASTE ELIMINATION

To initiate Lean, you need to identify the process activities that create value to the customer. Anything else is considered "waste" (Table 2.1). There are eight types of waste (*muda*):

1. **overproduction**: doing more than necessary
2. **inventory**: excess raw materials, end products that are stored, work in progress that has not been completed
3. **defects, errors**: waste in the form of time wasted for rework, extra capacity to redo the work, litigation, and so on
4. **motion**: unnecessary movements because supplies and tools are not easily accessible or visible
5. **extra processing**: doing more than the customer actually values
6. **waiting**: inactivity in a process because one or more activities have not been delivered in time
7. **transport**: unnecessary movement of materials during the process
8. **underutilization**: not distributing work properly to the people who can do the job

Healthcare is loaded with these wastes. Most healthcare workers will grossly underestimate the amount of inefficiency that can be taken out of their workday. The key is to get everyone in the organization to systematically find waste, make it visible, and eradicate it.

To continually identify and eliminate waste, organizations must learn to care about the little things. This means helping people see the waste around them and recognizing that eliminating waste will free them up to do more valuable and rewarding activities.

TABLE 2.1 THE EIGHT TYPES OF WASTE IN HEALTHCARE

Types of Waste	Examples	Causes
Overproduction	• Generating reports that are no longer used • Duplication of diagnostic tests • Preparing medications for a discharged patient	• No evaluation of reports' benefits • Insufficient attention paid to patients' records • Poor or late charting of patients' record information
Inventory	• Having a higher PAR level than needed for supplies • Medications having to be thrown out because of past expiration date	• Lack of rigorous ordering procedure • Clutter in cabinets making it difficult to see what is in the back
Defects	• Mislabeled specimen • Wrong diet given to a patient	• Batch printing of labels • Process failure
Motion	• Looking for blood pressure cuff to take patient's vital signs • Items not set up for easy use	• Cluttered work environment • Workstation design
Extra processing	• Asking the same question multiple times at registration desks • Requiring multiple approvals	• Customer voice not heard • Lack of respect for people's time • Outdated processes
Waiting	• Waiting to see the physician • Waiting to get test results	• Work imbalance • Inadequate capacity planning • Batch processing
Transport	• Transporting supplies from central area to patient care rooms • Transporting patients over long distances to see different providers	• Lack of local storage for commonly used supplies • Lack of coordination among care providers
Underutilization	• Manager performing tasks that can be done by support staff • Physician doing work that nurse can do • Fixing errors rather than caring for patients	• Lack of clarification of roles • Poor workflow design • Uneven workload • Low standards and poor accountability

Abbreviation: PAR, periodic automatic replacement.

LEAN PRINCIPLES

Womack and Jones (1996) identified five Lean principles used to examine any process (Figure 2.1; Lean Enterprise Institute, 2023a). When adopting Lean for the first time, leaders may wish to begin with a relatively simple, focused process so that employees can be trained on Lean methods. Prior to moving forward, they need to be sure that everyone involved in the process is on board and will contribute to the analysis and change, and that the parameters to gauge success are clearly articulated. As healthcare units become more experienced in Lean interventions, their leaders can adopt its holistic approach and implement ambitious projects to maximize quality and cost savings throughout their organizations (Tlapa et al., 2020a).

Identify Value

The customer of the process determines value. The product or service being delivered must be what is wanted, at the right time, and at the right price. The customer expects the same product or service to be delivered the same way, every time. Listening to the voice of the customer (VOC; Chapter 4) will help you understand what the customer values.

When a process is being reviewed through the Lean lens, you need to ask the question, "Are we providing what the customers want in the way they want it?" If not, ask "What needs to be changed?" Only a small fraction of the total time and effort in any activity actually adds value

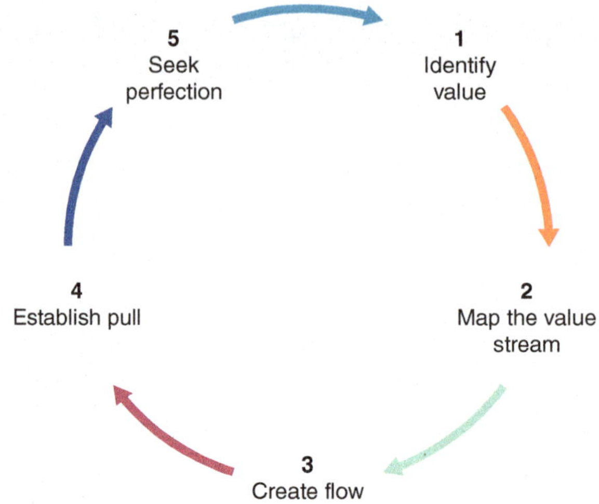

FIGURE 2.1 **Principles of Lean.**

Source: Lean Enterprise Institute. (2023a). *Lean thinking and practice*. https://www.lean.org/lexicon-terms/lean-thinking-and-practice/. Reprinted by permission from Lean Enterprise Institute.

for the customer. By clearly defining value for a specific product or service from the customer's perspective, all the non–value-added activities (waste) can be targeted for removal.

Map the Value Stream

Once you understand what your customer wants, the next step is to identify how you need to deliver it to them. The analysis and design of a process often starts with its graphical representation. A **value stream map (VSM)** depicts a process flow from a Lean perspective. It is understood that the process should create optimal value to the customer with high reliability and no, or minimal, waste. The VSM incorporates the activities that are valuable to the customer as well as those that are considered wasteful such as delays, errors, and unnecessary movements. The visualization of waste on the process map facilitates its subsequent elimination and thus aids in planning process redesign (Box 2.2). Although VSMs can be in digital form, it is sometimes easier for teams to collaborate on a VSM displayed on a wall (Figure 2.2). Team members will choose a scheme to represent the process steps and the weak points. For example, they can place sticky notes with different colors indicating value-added, non–value-added, needing improvement, and so forth.

BOX 2.2 QUALITY IN PRACTICE!

Identifying Waste at an Emergency Facility in Brazil

In emergency care facilities, overcrowding with long wait times and supply shortages is a common phenomenon. A VSM was developed to understand the flow for 30 nonemergent patients at an emergency referral unit in a large teaching hospital. For each patient, the process steps from admission to hospitalization or departure were identified and timed. Non–value-added time such as long waits and interruptions were considered as wasteful. A root cause analysis revealed that the principal reasons for waste were: (a) an imbalance between patient demand and personnel and room capacity, (b) system crashes, (c) poor distribution of work, (d) lack of materials used for patient risk classification, and (e) a poor referral process. Those issues became the focus of improvement efforts (de Barros et al., 2022).

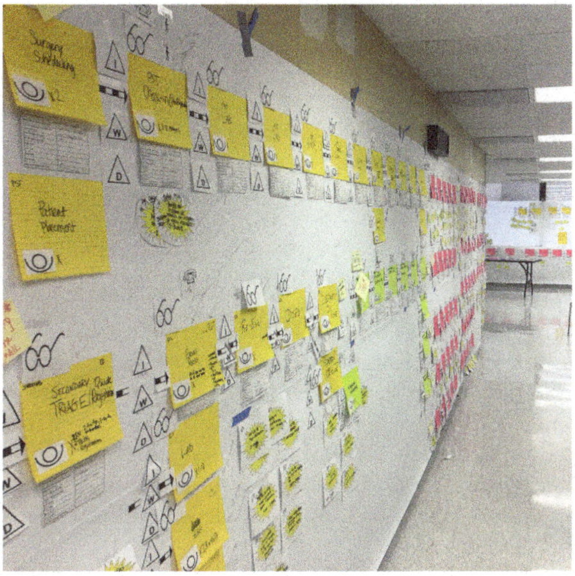

FIGURE 2.2 Value stream map showing process steps, waste, and opportunities for improvement.

Source: Photo credit: Dr. Robert Cavagnol.

Create Flow

The overarching theme in Lean is to create a smooth flow. Once the value to the customer is identified and the waste has been removed from the value stream, it is time to make the value-added steps flow with no disruptions (e.g., poor quality and rework, equipment breakdowns, convoluted processes, crowded workspace). To create flow, we must divorce ourselves from traditional thinking. We need to deconstruct the typical "departments" where activities are grouped by type and where batches of products, orders, documents, or people wait until resources are ready to process them. The more handoffs there are in the process, the more opportunities for errors, waits, and movements. Therefore, a simplification of the process through the elimination of steps is a good start. Then, rearranging the resources and workspace around the process sequence so that processing takes place in a continuous flow can proceed. Distances between the remaining process steps are meticulously documented, and every effort is made to reduce them. Physical layouts of the space may change as the non–value-added distances and disruptions in the flow are eliminated. The environment where activities are ongoing is also scrutinized to identify ways to do some "housecleaning" and make the use of the space more efficient. A tool used for this purpose is called the "**6S**" (Chapter 10).

Establish Pull

Before we discuss the concept of "pull" in Lean, let us talk about how traditional manufacturing processes work using the "**push system**." In a "push" environment, goods are produced without waiting for customer demand. For example, a hospital pharmacy may routinely make 100 saline IV bags per day. Why 100? Because it is the highest number of saline bags needed for patients in a day, and the pharmacy does not want to run out of bags. Because the hospital policy says that any IV bags not used in 24 hours must be discarded, many bags per day may be wasted. In a "push" system, process steps are executed independently, with little regard to the actual needs of the beneficiaries of their output. As a result, inventory accumulates, and materials may have to be discarded. When patients rather than materials or supplies are involved, they will have to wait (Figure 2.3).

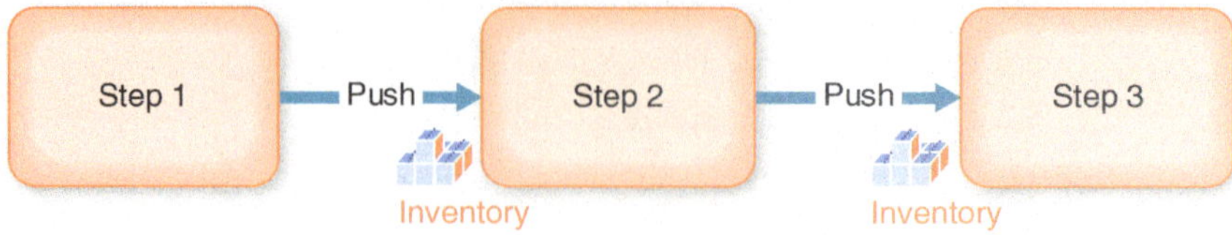

FIGURE 2.3 Push system.

The "**pull system**" principle is probably the most important logistical innovation of the TPS (Womack & Jones, 1996). "Pull" is the concept of producing a good or service in response to actual customer demand. The goal of "establishing pull" is to be highly responsive to customers' needs. The next person in the process is considered the "customer." Any demand (pull) from the downstream or "customer" process step triggers activity at the upstream or "supplier" process. Anything that is not used immediately or is waiting at any point in time to be processed at the next step is considered waste. A pull system allows materials, patients, documents, and so on, to flow smoothly from one step to the next; restocking takes place, but there is no overstocking; patients may wait, but for a short period of time.

No system is completely based on "pull." "Push" and "pull" must be used in tandem to produce a flow with minimal waiting between steps. In manufacturing, when a downstream process step initiates demand, a little bit of inventory must be available to meet that demand immediately (Figure 2.4). That little "slack" is consistent with a push system, but it is kept to a minimum. Whether we have a push or pull process, the real goal in Lean is "flow"—with downstream demand being promptly met by upstream supply. When you decrease the waste in the system, flow can happen.

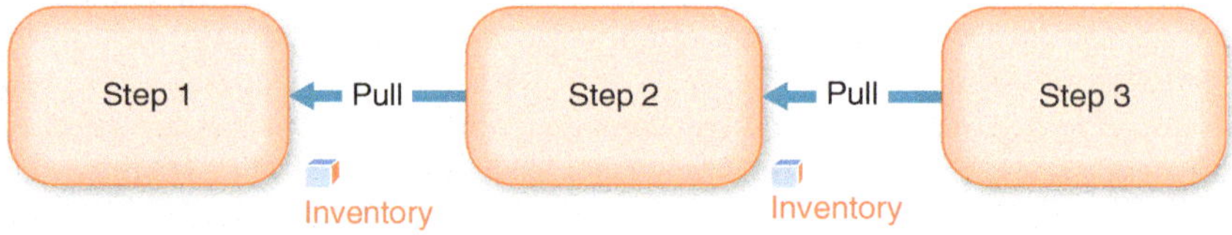

FIGURE 2.4 Pull system.

Just-in-Time

The pull system is consistent with the tightly coordinated processing system called **just-in-time (JIT)**. Under that system, materials, supplies, or patients move through the system exactly when they are needed, not early and not late. For example, Toyota ordered automobile parts in small quantities based on their short-term needs. The process was designed to ensure that a part would arrive just in time to be used, eliminating the need to keep it in inventory. Today, many healthcare organizations use a JIT system to eliminate the need to store excess supplies (Balkhi et al., 2022).

Central to the concept of JIT are visual aids. Good visual aids provide easy-to-understand information at a glance. As such, they help reduce miscommunication, a typical source of defects, delays, and other forms of waste. For example, with simple wallboards updated daily, healthcare professionals can get a quick look at the current status and performance trends and adjust their daily work accordingly (Exhibit 2.1). A team will usually review and discuss the information displayed on the board during the **daily huddle**, a short—10 to 15 minutes—meeting at the beginning of the workday to address progress toward performance goals and keep team members aligned and focused.

BRIGHT ANGEL MEDICAL CENTER 2.3

Mira Martinez, the health system COO, joined the ED director, Barbara Waters, to review their departmental visual management board posted outside the employee break room.

"Well, the good news is that we have nowhere to go but up," Mira said encouragingly. Barbara agreed. The performance of the ED was currently in the red or unacceptable range, and it was not even peak visit time yet.

"If you notice, the staff does not even look at the board anymore. They are so used to crises that they have become numb, even indifferent."

They brainstormed on the best way to encourage the ED staff to make better use of the visual management board and make progress. Mira shared the importance of creating the opportunity for small wins.

"I am with you," Barbara nodded. "Baby steps. At this point, we need to aim for progress over perfection."

When a system is highly dysfunctional, does it make sense to focus on small wins?

EXHIBIT 2.1 VISUAL MANAGEMENT TOOLS IN ED

Patient	Status	Triage
Smith	Stable	✓
Jenkins	Urgent	✓
Ramanathan	Stable	×
Merrick	Stable	✓
Danson	Urgent	⚠
Lee	Stable	×
Nguyen	Urgent	⚠

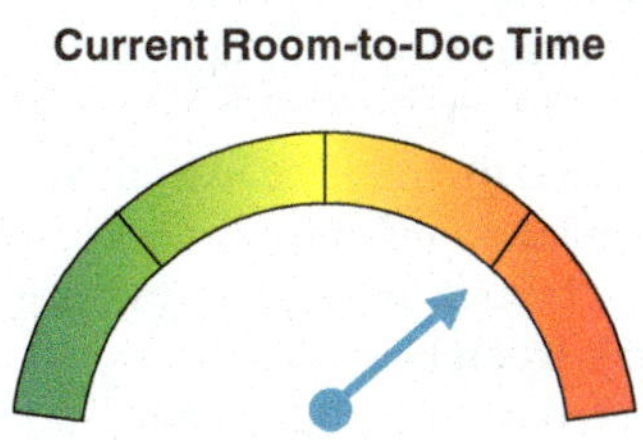

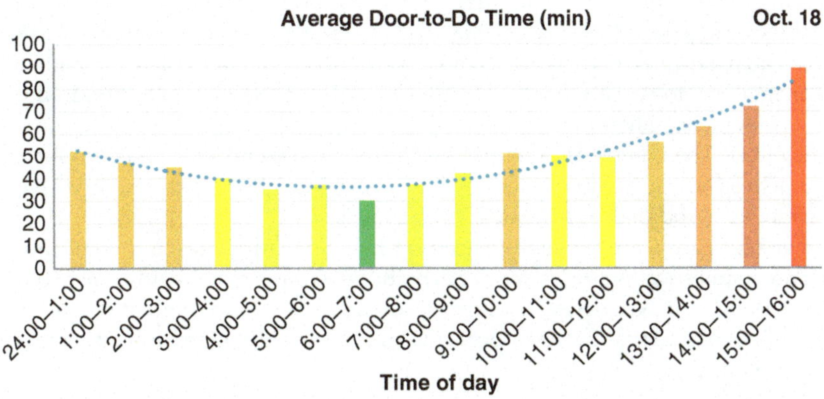

Seek Perfection

As we discussed in Chapter 1, the Deming Wheel (PDSA cycle) is the basis for continuous improvement. A Lean organization is always trying to achieve the perfect system, knowing that perfection is never attainable. Even after a process has been redesigned using the Lean methodology, people should begin to look at the process to see whether it can be refined further. The word for this continuous, incremental improvement in Japanese is *kaizen*. The term **kaizen** is derived from two

BOX 2.3 QUALITY IN PRACTICE!

Using Poka-Yoke to Prevent Medication Errors

In pediatrics, medication errors often occur when weights are recorded in the wrong units. To avoid this mistake, disabling the scale setting that enables multiple units is an easy and effective method to standardize procedures and prevent serious errors (Steele, 2019).

Japanese characters: *kai*, meaning "change," and *zen*, meaning "good." Kaizen emphasizes small, daily improvements as a way of life. Over time, these changes accumulate and amount to significant progress and even organizational transformation. At the core of kaizen is disciplined teamwork.

Poka-yoke, or "**mistake-proofing**" or "fail-safing," is a device or system that produces a signal before an error occurs so that corrective action can be taken. An example is the use of barcoding to identify patients. A barcode is placed on a patient's wristband. When an order for a medication is written, the order is connected with the patient's barcode. Before the nurse administers the drug, she checks the barcode that was printed on the medication dose and the barcode on the patient's wristband. If the barcodes do not match, the system alerts the nurse that the medication was not ordered for that patient. A medication administration error was prevented. Another example is the rule-based procedure in electronic health record systems that signals the potential for sepsis based on patients' vital signs and lab results.

Poka-yoking a process does not necessarily require technology (Box 2.3). For example, patients with asthma may be prescribed several different inhalers with similar names, but different dosages. Color-coding the plastic actuators is an effective way to ensure that patients promptly take the right inhaler when symptoms appear (Franklin, 2019).

Jidoka means "**automation with a human touch**." It is another TPS improvement activity that empowers employees to "stop the line" as soon as a problem occurs. The rationale is to detect problems *at the source* so that their root causes can be detected more quickly and accurately, and a more robust system can be put in place. In essence, everyone becomes a quality inspector. At the Johns Hopkins Hospital, when Dr. Peter Pronovost asked nurses to ensure that ICU physicians followed checklists and to report to him personally if the physicians refused to listen to them, he essentially instituted *jidoka*. He empowered all frontline workers to exercise their authority to stop mistakes as they were being made rather than wait until a patient's condition deteriorated and the causes became more difficult to detect (Pronovost & Vohr, 2010). Code blue is another *jidoka* situation in which a provider can activate an emergency alarm and prompt a care team to rush to a patient's bedside.

Lean management tools and practices should not be implemented individually. There is a strong body of evidence showing that the tools work together and that their combination has a synergistic effect. The combination is referred to as **Lean bundles** or "sets of interrelated and consistent practices which create efficient operations and combine best practices and concepts of Lean management" (Abdallah & Alkhaldi, 2019, p. 500).

To summarize, Lean is a philosophy based on five core principles and continuous improvement. There are many success stories about Lean implementations in healthcare: better health outcomes, improved patient experience, lower cost, smoother flow, and nimbler responses to changes in demand. This shows us that Lean supports the cumulative model in pursuing improvements in quality, cost, timeliness, and flexibility (Chapter 1).

SHORTCOMINGS OF LEAN IMPLEMENTATIONS IN HEALTHCARE

Despite two decades of implementations in healthcare, Lean is still in its infancy. Rigorous reviews of Lean adoptions in healthcare highlighted several approaches running counter to the Lean methodology and limiting its potential (Akmal et al., 2020; Shortell et al., 2021):

- A piecemeal rather than systems approach to Lean deployment. Most implementations are siloed and focused on individual departments or programs. Not only are they not integrated throughout the organization, but they also do not extend to the supply chain network, thereby transferring waste to other operations rather than eradicating it throughout the system (see Box 2.4).

BOX 2.4 QUALITY IN PRACTICE!

A Reconsideration of Lean After the COVID-19 Crisis

Lean supply chains call for a tight interdependence among their links. When major supply shortages occur, a lack of "slack" and a focus on low inventories can hamper a system's flexibility. This situation was especially acute at the height of the pandemic. In Dutch hospitals, two decades of Lean implementation emphasized cost reduction and efficiency. This approach ignored the risk of a pandemic and the need for sufficient ICU bed capacity, qualified staff pool, ventilators, supplies, and drug inventory. Consequently, scarce resources were pulled out of other facilities, such as nursing homes, with disastrous effects. Furthermore, many services such as elective surgeries and cancer screenings were canceled or postponed, aggravating patients' conditions. Drug shortages also contributed to rationing and poor, if not fatal, health outcomes (Kuiper et al., 2022).

The lesson to be learned is that quality should come first, not cost (see cumulative model in Chapter 1). Some capacity underutilization is a requirement of Lean and flow theory (Chapter 10). The Lean philosophy is not to blame for the shortage fiasco during the pandemic; its myopic implementation is.

- Overemphasis on tools and waste reduction with less consideration for continuous improvement and employee empowerment. Rather than pursuing the Lean philosophy and a culture transformation, healthcare organizations simply rely on the use of process improvement tools to obtain results. This approach limits the extent to which value can be created.
- Lack of a strategy or model for implementation. Lean is a direction, and it takes several years for an organization to become Lean. Unfortunately, many organizations conduct single, one-off interventions without ensuring their sustainability, thereby ignoring the philosophy of continuous improvement.

BRIGHT ANGEL MEDICAL CENTER 2.4

The executive team came into the quarterly board meeting exhausted from all the late-night meetings and prep sessions leading up to this critical discussion. They all knew that the stakes were high. Over the past 4 weeks, they had all met with their individual leadership teams to ensure the major problems facing the health system were identified. After multiple Gemba walks through the ED, they had seen how frustrated the staff was with patient complaints, inefficient schedules, missing supplies, unreasonable delays, poor training of new staff, and so forth. The ED was an aging facility, poorly equipped to handle a growing patient population.

The executive team's hard work paid off as the board agreed with the plans to focus attention on improving ED workflows while increasing throughput and patient experience scores. The board also considered approving funds to start planning for a free-standing ED on the other side of town or, at least, a major remodel.

"Great work, Kimberly," Stewart Baldrige praised, as they debriefed after the board meeting. "I'm really glad we were able to find some new members with diverse experience to help round out our board." With board alignment, they were ready to tackle the challenges in the ED and instill a new vision and culture.

SIX SIGMA

Six Sigma is a metrics-driven process improvement methodology that has the same general purpose as Lean—providing the customer with the best possible value. As Lean is focused on creating value and improving flow through a reduction of waste, Six Sigma focuses on eliminating defects and reducing variation. Six Sigma uses a rigorous approach to identify the root causes of problems and achieve predictable process output.

HISTORY OF SIX SIGMA

In the early and mid-1980s, Motorola engineers were not satisfied with the quality of their products. Bill Smith, Motorola's vice president and quality manager of the Land Mobile Product Sector, observed that the products with the least nonconformity during creation were also the most reliable on the field. Achieving "perfect" quality was therefore the overarching objective. He aimed to limit the defect rate to 3.4 defects per million opportunities—Six Sigma—by drastically reducing process variation. Besides eliminating defects, low variation would decrease overall costs and increase customer satisfaction. Smith and colleagues at Motorola developed a methodology to reduce the variability of their products. This data-driven, defect-reduction approach was called **DMAIC**: **Define–Measure–Analyze–Improve–Control**. The approach helped Motorola receive its first Malcolm Baldrige National Quality Award only 2 years after the inception of the Six Sigma program. It was later refined by other companies such as General Electric.

PRINCIPLES OF SIX SIGMA

Executing a process that brings a Six Sigma level of performance requires employees to identify any small deviations in the process almost immediately. At each step of the DMAIC methodology, qualitative and quantitative techniques and tools can help guide the process. Many of these tools are not unique to Six Sigma and are used in other methodologies, such as Lean. The application of Lean principles within the Six Sigma framework reflects the complementarity of both methodologies and has led to the synergistic appellation "Lean Six Sigma," a fact-based philosophy of improvement that prioritizes *doing it right the first time* rather than defect detection and correction. It boosts customer satisfaction and financial performance by reducing variation in output, waste, and lead time. It thus promotes a smooth flow and the application of standardized, best practices (American Society for Quality [ASQ], 2023).

Six Sigma depends on employees using standardized methods to identify problems and eliminate them. Six Sigma, a methodology originally based on statistics, has evolved from a metric used to measure product quality to a management philosophy that promotes collaborative problem-solving. Trained employees must examine statistical graphs, understand when there is a deviation from the standard, determine the root cause of failure, propose changes to prevent variation, and check to ensure the problem has been corrected. In this book, we will examine each stage in detail and describe the relevant tools and techniques. In doing so, we follow the framework for LSS Green Belt certification offered by ASQ. Note that the chapters covering the various tools and concepts are included in Figure 2.5. Also keep in mind that LSS is a system, not merely

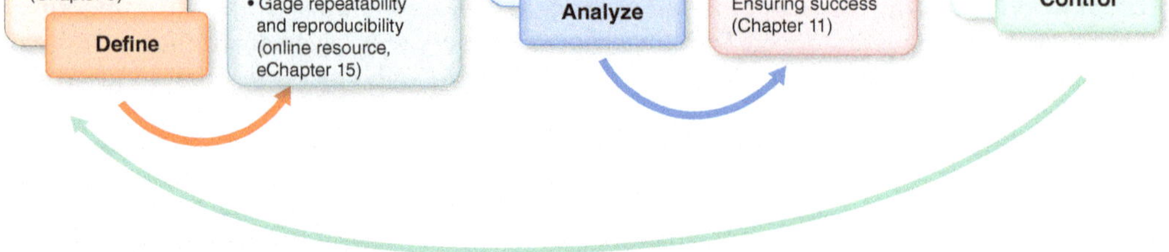

FIGURE 2.5 Define, measure, analyze, improve, and control stages and related chapters.

Abbreviations: VOC, voice of the customer; VOP, voice of the process.

a set of tools. This is why the quest for better value for the customer never ends, as shown by the loop-back from *Control* to *Define* new customer and stakeholder requirements.

Define—What Is the Process?

The first step is to define the process that is going to be improved. Process improvement projects often originate from someone's idea based on experience with the process and motivation to re-align it with customers' needs and wants.

At the *Define* stage, the scope and boundaries of a process are often nebulous. It is thus a good idea to develop a high-level map of the process that summarizes the inputs and outputs of a process in a table format. This exercise will facilitate process definition and requirements. A tool used for that purpose is **SIPOC** (Suppliers–Inputs–Process–Outputs–Customers). Creating a SIPOC diagram is a team effort involving all process stakeholders (Figure 2.6).

Once the process is fleshed out, it can be modeled with a simple tool like a flowchart or swim-lane diagram (Chapter 3). The latter is especially useful for processes affecting multiple departments or units because it displays all the major participants involved in performing the process.

For a process to deliver value to customers, it is necessary to define their specific requirements. Six Sigma leaders use multiple techniques, such as brainstorming, focus group interviews, and surveys (Chapter 4). Once the customer's desires are clarified, process indicators are defined, and the organization's required capabilities can be specified. Both customer and process requirements should be benchmarked against leading organizations to gauge the discrepancy between your organization's performance and top-class performers.

When projects are launched, a project charter is drafted to articulate why the project is being done, what the expected benefits are, what the scope is, who the team members are, what their roles will be, and the timeline for completion. This document is used as a communication tool by all members of the team (Chapter 5). Justifying the improvement project is part of the business case for action (Chapter 3). It is of utmost importance because it "sells" the need for change and

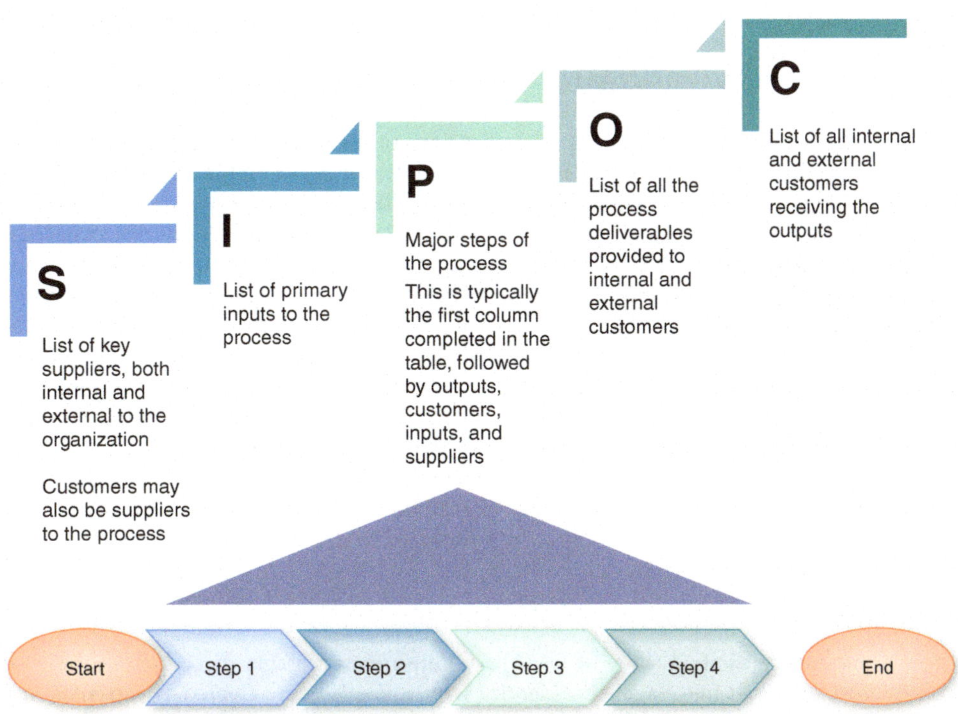

FIGURE 2.6 **SIPOC (Suppliers-Inputs-Process-Outputs-Customers) framework.**

helps secure the required resources from leaders. To substantiate the project timeline, the team can then proceed with a detailed list of all process activities and subactivities (work breakdown structure; see Chapter 5) and establish a schedule (Gantt chart or network diagram; see Chapter 5).

BRIGHT ANGEL MEDICAL CENTER 2.5

"The patient satisfaction survey data in the ED are indeed the worst!" Barbara muttered to herself as she reviewed the ED scores and patient comments. It was clear that something had to change. There was a knock at her office door.

"I heard you could use some help down here," remarked Olina Petrenko, the director of quality at Bright Angel. Olina and Barbara looked over several patient survey printouts together; after reading several of the comments, they both concluded that the long wait times were a major source of dissatisfaction. "Throughput seems to be where we need to focus. No doubt about it," said Barbara, "but there are just so many barriers to getting patients out of the waiting room. During our busiest time, we are holding six or eight patients waiting for admission to the hospital. That effectively cuts our capacity by 25%."

Olina nodded. "We will have to take a comprehensive look at the whole process and look for opportunities everywhere. I agree that the hospital being full is part of the issue, but there are also other issues that need our attention."

What other possible barriers to moving patients out of the waiting room and into an exam room exist?

Measure—Where Is the Waste and How Bad Is It?

Just as in Lean, Six Sigma uses value stream process mapping (Figure 2.2) as a valuable tool to track waste and outline all of the steps in the current process that will undergo improvement. Process activity charts and spaghetti diagrams also help uncover where bottlenecks occur, where mistakes are made, and where excess costs are incurred. The process must be mapped as it actually works, not how you think it should work. This is often difficult, particularly when there is significant variation in how different operators perform the work. Measuring the work of different people, at different times of the day, or on different days of the week is vital to understanding the variability within the process and to establishing current **throughput yields** as baselines. Data collection in Six Sigma is multipronged. It follows a preestablished plan and includes interviewing people, making firsthand observations (Gemba walks), asking questions, and poring over internal records. A variety of graphs and measures described in Chapter 7 can be quite useful to visualize and summarize process data. Careful sampling plans should be designed. Process distributions and their parameters should be obtained at this stage.

In Six Sigma, one of the data analysis objectives is to reveal the nature and extent of process variation. There are two types of variation: **nonrandom variation** and **random variation**. The former is caused by unusual phenomena that are external to the process. Once identified, they can be removed. The latter is inherent to the process, and only changes or improvements to the process can decrease it. Although there will always be some random variation, too much of it impairs **process capability**, that is, the ability to meet specific output requirements. In fact, Six Sigma quality demands that processes be *highly* capable, hence the need to decrease random variation through process improvements (Chapter 8).

Analyze—Why Is There Waste in the Process?

Data analysis is a very exciting stage of DMAIC because it transforms sheer metrics into useful, actionable information. At this stage, you identify why waste is being created at various points in the process. As always, it is a team effort that requires collective brainstorming. **Affinity diagrams** (Chapter 4) can help the team list all potential causes of waste and organize them into a **fishbone (or cause-and-effect or Ishikawa) diagram** (Chapter 9). Then, the team can drill down to the root cause(s).

TABLE 2.2 SYMPTOMS VERSUS ROOT CAUSES

Symptom	Root Cause
Employees do not know what they are doing.	The process is ambiguous and poorly defined.
The upstream processes give us junk to work with.	There is no feedback mechanism to communicate downstream processes' needs and expectations.
Nurses take days off when we need them most.	The scheduling system is based on providers' preferences rather than patient demand.
Patients never arrive on time.	The parking lot is too small to accommodate the patient volume.

Root cause analysis (RCA) can systematically uncover the underlying barriers to providing value-added services. The root causes are the fundamental breakdowns or failures in a process that, when corrected, prevent the recurrence of the problem. Each problem can be viewed as an opportunity to learn about the system. The reason for getting at the root cause(s) of a problem is that they reveal the true nature of the problem and thus make it worthwhile to identify and implement sensible solutions. If we do not know the root causes, we will waste time and resources trying to correct symptoms, rather than addressing fundamental issues. Examples of symptoms versus root causes are provided in Table 2.2.

When you go to the doctor's office, care providers try to find the root cause of your problem. For example, if you go in complaining of pain in your hand, the doctor will ask many questions and look at your hand carefully. Likely, the doctor will order an x-ray to be sure that there are no broken bones. The doctor is actually looking for the root cause of your problem, resulting in pain. The doctor could easily give you pain medications, but if a bone is broken, the pain medicine will only mask the symptoms, and the problem will not be fixed.

When performing an RCA, you should assume that things are done incorrectly. Keep questioning what is taking place. A simple root cause tool is the "**5 Whys**." It involves asking the question "Why?" at least five times to get to the root cause of a problem (Figure 2.7). Another important tool covered in Chapter 9 is the **failure mode and effects analysis (FMEA)** designed to identify all potential failure points in the process.

Sometimes, more sophisticated tools or techniques are required. For example, a scatterplot or correlation analysis will shed light on the extent to which various factors or causes such as patient engagement and surgeon experience influence a patient's recovery period. Furthermore, some hypotheses regarding means, proportions, and other parameters can be tested to sharpen our understanding of how some process characteristics influence value and performance. Please note that statistical analysis can only show associations, not causation. **Controlled experiments** are the only research design methodologies capable of demonstrating an actual "cause-and-effect" relationship between factors and outcomes without the interference of other variables that may influence those outcomes. Thorough and rigorous analysis during the *Analyze* phase should offer a blueprint for improvements.

Improve—How to Eliminate Waste?

Not only should successful changes prevent problems from occurring again, but they should also bring the organization or process closer to the targeted **benchmark** (Chapter 4). Although lofty goals are commendable, they should not become obstacles to pragmatism. What appears to be the best solution is not always workable, and your team must brainstorm to identify alternatives that are aligned with the organization's culture and compatible with available resources. When you evaluate proposed changes, you will have to think through their effects, including the unintentional consequences of making these changes. Cost-benefit analyses are often conducted at this point to help select the most promising, yet achievable, improvement solution or bundle. Actual experiments can be conducted to verify the viability of these proposals. As mentioned earlier, experiments will enable you to assess the impact of a given solution on outcomes without the "noise" of other variables. However, for practical or ethical reasons, experiments may not be

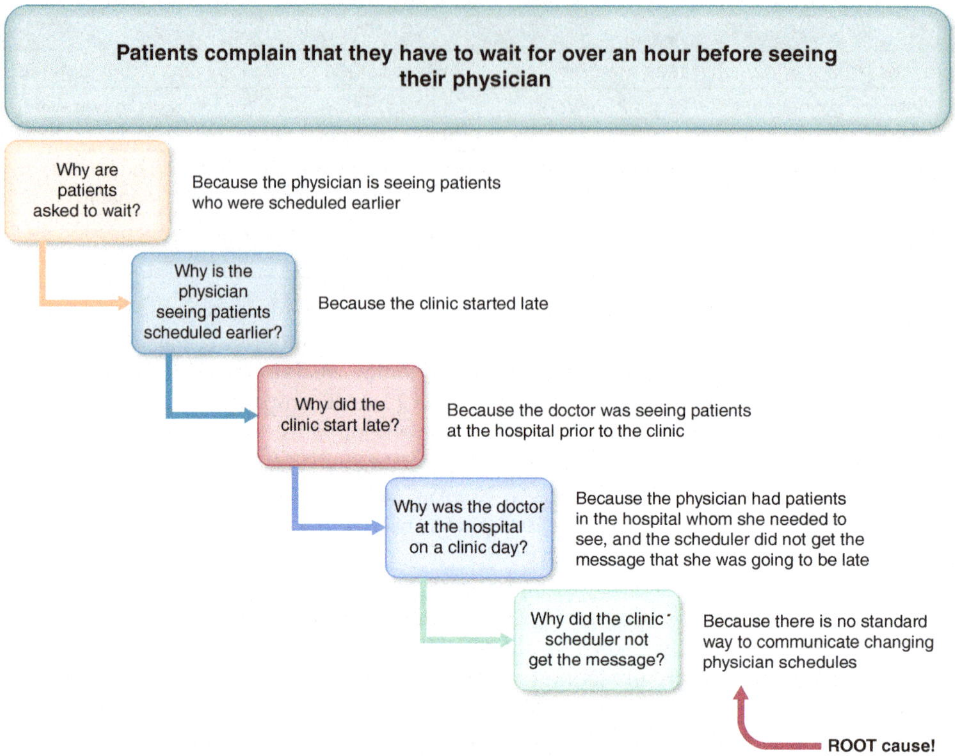

FIGURE 2.7 The 5 Whys.

possible. Fortunately, improvement alternatives can be simulated to gauge their impact on performance and resources ahead of their implementation. Accordingly, they save time and money and reduce the risk of faulty improvements.

Lean and process design principles (Chapter 10) offer an extensive repertoire of solutions aimed at creating flow. They help build robust processes that support the creation of value for the customers of the process. They rely on employee empowerment and technology to be on the lookout for problems, expose them, and mistake-proof the system to prevent their reoccurrence. The design principles also aim to reduce process variation. To reduce variation, a common solution is standardization. How can standardization be achieved in a high-variety service environment such as healthcare? With checklists! **Checklists** are lists of actions that must be performed to reach a successful outcome. In healthcare, they are grounded in evidence-based medicine or best practices (Box 2.5). They ensure that the exact, same proven steps are always followed uniformly across individuals.

Processes involve workflows. Often, improvements will require layout changes that support rather than impede the workflow. Layouts that minimize unnecessary movements, facilitate interactions among selected providers, and are patient-friendly certainly contribute to the eradication of waste and variation.

Once an improvement is decided upon, you should pilot the change to uncover other problems that may arise as a result of the change. If the pilot shows that the change improves the process so that fewer variations or defects are produced, you may want to use simulation again to see the impact of the change(s) on a larger scale (Chapter 11). The results might suggest additional modifications or refinements before expanding the implementation of the change(s). At this stage, Gantt charts (Chapter 5) can help keep track of activities and timelines for

BOX 2.5 QUALITY IN PRACTICE!

Standardizing With Checklists

In 2001, Peter Pronovost, a critical care specialist at Johns Hopkins Hospital in Baltimore, Maryland, decided to see whether checklists, like those used in aviation, could improve the reliability of care in the ICU. He chose to focus on one process, the insertion of central venous catheters (CVCs) in patients. Taking care of patients in an ICU setting is very complicated. In fact, previous research showed that to take care of a critically ill patient, 178 individual actions were required per day, many of which needed to be performed in a specific sequence. The same research also found that although only 1% of the individual actions were incorrectly performed, they added up to one to two errors per patient per day! Pronovost decided to see whether a five-step checklist could decrease the error rate when inserting CVCs. The five steps were simple:

1. Wash hands with soap.
2. Clean the patient's skin with chlorhexidine antiseptic.
3. Use sterile drapes that cover the entire patient.
4. Wear a sterile mask, hat, gown, and gloves.
5. Put a sterile dressing over the catheter insertion site once the line is placed.

When the checklist was first tried, a review of CVC placements for 1 month showed that physicians skipped at least one step in more than a third of patients. The next step was to give nurses the authority to stop the procedure if they saw them skip a step on the checklist. After 1 year, the infection rate of CVCs in place for over 10 days went from 11% to zero.

Pronovost observed that the checklists provided two main benefits. One, they helped with memory recall, especially when mundane tasks are being done and many chaotic events are going on all around you. Two, checklists provided explicit instructions on the expected steps to be taken in the process. This prompted physicians and nurses to talk about the clinical evidence that supported each step in the complex process. Checklists established a higher standard of baseline performance (Gawande, 2007).

improvement. Following the progress of the process improvement with performance metrics (e.g., throughput yield) and tools (e.g., comparative control charts, dashboards, general process charts) can demonstrate that the changes made are actually producing positive results. By the end of the *Improve* step, you should be able to document that the process was actually enhanced by your actions and get ready to deploy the improvement on a larger scale, that is, the *Act* part of the Deming Wheel (Chapter 1). The improvement is now the new standard.

Control—How to Keep Waste at Bay?

All of your work that has gone into identifying the root causes of a problem and improving the process will be lost if you do not monitor results. Statistical process control (SPC) is one method of monitoring results and identifying variation patterns before processes become unstable. Dashboard metrics help you track and document successes and failures. Visual management tools continuously display performance on key metrics and trigger swift responses when changes occur. In all the preceding cases, information must be timely. **Total productive maintenance (TPM)**, a Lean tool that engages everyone to monitor the equipment when using it, also offers the opportunity to control the process by getting everyone involved in making sure that equipment-related disruptions are minimized. Sticking to the rules set forth by 6S is another way to control the process and sustain the improvement. A **control plan** and **standard operating procedures (SOPs)** will assist all process players in avoiding the return to the "old ways" of doing things.

THE A3 REPORT

To organize and document the DMAIC steps in a process improvement project, teams complete an A3 report. The **A3 report** is a one-page document that summarizes the various activities and findings in a Six Sigma project (Figure 2.8). It usually includes:

- the background: a short description of the problem and its importance;
- the current conditions: visual depictions of the problem and appropriate metrics;
- the analysis: methods used to identify the root causes of the problem;
- the target condition: objective of considered intervention(s);
- recommendations: proposed interventions;
- implementation plan: tasks, responsibilities, and schedule for completion;
- follow-up: tasks to be performed to maintain benefits of intervention; and
- results report: evaluation of intervention with appropriate metrics.

For complex projects, more detailed reports are necessary. This documentation will provide the blueprint for future action and help you start responding to other problems in a constructive way. Through this continuous group problem-solving, you learn what works in your organization and help build a culture of teamwork (Box 2.6). Since continuous improvement is an ongoing pursuit, it is vital that frontline employees identify further areas that need improvement. Suggestion boxes or wallboards where people post ideas are good vehicles to get everyone involved as long as proposals are considered seriously and get a fair chance of being implemented.

THE LEARNING CULTURE IN SIX SIGMA AND KEY PLAYERS

The power of Six Sigma to create a culture of continuous improvement lies in the combination of changing the way work gets done and teaching people to collaboratively solve problems. Implementing the methods of Six Sigma throughout an organization requires a serious business commitment. There needs to be a dedicated staff overseeing the steps of Six Sigma daily, and everyone in the organization must follow the DMAIC framework. The top professionals who drive the changes in a Six Sigma organization are listed in Figure 2.9.

Executive sponsor or champion. This is often a clinical leader or senior manager who assigns the project, ensures that resources are available, sets a timeline for completion, and ensures accountability for implementation. They will remove any roadblocks for the teams to guarantee successful project implementation.

Master Black Belts. They have extensive quantitative skills and Six Sigma experience, which enables them to monitor, review, and mentor Black Belts and Green Belts across projects. They develop important metrics and formulate the strategic course of the projects.

Black Belts. They devote all of their time to Six Sigma projects. They have extensive training in statistics, quality tools, project management, and soft skills. They may lead several DMAIC projects across organizational areas in which they have no prior work experience. Their soft skills repertoire is important to get to know the people and the process needing improvement.

Green Belts. They provide assistance in data collection and analysis for Black Belt projects. They are also leaders of Green Belt projects, that is, DMAIC projects in areas where they are subject matter experts.

Yellow Belts. They are project team members who know the process well and are responsible for completing specific project benchmarks. Yellow Belts are often in charge of data collection and project monitoring. They assume Six Sigma responsibilities in addition to their regular roles in the organization, but may be temporarily assigned to a project on a full-time basis.

White Belts. They have very basic Six Sigma training. They assist in local problem-solving, but are not full members of the project team.

In addition to understanding the methods of Six Sigma, key players need to have the communication and leadership skills to involve and communicate with everyone on the team. They must be able to pull together multifunctional teams to focus on the problem. Having a team with diverse skills and experiences increases the likelihood of identifying variations and developing creative solutions.

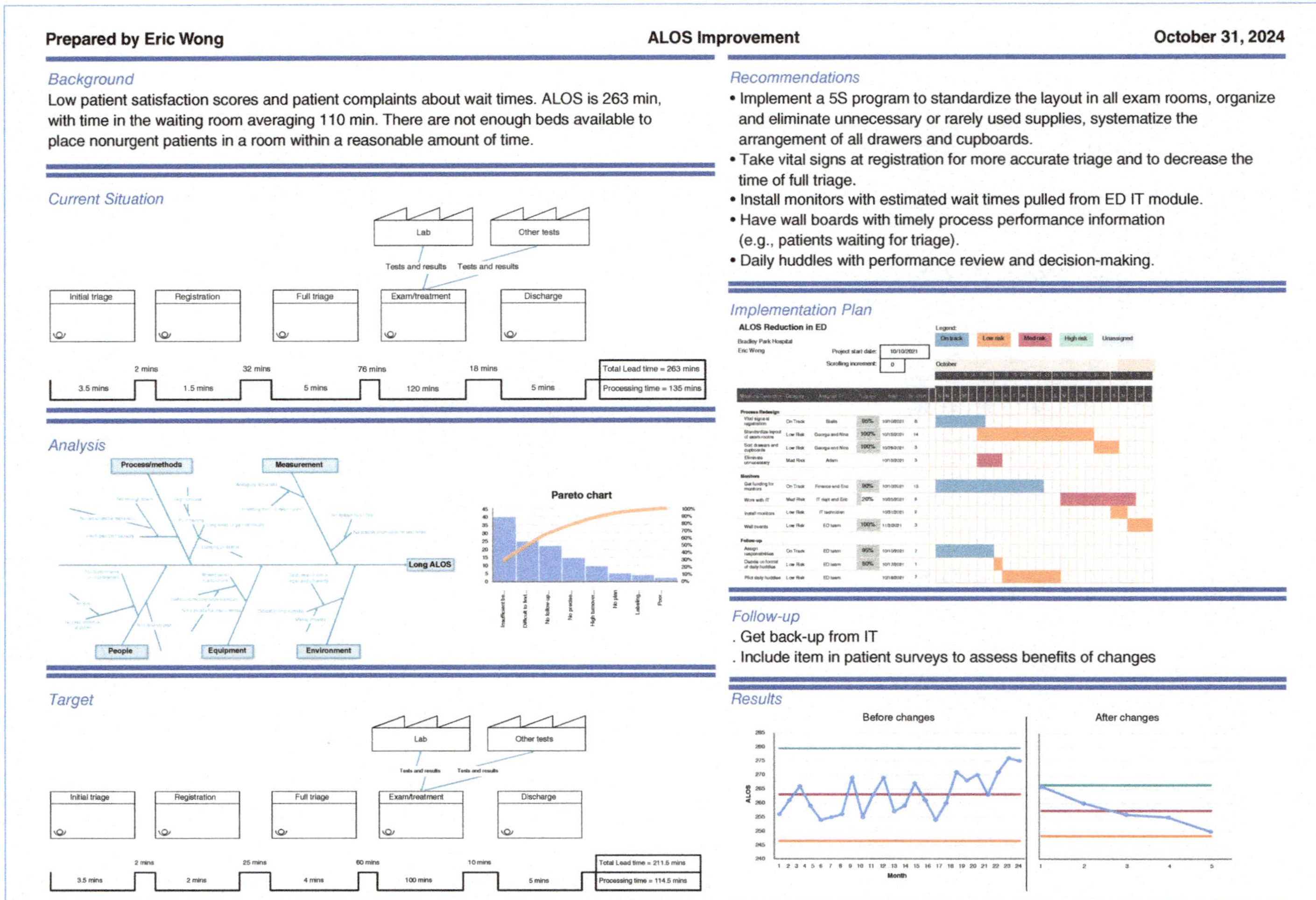

FIGURE 2.8 An example of a complete A3 report.

Abbreviations: ALOS, average length of stay; IT, information technology.

BOX 2.6 QUALITY IN PRACTICE!

Reducing Pharmacy Medication Errors With Lean Six Sigma in a Thai Public Hospital

Despite pharmacists' efforts to detect and correct medication errors before dispensation, the problem remains too widespread. In a 508-bed hospital in Thailand, the dispensing process by the inpatient pharmacy was targeted for improvement. A project team comprising the pharmacy head, two pharmacists, and three technicians was formed. The *Define* phase revealed that errors primarily occurred because: (a) medication orders were entered incorrectly into the electronic system, and (b) medications were selected incorrectly by the pharmacy technicians. During the *Measure* phase, the problems were quantified, and the average dispensing error proportion was determined to be 0.18%. The *Analyze* phase identified a series of potential causes of incorrect order entry and incorrect selection. The 5 Why analysis helped drill down to the root causes of the problems: lack of delivery guidelines, lack of criteria to send medication errors to the pharmacy, and misinterpretation of handwritten medication orders by nurses before sending them to the pharmacy. During the *Improve* phase, the team brainstormed and redesigned the processes to submit, process, and deliver orders. SOPs were developed, and SPC was implemented in the *Control* phase to ensure sustained improvement (Trakulsunti et al., 2022).

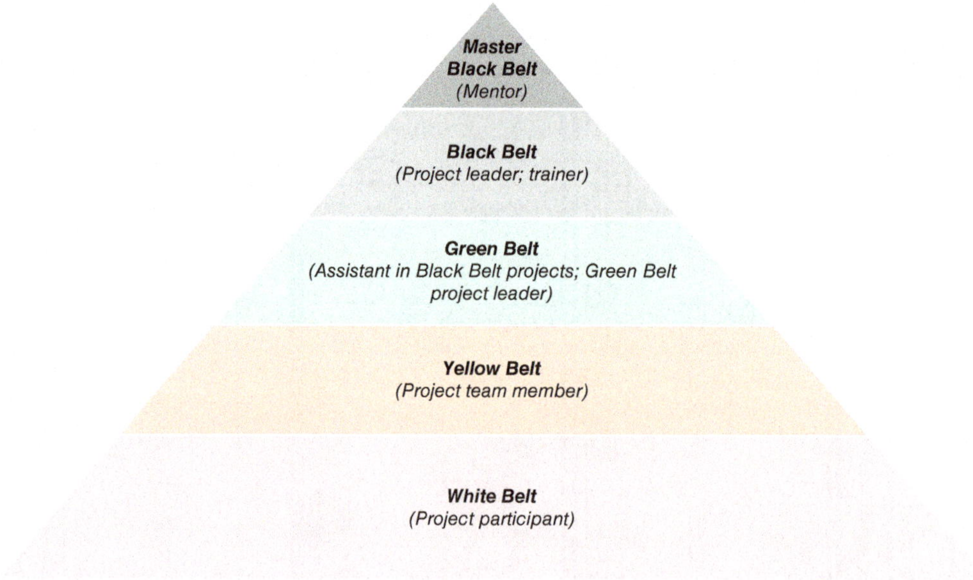

FIGURE 2.9 Six Sigma roles' pyramid.

BENEFITS OF LEAN AND SIX SIGMA

Different organizations may choose one methodology over the other, but neither is considered "best." Although each methodology can be deployed by itself for a specific problem to which it is especially well suited, there is a trend toward the fusion of Lean and Six Sigma, LSS, at the organizational level. The combination of both methodologies outperforms either one by itself (Tlapa et al., 2020b). If only Lean was pursued, processes that are not in statistical control would be considered acceptable. At the same time, with Six Sigma only, we might not be able to increase the fluidity of the process, reduce inventories, increase workforce flexibility, establish pull, and induce cultural change (Hamilton, 2018). Organizations that adopt an LSS methodology and culture achieve significant benefits. In a systematic review of the literature, the integration of both methodologies was shown to yield the following benefits (McDermott et al., 2022):

- better operational and financial performance (reduced costs and higher profits);
- better quality (improved customer satisfaction and service; fewer medical and prescription errors);
- improved timeliness (reduced patient wait times; low turnaround times);
- improved employee morale and engagement; and
- higher safety.

In healthcare, the quality of services rendered depends a lot on human skills. If LSS methodologies are followed and cultures are built around process improvement, there will be improved communication and skill development throughout the organization, in addition to the aforementioned benefits.

ETHICAL SCENARIO 2.1

Overutilization and Defensive Medicine

Physician practices vary across the United States, and some doctors in private practice have access to revenue from what are referred to as "ancillary services." Most commonly laboratory tests and imaging studies, these additional services are billable to insurance and result in added income for some physician practices. When physicians are reimbursed based on the volume of tests they order, that can lead to "overutilization" of these services. Overutilization is a source of waste in the U.S. healthcare system and is a contributing factor to the high cost of healthcare when compared with other countries. Defensive medicine, which is when physicians order a battery of tests to avoid lawsuits due to ordering tests to rule out every conceivable condition, is another contributor to the high cost of care.

What are the ethical concerns when physicians share in the revenue generated by ordering lab and x-ray tests?

Who benefits from overutilization?

What impact does the malpractice system have on overutilization?

SUMMARY

The continuous improvement methodologies of Lean and Six Sigma developed separately in the manufacturing sector. However, both are now used extensively in healthcare. The Lean principles of (a) identify value, (b) map the value stream, (c) create flow, (d) establish pull, and (e) seek perfection are designed to drive "waste" out of the system and improve process flow. Six Sigma's principles of DMAIC are focused on decreasing variation to enhance process effectiveness. Lately, especially in large healthcare organizations, Lean and Six Sigma have merged and share tools. In fact, if you look at the principles of Lean and Six Sigma side by side, you will see many similarities. Mapping the value stream, eradicating waste, and creating a smooth, predictable, robust, and defect-free process flow mesh together to build a culture of continuous improvement and focus efforts on creating value for the customer.

Through reductions in waste and variation, LSS not only improves quality, but it also lowers costs and facilitates timely care delivery. The expanded skill repertoire of the individuals involved in these projects fosters greater flexibility. In improving processes on multiple fronts, LSS boosts performance not only in quality, but also in the other competitive priorities presented in Chapter 1.

CERTIFICATION TIPS

There are many organizations offering LSS certification. Some of the most popular ones include:

- The Council for Six Sigma Certification

- Six Sigma Global Institute
- International Association for Six Sigma Certification
- ASQ
- Lean Six Sigma Institute
- 6Sigma.us

Each one offers a similar set of online courses. However, the courses are not free. Of course, you do have the option to study on your own and bypass the organization-sponsored training programs. If you feel adequately prepared, you may simply register for the certification exams. Make sure that you research the reputation of the certifying organization and its relevance in the country where you work. Several colleges and universities also provide certification training; this could affect your selection of the certification provider as well, especially if you value their educational formats.

You will find that the topics covered in LSS certification and Six Sigma certification are quite similar. This reflects the trend of combining the principles and tools of these two methodologies. However, be aware that Six Sigma is more technical and requires already stable processes. If you work for an organization that is not ready for Six Sigma implementation, you may want to opt first for Lean certification.

Now, is LSS certification right for you? Before you make a decision, you need to ask yourself:

- Is the LSS certification valued in your field and/or industry?
- Would another type of certification such as Project Management Professional certification be more useful at this stage?
- Do you feel capable of skipping some belt levels and sign up right away for, let's say, Black Belt certification (more bang for your buck)?
- Do you currently have the time and resources to study for the exams? Will your employer be supportive in that respect?

KEY TERMS

Lean
Waste
Gemba walk
Four Conversations
Value stream map (VSM)
6S
Push system
Pull system
Just-in-time (JIT)
Daily huddle
Kaizen
Poka-yoke (mistake-proofing)
Jidoka (automation with a human touch)
Lean bundle
Six Sigma
DMAIC (Define–Measure–Analyze–Improve–Control)
SIPOC (Suppliers–Inputs–Process–Outputs–Customers)
Throughput yield
Nonrandom variation
Random variation
Process capability
Affinity diagram
Fishbone (or cause-and-effect or Ishikawa) diagram
Root cause analysis (RCA)
5 Whys
Failure mode and effects analysis (FMEA)
Controlled experiment
Benchmark
Checklist
Total productive maintenance (TPM)
Control plan
Standard operating procedures (SOPs)
A3 report
Executive sponsor or champion
Master Black Belts
Black Belts
Green Belts
Yellow Belts
White Belts

REVIEW QUESTIONS

1. What is culture in general, and what is a Lean culture in particular?
2. What is a Gemba walk? Why is it important?
3. What are the four types of conversation? Briefly describe each one.
4. Name the eight types of waste (Lean methodology) and give an example of each in healthcare.

5. List the Lean principles and explain how each one is used to examine/improve a process.
6. Why is flow important in Lean?
7. What are the differences between push and pull systems?
8. Give an example of a JIT system. Explain why it is beneficial.
9. What is poka-yoke? Name three examples of its use in healthcare.
10. What are Lean bundles? Why are they more effective than isolated Lean activities?
11. What are some of the shortcomings of Lean implementations in healthcare?
12. What are the steps in Six Sigma?
13. What is a root cause and how do you identify it? Give an example.
14. What is the purpose of an A3 report and what are its various parts?
15. What are the various roles of people involved in Six Sigma projects?
16. What are the benefits of an integrated LSS methodology?

LEARNING ACTIVITIES

1. Conduct a mock interview (two students) on video. One student (the interviewer) interviews the current president of the American Medical Association (AMA; the interviewee). Main topic of the interview: Can the implementation of Lean Six Sigma in healthcare benefit patients? Can it hurt? If so, How? Hint: Do some research on the interviewee's background before conducting the interview.
2. Do a Pecha Kucha presentation (20 slides, 20 seconds for each slide) on how the implementation of LSS in healthcare can benefit patients.
3. Identify the most wasteful activity in your workday. Why is it happening? What can you do about it?
4. Think like a leader: Determine how you would motivate your staff to engage in process improvements.
5. Go to http://archive.ahrq.gov/professionals/quality-patient-safety/patient-safety-resources/resources/mistakeproof/mistake8.html. Explain why barcoding of specimens or drugs can be considered a method of poka-yoke. Name one mistake that can come with barcoding.
6. Describe a way to poka-yoke your morning routine so that you wake up on time and remember to take your cell phone to work.
7. Select a process in your organization and develop a SIPOC chart.
8. Is LSS certification right for you? Explain why or why not.

SPRINGER PUBLISHING CONNECT™

A robust set of instructor resources designed to supplement this text is located at **http://connect.springerpub.com/content/book/978-0-8261-7976-0.** Qualifying instructors may request access by emailing **textbook@springerpub.com**.

REFERENCES

Abdallah, A. B., & Alkhaldi, R. Z. (2019). Lean bundles in health care: A scoping review. *Journal of Health Organization and Management*, *33*(4), 488–510. https://doi.org/10.1108/JHOM-09-2018-0263

Akmal, A., Greatbanks, R., & Foote, J. (2020). Lean thinking in healthcare: Findings from a systematic literature network and bibliometric analysis. *Health Policy*, *124*(6), 615–627. https://doi.org/10.1016/j.healthpol.2020.04.008

American Society for Quality. (2023). *What is Lean Six Sigma*? https://asq.org/quality-resources/six-sigma

Antony, J., Sunder, V. M., Sreedharan, R., Chakraborty, A., & Gunasekaran, A. (2019). A systematic review of Lean in healthcare: A global perspective. *International Journal of Quality & Reliability Management, 36*(8), 1370–1391. https://doi.org/10.1108/IJQRM-12-2018-0346

Balkhi, B., Alshahrani, A., & Khan, A. (2022). Just-in-time approach in healthcare inventory management: Does it really work? *Saudi Pharmaceutical Journal, 30*(12), 1830–1835. https://doi.org/10.1016/j.jsps.2022.10.013

de Barros, L. B., Caldas, L. P., Bohomol, E., Sarantopoulos, A., Minatogawa, V., & Gasparino, R. C. (2022). Evaluation of waste related to the admission process of low-complexity patients in emergency services, in light of the Lean healthcare philosophy. *International Journal of Environmental Research and Public Health, 19*, 7044. https://doi.org/10.3390/ijerph19127044

Ford, H., & Crowther, S. (1922). *My life and work*. Doubleday.

Ford, J., & Ford, L. (2009). *The Four Conversations: Daily communication that gets results*. Berrett-Koehler Publishers, Inc.

Franklin, R. (2019, September 18). *Mistake proof your practice to avoid medical errors*. Mobius MD. https://mobius.md/2019/09/18/mistake-proof-your-practice-to-avoid-medical-errors

Gawande, A. (2007, December 10). The checklist. *The New Yorker*. http://www.newyorker.com/reporting/2007/12/10/071210fa_fact_gawande

Graban, M. (2019). Lean: Breaking down barriers for the sake of improvement. *International Journal for Quality in Health Care, 31*(S1), 1–2. https://doi.org/10.1093/intqhc/mzz112

Hamilton, L. (2018). *Lean, Lean Six Sigma, and the clinical laboratory*. Medical Laboratory Observer. https://www.mlo-online.com/home/article/13009430/lean-lean-six-sigma-and-the-clinical-laboratory

Hunter, J. (2013). *Deming and Lean: Disparities and similarities*. The W. Edwards Deming Institute. https://deming.org/deming-and-lean-the-disparities-and-similarities

Kuiper, A., Lee, R. H., van Ham, V. J. J., & Does, R. J. M. M. (2022). A reconsideration of Lean Six Sigma in healthcare after the COVID-19 crisis. *International Journal of Lean Six Sigma, 13*(1), 101–117. https://doi.org/10.1108/IJLSS-01-2021-0013

Lean Enterprise Institute. (2023a). *Lean thinking and practice*. https://www.lean.org/lexicon-terms/lean-thinking-and-practice

Lean Enterprise Institute. (2023b). *What is Lean?* https://www.lean.org/explore-lean/what-is-lean

McDermott, O., Antony, J., Bhat, S., Jayaraman, R., Rosa, A., Marolla, G., & Parida, R. (2022). Lean Six Sigma in healthcare: A systematic literature review on motivations and benefits. *Processes, 10*(10), 1910. https://doi.org/10.3390/pr10101910

McKinsey & Company. (2017). *The work of leaders in a Lean management enterprise*. https://www.mckinsey.com/capabilities/operations/our-insights/the-work-of-leaders-in-a-lean-management-enterprise

Pronovost, P., & Vohr, E. (2010). *Safe patients, smart hospital: How one doctor's checklist can help us change health care from the inside out*. Hudson Street Press.

Shortell, S. M., Blodgett, J. C., Rundall, T. G., Moshe Henker, R., & Reponen, E. (2021). Lean management and hospital performance: Adoption vs. implementation. *The Joint Commission Journal on Quality and Patient Safety, 47*(5), 296–305. https://doi.org/10.1016/j.jcjq.2021.01.010

Steele, C. (2019). *Poka yoke examples you need to know*. GoSkills. https://www.goskills.com/Lean-Six-Sigma/Resources/Poka-yoke-examples

Tlapa, D., Zepeda-Lugo, A. A., Tortorella, G. L., Baez-Lopez, Y. A., Limon-Romero, J., Alvarado-Iniesta, A., & Rodriguez-Borbon, M. I. (2020a). Effects of Lean healthcare on patient flow: A systematic review. *Value Health, 23*(2), 260–273. https://doi.org/10.1016/j.jval.2019.11.002

Tlapa, D., Zepeda-Lugo, A. A., Tortorella, G. L., Baez-Lopez, Y. A., Limon-Romero, J., Alvarado-Iniesta, A., & Rodriguez-Borbon, M. I. (2020b). Effects of Lean healthcare on patient flow: A systematic review. *Value Health, 23*(2), 260–273. https://doi.org/10.1016/j.jval.2019.11.002

Trakulsunti, Y., Antony, J., Edgeman, R., Cudney, B., Dempsey, M., & Brennan, A. (2022). Reducing pharmacy medication errors using Lean Six Sigma: A Thai hospital case study. *Total Quality Management & Business Excellence, 33*(5–6), 664–682. https://doi.org/10.1080/14783363.2021.1885292

Virginia Mason Franciscan Health. (2023). *VMPS success stories*. https://www.vmfh.org/about-vmfh/research-care-quality/virginia-mason-production-system/vmps-success-stories

Virginia Mason Institute. (2021, August 31). *What is Lean healthcare?* https://www.virginiamasoninstitute.org/what-is-lean-health-care

Womack, J. P., & Jones, D. T. (1996). *Lean thinking: Banish waste and create wealth in your corporation*. Simon & Schuster.

PART II

DEFINE—What Is the Process?

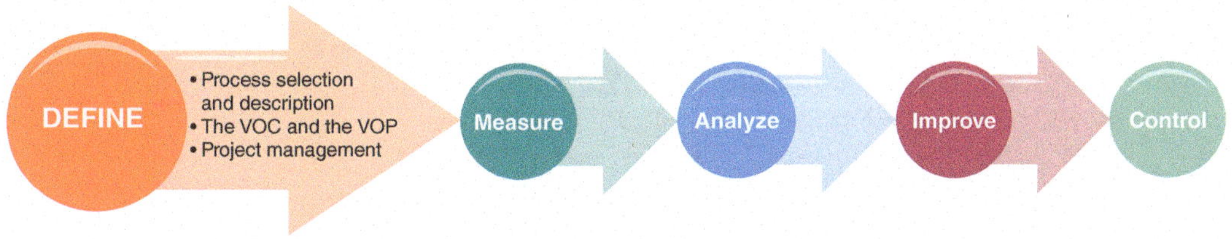

CHAPTER 3

PROCESS SELECTION AND DESCRIPTION

BRIGHT ANGEL MEDICAL CENTER 3.1

Barbara Waters knocked on the office door of the ED medical director, Dr. Hana Aoki. The door was ajar, revealing Dr. Aoki sitting at her desk with her head in her hands. She looked up as Barbara peered in.

"Everything ok in here?" asked Barbara.

"No," Dr. Aoki replied, "it is far from ok. Our patient left without being seen rate is through the roof, patients are complaining, and our staff turnover is the highest it's ever been."

Barbara took a deep breath. "Look, I am feeling a little discouraged, too. That's why I asked Olina and the chief medical officer for help. We are scheduled to meet with them in the ED conference room in 10 minutes. Let's think about how they can help us."

Barbara and Dr. Aoki chatted as they made their way to the conference room.

"Good morning," shouted Dr. Tibbets from across the conference room as he waved them in.

Barbara and Dr. Aoki sat down and noticed several charts, graphs, and other papers spread out across the conference room table.

Olina spoke up, "We all agree that increasing throughput is our top priority. If we can get patients in and out faster, wait times will decrease and patient experience scores will go up. Any other opportunities for improvement?"

Dr. Tibbets asked, "What about our nursing team? I'm hearing that we have over 50% traveling nurses down here. Is that accurate?"

"Unfortunately, it is," said Dr. Aoki, "and it shows. We need to improve the work environment so that we can retain our great nurses. Barbara and I have identified so many problems . . . . We just don't know where to start."

Olina nodded. "First things first. Let's get to know the process we want to improve," she said.

Have you had reasons to be dissatisfied when going to see a doctor? What were those reasons?

LEARNING OBJECTIVES

After reading this chapter, you will be able to:

- Identify processes that are good candidates for improvement.
- Make a strong business case for action.
- Develop a Suppliers–Inputs–Process–Outputs–Customers (SIPOC) diagram.
- Identify the customer(s) and supplier(s) of a process step.
- Recognize the value chain in a process.
- Model a process using different tools.

INTRODUCTION

Chapter 2 provided a framework of the successive phases of a process improvement project. Accordingly, we will start with the *Define* phase and identify the process that we want to improve. Which processes need improvement? All of them, but some more than others. In order to deploy our resources effectively, we need to prioritize our efforts. From Chapter 1, we know that strategic alignment throughout the organization is critical. Therefore, we need to select a process improvement project that will contribute substantially to the achievement of the organizational strategy. Once the project is selected, the process scope and boundaries will need to be identified. All stakeholders should be involved in this process. We will revisit the SIPOC diagram (Chapter 2) in more detail for this purpose.

WHY IS THIS MATERIAL USEFUL?

In our constant quest for increasing value, we want to ensure that we will not allocate our resources to efforts that will yield minimal benefits. Rather, we want to "get the most bang for our buck" when we improve a process. Learning how to select a process improvement project and justify it is the first step. The second step is to define the process that will be improved, identify all its steps, and model the sequence of activities in the process. Process models give project stakeholders a clear "picture" of the process and a common frame of reference to facilitate collaboration.

SELECTING A PROJECT FOR IMPROVEMENT

Which process is going to be improved? Based on your experience with several processes at work, you may already have a pretty good idea of which ones fail to meet customers' expectations and desires. However, it takes more than an idea or hunch to select a good candidate for improvement. Only processes that meet the following criteria should be considered for upgrade and redesign:

- **Importance**: These processes are critical in supporting the strategy and have the potential to create the most value for customers.
- **Dysfunction**: These are processes with poor performance (Table 3.1). These processes generate waste and do not minimize the chances for errors.
- **Feasibility**: These processes have the most potential for successful improvement in terms of cost, process owners' commitment, project team's skills and experience, and scope. If a process is highly dysfunctional but current resources do not permit its improvement, it would be futile to consider it as a candidate. If the **process owners**, that is, people performing the process, are not interested in improving it or are suspicious of the project champion's or leaders' motivations, they will resist the proposed change. Their buy-in must thus be secured before undertaking any improvement project. Some process improvements may require highly technical expertise (e.g., new information system). If the project team lacks the knowledge and skills to fully participate in the redesign, the improvement is doomed to failure. Finally, if the scope of a project is too broad, the project's requirements will be difficult to pin down, and its execution will be marred by delays and cost overruns, thereby increasing the chances that leaders will pull the plug (Figure 3.1).

TABLE 3.1 INDICATORS OF DYSFUNCTIONAL PROCESSES

Warning Sign	Problem
Redundant data and activities	Subjective fragmentation of a process; too many handoffs
Inventory, wait	Uncertainty and variability in the process
Excessive number of checks and rechecks	Fragmentation; too many handoffs
Rework	Lack of standards or specifications; inadequate feedback and communication along the process
Complex, convoluted processes with numerous exceptions	Process that "grew" as new patients, services, and procedures were added over time

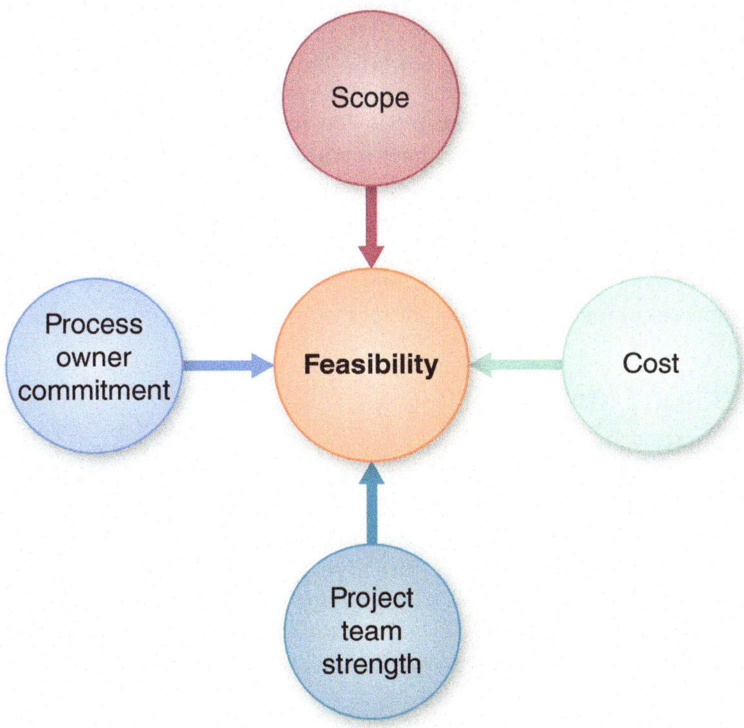

FIGURE 3.1 Feasibility elements for process improvement candidate.

BUSINESS CASE FOR ACTION

A process improvement is a project (Chapter 5). Like most projects, process improvements face many obstacles, the most daunting one being people's natural resistance to change. Individuals performing the process will feel that it works just fine the way they do it, or they will fear that efficiency gains will come at the expense of their job, power, or autonomy; people working upstream and downstream of the process will resent the adjustments they may have to make in their routines; and upper management will require evidence of substantial improvement in the bottom line. It is, therefore, very important to develop a **business case for action**, a document or presentation that makes a compelling, clear, and concise argument for change and the resources to implement it. For process improvements, a business case for action should comprise five short sections (Cassidy & Guggenberger, 2002):

1. **Business environment.** As processes are supposed to support the organizational strategy, the business case for action should identify the environmental pressures that justify change. For example, wait times at a competing hospital's ED are 10 minutes shorter, on average.
2. **Problem.** The problem(s) stemming from the current process should be clearly articulated. For example, wait times are very long during certain times of the day when patient volume is higher.
3. **Diagnosis.** The reasons for the process's dysfunction should be listed and briefly explained. In the case of long wait times, a diagnosis could refer to (a) poor triage hindering a rapid and smooth flow of patients through the ED, (b) lack of provider capacity at peak times, and (c) inappropriate layout.
4. **Cost of inaction.** This section warns the various **stakeholders**—people with a vested interest in the process (suppliers, employees, customers) and its performance (Munro et al., 2022)—of the consequences of maintaining the status quo in terms of lost business, loss of reputation, missed opportunities, and/or excess cost. Left alone, the processes in the ED would result in (a) an increase in left-without-being-seen (LWBS) cases (lost revenue); (b) low patient satisfaction scores (lower reimbursements by Medicare, unfavorable contracts with payers); (c) tarnished reputation (lost opportunities for future revenue); (d) increased turnover (higher staffing costs) and, even worse, poor medical outcomes because of delayed treatment (litigation costs).
5. **Objectives.** The objectives section should list the tangible and intangible benefits to be derived from the improvement. In the ED example, redesigned processes might reduce wait times by 15 minutes on average, decrease LWBS cases by 30%, improve providers' morale and productivity, and increase competitiveness for future business.

BENEFITS/EFFORT MATRIX

Senior leaders will be presented with a multitude of worthy improvement projects. The projects that make the final cut should justify the time and resources expended in their implementation. A **benefits/effort matrix** is a useful tool to display the values of potential projects based on an assessment of the efforts and benefits they involve (Table 3.2). Projects with high benefits and low efforts present the most attractive opportunities and should be prioritized. Conversely, projects with low benefits and high efforts should be discarded unless they are necessary to comply with regulations. Projects with low costs and low-to-medium benefits may be suitable contenders for kaizen events, that is, short-term improvement initiatives (Dyer, 2022).

You may recall from Chapter 1 that Bright Angel Medical Center (BAMC)'s ambulatory surgery center and ED were in need of improvement. After doing a SWOT analysis, Kimberly Mitchell and her team tended to favor the ED because increasing its throughput offered a better strategic fit. Using a benefits/effort matrix, they would also realize that even though both

TABLE 3.2 TYPES OF EFFORTS AND BENEFITS

Efforts	Benefits
Personnel requirements	Strategic fit
Capital investment	Financial benefit (extra revenue, lower cost)
Project duration	Added value to service
Project risk	Faster delivery
Buy-in from stakeholders	Increased flexibility
	Fewer errors

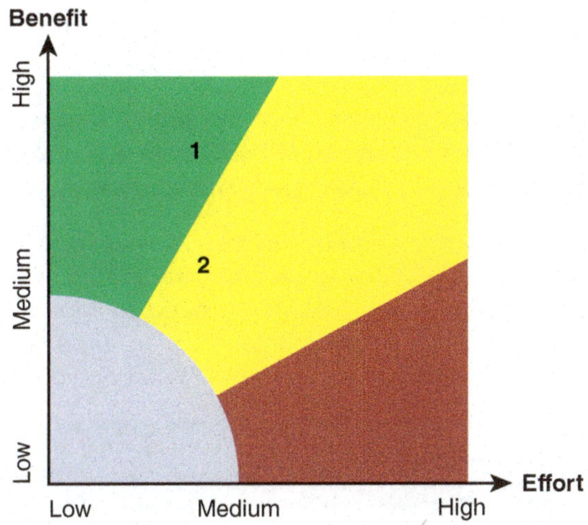

FIGURE 3.2 **Benefits/effort matrix for Bright Angel Medical Center.**

Legend: Project 1: ED; Project 2: Ambulatory Surgery Center

Source: Picture cropped from: https://www.isixsigma.com/project-selection-tracking/selecting-best-business-process-improvement-efforts

improvement projects require a substantial amount of effort, the ED project is more promising in terms of financial benefits: higher revenue and lower costs with fewer, if any, travel nurses (Figure 3.2)

DESCRIBING THE PROCESS

Once an improvement project has been selected, it is time to delineate what exactly needs to be improved. How do you start? It seems like an overwhelming task with no end in sight. First, get the big picture. Develop a high-level view of the process requiring improvement and identify its inputs, outputs, and boundaries.

HIGH-LEVEL VIEW

As mentioned in Chapter 2, the SIPOC diagram (Figure 2.6) is a useful tool for this purpose. You may think that it might be difficult to identify suppliers before knowing the process steps. You are right! In practice, process improvement project teams often follow this sequence to complete the SIPOC, or POCIS, diagram:

1. **Process**. Identify 4 to 5 high-level steps in the process.
2. **Outputs**. List all the process outputs.
3. **Customers**. List the internal and external customers of the process.
4. **Inputs**. Determine all the inputs and resources that will be necessary to carry out the process.
5. **Suppliers**. Identify the internal and external suppliers of the inputs and resources.

Some teams opt for a more customer-driven approach and begin by identifying the customers of the process, then the outputs, process steps, inputs, and suppliers. This method is referred to as "COPIS." Irrespective of the method selected, the result is a diagram that defines the process, its stakeholders, and what it takes to get the outputs desired by customers. Furthermore, the SIPOC recognizes that a process often extends beyond a work area, department, or organization. It thus promotes an integrated systems view that calls for optimizing and coordinating the entire process.

The SIPOC high-level process view is a good starting point to describe the process, but often it is not sufficient to understand what needs to be done to improve it. In the next sections, we delve into some of the SIPOC elements in more detail.

BRIGHT ANGEL MEDICAL CENTER 3.2

Olina Petrenko knocked on Dr. Aoki's door. "Come in," said a tired voice.

Olina walked toward the desk with a smile on her face. "I am happy to report we have made some progress. We developed a SIPOC diagram and, after talking with the ED staff, we came up with a preliminary description of the process we need to improve (Exhibit 3.1). We just used the COPIS sequence because it made brainstorming easier for the team," she said cheerfully while placing a piece of paper on the desk. "What do you think, Dr. Aoki?"

EXHIBIT 3.1 COPIS DIAGRAM FOR BAMC'S ED THROUGHPUT IMPROVEMENT PROJECT

Customers	Outputs	Process	Inputs	Suppliers
Patients	• Effective care delivery • Emergency access • Value • Respect	• Registration • Triage • Diagnosis • Treatment • Discharge/ Admission/ Transfer	• Supplies • Medication • People • Equipment • Technology	• Medical supply companies • Educational institutions • Community • Device manufacturers • Software companies
Staff	• Skill utilization • Autonomy • Proper use of time • Compensation	• Hire • Train • Promote	• LSS trainers	• Internal LSS mentors and trainers • Consultants
Community	• Employment • Access to care	• Based on above	• People	• Recruiters • Health system
Payers	• Value • Documentation	• Waste analysis • Error reduction • Accurate and prompt filing	• People • Technology	• Internal LSS mentors and trainers • Software companies
Joint Commission	• Performance • Documentation • Improvement	• Systematic data collection • Analysis • Reporting • Improvement planning	• People • Technology	• Internal LSS mentors and trainers • Software companies

Abbreviations: BAMC, Bright Angel Medical Center; LSS, Lean Six Sigma.

Dr. Aoki glanced at the diagram and seemed unimpressed. "Well, it is a start," she said without looking up. "Keep up the good work."

How would you describe Dr. Aoki's attitude? Can it affect the project's success? Discuss.

Why would the COPIS sequence make it easier for a team to brainstorm?

CUSTOMERS

For many businesses, it is easy to identify the customer: patrons in a restaurant, shoppers in a clothing store, readers in a library, and so on, but who is the "customer" in healthcare? Although the patient is the ultimate customer, there are many processes and steps required to care for patients that involve multiple customers. All entities mentioned in Table 3.3 are major customers of the healthcare system. If you consider treatment, the customer is the patient. If you examine the delivery of supplies to the operating room, the customers are the doctors and nurses. In the case of billing, the customer is an insurance company, an individual, or a third-party administrator. In fact, we could consider accrediting agencies as customers of the providers' quality reports.

Now, let us consider these customers' different expectations. In the following paragraphs, we elaborate on each one's perspective.

Patients' Perspectives

As healthcare *consumers*, individuals may focus on the costs of their care, especially when choosing a plan. However, as *patients*, quality is their primary concern. They form perceptions about their healthcare experiences during care delivery and about outcomes after care delivery. They are sensitive to their provider's expertise, courtesy, attentiveness to their needs, and respect for their time. They also appreciate the appearance, atmosphere, and ease of access to the facilities. With regard to health outcomes, patients often evaluate their results in terms of well-being (e.g., less pain or increased mobility). These perceptions are subjective; they are shaped by personal feelings, opinions, or outlook on life. For example, Patient A may feel that a 10-minute wait is acceptable, whereas Patient B finds it intolerable. Patient C may be delighted to walk unassisted for 20 minutes 1 month after knee surgery, whereas Patient D may wish to run a half marathon.

Providers' Perspectives

Providers are most interested in the process of providing care and in its clinical outcomes. The patient's health is their top priority. As a result, they may distrust cost reduction programs, which, in their views, may be threats to both patient safety and their incomes. They often clash with hospital administrators, who have a more business-oriented perspective of healthcare delivery and want to balance costs and quality. Some providers may also be skeptical of the importance of the patient's experience, the subjective elements of which seem less relevant than sound, objective clinical indicators. They prefer to evaluate patients' care and health against "hard" measures with well-established standards: blood pressure, mortality rate, readmissions,

TABLE 3.3 CUSTOMERS IN HEALTHCARE

Customers	Examples
Patients	• Young patients wanting convenient access to clinic • Older patients with diabetes having difficulties with transportation
Providers and administrative staff	• Community physicians or clinics referring patients to your hospital • Physicians sending specimens to your laboratory • Nurses in the ICU receiving patients admitted through the ED • Bed control staff needing information when a patient is discharged
Third-party payers	• Managed care organizations contracting with physician • Self-insured employers contracting with third-party administrators • Centers for Medicare & Medicaid Services
External reviewers	• Accreditation agencies • Certification organizations • Award organizations

patient falls, percentage of time a prophylactic antibiotic was received within 1 hour prior to surgical incision, and so on.

Third-Party Payers' Perspectives

Third-party payers are interested in both quality and efficiency. They do value positive clinical outcomes, but they are wary of costly, new treatments and procedures, the effectiveness of which may not be superior to older alternatives. As a result, they are often at odds with both patients and providers as they may deny coverage of treatments preferred by these two parties (Rosenthal, 2023). Insurers and self-insured employers have been at times vocal in emphasizing evidence-based practice and cost-effectiveness of multiple treatment options.

Some payers may welcome innovative options that they consider cost-effective in the long run. They may cover alternative treatments such as homeopathy, acupuncture, and restorative yoga. They may also offer incentives to participate in nutrition counseling and smoking cessation programs. They may even encourage treatment away from home (another city or country) if the value proposition is favorable and often pay for a companion to stay with the patient in a hotel in the destination city (Box 3.1).

Accrediting Agencies

Accrediting agencies such as The Joint Commission can also be considered customers of healthcare organizations. Among other things, they review information and documents prepared by these organizations to evaluate their performance and adherence to patient safety and quality of care standards (The Joint Commission, 2024).

PROCESS STEPS

Let's take a closer look at the process steps on BAMC's SIPOC diagram. They are purposely broad. In fact, they are major subprocesses or modules. Let us focus on the patients as customers, and disaggregate each of the subprocesses into individual steps (Table 3.4). To do so, the team should:

- Specify the starting and ending points of the process, that is, its boundaries.
- Follow multiple flow units through the entire process.
- List all the steps in their sequence.

BOX 3.1 QUALITY IN PRACTICE!

Walmart's Centers of Excellence Program

Walmart, the largest employer in the world, is self-insured for healthcare. It has encouraged its employees across the country to use Centers of Excellence (COE; health systems and hospitals that provide highly specialized treatment, procedures, and surgeries for complex conditions). COEs are made up of highly skilled experts dedicated to providing comprehensive, interdisciplinary care in specific therapeutic areas. In 2015, Walmart partnered with Mayo Clinic to establish an oncology COE for its employees. Today, the program has expanded to encompass 18 medical care partners in multiple specialties: heart surgery, weight loss surgery, spine surgery, cancer treatment, hip and knee replacements, organ and tissue transplants, and fertility treatments. The reason that Walmart is interested in paying for its employees to travel to these centers is that the care is deemed exceptional, with fewer complications and unnecessary procedures, and more cost-effective. Although many companies cannot replicate the Walmart model, it may provide a roadmap for large employer healthcare benefit design in the years to come (Emerson, 2022).

TABLE 3.4 SUBPROCESSES AND STEPS

Improving ED Throughput	
Subprocess	**Individual Steps**
1. Registration	• Patient checks in/ Patient arrives by ambulance • Initial triage • Patient's information and primary complaints are entered
2. Triage	• Verify patient information • Collect additional patient information • Examine observable signs (e.g., bruise, burn) • Take vital signs • Determine ESI level • Request immediate rooming if necessary
3. Initial assessment	• Examine patient • Order diagnostic tests if necessary (other subprocesses follow) • Review test results • Make diagnosis
4. Treatment	• Initiate treatment • Reassess condition

5. Disposition	• Discharge:
	  • Place discharge order
	  • Prescribe medications
	  • Provide discharge instructions
	• Admission:
	  • Contact admitting service
	  • Request bed
	• Transfer:
	  • Contact transfer center
	  • Request bed
	  • Arrange transport

Abbreviation: ESI, Emergency Severity Index.

ON THE JOB! INTERVIEW VIDEO 3.1

Sharon Erickson
Quality and Patient Safety Manager in Ambulatory Care

Creating Action Based on Data
SIPOC
Including all stakeholders
Creating buy-in
Combination of failure mode and effects analysis (FMEA) and root cause analysis (RCA)

1. What are the advantages of using the SIPOC tool?
2. What is the goal of asking the five "whys" during a risk priority numbering exercise?
3. Utilizing the frequency, severity, and detectability tool allows the team to create a risk priority number. Discuss the value of having a score assigned to each of the various root causes.

The interview is available online by visiting www.springerpub.com/courseconnect. See inside front cover and tear-out card for CourseConnect details.

PROCESS MODELING

When looking at Table 3.3, we see that the customer of a process step may become the supplier for the next step. One simple way to identify the customers of a process is thus to adopt the **"next process" concept**: view the customer as the beneficiary of the next step in the process of healthcare delivery. The next process concept therefore captures the perspective of a customer-driven value chain and enables us to determine value-added requirements for each activity. Process modeling helps you visualize the process and the transitions of responsibility or handoffs between people.

A **process model** is essentially a simplified, graphic representation of a process. Modeling can be accomplished at various levels of detail. The model can be a simple diagram depicting the basic workflow of the activities comprising the process. The diagram can be refined to include the players as well as the various points of "waste" in the process. At its most advanced state, the process model is a sophisticated simulation model that mimics the existing, or planned, process and generates performance measures based on its configuration.

FLOWCHART

The analysis and design of a process often start with its depiction. There are many established, as well as original, diagramming conventions available for the purpose. A popular one is a **flowchart**. A flowchart shows the movement of a **flow unit** through the process. A flow unit refers to a transient entity that enters the process, goes through a sequence of activities, and exits the process (Laguna & Marklund, 2019). Depending on the context, the flow unit could be a patient, a lab order, a medical record, or a purchase requisition. The flowchart displays the progress of the flow unit through the process steps (Table 3.4) as a left to right (or top to bottom) arrangement of symbols (Figure 3.3) from the starting to the ending points. It can show loops when rework needs to be done, decision points, alternative paths or routings, and activities that can be performed in parallel, independently from one another. Once the process is diagrammed, all process owners should verify its accuracy. Let us consider the ED patient flow at BAMC. The flow unit is the patient, and the process consists of 16 steps (Figure 3.4). The patients arrive either via an ambulance or private vehicle. Then they go through a multistep process: initial assessment, laboratory or radiology workup, diagnosis, treatment, and then disposition. Note the key decision points in the process influence the logical sequence of steps.

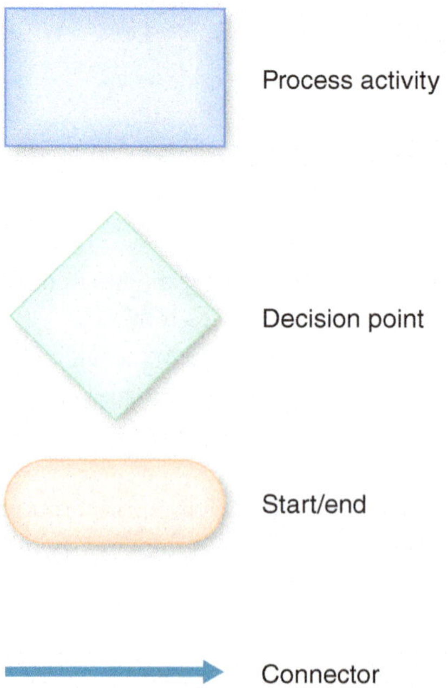

FIGURE 3.3 Basic flowchart symbols.

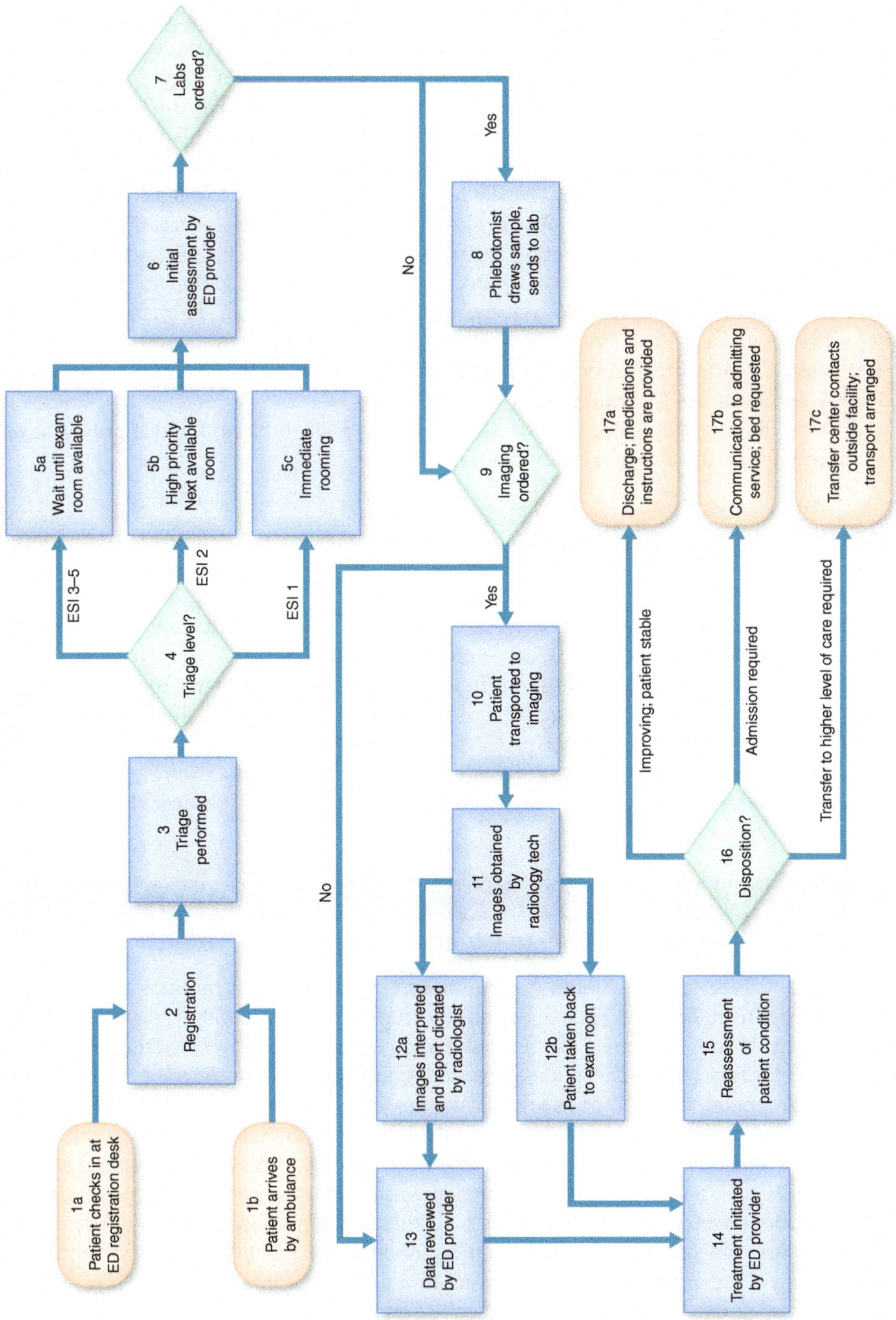

FIGURE 3.4 Flowchart of current patient flow.

Abbreviation: ESI, Emergency Severity Index.

SWIMLANE DIAGRAM

A **swimlane diagram** is a type of flowchart that identifies all the players in the process. It is composed of several bands or lanes, each one corresponding to a participant or player in the process. This information is useful when determining the various resources involved in performing the process; it also hints at the subprocesses performed by the players (Box 3.2). In our example, ordering lab tests would trigger a series of subactivities, such as retrieving a patient record, assigning a phlebotomist, labeling samples, analyzing, and logging the results. Figure 3.5 extends the basic flowchart for a patient arriving at the ED in a private vehicle (see Figure 3.4) by indicating the roles played by specific individuals/departments in the process. The registration clerk checks in the patient. The triage nurse takes the patient's vital signs and determines the patient's Emergency Severity Index (ESI) classification. The ED provider assesses the patient's condition, orders lab and/or imaging tests when appropriate, reviews the test results, initiates treatment, reassesses the patient's condition, and decides whether the patient should be discharged, admitted, or sent to another facility. The phlebotomist draws a blood sample and sends it to the lab (subprocess not depicted for simplification). The radiology technician takes the images. The radiologist reviews the images and dictates a report. Depending on the patient's disposition, a nurse performs the discharge process, the admitting service requests a hospital bed, or the transfer center contacts another facility and arranges for transport.

Once a process has been depicted, it becomes easier to understand it and detect potential weak spots. A good tool for this purpose is the 5w2h framework.

THE 5W2H FRAMEWORK

Originally used for benchmarking, the **5w2h framework** also contributes to the description of the process by asking pertinent questions (who, what, when, where, why, how, and how much) and identifying improvement opportunities. Typically, the process improvement team will consult multiple sources of information to answer these questions. Interviews of process participants, internal documents, and video recording of the process in action may prove useful in painting an accurate and comprehensive picture of the process. Sometimes, a broad 5w2h framework involves the entire process. Preferably, each process step is scrutinized. Table 3.5 focuses on one subprocess and indicates how ordering and performing imaging tests should be questioned and evaluated for redesign.

BOX 3.2 QUALITY IN PRACTICE!

Improving School Nurses' Access to Children's Electronic Records

When treating children, school nurses need access to their medical records to ensure the best possible health outcomes. This is especially true for children with chronic conditions who might end up in the ED unless the school nurses know about their medical history and care plans. Unfortunately, obstacles such as federal regulations and inefficient communication systems between pediatricians' offices and school nurses have traditionally prevented nurses from accessing up-to-date information in a timely manner. The "Colorado Connect School Nurses Program" enables school nurses to view, not edit, some of the children's electronic health records (EHR). In a study of the program's effectiveness, the complex approval process to access a student's EHR was depicted in a swimlane diagram showing the interactions among the hospital, the school, and the parent/guardians. The sample consisted of students suffering from severe allergies, asthma, seizures, and type 1 diabetes. The findings revealed that school nurses' access to the EHR dramatically curtailed the number of ED visits and hospitalizations (Baker et al., 2022).

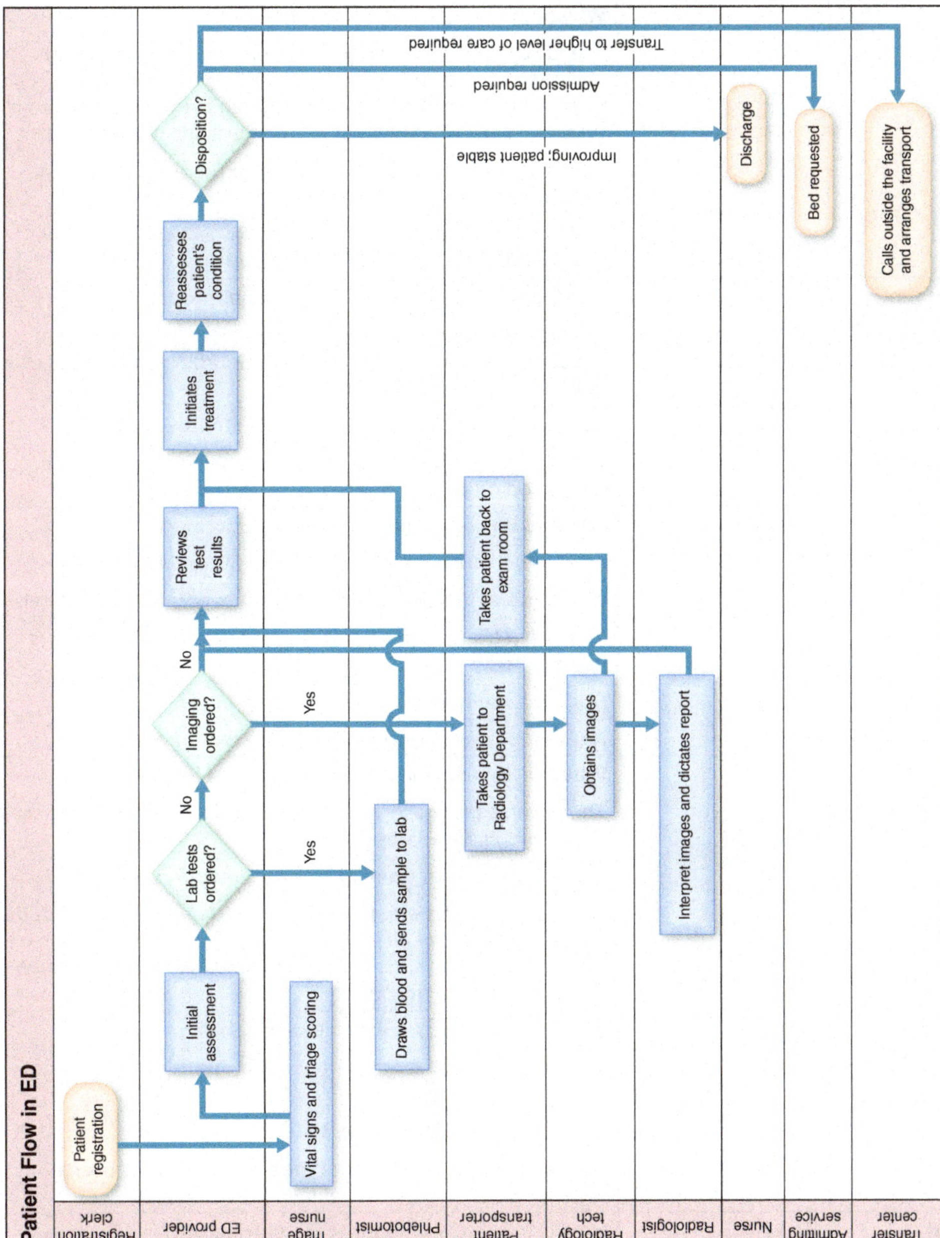

FIGURE 3.5 Swimlane diagram of current patient flow.

TABLE 3.5 5W2H FRAMEWORK FOR OBTAINING A RADIOLOGIC STUDY IN THE ED

Classification	5w2h Questions	Description
People	Who?	**Who is performing the activity/subprocess?** The ED provider, the patient transporter, the radiology technician, and the radiologist. **Why are these people doing it?** The ED provider must give the order and evaluate the results. The patient transporter must take the patient to the Radiology Department. The radiology technician must take the images. The radiologist must examine the images, diagnose, and dictate a report. ***Could/should someone else perform the activity/subprocess? Could fewer people be involved?*** *The patient transporter would not be needed if the patient did not have to go to another department.*
Subject matter	What?	**What is being done in this activity/subprocess?** Orders are placed; transport is requested and performed; images are taken and checked for accuracy; images are evaluated and report is dictated. ***Can the activity/subprocess in question be eliminated?*** *The subprocess itself cannot be eliminated, but it can be shortened by eliminating the transport activity.*
Sequence	When?	**When is this activity/subprocess performed?** After preliminary assessment by the ED provider. **When is the best time to perform this activity/subprocess?** *Immediately after lab tests are drawn and/or after order is placed.* ***Does it have to be done at a certain time?*** *As soon as possible after the initial assessment.*
Location	Where?	**Where is this activity/subprocess carried out?** The order is placed in the exam room. The images are taken in the Imaging Department. ***Does it have to be done at this(ese) location(s)?*** *Yes for placing orders. For CT scan, MRI, and ultrasound, the images must be taken in the Imaging Department. X-rays can be done portably in the ED to save time, sometimes though at the expense of quality.*
Purpose	Why?	**Why is this activity/subprocess needed?** Radiology studies are done to support or rule out various diagnoses. ***Clarify and justify its purpose*** *Radiology studies are part of the overall comprehensive workup to complete the evaluation of the patient.*
Method	How?	**How is the activity/subprocess carried out?** The patient transporter takes the patient to the Imaging Department. The radiology tech performs the radiologic exam of the patient using the appropriate equipment based on the test ordered. Images are captured digitally and transmitted to the radiology reading room for evaluation by the radiologist. The radiologist interprets the images and dictates a report which appears in the medical record for use by other clinicians for the diagnosis of the patient.

(*continued*)

TABLE 3.5 5W2H FRAMEWORK FOR OBTAINING A RADIOLOGIC STUDY IN THE ED (*CONTINUED*)

Classification	5w2h Questions	Description
		Is this the best way or are there alternatives? *Transport to and from the Imaging Department can be eliminated if x-rays are taken with a portable machine. Transport time, wait time in the Imaging Department, and wait time to read the exam can be reduced. Time spent in the Imaging Department is wasted if the patient has to wait on others completing their exams.*
Cost	How much?	**How much does it currently cost?** The cost is based on the time spent by the transporter, the radiology tech, and the radiologist as well as the capital depreciation of the equipment. Lower reimbursements due to poor patient satisfaction scores and lost revenue due to limited throughput with long visit times. ***What would the tentative cost be after improvement?*** *Elimination of transport would get rid of that wage cost.* *Patient satisfaction scores would increase, and lost revenue would decrease.*

BRIGHT ANGEL MEDICAL CENTER 3.3

Olina Petrenko printed copies of the ED workflow, swimlane, and 5w2h framework for everyone in the meeting.

"This is great work," exclaimed Dr. Tibbets, "the flowchart really helps us see the convolutedness of this process and where we should start to focus our attention. The swimlane also shows the large number of handoffs and how coordinating all aspects of care becomes tricky."

Dr. Aoki was fixated on the 5w2h framework. "Our patients spend a lot of time going to and from the Imaging Department. We need to look at this in more detail."

Barbara jumped in, "I was just in the ED and everyone was hustling. No one is lounging around, staring at their phones. I don't know how we could work any faster."

Olina smiled. She had led other teams through a similar exercise and she knew that it was hard to see how to improve without scrutinizing the facility space and all the wasted steps in the workflow. "You are correct, Barbara. We aren't going to ask anyone to work faster. That could actually make conditions worse and be a safety issue. What we want to do is remove wasted time and unnecessary steps in the process. That is where most of the efficiency comes from. That and improving the layout of the ED. For example, the patient discharge instructions only print up front at registration. The nurses are wasting hours every day walking back and forth to collect that paperwork and deliver it to patients. That is just one example of how we can improve the workflow."

Dr. Tibbets was pleased with what he was hearing. He knew they had the right leadership around the table to fix this issue. "We are missing one key element here before we start making any changes. Frontline employees. Those are people doing the work and they are the best positioned to know what is not working well. Too often, leaders institute changes without including input from the frontline. That is a critical mistake we need to avoid."

The group nodded in agreement. "Let's get after it," Barbara said with excitement. She couldn't wait to uncover and solve all the problems in the ED.

Why is it a good idea to represent a process graphically?

ETHICAL SCENARIO 3.1

Selection of Pet Projects

Health system leaders need to prioritize their projects or initiatives to drive improvements. This is due to the time and resource constraints that impact us all. The process that leaders follow to select projects is important. It needs to be transparent and aim for the health system's and community's best interests. Occasionally, leaders can deviate from these guiding principles when they have an attachment to a certain project. Depending on the position of the leader in the organization, undue influence can be applied to prioritize a pet project above the greater needs of the health system.

How can the selection of a pet project impact the morale of the workforce?

What is the impact of executives selecting projects that may be important to them as individuals but not to the community?

SUMMARY

The beginning of a project is always overwhelming. This chapter offers tools and tips to increase the likelihood that process improvement efforts will be well spent. Criteria for project candidacy are provided: importance, dysfunctionality, and feasibility in terms of scope, cost, team strengths, and process owner acceptance and commitment. The candidates are then evaluated and placed on a benefits/effort matrix to prioritize them. Once the project has been selected, the process(es) it involves is(are) described. The recommended approach is to start with a high-level, comprehensive view of the process, then identify all the steps and graph the process flow in order to facilitate process understanding, visualize handoffs, and detect potential weaknesses.

CERTIFICATION TIPS

This chapter is the first part of the *Define* phase in the DMAIC (Define–Measure–Analyze–Improve–Control) framework. In addition to the material presented in this chapter, we recommend that you do the following items for the *Define* section of the exam:

- Understand when the DMAIC methodology is appropriate: https://www.learnleansigma.com/improvement-methodology/dmaic-vs-dmadv.
- Review the parts of a process and boundaries (Chapter 1) and the elements of a SIPOC diagram (Chapter 2).
- Differentiate between process owners and stakeholders.
- Understand how processes support an operations strategy which is aligned with the business strategy (Chapter 1).
- Remember that systems thinking is important to understand how one step in the process affects the next one, and potentially, all downstream steps.
- Recognize the different contributions of flowcharts and swimlane diagrams and know how to develop each one.

KEY TERMS

Process owner
Business case for action
Stakeholder
Benefits/effort matrix
Next process concept
Process model
Flowchart
Flow unit
Swimlane diagram
5w2h framework

REVIEW QUESTIONS

1. What are the criteria used to identify processes that are candidates for improvement? Explain each one briefly.
2. What are the warning signs of dysfunctional processes? What do they signal?
3. What is a business case for action? What are its elements?
4. What is a benefits/effort matrix and what is its purpose?
5. What is the difference between process owners and process stakeholders?
6. What are the differences between a SIPOC diagram and a list of process steps?
7. How does one develop a list of process steps?
8. Differentiate among the quality expectations of patients, providers, and third-party payers.
9. What is a flowchart? What does it show?
10. What is a swimlane diagram? What does it show?
11. What is a 5w2h framework? What is its purpose?

SOLVE BRIGHT ANGEL MEDICAL CENTER'S PROBLEMS

1. The following are the evaluation scores of a series of projects.

Project	Benefits (Low: 1; Medium: 2; High: 3)	Effort (Low: 1; Medium: 2; High: 3)
A	3	2
B	2	2
C	1	3
D	2	3
E	1	1
F	3	3

a. Place them on the benefits/effort matrix that follows:

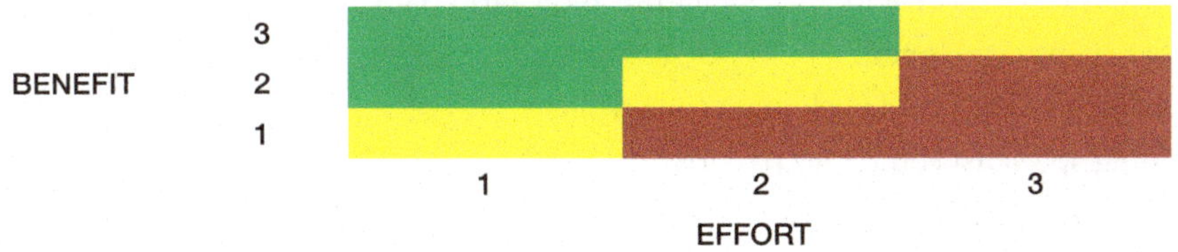

b. Determine which one(s) you would undertake as DMAIC projects and why.

2. The following are the evaluation scores of a series of projects.

Project	Benefits (Low: 1; Medium: 2; High: 3)	Effort (Low: 1; Medium: 2; High: 3)
A	1	1
B	3	1
C	2	2
D	3	2
E	1	3
F	2	1

a. Place them on the benefits/effort matrix that follows:

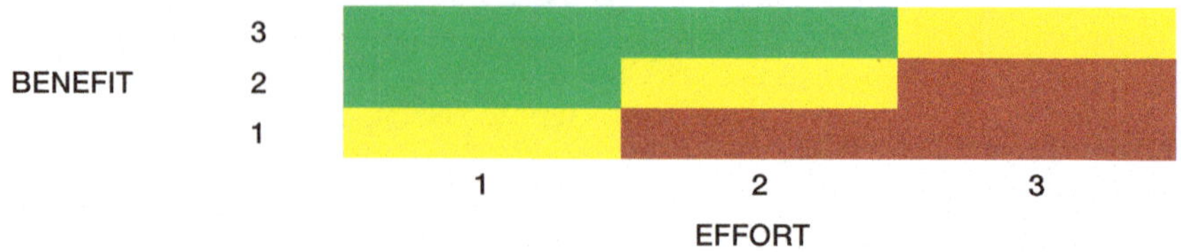

b. Determine which one(s) you will *not* undertake and why *not*.

3. These are the steps for patients making appointments at an Urgent Care clinic using an online system:
   - Patient registers on the MyAppointment system.
   - Patient arrives at Urgent Care.
   - Patient checks in/fills out paperwork.
   - Patient is triaged.
   - Patient is taken to exam room.
   - Exam is performed.
   - Doctor places orders for discharge.
   - Nurse discusses discharge paperwork.
   - Nurse marks patient as discharged in hospital chart.
   - Registration clerk marks patient as discharged on MyAppointment system.
   - Patient leaves Urgent Care.
     a. Develop a SIPOC diagram.
     b. Develop a flowchart of the process.
     c. Develop a swimlane diagram of the process.
4. These are the steps involved in the specialty medication referral process:
   - Provider sends referral to specialty pharmacy.
   - Pharmacy verifies patient's insurance coverage.
   - Billing specialist identifies prior authorization form needed.
   - Form is faxed to provider for signature and chart note.
   - Documents are signed.
   - Documents are faxed back to pharmacy.
   - Billing specialist completes paperwork.
   - Documents are faxed to insurance company.
   - Reviewer makes decision for coverage.
   - Documents are faxed back to pharmacy.
   - Pharmacy verifies prescription order.
   - Pharmacy fills prescription order.
     a. Develop a SIPOC diagram.
     b. Develop a flowchart of the process.
     c. Develop a swimlane diagram of the process.
5. These are the steps of the thyroid biopsy process:
   - Patient is brought to exam room.
   - Nurse takes vitals.
   - Technician performs ultrasound to locate the thyroid nodule.

- Patient is moved to procedure room.
- Consent form is signed.
- Physician applies local anesthesia.
- Fluid and tissue samples are drawn from nodule.
- Patient is monitored after biopsy.
- Patient is taken to checkout.
- Patient checks out.
- Procedure room is cleaned.
- Samples are sent to lab.
  a. Develop a SIPOC diagram.
  b. Develop a flowchart of the process.
  c. Develop a swimlane diagram of the process.

LEARNING ACTIVITIES

1. Read the transcript of the following interview of Lisa Woods, vice-president, physical and emotional wellbeing, at Walmart: https://workology.com/episode-381-benefits-and-centers-of-excellence-with-lisa-woods-from-walmart.
   According to Ms. Woods,
   a. What are Walmart's reasons for having COE? Are those compatible with the idea of value? Why or why not?
   b. Are new service offerings like fertility services a value proposition for Walmart? Discuss.
   c. What do you think Walmart should do to enhance their COE program?
2. In your department, identify three processes that are dysfunctional and answer the following questions:
   a. Why is each one dysfunctional? Are you completely sure? Why or why not?
   b. To develop a business case for action for each project, what additional information would you need?
   c. Which one of the three projects has the best chance to be selected for improvement? Why?
3. For one of the processes identified in Question 2, develop a 5w2h framework for the overall process.

REFERENCES

Baker, C., Lorestro, F., Jr., Pickett, K., Samay, S. S., & Gance-Cleveland, B. (2022). Facilitating health information exchange to improve health outcomes for school-aged children: School nurse electronic health record access. *Applied Clinical Informatics*, *13*(4), 803–810. https://doi.org/10.1055/a-1905-3729

Cassidy, A., & Guggenberger, K. (2002). *A practical guide to information systems process improvement*. CRC Press.

Dyer, L. (2022, April 6). *The benefit effort matrix—A tool to determine where to apply your resources*. Pyzdek Institute. https://www.pyzdekinstitute.com/blog/six-sigma-tools/the-benefit-effort-matrix-a-tool-to-determine-where-to-apply-your-resources.html

Emerson, J. (2022). *The 18 health systems Walmart sends its employees to for care in 2022*. Becker's Hospital Review. https://www.beckershospitalreview.com/strategy/the-18-health-systems-walmart-sends-its-employees-to-for-care-in-2022.html

Laguna, M., & Marklund, J. (2019). *Business process, modeling, simulation, and design* (3rd ed.). Routledge.

Munro, R. A., Ramu, G., & Zrymiak, D. J. (2022). *The ASQ certified Six Sigma Green Belt handbook* (3rd ed.). ASQ Quality Press.

Rosenthal, E. (2023, May 28). *Analysis: Health insurance claim denials are on the rise, to the detriment of patients*. PBS NewsHour. https://www.pbs.org/newshour/health/analysis-health-insurance-claim-denials-are-on-the-rise-to-the-detriment-of-patients

The Joint Commission. (2024). *About our standards*. https://www.jointcommission.org/standards/about-our-standards

CHAPTER 4

THE VOICE OF THE CUSTOMER AND THE VOICE OF THE PROCESS

BRIGHT ANGEL MEDICAL CENTER 4.1

Barbara Waters and Olina Petrenko met for a working lunch to discuss the major issue facing the ED.

"I'm a little overwhelmed," Barbara shared. "I know it always starts with the patient. Our ED length of stay is probably twice what it should be. The patients keep complaining mostly about the wait times in the surveys, but there are several other issues, and I'm not sure they are related to throughput. Are we on the right track?"

"Listen," Olina encouraged, "we can figure this out. Let's look at what patients want the most and see if our process metrics even capture those wants. Without these metrics, we are all in the dark."

Have you ever been to the ED? Compare your expectations and actual experience of the service rendered.

LEARNING OBJECTIVES

After reading this chapter, you will be able to:

- Differentiate between *quality* and *excellent quality.*
- Develop the house of quality (HOQ).
- Capture the voice of the customer (VOC) with subjective measures.
- Distinguish between qualitative and quantitative research data collection methods.
- Understand the dynamic nature of quality improvements through the lens of the Kano model.
- Translate the VOC into the voice of the process (VOP) by developing internal, objective quality indicators.
- Develop a critical-to-quality (CTQ) tree.
- Describe the various purposes of quality measures in healthcare.
- Understand the concept of cascading dashboards.

INTRODUCTION

Let us go back to the first question we asked you in Chapter 1: What does quality healthcare mean to you? There was not a unique answer. Healthcare quality has indeed many facets, which make it difficult to pin it down precisely. Further complicating the issue, different groups of people perceive *quality* differently. Healthcare providers tend to view quality exclusively in terms of processes and clinical outcomes, whereas patients focus on the quality of their experience, *in addition* to the outcomes. The payers (i.e., health plan sponsors of insurance companies, such as employers, unions, and government agencies) insist not only on excellent health outcomes but also on efficiency. Besides the multidimensionality of the concept itself, this plurality of perspectives regarding its meaning magnifies the difficulty of building a coherent healthcare quality system. Yet, this challenge was one of the Affordable Care Act (ACA)'s imperatives (White House, 2010). By requiring public reporting of providers' performance on key quality indicators and penalizing providers for poor performance, the ACA, private insurers, and state governments put quality at the forefront of the healthcare policy. In this chapter, you will begin to develop a quality system in a healthcare organization.

WHY IS THIS MATERIAL USEFUL?

As per the cumulative model (Chapter 1), quality provides the foundation for achieving excellence. Customers ultimately define what quality should be, which is why it is important to capture their voice and design quality systems aligned with, or even exceeding, customers' expectations. These expectations are then translated into observable, objective quality indicators that help an organization gauge and track its performance systematically.

WHAT IS QUALITY?

Who defines quality? The customer! If customers are responsible for defining the quality they want, providers of the product/service are responsible for delivering that quality. As a result, a broad, common definition of **quality** involves *meeting customers' expectations of product/service characteristics.* There are two important elements in these definitions: (1) the customers and (2) their expectations. In Chapter 3, you saw that customers are the beneficiaries of a process, or even process step, output. Therefore, there are many different customers with different expectations. As healthcare professionals, your challenge is to develop and improve the processes that will produce **excellent quality**, which means *exceeding* customers' expectations. In order to do so, you need to ensure that your processes create the quality your customers deserve. You must also deliver that quality every time. According to Lean Six Sigma (LSS) principles (Chapter 2), that means *doing it right the first time.*

The **house of quality (HOQ)** provides a useful framework to define quality more precisely and build it into the system.

THE HOUSE OF QUALITY

In our quest to develop and manage a quality system, we must ensure that all processes are developed and managed to satisfy customers' needs. **Quality function deployment (QFD)** is a systematic approach to incorporate these needs into each step of a process, that is, deploy quality into the design of a process. The tool used in QFD to merge the **voice of the customer (VOC)** with the **voice of the process (VOP)** is the HOQ. The HOQ is a matrix that depicts clear relationships between customer and process requirements (Figure 4.1). Building the house comprises several steps. The first step involves asking customers what they want.

1. **Capture the customers' requirements (VOC).** This can be done informally through discussions and/or formally through other methods of data collection, such as surveys or structured interviews. The **Kano model** (Figure 4.3) or customers' ratings in a questionnaire can be used to determine the importance of each required service feature. These customers' requirements and their relative importance are the inputs into the HOQ. In our example, patients presenting to the ED want to be seen by the physician promptly after arrival, be diagnosed and treated

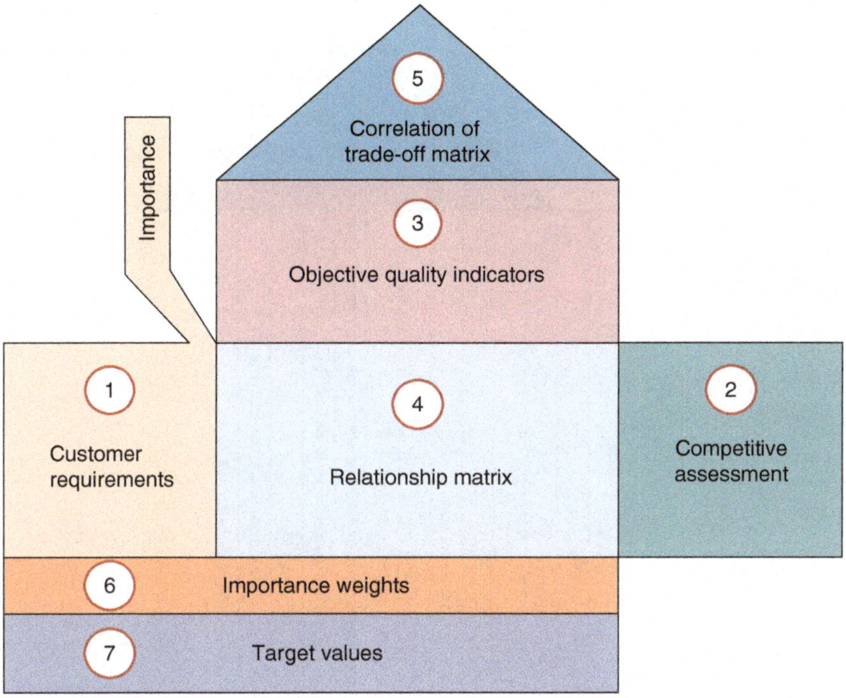

FIGURE 4.1 Overview of the HOQ.

Abbreviation: HOQ, house of quality.

Source: Russell, R. S., & Taylor, B. W. (2023). *Operations and supply chain management* (11th ed.). Wiley. Copyright © 2023, 2019, 2016, 2014, 2011, 2008, 2005.

correctly, receive clear discharge instructions, and so forth. However, even though they value clean facilities, they view a correct diagnosis as the most important requirement (Figure 4.2).

2. **Conduct a competitive assessment by comparing your performance to your competitors' on the various customer requirements.** Access to the national norms of a patient satisfaction database, or the Centers for Medicare & Medicaid Services (CMS) databases on Care Compare on Medicare.gov, will facilitate this task. In our example, we see that the Bright Angel Medical Center (BAMC) ED performs well in terms of cleanliness. For those attributes in which BAMC surpasses the competition, a design change may not be necessary. For those in which it trails the competition, change is imperative. If considered important to customers, these attributes (e.g., understanding follow-up care, correct diagnosis, respect, minimal wait, and prompt admission after diagnosis) are at least order qualifiers, and not being on par with the competition may result in revenue losses.
3. **Translate the customer's requirements (VOC) into observable process requirements (VOP).** At this point, the perceptual measures obtained from the customer are converted into objective **quality indicators** that are **critical to quality (CTQ)**, that is, essential to meet customers' quality requirements (Figure 4.4). Indicators are operationalized definitions of quality; they can be observed, measured, and tracked consistently by the service provider. For example, correct diagnosis can be measured by: (a) mortality ratio, (b) percentage of return visits for the same condition within 72 hours, and (c) percentage of prescription changes for the same condition within 72 hours. It is a good idea to generate a large number of indicators because some of them might be discarded later if deemed less adequate than others in capturing the VOC.
4. **Indicate the strength of the relationship between a given customer requirement and an observable quality indicator in the relationship matrix.** This can be done with a number or a symbol (see Figure 4.2). In our example, the door-to-doc time is a stronger indicator of the patient's wish to be seen promptly than the door-to-triage time because the patient will likely

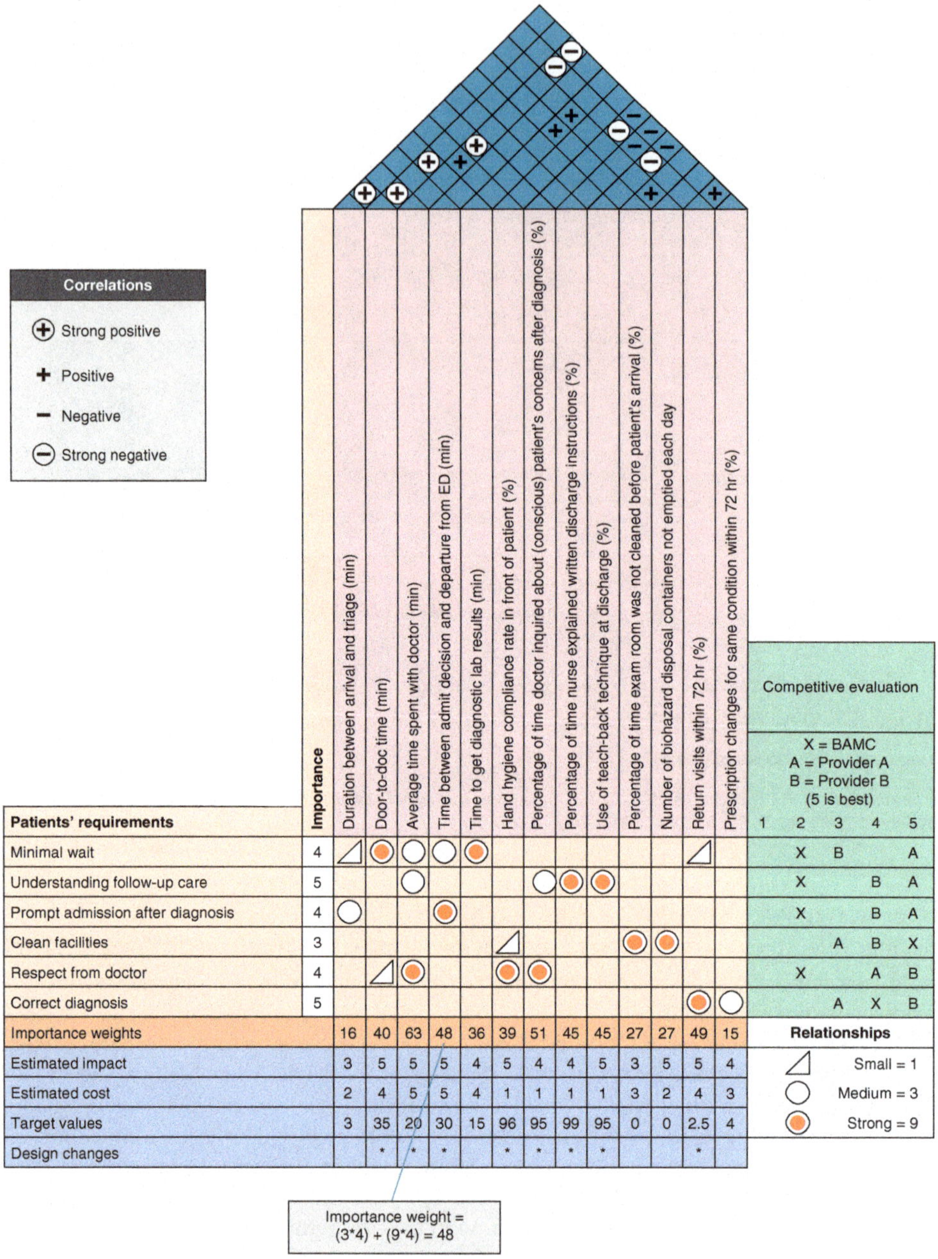

FIGURE 4.2 House of quality (HOQ).

wait longer in both the waiting room and the exam room before being seen by the physician. Although the door-to-triage time is a "weaker" indicator, it should not be discarded at this point as it may reveal an important source of delay before the physician sees the patient.

5. **Determine the correlations or trade-offs between pairs of indicators.** Achieving excellence in one indicator may reinforce or hinder performance on another because they are interrelated. For example, increasing the average time of doctor–patient interaction would decrease the number of patients seen in a day, which would contribute to further congestion and longer door-to-doc times at the ED. However, superficial exam and diagnosis may impact the percentage of return visits for the same condition. Considering all this information is necessary to build the most effective and efficient processes.

6. **Compute the indicators' importance weights.** This is done by multiplying the importance rating of a customer requirement by the strength of the relationship between the requirement and an indicator and summing through all customer requirements. See example in Figure 4.2
7. **Determine the target value for each indicator, and the cost and impact of achieving that target value.** Generally, process design improvements will be called for if:
   a. The provider is trailing the competition in areas customers consider important (e.g., correct diagnosis, minimal wait).
   b. The impact of a change exceeds its cost. In our example, BAMC may already be a leader in terms of cleanliness, but it falls really short in seeing and admitting patients promptly, understanding follow-up care, and in showing patients signs of respect (see Figure 4.2). The cost of improving timeliness requires major costly changes, but the costs of showing signs of respect and improving the understanding of follow-up care are relatively small compared to their impact. Although all these improvements are necessary, the last two are easy to achieve with training and reminders.

THE KANO MODEL

Besides survey ratings, a useful tool to help us determine the importance of customers' requirements (Step 1) is the **Kano model**. In the end, patients—the ultimate customers in healthcare—are often the ones who define quality, and we should "wow" them. The Kano model reminds us that value to the customer is the overarching goal.

Developed by Dr. Noriaki Kano, the Kano model argues that from a customer perspective, more is not always better. It does not necessarily run counter to the argument that organizations should exceed customers' expectations, but it highlights the fallacy of introducing improvements that customers do not particularly value. The Kano model is based on three levels of quality: basic, performance, and excitement (Figure 4.3).

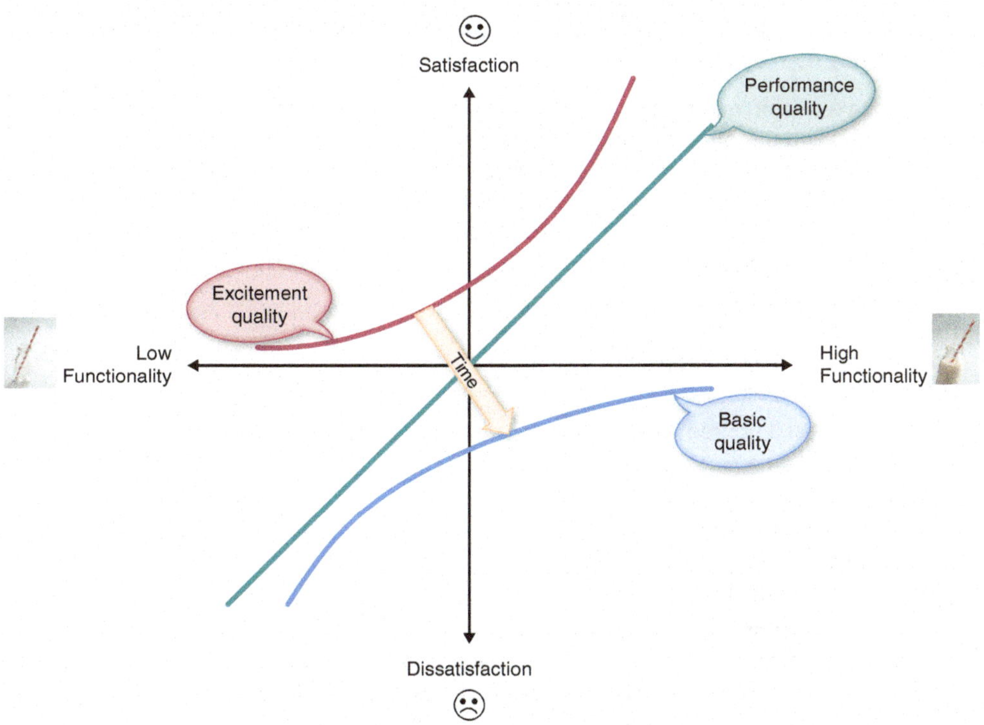

FIGURE 4.3 The Kano model.

Basic quality is associated with customer requirements that are essentially order qualifiers (see Chapter 1) or "must haves." In other words, they represent customers' basic expectations of a product or service. Although they do not result in satisfaction when present, they do produce dissatisfaction if not present and could then lead to the loss of business. Examples of basic quality include clean waiting rooms or physicians washing their hands before examining a patient.

Performance quality refers to customer requirements that produce satisfaction proportionally to their level of appeal. These are the "wants" that customers express in the VOC. Whether they trigger satisfaction or dissatisfaction depends on the extent to which they are present. The ease of making an appointment with a primary care physician or a 5- to-10-minute wait time in the waiting room are examples of performance quality. If patients can get same-day appointments or wait only a couple of minutes, their satisfaction will increase.

Excitement quality goes beyond customers' expectations. It exceeds them in a meaningful way. The quality attributes are sometimes referred to as "delighters." They represent the extras or order winners described in Chapter 1 and always generate satisfaction because they are unexpected. For instance, an endodontist offering free patient drop-off after a procedure or a hospital offering free valet parking to ED patients would generate excitement quality.

With time, as shown by the arrow pointing down in Figure 4.3, delighters become wants, and wants become must haves. This is why healthcare organizations must systematically capture the VOC and identify patients' changing needs and wants. Although the principles of questionnaire design presented in Appendix 4.1 still apply, the format of questions and answer scale is specific in a Kano survey (see Box 4.1). Once the VOC has been translated into the VOP, organizations can track their ability to meet customers' requirements or wants. Improving the delivery of customers' wants should be pursued as long as the benefits outweigh the costs because more is better. Excitement factors can be expensive to deliver. However, even small improvements can yield substantial increases in satisfaction. As long as they are cost-effective, improvements on these factors should be pursued because they ultimately generate customer loyalty and recommendations to other, potential customers. As for basic needs, they must be met but not necessarily improved since they are unlikely to produce extra value to the customer. For those needs, more is not better.

BOX 4.1 QUESTION AND ANSWER FORMAT IN KANO SURVEY

Developing a Kano Survey

In a Kano survey, each feature should be evaluated with two questions, one positive (presence of functionality) and the other negative (absence of functionality). The answer categories must include the full spectrum from pleasure to avoidance of displeasure: I like it, I expect it, I am neutral, I can tolerate it, I dislike it. Multiple variations in wording exist. See the following example:

How do you feel if the hospital offers free valet parking to patients arriving at the ED?

- This would be very helpful to me.
- This is a basic requirement for me.
- This would not affect me.
- This would be a minor inconvenience.
- This would be a major problem for me.

How do you feel if no free valet parking is offered to patients arriving at the ED?

- This would be very helpful to me.
- This is a basic requirement for me.
- This would not affect me.
- This would be a minor inconvenience.
- This would be a major problem for me.

Once these questions are asked, an evaluation table needs to be developed to categorize the feature as attractive, performance, or must-be. More detailed coverage of the evaluation and analysis process can be found in *The Complete Guide to the Kano Model* (https://foldingburritos.com/blog/kano-model; Zacarias, 2015).

THE CRITICAL-TO-QUALITY TREE

Another useful tool to assist in the development of the HOQ is the **CTQ tree** (Figure 4.4). A CTQ tree can help generate important, objective performance requirements or CTQs from the VOC (Step 3). CTQs are thus observable and measurable characteristics of a process or its outputs whose specification limits (Chapter 8) must be met in order to satisfy the

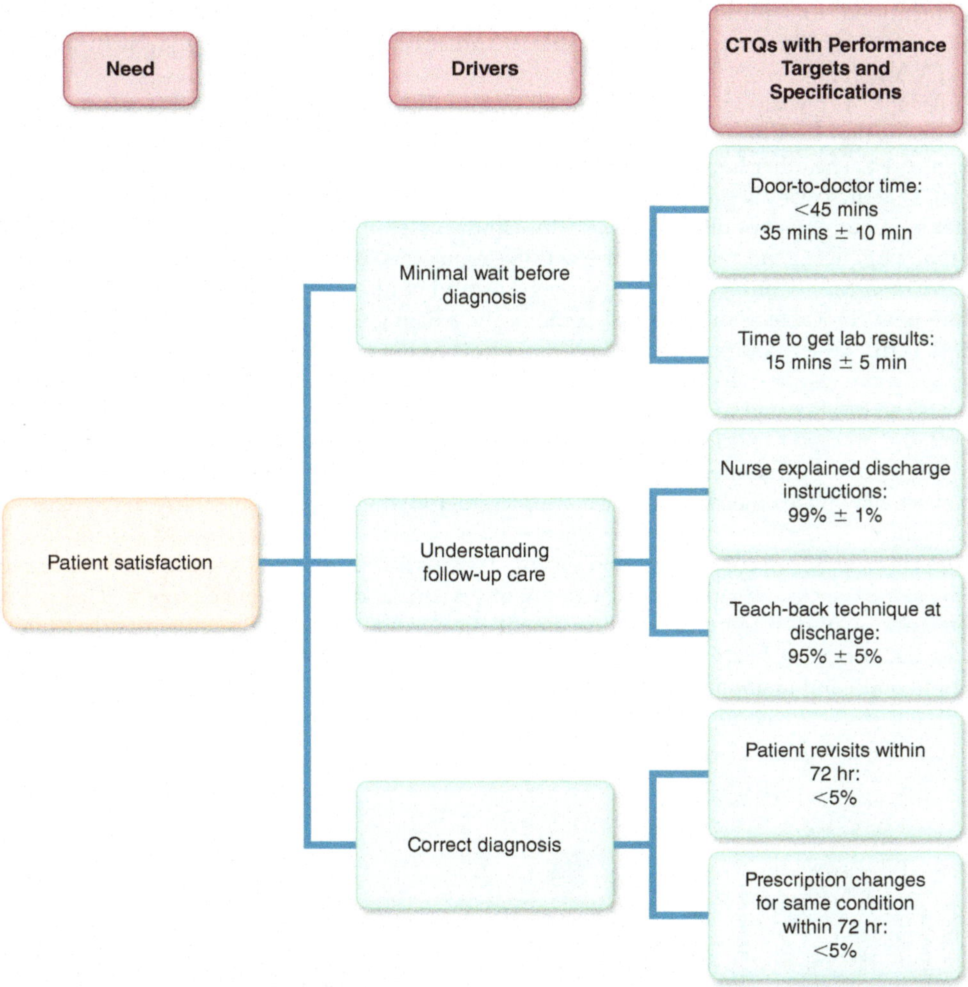

Steps	Explanation	Example
1. Define service characteristics from customers' perspective	Describe some feature of the service	Patients want minimal wait time before being seen by a doctor
2. Develop objective, quantitative measures, or indicators	Define how the product or service's characteristic can be translated into an observable,quantitative indicator	Door-to-doctor time
3. Develop targets	Specify the target value for the indicator	35 min
4. Establish specification limits	State how much variation from the target will be tolerated	± 10 min

FIGURE 4.4 Partial CTQ tree for BAMC.

Abbreviations: BAMC, Bright Angel Medical Center; CTQ, critical to quality.

customer. In order to make a CTQ tree, you articulate the need expressed in the VOC. In this case, the need is high patient satisfaction. You then determine the drivers that can affect performance outcomes. For example, in our HOQ (Figure 4.2), minimal wait, understanding follow-up care, and correct diagnosis are three patient requirements that are deemed important or very important, but BAMC lags behind the other competitors. In the next step, observable and measurable quality indicators are generated. If you integrate this process with the HOQ, the strength of the relationship between these indicators and the drivers is determined, and importance weights are computed. The strong indicators can then be used to specify performance targets (Step 7) and specification limits (DeLayne Stroud, 2010; MindTools, 2023).

To ensure a consistency of purpose at all levels of quality deployment, QFD relies on a series of matrices that look like interconnected houses (Figure 4.5). The first house is the *HOQ* shown in Figure 4.2. The other houses provide the structure to carry out the design changes proposed in the HOQ at increasingly greater levels of detail. Based on Figure 4.2, if BAMC decides to meet the customer requirement of minimal wait before initial assessment at the ED, it will need to decrease the time patients spend waiting in the waiting room and/or the exam room. The second house, *resource requirements*, analyzes which resources would be affected by such changes. We might have to hire new clinical staff or "free up" some of the existing resources by automating some activities. In turn, these resource changes become inputs to the next house, *process planning*. With new inputs, a more responsive process with fewer or simplified steps can be designed, and human resources can be allocated to patients more efficiently. However, the adoption of more streamlined, automated processes requires a fourth house, *quality plan*, where specific instructions for training, software updates, equipment maintenance, and process control can be developed. The succession of houses maximizes the chances for a seamless deployment of customer-driven changes in the organization.

QFD is an excellent communication system. It helps multidisciplinary groups to interact, focus on the same issues, and agree on measurement systems and performance targets. It can serve as a reference point during process improvement efforts and can be upgraded regularly (Russell & Taylor, 2023). Several healthcare organizations or departments have used or adapted the methodology to build and maintain a coherent quality system (Box 4.2).

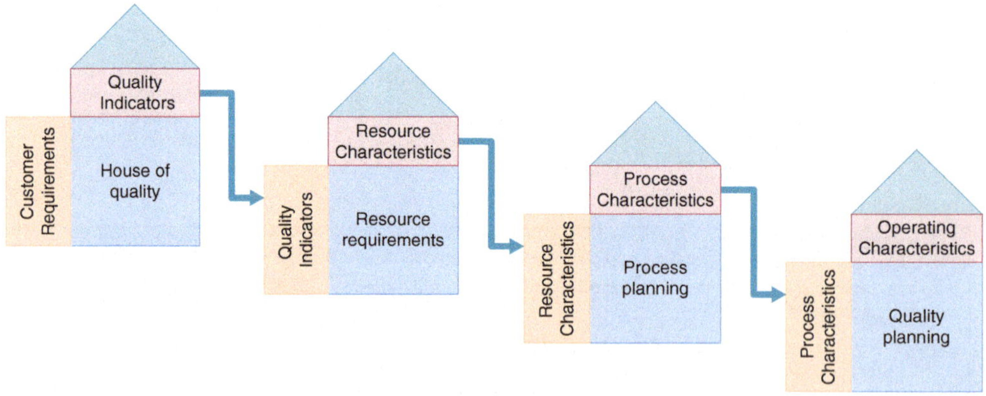

FIGURE 4.5 Connected HOQ.

Abbreviations HOQ, houses of quality.

Source: Russell, R. S., & Taylor, B. W. (2023). *Operations and supply chain management* (11th ed.). Wiley. Copyright © 2023, 2019, 2016, 2014, 2011, 2008, 2005.

BOX 4.2 QUALITY IN PRACTICE!

Quality Function Deployment to Improve Quality in Radiology Centers

QFD was used to develop a quantitative assessment framework for the improvement of services in radiology centers. The project involved the following steps (Gavahi et al., 2023):

1. The voice of patients—customers—was obtained via surveys, experts' opinions, and literature review to uncover their service expectations.
2. The voice of the experts—professors, hospital professionals, and radiologists—was obtained via observations and interviews to obtain stakeholders' required service elements: equipment, computer system, air conditioning, scheduling, staffing needs, and reporting (Note: These are not objective indicators!)
3. Patients' requirements were prioritized according to the total mean scores obtained from the surveys.
4. The relationships (trade-offs) between the service elements were determined.
5. The experts determined the relationship between patients' requirements and the service elements. A *subset* of the relationship matrix is shown in the following table.

			Voice of Experts: Service Elements						**Weight *(1–5)***
Voice of Patients: Customer Requirements		**Importance Rating**	**A**	**B**	**C**	**D**	**E**	**F**	
Tangibles	CR1	14	9	0	3	1	0	0	4.04
	CR3	20	0	0	9	3	0	9	3.40
Reliability	CR10	17	0	1	0	3	0	0	3.70
	CR11	2	0	9	0	1	0	0	4.70
Responsiveness	CR13	22	0	0	0	9	0	1	3.20
	CR14	8	0	0	1	0	0	0	4.54
Assurance	CR22	13	0	0	9	0	0	0	4.14
Empathy	CR23	12	0	0	1	0	0	0	4.28
	CR24	21	0	0	9	0	0	0	3.22
Importance weights			36.36	74.08	79.02	234.68	41.88	58.16	

A = hygiene and cleanliness; B = timetable of services; C = air conditioning; D = customer care; E = comfort of waiting room; F = scheduler's speed and knowledge.

6. Patients' satisfaction with their requirements was assessed.
7. The importance/satisfaction relationship was analyzed to target improvements.

The Delphi technique was used to identify and eliminate suggestions for improvements that closed the gap between importance and satisfaction.

BRIGHT ANGEL MEDICAL CENTER 4.2

"What's this HOQ diagram that I am hearing so much about?" asked Barbara as she walked into the ED conference room. Dr. Aoki had arrived a few minutes before and found Olina spreading some printed pages out on the table.

"Wow. Looks detailed," she said as she sat down next to the pair.

Olina started, "This helps us focus on the VOC. We can use our patient satisfaction surveys to determine the importance of several of these items to our patients."

"You mean the patient dissatisfaction surveys?" asked Dr. Aoki sarcastically.

(continued)

BRIGHT ANGEL MEDICAL CENTER 4.2 (*CONTINUED*)

"Very funny, Dr. Aoki," Olina continued. "We translate the patient requirements into process indicators using the critical-to-quality outputs. That allows us to track and trend improvements over time. We can't track all possible indicators, but this will allow us to evaluate various options and gauge trade-offs, taking effort and other factors into account."

"I love it!" said Barbara enthusiastically.

What is there to "love" in an HOQ?

THE VOICE OF THE CUSTOMER

The HOQ starts with the VOC. Let us expand on this important driver of quality deployment. For the following discussion, we continue to focus on the patient as the customer. How do we define our customers? By asking *who* they are and *what* they want.

The first question—who they are—can be answered with **demographics**, which is information about age, sex, income, education level, race, ethnicity, place of residence, and so on. It can also be answered with a group classification such as patient-provider-payer (see Chapter 3), veteran versus non-veteran status, and so on. These types of identifiers are basically external descriptions of an individual. They are often straightforward, and, when asked, customers can provide them easily because they are part of their administrative records.

The second question—what they want—is more intrusive because it deals with **psychographics**, which is information about people's psychological characteristics such as beliefs, attitudes, values, fears, preferences, needs, and wants. These are internal, personal descriptions of an individual. They are subjective and more difficult to capture, but they are extremely important for providers to consider. Patients, for example, care how providers interact with them and note when they are dismissed or are not taken seriously. As a result, physicians and other caregivers must enter the patient relationship in a mutually respectful way. This type of interaction forms the basis for "patient- and family-centered care" (PFCC; Institute for Patient- and Family-Centered Care, 2023). PFCC is characterized by a two-way partnership that values the opinions, beliefs, attitudes, and wishes of patients and their families as advisors. Some clinicians may be skeptical because they fear that they must spend more time (and lose money) listening to patients and their families. However, when PFCC is done well, the overall resources spent on a patient's care are usually less while the patient and family satisfaction with the experience is greatly enhanced (Box 4.3). Together, providers, patients, and families *co-create* value.

BOX 4.3 QUALITY IN PRACTICE!

Family Presence Expert Panel at Saskatchewan Health Authority

COVID-19 placed serious restrictions on family visitations to long-term care residents and acute care patients, causing loneliness, isolation, and loss of support. To address this problem, the Saskatchewan Health Authority (SHA) created the Family Presence Expert Panel (FPEP). The panel includes healthcare professionals, leaders, and resident and family partners. It created a policy that ensures that at least one family member or friend is part of the care team for each resident or patient. This approach is perfectly aligned with PFCC and makes family members active participants in providing care to their loved ones. In 2022, the FPEP was the recipient of the Institute for Patient- and Family-Centered Care's Partnership Award. The award recognizes innovative partnerships among patients, families, and healthcare professionals (SHA, 2022)

ON THE JOB! INTERVIEW VIDEO 4.1

Jami Momberger
Senior Director of Care Experience

Humanizing Healthcare
Importance of measuring patient experience
Patient-centered care
Talking less and listening more
Leading with empathy

1. Jami discusses the Hospital Consumer Assessment of Healthcare Providers and Systems (HCAHPS) survey that is utilized in hospitals to evaluate patient experience. What does this survey measure?
2. List some strategies that hospitals and health systems can deploy to improve their patient experience scores.
3. Jami shares a framework, "humanizing healthcare," to provide a better experience for patients. What are the four elements that her team uses to improve how patients experience care?

The interview is available online by visiting www.springerpub.com/courseconnect. See inside front cover and tear-out card for CourseConnect details.

DATA COLLECTION METHODS

Both qualitative and quantitative research data collection methods can be used to capture the VOC. The most common **qualitative research data collection methods** include observation, **focus group interviews**, and **unstructured** and **semistructured personal interviews**. Their purpose is to generate deep insights into a particular phenomenon through visual analysis or open-ended communication. They are especially useful for new issues or services that have never been examined before. One of their greatest advantages is flexibility in exploring issues and eliciting responses. For example, the interviewer can clarify or rephrase a question as needed, alter the sequence of the questions based on participants' answers, and probe for further information. On the other hand, these data collection methods tend to be expensive, require a skilled and unbiased interviewer/observer, and have low generalizability. A summary of each method's advantages and disadvantages is presented in Table 4.1.

TABLE 4.1 ADVANTAGES AND DISADVANTAGES OF THREE QUALITATIVE RESEARCH DATA COLLECTION METHODS

Method	Advantages	Disadvantages
Observation	• Low cost • Easy to perform	• Limited to observable behavior • Subjective and difficult interpretation of behavior • Limited generalizability
Focus group interview	• Rich insights • Small sample size • Dynamic brainstorming through multiperson interactions • Flexible	• Moderate to high cost • Skilled moderator is required • Limited generalizability • Potential for groupthink
Personal interviews	• Very rich insights • Very flexible	• High cost • Labor-intensive • Time-consuming • Skilled interviewer is required • Limited generalizability

Affinity Diagram

Because the data obtained through qualitative research data collection methods are textual or visual, their codification and summarization are difficult. One popular tool to organize and make sense of these data is the affinity diagram. Affinity diagrams encourage people to think creatively about new concepts and/or to organize large amounts of language data (ideas, opinions, problems, etc.) into logical groupings. They can thus be used to categorize and analyze participants' ideas in focus group interviews, as well as respondents' open-ended feedback in questionnaires. To develop an affinity diagram, a team should follow the given steps (American Society for Quality, 2024):

STEP 1: Generate ideas and write them down on separate sticky notes.

STEP 2: Display the notes on a wall, board, or table.

STEP 3: Sort ideas into related groups until all ideas have been placed into groups. Ungrouping and regrouping ideas may occur, and this is a normal part of the process.

STEP 4: For each group, develop a meaningful title that captures the relationship among all ideas in the group. If there is a relationship between two or more groups, place the groups under a "super group" title.

STEP 5: Draw the finished affinity diagram.

Figures 4.6 and 4.7 show Steps 1 and 5 in the creation of an affinity diagram of the reasons why patients may not take their medications as prescribed.

Whereas qualitative research methods focus on deep exploration, quantitative research methods seek support/disconfirmation of specific hypotheses about phenomena, information about customers' opinions, or knowledge about trends or patterns. **Quantitative research data collection methods** are typically structured, and therefore less flexible. They involve the review of existing records or reports (e.g., patients' blood pressure in electronic health records) or the administration of surveys with mostly close-ended questions via mail, phone interviews, or electronic media.

In healthcare, the **Consumer Assessment of Healthcare Providers and Systems (CAHPS)** and SERVQUAL are well-known, structured survey instruments to help you capture patients' experience. Some vendors also offer their proprietary instruments along with a gamut of survey administration and data analysis services (e.g., Press Ganey and Professional Research Consultants).

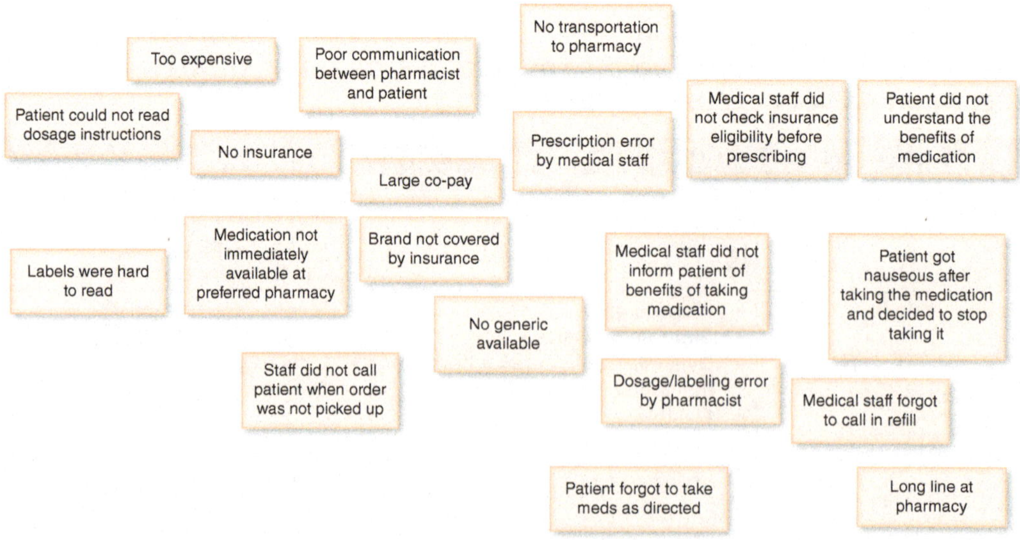

FIGURE 4.6 Idea generation.

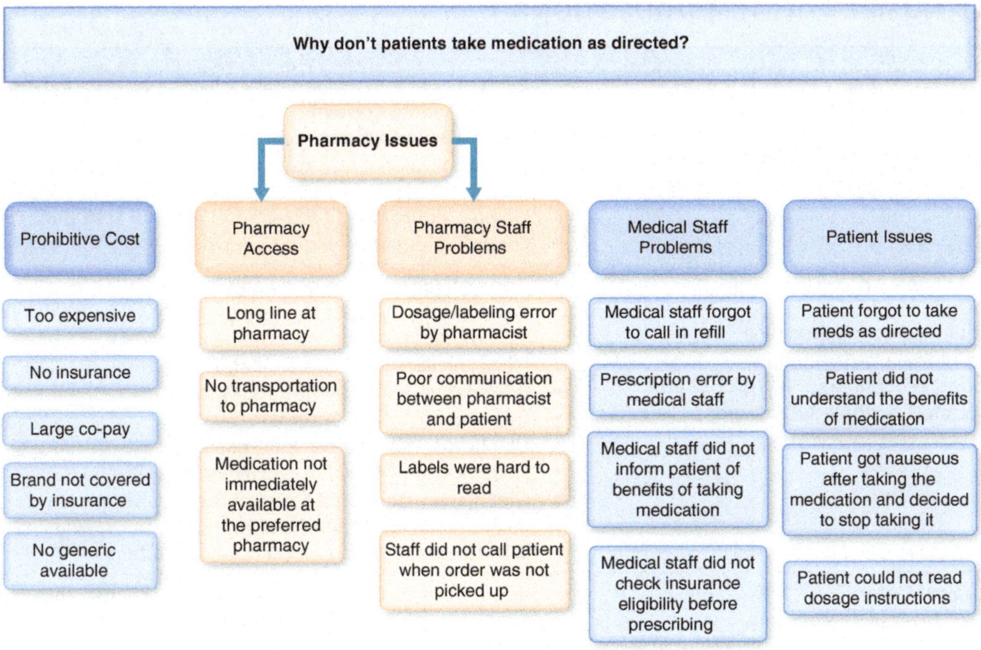

FIGURE 4.7 Affinity diagram.

CONSUMER ASSESSMENT OF HEALTHCARE PROVIDERS AND SYSTEMS SURVEY INSTRUMENT

In response to a lack of information regarding the quality of health plans from a consumer perspective, the Agency for Healthcare Research and Quality (AHRQ) introduced the CAHPS program in 1995. Several research organizations—known as the CAHPS Consortium—collaborated to develop and test standard instruments for enrollees to rate the quality of their plans. The purpose was to collect massive amounts of data and produce reports that health consumers could use in comparing and selecting plans against a predetermined set of criteria. Over the years, the program's scope was expanded to other health services provided in physicians' offices, hospitals, nursing homes, hospices, dialysis centers, behavioral health facilities, and patients' homes (AHRQ, 2023). The surveys are administered to random samples of adult patients; they are *not* limited to Medicare beneficiaries.

The perceived quality of care is a multidimensional construct. In other words, several conceptual elements make up its domain. Therefore, a survey instrument should measure all these elements to render a valid account of a patient's experience of care. The core quality elements measured in various CAHPS instruments are presented in Table 4.2. Supplemental measures, such as the Patient-Centered Medical Home (PCMH) item set, are available as well. The adult version of the PCMH item set complements the list of topics covered in the Clinician & Group Survey with questions about access, coordination, self-management support, and comprehensiveness of care.

As a member of the CAHPS Consortium, CMS collects Hospital Consumer Assessment of Healthcare Providers and Systems (HCAHPS) data from all hospitals serving Medicare recipients. After eliminating incomplete surveys and surveys from ineligible patients, it calculates the provider's **"top box" score** for each set of measures. The "top box" score is the percentage of a provider's patients who selected the most positive response to the HCAHPS survey items. For the **hospital value-based purchasing (VBP) program** (see Table 4.5, later in this chapter), CMS adjusts some of the scores for patient mix and survey mode and calculates a Patient Experience of Care Domain Score.

TABLE 4.2 SELECTED CAHPS SURVEYS WITH QUALITY MEASURES AND NUMBER OF ITEMS/QUESTIONS

Survey Instrument	Measures
Clinician & Group, Version 3.1 https://www.ahrq.gov/cahps/surveys-guidance/cg/about/survey-measures.html	• Getting timely appointments (3 items) • Providers' communication with patients (4 items) • Providers' use of information to coordinate patient care (3 items) • Helpful, courteous, and respectful office staff (2 items) • Overall rating of provider (1 item)
Hospitals—Adult (HCAHPS) https://www.hcahpsonline.org/globalassets/hcahps/updated-hcahps-survey/proposed-updated-hcahps-survey-.pdf	• Communication with nurses (3 items) • Communication with doctors (3 items) • Communication about medicines (2 items) • Responsiveness of hospital staff (2 items) • Information about symptoms (1 item) • Care coordination (3 items) • Discharge information (2 items) • Restfulness of hospital environment (3 items) • Cleanliness of hospital environment (1 item) • Overall hospital rating (1 item) • Willingness to recommend hospital (1 item)
Surgical Care https://www.ahrq.gov/cahps/surveys-guidance/surgical/about/survey-measures.html	• Information to help prepare for surgery (2 items) • Surgeon's communication before surgery (4 items) • Surgeon's attentiveness on day of surgery (2 items) • Information to help recover from surgery (4 items) • Surgeon's communication after surgery (4 items) • Helpful, courteous, and respectful staff at surgeon's office (2 items) • Overall rating of surgeon (1 item) • Communication with the anesthesiologist (3 items) • Overall rating of anesthesiologist (1 item)
Nursing Home (Family Member) https://www.ahrq.gov/cahps/surveys-guidance/nh/about/survey-measures.html	• Nurses/aides' kindness toward resident (5 items) • Help with eating, drinking, and toileting (3 items) • Information to and involvement of respondent (6 items) • Staffing, care of belongings, and cleanliness (7 items) • Overall rating of nursing home (1 item)
Home Health Care https://homehealthcahps.org/Portals/0/HHCAHPS_steps_calculate_composites.pdf?ver=2016-11-07-101103-157	• Care (4 items) • Communication between providers and patients (6 items) • Specific care issues (7 items) • Overall rating of care provided by the agency (1 item) • Willingness to recommend the agency (1 item)

Abbreviations: CAHPS, Consumer Assessment of Healthcare Providers and Systems; HCAHPS, Hospital Consumer Assessment of Healthcare Providers and Systems.

In 2015, CMS added the HCAHPS Star Ratings to the Hospital Compare website. The Star Ratings summarize survey responses for each HCAHPS set of measures and present these in a format that is easy for consumers to understand. A Summary Star Rating also appears on Hospital Compare. HCAHPS Star Ratings are updated quarterly.

Because of their significant role in public reporting in general and in the Medicare program in particular, CAHPS surveys are the standard adopted by most providers. However, capturing patient experience is not limited to the measures provided in these regulatory surveys (Box 4.4). Hence, other instruments may be used to complement CAHPS surveys.

BOX 4.4 QUALITY IN PRACTICE!

Using a Chatbot to Improve Bedside Manners

Less than 72 hours after the release of ChatGPT's free version, doctors were using it to express more compassion in their communication with patients. Empathy is a dimension of quality that patients highly value. This is especially true for those who are terminally ill and their families.

A doctor whose friend had advanced cancer asked ChatGPT to generate a script about the lack of effective treatments for her situation. ChatGPT offered the following words:

> *"I know this is a lot of information to process and that you may feel disappointed or frustrated by the lack of options . . . I wish there were more and better treatments . . . and I hope that in the future there will be."*

Wanting to help a patient suffering from a chronic inflammatory disease, another doctor asked ChatGPT to write a letter of appeal to an insurance company that had denied coverage for an expensive drug. The letter was so persuasive that the insurer decided to grant the request. Many providers agree that ChatGPT is by no means perfect, but it is certainly worth a try (Kolata, 2023).

SERVQUAL SURVEY INSTRUMENT

Originally developed in 1988 and revised in 1991, **SERVQUAL** is an instrument measuring the major facets of service quality (Parasuraman et al., 1991):

1. **Tangibles**: Physical facilities, professional appearance of personnel, equipment
2. **Reliability**: Ability to perform the promised service dependably and accurately
3. **Responsiveness**: Willingness to help customers and provide prompt service
4. **Assurance**: Knowledge and courtesy of employees and their ability to inspire trust and confidence
5. **Empathy**: Caring, individualized attention given to customers

As you can see, there are overlaps between CAHPS and SERVQUAL. Nevertheless, items in SERVQUAL can be used to collect supplemental data on patients' opinions regarding professionalism of employees, billing accuracy, knowledge of staff, and degree of personal attention. Just like CAHPS instruments, SERVQUAL uses multiple items/questions to tap one measure, and the ratings on the items are later aggregated for each measure. Adaptations of SERVQUAL for healthcare services are publicly available (e.g., Babakus & Mangold, 1992; Sharifi et al., 2021).

SERVQUAL was tested in multiple consumer samples before its publication and has been used extensively in academic research. Although the psychometric properties of the scale are not perfect, there is a general consensus that SERVQUAL provides a comprehensive measurement of consumers' perceptions of service quality.

In summary, patients may not be able to assess the clinical quality of the care they receive, but they can voice their opinion about their experience of care. These opinions or perceptions constitute the VOC (Figure 4.8), which is often captured in standardized questionnaires. The CAHPS and SERVQUAL instruments were developed by experts and were tested extensively. We recommend that you use them or adapt them whenever appropriate. However, you may have to develop a customized questionnaire for a specific purpose. For example, you may want to survey patients on a new, online scheduling system, or ask employees about their opinions on the existing patient referral system. In that case, the principles of questionnaire design presented in Appendix 4.1 will prove useful.

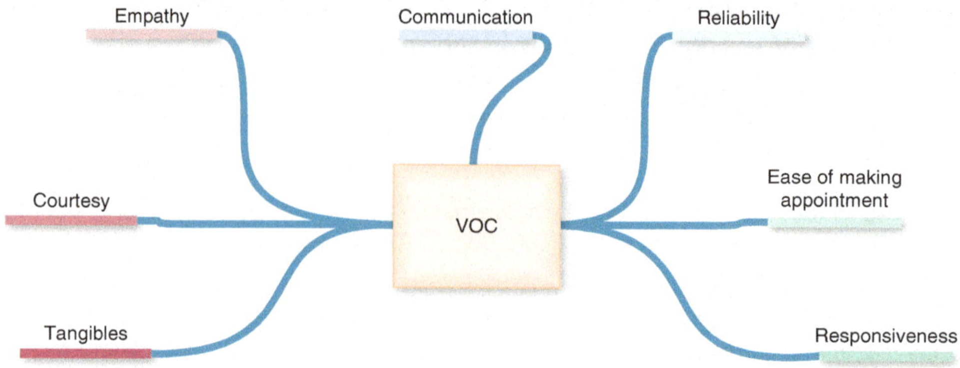

FIGURE 4.8 Dimensions of perceived healthcare quality.

Abbreviation: VOC, voice of the customer.

BRIGHT ANGEL MEDICAL CENTER 4.3

Barbara walked into the boardroom. The entire executive team was already seated, and Kimberly Mitchell welcomed her to their weekly meeting. "Let's jump right in. Mira gave me some advanced notice that you are bringing new ideas about capturing our patients' experience."

"Thank you for the invitation today," Barbara started. "We all know that our patients are not receiving the care nor experience that they deserve or that we strive to provide in our ED. The CAHPS scores for the ED indicate long waits, low respect from doctors, and poor understanding of follow-up care. We believe that when doctors are overwhelmed, they do not give patients the attention and compassion they need, which explains the perception of lack of respect. Yet, at other times, physicians are idle, but we are holding patients who are waiting to be admitted or even discharged. When that happens, you guessed it, patients are stuck in the waiting room for long periods of time. Many give up and leave. We believe that making the process more efficient and improving the layout will create a better flow, decrease wait times, and make it easier for providers to establish some rapport with their patients."

"What about follow-up care?" Michael Chen, the chief nursing officer, asked.

"That's what I really wanted to talk to you about," Barbara said. "This is an issue we'd like to understand better. We have worked with our quality team to develop custom surveys: one for our patients and one for our nurses. These will help us identify areas where we are deficient and take remedial actions."

Kimberly Mitchell crossed her arms, "Good idea. Better to know what is really going on than making assumptions."

Samantha Enapay, the chief human resources officer, joined in, saying, "I agree, and talking about what is really going on, Barbara and I have met several times to find ways to make the staff feel better supported and to incorporate nurses and techs into a leadership council that can inform the decisions we are making."

Barbara nodded, "I even asked your newest board member, Emily Bates, for suggestions. She recommended that I have annual, one-on-one conversations with every single employee and solicit their input."

The meeting continued for another 45 minutes with a robust discussion around costs for renovating the ED. All seemed satisfied when they left.

What do you think of Barbara's plan to survey patients and staff on follow-up care?

THE VOICE OF THE PROCESS

As per the HOQ, once customers' needs have been identified, they need to be translated into objective, process quality measures known as indicators. As you will recall, those are CTQs. Indicators are purely quantitative; they represent actual numbers: number of patient falls per 1,000 bed-days, average temperature in operating room (OR), percentage of times discharge instructions were not given in a particular month, and so on. They should also have clear and precise operational definitions to avoid confusion (e.g., number of urinary tract infections per 1,000 catheter days instead of number of infections). In his seminal article, "Evaluating the Quality of Medical Care," Donabedian (1966), a physician and the father of quality assurance in healthcare, argued that quality indicators should measure performance along the three stages of the healthcare delivery system: input, process, and output. Accordingly, his measurement model—often called the "Donabedian triad" (Figure 4.9)—features three types of quality indicators: structure, process, and outcomes. This is also the way we describe the dimensions of the VOP (Figure 4.10), although *theoretically*, it only focuses on process indicators. Our rationale is that a productive system involves the transformation—or processing—of inputs into outputs (see Chapter 1). Better inputs lead to better processes which, in turn, lead to better outputs; they are intrinsically linked.

STRUCTURE

Structural indicators measure the quality of what went into the care process (input). They include facilities, equipment, human resources, managerial talent, organizational culture, and so on. The metrics help answer questions such as: Is our staff trained well? Is the facility well maintained? Is the technology up-to-date and reliable?

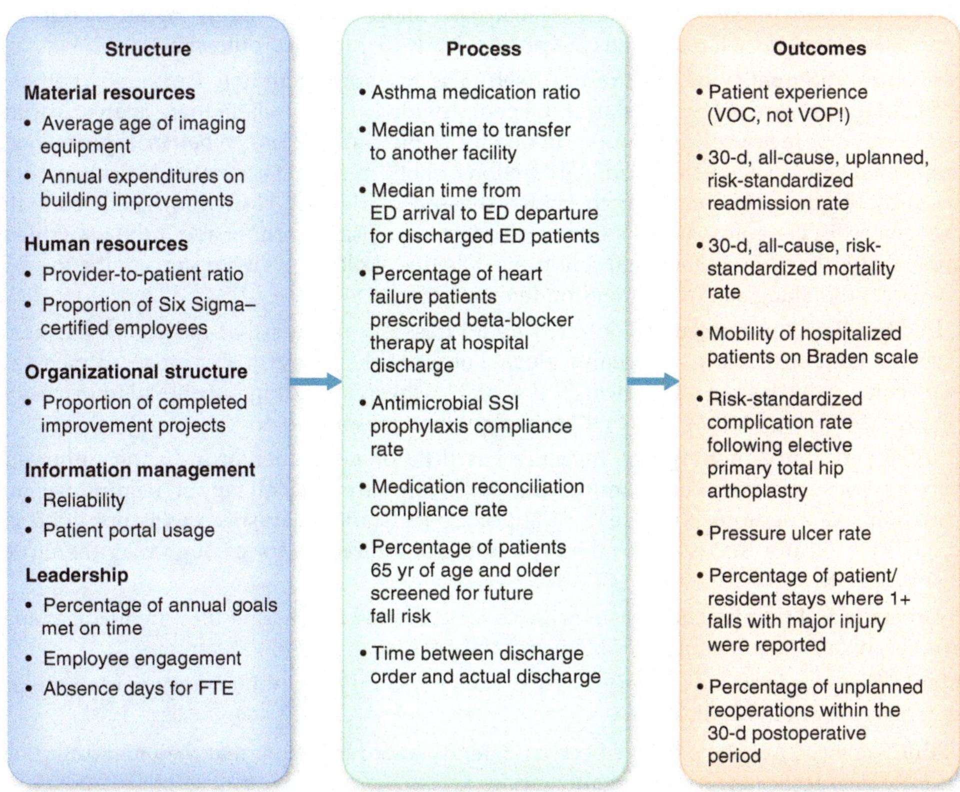

FIGURE 4.9 The Donabedian triad.

Abbreviations: FTE, full-time equivalent; SSI, surgical site infection; VOC, voice of the customer; VOP, voice of the process.

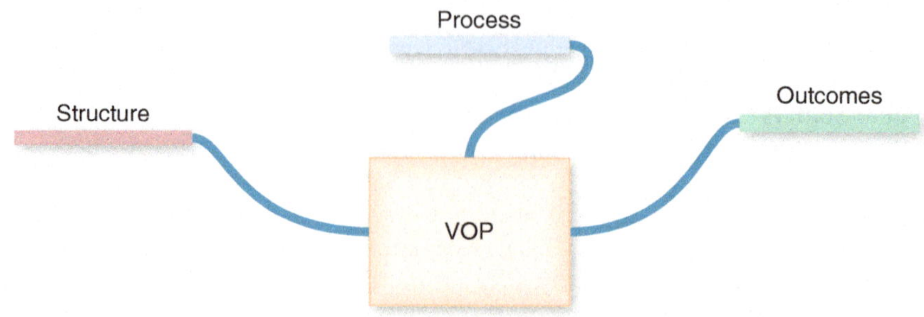

FIGURE 4.10 **Dimensions of objective healthcare quality.**

Abbreviation: VOP, voice of the process.

PROCESS

Process indicators measure the quality of how the process is being performed. Many of the process indicators reflect whether evidence-based procedures have been followed. Are patients with diabetes getting tested to see whether their glucose level is high? Are patients with heart disease being treated with the proper medication? Has a "safe surgery" checklist been used?

Ideally, high compliance with process measures should lead to better outcomes, but it is not always the case. Indeed, the value of the indicators themselves needs to be scrutinized and the following criteria met (AHRQ, 2018; Chassin et al., 2010):

1. **Evidence-based:** There is a strong evidence base (more than one study; mostly randomized controlled trials) showing that the care process leads to improved outcomes.
2. **Reflecting the quality of the process itself:** The measure accurately captures whether the evidence-based care process has, in fact, been provided. This is where there is great variation in the value of measures to capture the quality of the care process. Whether aspirin was administered after an acute myocardial infarction or not ("yes/no") accurately reflects the action taken by the nurse to comply with evidence-based guidelines. However, whether a patient was given discharge instructions or not (also "yes/no") says nothing about the way this was done, that is, handing out an instruction sheet versus explaining all the steps of the discharge process and making sure the patient understands them.
3. **Directly related to outcome:** The measure addresses a process that influences the desired outcome with only a few intervening steps. For example, properly administered medication that achieves the desired effect meets this goal. However, providing nutritional information to a patient believing that the effect will be weight loss does not.
4. **Proven safe:** Implementing the measure has little or no chance of inducing unintended, adverse consequences. For example, the practice of treating all upper respiratory infections with an antibiotic could lead to antibiotic-resistant organisms and is not good care. A quality indicator that captures the prescribing of antibiotics for a cough may therefore be inappropriate.
5. **Systematic and timely:** The measures are collected continuously, and they are made available in a timely fashion to enable corrective action if needed.
6. **Stable:** The measures are endorsed by the National Quality Forum and are not scheduled to be replaced by better indicators.
7. **Valid:** The measures should have been sufficiently tested to ensure that they measure process performance accurately across organizations.

If process indicators meet these seven criteria, they are more likely to lead to better clinical outcomes.

OUTCOMES

In principle, **outcome indicators** measure the end result of the care process (output). Did the patient improve? Did the patient's glucose level remain under control? Was the patient satisfied with the care experience? Note that patient experience is the VOC (not an objective indicator), but it is an outcome of structural variables and care processes. If the healthcare personnel are highly qualified, the facilities are state-of-the-art, and patients are treated with compassion, respect, and efficiency, then their satisfaction will likely increase.

Although outcomes are assumed to be unambiguous and easy to determine objectively, they may not always be a reflection of the quality of care provided at the process stage. For example, a patient may die (bad outcome) while given the best possible care. Unfortunately, the patient was terminally ill, and her condition had no chance for improvement, given the current state of science. Many providers have voiced their opposition to several outcome measures, such as mortality rate, because they question the method for risk adjustment (Box 4.5). It is important to remember that if poor quality measures are chosen, resources are wasted. However, when good quality measures are chosen, healthcare organizations can make significant advances in the quality of patient care, as will be shown in the next section.

THE VITAL FEW

The steady proliferation of indicators, both voluntary and mandatory, can be overwhelming to hospitals and health systems (Dunlap et al., 2016). Over the years, several bodies, including insurers, government agencies, and international healthcare organizations, have proposed "core sets" of measures for performance tracking and reporting (WHO Working Group, 2020).

Since 2011, the National Quality Forum's Measure Applications Partnership (MAP) has advised the Department of Health & Human Services (HHS) on the selection of appropriate health quality

BOX 4.5 FAQs

Many countries use in-hospital mortality as an outcome measure of healthcare quality. Do you think it is a good measure? Why or why not?

Linking hospital mortality with quality presumes that death represents a failure and does not take into account that patients may come to the hospital for their end-of-life care. Thus, hospitals that have a higher number of terminally ill patients (higher risk) would look like they have poorer care.

Because outcome measures require adjusting for the severity of underlying medical problems, the way these measures are "adjusted" can change the outcome significantly. Some hospitals with better mortality ratios according to one method may show worse mortality using another method (Gattellari et al., 2019; Tabbutt et al., 2019).

measures for federal programs. In 2014, it created groups of "high impact" measures that could be used for public reporting, performance-based payments, and identification of areas needing improvement. These groups promoted the use of the same measures for multiple purposes and across different external entities, thereby alleviating the measurement burden for the provider (National Quality Forum, 2014). In 2017, HHS reaffirmed the need to reduce data collection and identify top priorities for quality measurement and management. In addition, it urged shifting the emphasis away from process measures toward outcome measures. Accordingly, it launched the Meaningful Measures initiative for CMS. This interdisciplinary work covered the following eight priorities (CMS.gov, 2023):

1. Deliver patient-centered care.
2. Make care safer by reducing preventable harm and building a safety culture.
3. Promote effective prevention and treatment of chronic disease and its complications.
4. Provide seamless care coordination with optimal interoperability and smooth transitions of care.
5. Promote equity in care quality so that everyone can attain optimal health.
6. Make care affordable and efficient.
7. Emphasize wellness and prevention in public health.
8. Promote screening and treatment for mental health and substance abuse.

MAP supports the Meaningful Measures initiative. Each year, it reviews the new measures under consideration by CMS and provides feedback to HHS.

USE OF QUALITY MEASURES

Quality metrics are useful indicators of a healthcare system's health that give leverage to government and regulatory entities, commercial payers, patients, and the care providers themselves.

THE OVERALL HOSPITAL QUALITY STAR RATING

In addition to the star rating for HCAHPS, Care Compare provides an **overall hospital quality star rating** for eligible hospitals. The overall rating is a single, aggregate measure of quality combining patient experience, process, and outcomes measures. In other words, it includes both subjective and objective measures. The five measure groups and their respective weights in determining the hospital overall rating are shown in Table 4.3. The overall score for a hospital is the weighted average of its scores in each group (CMS, 2024).

What happens if a hospital does not report measures in one or more groups? In that case, the group is considered missing, and the weight of the missing group is redistributed across the other groups. Although the majority of hospitals get a 3- or 4-star rating, only 8% of those reporting achieve the top, 5-star score (Table 4.4; CMS, 2024).

TABLE 4.3 MEASURE GROUPS AND WEIGHTS FOR OVERALL HOSPITAL QUALITY STAR RATING

Type of Measure	Measure Group	Weight (%)
VOC	Patient experience	22
Process	Safety of care	22
	Timely and effective care	12
Outcomes	Readmission	22
	Mortality	22

Abbreviation: VOC, voice of the customer.

TABLE 4.4 NATIONAL DISTRIBUTION OF OVERALL HOSPITAL QUALITY STAR RATINGS (JULY 2024 RESULTS)

Overall Rating	Number of Hospitals (N = 4,658, %)
*	277 (5.9)
**	595 (12.8)
***	828 (17.8)
****	766 (16.4)
*****	381 (8.2)
N/A	1,811 (38.9)

HOSPITAL VALUE-BASED PURCHASING PROGRAM

The VBP program under CMS rewards acute care hospitals for the quality and efficiency of care provided in the inpatient hospital setting (CMS.gov, 2024). The way the program works is that 2% of the payments for all of the participating hospitals are withheld and redistributed to the hospitals based on their performance on a set of quality and cost measures in four domains: clinical outcomes, person and community engagement, safety, and efficiency and cost reduction. The measures and the weights reflecting the importance of each domain in determining performance are shown in Table 4.5. By tying payments to health outcomes, patient experience, safety, and efficiency (incentive payments for performance achievements or performance improvements; penalties for poor performance), VBP attempts to unify the patients', providers', administrators', and payers' interests. As the government agency that pays for healthcare services for all Medicare or Medicaid recipients, CMS has huge power over the U.S. healthcare enterprise, and it is using this power to transform care.

BRIGHT ANGEL MEDICAL CENTER 4.4

Barbara opened her ED huddle with a brief summary of the problems encountered the previous week. "Last Tuesday, we had a patient who almost died while in the waiting room. That should never happen again. Patients come here to receive rapid and high-quality care. The most important thing to them is that we get their diagnosis and treatment right. But wait times are also important. Therefore, I asked our IT people to create an electronic wallboard with important indicators in the ED. I thought about wait times, number of patients waiting, left-without-being-seen (LWBS), and discharge status. Those would be refreshed throughout the day."

One of the nurse managers approved, "This would help visualize what is going on in the ED and help us be more responsive."

Barbara nodded, "That's the intent. However, I just suggested these indicators. Put some thought into what you want to track at all times. We'll discuss that during our next huddle. Please bring your best thinking."

In your opinion, what indicators should be displayed on the ED wallboard?

LEAPFROG

The Leapfrog group is a nonprofit organization founded in 2000 by large employers aiming to improve the quality, safety, and affordability of healthcare in the United States. The unavailability of data on healthcare quality along with the prevalence of preventable medical errors revealed in the Institute of Medicine (IOM; 1999) report, *To Err Is Human*, motivated the group to make transparency the driving force for improvement. With access to information, people could make decisions

TABLE 4.5 VBP: QUALITY DOMAIN WEIGHTS FY 2025

Domain	FY 2025 Weight (%)
Clinical Outcomes • Acute myocardial infarction 30-d mortality • Coronary artery bypass graft surgery 30-d mortality • COPD 30-d mortality rate • Heart failure 30-d mortality rate • Pneumonia 30-d mortality • Total hip arthroplasty/Total knee arthroplasty complication rate	25
Person and Community Engagement • Communication with nurses • Communication with doctors • Responsiveness of hospital staff • Communication about medicines • Hospital cleanliness and quietness • Discharge information • Care transition • Overall rating of hospital	25

Safety
• Catheter-associated urinary tract infection
• Central line-associated bloodstream infection
• *Clostridium difficile* infection
• Methicillin-resistant *Staphylococcus aureus*
• Surgical site infection
  • Colon surgery
  • Abdominal hysterectomy
• Severe sepsis and septic shock: management bundle
	25

Efficiency and Cost Reduction • Medicare spending per beneficiary	25

Abbreviations: COPD, chronic obstructive pulmonary disease; FY, fiscal year; VBP, value-based purchasing.

about healthcare, and employers could reward top-performing providers and thus promote high-value care. Today, its programs include (The Leapfrog Group, 2024):

- The Leapfrog Hospital Survey, which evaluates safety, quality, and efficiency. Participation is voluntary, and the performance results are published on the Leapfrog website.
- The Leapfrog Hospital Safety Grade, which evaluates around 3,000 hospitals on safety performance and assigns a consumer-friendly letter grade.
- The Leapfrog VBP Program, which assists health plans, self-insured employers, and third-party administrators in identifying high-value hospitals. A VBP value score is generated from the Hospital Survey results. This score can be used to rank hospitals and establish benchmarks for financial rewards and incentives.
- The Leapfrog Ambulatory Surgery Center Survey, which enables ambulatory surgery centers to voluntarily submit their answers to questions on facilities, staff, procedure volume, safety, and patient experience.

As you can see, there is much overlap between the CMS and The Leapfrog Group programs. In fact, many of the measures used in the Leapfrog Hospital Survey are the same as those used by CMS, the Centers for Disease Control and Prevention, and The Joint Commission.

Besides reporting, indicators can also be used to gauge and track specific improvement areas (Box 4.6). Benchmarking, the balanced scorecard, and dashboards fulfill that purpose.

BENCHMARKING

Although it is tempting to select indicators that showcase the areas in which you excel—the *feel-good* factor—it is much more productive to track indicators that highlight your weaknesses so that you can focus on improvements in areas critical to your competitiveness. **Benchmarking** is a useful

BOX 4.6 QUALITY IN PRACTICE!

The National Surgical Quality Improvement Program Uses Measures to Improve Surgical Care

In 2004, the American College of Surgeons (ACS) extended the National Surgical Quality Improvement Program (NSQIP) a quality program first developed in the Veterans Administration Hospitals, to private sector healthcare institutions. The program was "the first nationally validated, risk-adjusted, outcomes-based program to measure and improve the quality of surgical care." In each hospital, pre- and postoperative data are collected on a random sample of patients' charts. Data are entered into a national database so that other hospitals can view the information and compare their outcomes with those of top-performing hospitals. Conference calls between surgeons provide a forum to learn from others and adopt best practices. Today, more than 600 hospitals in the United States and 50 outside the country participate in the program. The ACS NSQIP program received the 2014 John M. Eisenberg Patient Safety and Quality Award in the category of Innovation in Patient Safety and Quality (ACS, 2023).

tool to help you identify opportunities for improvement. Benchmarking involves comparing your organization's performance to the best organization's performance in a particular industry or a particular process in order to identify and follow best practices. The key word is "best." You are not simply gauging your performance against your competitors (i.e., competitive analysis); rather, you are evaluating yourself against the top performer in a given field. Similarly, a benchmark is not an aggregate performance target derived from averaging indicator values for multiple organizations. On the contrary, a **benchmark** is the score achieved by one organization: the leader. Indicators for which the difference between the score set by the leader and your own tends to be large are natural candidates for selection, as long as they are aligned with your strategic goals.

A logical tool to aid in the selection of improvement-focused indicators is the HOQ discussed earlier (Figure 4.2). The indicators most strongly related to customer requirements certainly demand the provider's full attention. In the BAMC example, this would include door-to-doc time, time spent with physician, time between admit decision and departure from ED, and return visits for the same condition within 72 hours. All of them have higher importance weights.

BALANCED SCORECARD

In order to assess whether the organization is on track to meet its strategic objectives, it must have an effective performance measurement system. The **balanced scorecard** displays a balanced view of organizational performance. In their seminal article on the balanced scorecard, Kaplan and Norton (1992, p. 72) gave a perfect analogy: "The balanced scorecard is like the dials in an airplane cockpit: it gives managers complex information at a glance." It allows for monitoring of different performance metrics often called **key performance indicators (KPIs)** simultaneously from four different angles: the organization's ability to (1) create value for its customers, (2) manage its internal processes to meet customers' expectations, (3) innovate and improve, and (4) generate financial growth and strength (Kaplan & Norton, 1992, 1996). Note that the balanced scorecard reflects the collaboration of all functional areas on overall performance. For example, creating value for customers requires Marketing's capture of the VOC. Likewise, Human Resources (HR) promotes a culture of innovation and improvement through employee selection, training, and development. Operations (and therefore quality) relies on Marketing's and HR's contributions to design, manage, and control the processes that enable the creation of value and eventually lead to financial performance (Figure 4.11). The scorecard brings people together to understand what is strategically important and, therefore, connects the business strategy with the functional strategies.

The balanced scorecard has evolved over the past few decades and has seen significant adoption within the healthcare industry. At a minimum, it is used as a monitoring system to track progress and watch areas that need improvement. In its fullest form, it is a strategy management tool used for mapping functional activities and resources to strategic objectives focused on value creation (Kaplan & Norton, 2008).

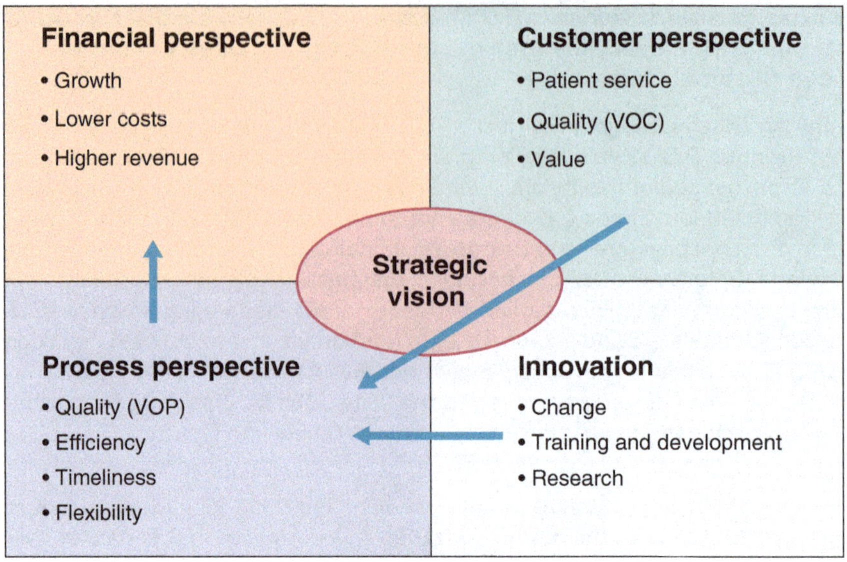

FIGURE 4.11 Balanced scorecard with synergistic effects.

Abbreviations: VOC, voice of the customer; VOP, voice of the process.

DASHBOARDS

A **dashboard** is a visual tool that also tracks KPIs over time. Dashboards cascade down from strategic to operational performance to maintain a consistent and unified strategy throughout the organization (Gartner & Lemaire, 2022).

1. **Strategic dashboards** monitor the achievement of strategic objectives in each functional area (e.g., in Operations, readmission rates and patient satisfaction for *quality*; average cost per discharge for *cost*). They emphasize performance management and the actions necessary to accomplish long-term goals through coordination and collaboration. Executives review the KPIs at monthly meetings.
2. **Tactical dashboards** track specific departmental measures and processes (e.g., readmission rates for thoracic surgery, wait times in preoperative holding areas, average cost per discharge in the ED). They focus heavily on analysis and enable users to search for the root causes of alert situations (e.g., factors contributing to high wait times in preoperative holding areas). KPI values on tactical dashboards are usually updated daily or weekly (Karami et al., 2013).
3. **Operational dashboards** track real-time data in specific processes (e.g., lab turnaround time, current ED occupancy, times from arrival to discharge in ED). They emphasize monitoring and signal alerts for quick intervention.

There are hundreds of measurements that determine your car's functioning and performance. Nevertheless, only a few critical gauges are displayed: speedometer, tachometer, fuel, temperature, and oil pressure. The same is true for a dashboard: It only displays the "vital few" measurements that are the strongest indicators of performance.

We focused on the organizational, strategic quality dashboard (Table 4.6) and cascaded it down to the tactical (Table 4.7) and operational (Table 4.8) levels. The quality dashboard in Table 4.6 displays several quality indicators in the process, outcomes, and patient experience areas at the organizational level. Some of the indicators in Table 4.6 (e.g., hand hygiene compliance rate, mortality ratio, readmission rate, understanding care when leaving the hospital) are also tracked at the ED level (Table 4.7). Finally, the indicators that are collected and tracked in real time are presented in Table 4.8 in a tabular format. We used the Tableau software to generate the wallboard shown in Figure 4.12. This powerful software helps create highly interactive dashboards, but you can also use Microsoft Excel to develop interactive dashboards (see Quality Dashboard data set in the online student resources). As you can see, BAMC's performance is dismal: a sea of red!

TABLE 4.6 STRATEGIC QUALITY DASHBOARD AT BAMC

Measures	FYTD Actual	FY Target	Jan	Feb	Mar	Apr	May	Jun	Jul	Aug	Sep	Oct	Nov
Process													
Heart failure patients prescribed beta-blocker therapy at discharge (%)	80.3	>90	91	93	89	87	80	77	74	73	70	79	70
Antimicrobial SSI prophylaxis compliance rate (%)	83.6	>95	92	96	72	80	82	84	80	83	80	82	89
Time between discharge order and actual discharge (hours)	7.7	<4	12	10	9.2	8.2	8	7.6	6	5	7	4	8
Hand hygiene compliance rate (%)	88.6	>95	95	74	82	76	86	90	92	95	97	98	90
Travel nurses FTEs	61.8	<60	63.2	64.2	66.3	61.2	59.3	59.7	60	61.2	61.8	60.8	62.1
Outcomes													
# of CLABSI	13	0	1	1	2	2	0	0	0	1	1	2	3
# of CAUTIs	9	0	0	1	1	0	1	0	2	1	1	0	2
# of VAPs	5	0	0	2	0	1	1	0	0	0	0	0	1
# of HACs	22	0	2	3	3	0	3	3	2	0	2	3	1
Fall with injury rate (per 1,000 patient days)	8	<6	12	9	10	11	8	7	8	6	5	7	5
ALOS (days)	4.2	<3.8	4.6	4.5	4.3	4.4	4.5	4.2	3.8	3.5	4	4.3	4.2
Mortality ratio—All cause (O/E)	1.1	<1	1	0.9	0.9	1.1	1.1	1.1	1.2	1.1	1.2	1.2	0.9
All-cause, 30-d readmission rate (%)	11.3	<8	9	10	14	12	13	10	15	8	9	11	13
Heart failure, 30-d readmission rate (%)	15.8	<12	20	20	18	15	18	14	16	12	17	11	13
Patient Experience													
Overall (% top box)	80.3	>80	79.4	81.6	82.7	79.8	82.2	78.4	81.9	80	78.2	79.7	79.2
Doctors listening carefully (% top box)	46	>60	38	34	30	36	45	55	60	45	50	55	58
Courtesy and respect from doctors (% top box)	54.8	>60	40	42	52	50	56	62	58	65	62	57	59
Nurses listening carefully (% top box)	58.5	>60	48	50	58	60	62	60	66	62	59	61	58
Courtesy and respect from nurses (% top box)	57.5	>60	45	48	61	60	60	59	63	62	57	61	57
Understanding care when leaving hospital (% top box)	76.9	>85	55	56	83	81	79	80	80	86	82	83	81

Abbreviations: ALOS, average length of stay; BAMC, Bright Angel Medical Center; CAUTI, catheter-associated urinary tract infection; CLABSI, central line-associated bloodstream infection; FYTD, fiscal year to date; HAC, hospital-acquired condition; FTE, full-time equivalent; SSI, surgical site infection; VAP, ventilator-associated pneumonia.

TABLE 4.7 TACTICAL QUALITY DASHBOARD AT BAMC'S ED

Measures	FYTD Actual	FY Target	Jan	Feb	Mar	Apr	May	Jun	Jul	Aug	Sep	Oct	Nov
Process													
t-PA infusion rate for stroke, when indicated (%)	88	>95	78	80	84	86	92	88	96	97	90	88	89
Door-to-doc time (min)	102.7	<45	75	80	81	94	95	100	112	110	120	128	135
Door-to-balloon time for STEMI (min)	99	<90	120	90	90	89	96	104	102	103	100	97	98
Time between discharge order and actual discharge (min)	25.5	<10	10	9	28	26	20	21	45	42	22	27	31
CT scan use for pediatric patients with abdominal pain (%)	63.4	<30	80	84	66	64	62	40	72	51	61	62	55
Hand hygiene compliance rate (%)	87.4	>95	97	96	87	76	86	90	95	82	88	84	80
Chart closure (% in 24 hr)	87.7	>95	95	89	84	82	86	88	90	96	94	81	80
Travel nurses FTEs	21.9	<20	18.3	19.7	21.2	21.3	22.2	22.2	22.4	25.1	22.6	23.2	22.4
Outcomes													
Mortality ratio—All cause (O/E)	0.99	<1	0.9	0.8	0.9	1.1	1.1	0.9	1.1	1.1	1.2	0.9	0.9
All-cause, 72-hr return to ED (%)	7.5	<5	10	12	7	6	8	5	4	4	7	8	11
Average time from ED arrival to ED departure for discharged patients (min)	281.1	<150	155	185	257	265	285	275	285	330	325	345	385
Average time from ED arrival to ED departure for admitted patients (min)	339.7	<200	232	255	285	330	325	385	390	382	353	375	425
LWBS (% of arrivals)	4.2	<2	2.2	2.3	2.6	3	3.6	3.7	4.1	6	5.5	6.2	6.4
Patient Experience													
Overall (% top box)	80.1	>80	80.1	79.1	79.4	81.6	75.4	79.8	82.2	78.4	82.9	81	80.9
Doctors listening carefully (% top box)	42.1	>60	36	40	30	42	57	44	42	41	46	36	49
Courtesy and respect from doctors (% top box)	55	>60	50	60	67	55	60	44	48	54	58	50	59
Nurses listening carefully (% top box)	53.9	>60	65	67	56	50	51	50	55	59	47	44	49
Courtesy and respect from nurses (% top box)	57.7	>60	52	60	61	67	62	60	65	57	52	48	51
Understanding care when leaving hospital (% top box)	73.5	>85	86	85	80	68	70	71	76	78	63	62	70

Abbreviations: BAMC, Bright Angel Medical Center; FTE, full-time equivalent; FYTD, fiscal year to date; LWBS, left-without-being-seen; STEMI, ST-segment elevation myocardial infarction.

TABLE 4.8 OPERATIONAL QUALITY DASHBOARD ED—DECEMBER 1, 2024

Measures	Target	8:00	9:00	10:00	11:00	12:00	13:00	14:00	15:00	16:00	17:00	18:00	19:00	20:00
Number of patients waiting in waiting room	<10	12	14	11	18	20	21	18	20	22	26	27	25	25
ED LOS (min)	<180	140	145	150	162	180	205	252	261	280	300	310	340	360
Room-to-doc time <20 min (%)	>90	91	92	86	82	87	78	72	64	79	83	68	51	58
Average wait time in waiting room (min)	<50	58	62	74	61	76	68	65	81	79	125	140	135	168

Abbreviations: LOS, length of stay.

ED Patient Flow

Treated within 4 hr: 32% **Patients waiting now: 19%** **Boarded: 6%**

Discharge status

Patient	Time waiting for discharge
Sulaiman, H	22
Gounder, L.	10
Shriver, P.	5
Lowell, M.	25
McMillan, T.	30
Li, W.	1
Sun, W.	8
Russo, G.	12

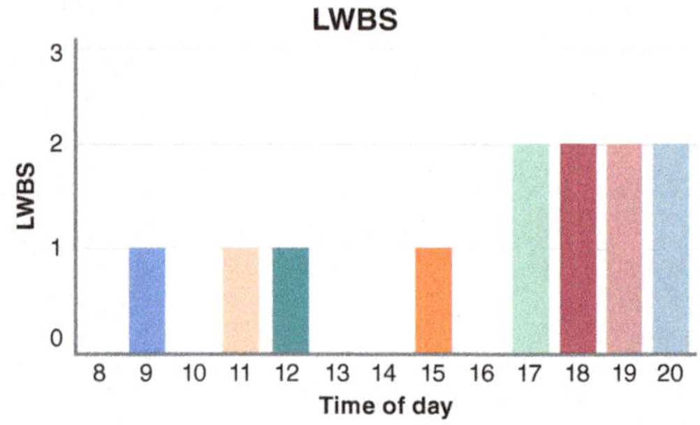

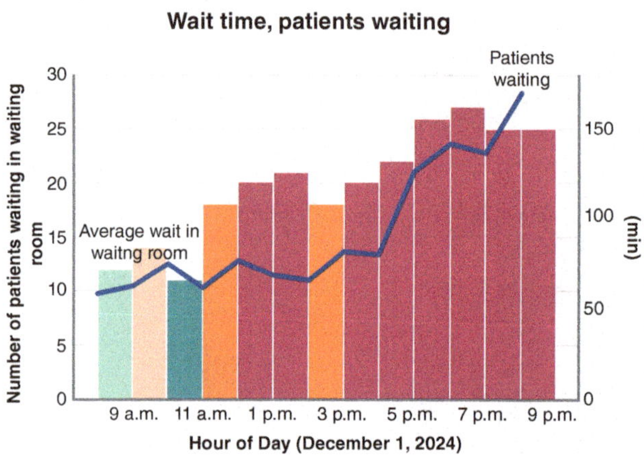

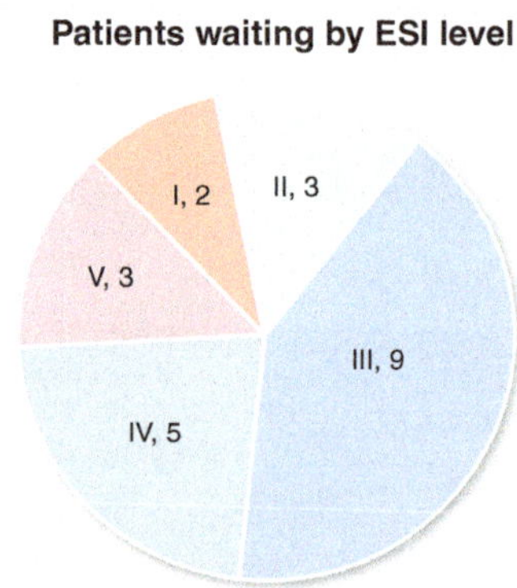

FIGURE 4.12 Wall board ED—December 1, 2024.

Abbreviations: ESI, Emergency Severity Index; LWBS, left-without-being-seen.

The idea behind tracking quality performance with dashboards is to identify weaknesses and performance shifts quickly and take remedial action before the situation becomes a crisis. Once a dashboard signals a problem area, several quality tools can be used to examine the problem, identify its roots, prioritize them, and therefore set the stage for improvement.

BUILDING THE A3 REPORT

The A3 report was introduced in Chapter 2. As the BAMC team advances through the various stages of the project, we will populate this document. So far, the team has described the problem and made a case for action. Figure 4.13 displays the current progress.

Prepared by Adeleke Mensah **ED Throughput** **December 1, 2024**

Background

Low patient satisfaction scores and high LWBS. ALOS in the ED is over 6 hr. Average wait time in early evening exceeds 2 hr. Delays to get x-rays and lab results. High readmission rates within 72 hr. Boarding issues. Poor patient experience with providers.

FIGURE 4.13 Problem background on A3 report.

Abbreviations: ALOS, average length of stay; LWBS, left-without-being-seen.

ETHICAL SCENARIO 4.1

Opioid Misuse and Abuse

Opioid misuse and abuse are a national crisis in the United States. In the late 1990s, the American Pain Society advocated to have pain categorized as the fifth vital sign in response to perceived lack of adequate pain recognition and treatment. A decade later, questions about adequate pain control were embedded in patient satisfaction surveys. These measures, combined with aggressive marketing campaigns launched by a few pharmaceutical companies, contributed to the explosion in opioid prescriptions and subsequent consumption by the American public. Physicians, particularly in the ED, are faced with the dilemma of satisfying patients versus following best practices. Doctors can feel pressure related to satisfaction surveys and the fear of being "penalized" by patients who are asking for opioids without appropriate indications.

If you were an emergency physician, how would you reconcile best practice and patient satisfaction?

SUMMARY

In this chapter, you learned that the customers of a process define the meaning of quality. This is the VOC. The VOC reflects opinions and perceptions regarding the service provided. The HOQ helps ensure that the VOC remains heard by providing a framework that "translates" customer requirements into process characteristics or quality indicators, that is, the VOP (Figure 4.14). As opposed to the VOC, which reflects opinions and perceptions, the VOP is a set of objective measures or indicators capturing the quality of the inputs (structure), processes, and outputs (outcomes) of healthcare delivery. Both subjective and objective quality measures are used for external reporting: Overall Hospital Quality Star Rating, VBP program, Leapfrog, and so on. They also play an important role in targeting and tracking improvement areas: benchmarking, balanced scorecard, and dashboards.

CERTIFICATION TIPS

Just like in this book, the VOC is covered in the *Define* phase of the certification exam. The HOQ is labeled as "the QFD matrix" because the terms "QFD" and "HOQ" are viewed as interchangeable. We only covered CTQ in this chapter, but certification materials also refer to CTX (X = quality, cost,

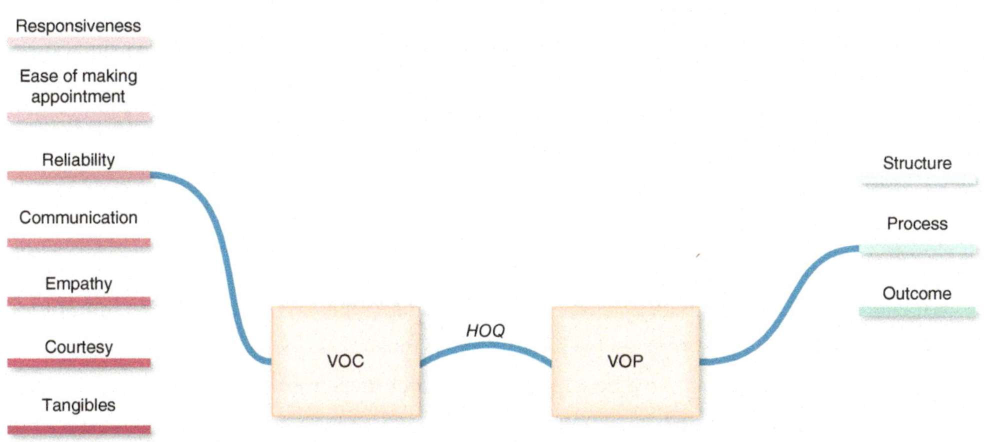

FIGURE 4.14 Mind map of translation of VOC into VOP.

Abbreviations: VOC, voice of the customer. VOP, voice of the process.

safety, etc.). Because the general American Society for Quality (ASQ) certification does not focus on healthcare specifically, there is no discussion of the types of indicators listed in the Donabedian triad. For certification purposes, indicators become more relevant at the Measure and Analyze phases. In other words, capturing the VOC via surveys and focus group interviews and translating it into product/service design specifications—VOP in this chapter—is what you need to know for certification. You are required to know and *apply* (when and how to use) these concepts.

ASQ also distinguishes between technical and competitive benchmarking and covers the benchmarking procedure: https://asq.org/quality-resources/benchmarking. You need to *understand* these concepts.

KEY TERMS

Quality
Excellent quality
House of quality (HOQ)
Quality function deployment (QFD)
Voice of the customer (VOC)
Voice of the process (VOP)
Kano model
Quality indicators
Critical to quality (CTQ)
CTQ tree
Demographics
Psychographics
Qualitative research data collection methods
Focus group interview
Unstructured personal interview
Semistructured personal interview
Quantitative research data collection methods
Consumer Assessment of Healthcare Providers and Systems (CAHPS)
Top box score
SERVQUAL
Tangibles
Reliability
Responsiveness
Assurance
Empathy
Structural indicators
Process indicators
Outcome indicators
Overall hospital quality star rating
Benchmarking
Benchmark
Balanced scorecard
Key performance indicator (KPI)
Dashboard

REVIEW QUESTIONS

1. What is the difference between quality and excellent quality?
2. What is QFD? What is the HOQ?
3. What are the seven steps involved in building the HOQ?
4. What is the purpose of a CTQ tree?
5. What is the VOC?
6. What is the difference between demographics and psychographics? Give two examples of each one.
7. What is the Kano model? What happens to "delighters" over time?
8. Differentiate between qualitative and quantitative research data collection methods.
9. What is the purpose of an affinity diagram?
10. What is the VOP?
11. What are the three types of objective quality indicators?
12. What is the overall hospital quality star rating? What groups of measures does it combine?
13. What is the hospital VBP program? What groups of measures does it include?
14. What is the difference between a benchmark and benchmarking?
15. What is the Leapfrog Group?
16. What are the various types of dashboards?
17. Explain the concept of "cascading dashboards."

SOLVE BRIGHT ANGEL MEDICAL CENTER PROBLEMS

All chapter-specific data from the following problems are provided as Excel files which may be accessed via the show supplementary tab (Student Material) available online by visiting www.springerpub.com/courseconnect. See inside front cover and tear-out card for CourseConnect details.

1. One of the surgeons at BAMC would like to complement the CAHPS survey with some additional measures pertaining to reliability (as defined in SERVQUAL). Generate a few questions that would tap this dimension of patient experience.
2. Assume there are two quality indicators: (1) time in the waiting room and (2) duration between appointment time and doctor's arrival in exam room. Which one is a better indicator of quality? Why?
3. Several of the orthopedic surgeons are brainstorming to develop process indicators to measure responsiveness (as defined in SERVQUAL). They have solicited your help for this task. Help them develop such indicators.
4. Following a survey of the administrative staff involved in sending and receiving referrals for fractures, the office manager of BAMC's orthopedic clinic is trying to translate customer requirements into process characteristics. Help him accomplish this task and develop a CTQ tree based on the following data:

Administrative Staff's Requirement	Importance Rating (1–5)
Referral forms are standardized	5
Providers sending the referrals receive timely patient follow-up instructions	2
Referrals are sent to the correct clinic	4
After referral, appointments are made promptly	4

5. Based on the following relationship matrix, compute the importance weights. Which indicators are most important?

		Indicators							
		1	2	3	4	5	6	7	8
Customer requirement	Importance								
A	5	◉			◉				△
B	4		◉				◉		△
C	3	◉	○				◉	○	
D	2			△	◉		△		○
E	3		○			△		◉	
F	2	△	◉	△					
Importance weights		?	?	?	?	?	?	?	?

6. Based on the following relationship matrix, compute the importance weights. Which indicators are most important?

		Indicators						
		1	2	3	4	5	6	7
Customer Requirement	Importance							
A	4	○	◉	△		○		
B	5	○		△		◉		◉
C	5	◉	◉		△			○
D	3		○	○		○	◉	◉
E	2				◉	△	◉	
F	3	△		◉	◉	○		
Importance weights		?	?	?	?	?	?	?

7. The BAMC culinary staff has been asking children in the pediatric unit what they would like to eat on Thanksgiving Day. Here are their responses. Organize them into an affinity diagram. (Use sticky notes or the affinity diagram template provided in the online student resources.)

Turkey	Peas	Mashed potatoes	Green beans	Ham	Duck	Roast beef	Sweet potatoes
Fish sticks	Carrots	Plums	Pretzels	Noodles	Hamburger	Apple *pie*	Chips
Pumpkin pie	Ice cream	Cranberries	Chocolate cake	Bread pudding	Broccoli	Corn	Spinach
Squash	Shrimp	Strawberry pie	Corn bread	Chicken nuggets	French fries	Hot dogs	Croissants
Pork chops	Won tons	Fajitas	Steak	Refried beans	Cheetos	Potato salad	Tomato salad
Rice	Lamb chops	Tomato soup	Bratwursts	Cabbage	Baguette	Candy	Cauliflower
Egg rolls	Garlic bread sticks	Marshmallows	Cheese cake	Banana pudding	Spring rolls	Beef burritos	Popcorn
Tandoori chicken	Chocolate mousse	Chocolate pudding	Chicken curry	Irish stew	Stuffing	Chicken pot pie	Fish tacos

8. Access the Quality Dashboard data set in the online student resources and click on the "Bundle Compliance" tab at the bottom of the workbook.

- From October 2017 to December 2020, did the whole health system (BAMC) improve over time in terms of central venous line care bundle compliance? In which months were there typically dips in performance?

- From October 2017 to December 2020, check the performance of each unit (ICU, Medical/ Surgical, cardiac intensive care unit [CICU], and Orthopedics) in terms of Fall prevention safety bundle compliance. What do you notice in terms of variability? Can you explain it?

9. Access the Quality Dashboard data set in the online student resources and click on the "Hand Hygiene" tab at the bottom of the workbook.

   - From October 2017 to December 2018, compare the performance of the four units (ICU, MSG, CICU, and Orthopedics) in terms of hand hygiene compliance. Which units tended to perform worse than the others? Did they improve their performance subsequently?

LEARNING ACTIVITIES

1. Identify service features that would provide basic, performance, and excitement quality for a root canal performed at your endodontist's office.
2. Translate the VOC into VOP! Download the HCAHPS survey from the CMS website (https://hcahpsonline.org/en/survey-instruments) and develop an indicator for each questionnaire item.
3. Notice that most quality measures in the CAHPS surveys include multiple questions or items. Why?
4. Access the CAHPS survey for EDs (https://www.cms.gov/data-research/research/consumer-assessment-healthcare-providers-systems/emergency-department-cahps.) What are the domains and questions?
5. Compare CMS's and the Leapfrog Group's VBP programs. What conclusions can you draw?
6. Do you think that listening to the patient leads to better outcomes? Explain.
7. What eligibility criteria determine whether hospitals can receive an overall hospital quality star rating?
8. Go to https://www.medicare.gov/hospitalcompare/search.html and compare providers in your market. Which one would you choose and why? Do you think the data are relevant to all patients? Why or why not?
9. Look at the quality dashboard (see Table 4.7). Can you identify other quality indicators that would be appropriate?
10. With some of your classmates, brainstorm about the best features of your degree program. Organize your ideas in an affinity diagram and propose some marketing themes to the program director.`
11. In his book, *Telltale Hearts*, Dr. Schillinger stresses the importance of listening to the patient's story. How does that complement a description of the patient's symptoms? (https://www.nytimes.com/2024/08/03/health/schillinger-telltale-heart.html)

REFERENCES

Agency for Healthcare Research and Quality. (2018, November). *Key questions when choosing health care quality measures.* U.S. Department of Health & Human Services. https://www.ahrq.gov/talkingquality/measures/measure-questions.html

Agency for Healthcare Research and Quality. (2023). *The CAHPS program.* U.S. Department of Health & Human Services. https://www.ahrq.gov/cahps/about-cahps/cahps-program/index.html

American College of Surgeons. (2023). *ACS NSQIP: History*. https://www.facs.org/quality-programs/data-and-registries/acs-nsqip/about-acs-nsqip/history

American Society for Quality. (2024). *What is an affinity diagram?* https://asq.org/quality-resources/affinity

Babakus, E., & Mangold, W. G. (1992). Adapting the SERVQUAL scale to hospital services: An empirical investigation. *Health Services Research, 26*(6), 767–786.

Centers for Medicare & Medicaid Services. (2024). *Overall hospital quality star rating*. https://data.cms.gov/provider-data/topics/hospitals/overall-hospital-quality-star-rating

Chassin, M. R., Loeb, J. M., Schmaltz, S. P., & Wachter, R. M. (2010). Accountability measures—Using measurement to promote quality improvement. *New England Journal of Medicine, 363*(7), 683–688. https://doi.org/10.1056/NEJMsb1002320

CMS.gov. (2023). *Cascade of meaningful measures*. Centers for Medicare & Medicaid Services. https://www.cms.gov/medicare/meaningful-measures-framework/cascade-measures

CMS.gov. (2024). *The hospital value-based purchasing (VBP) program*. Centers for Medicare & Medicaid Services. https://www.cms.gov/medicare/quality/value-based-programs/hospital-purchasing

DeLayne Stroud, J. (2010). *Defining CTQ outputs: A key step in the design process*. ISIXSIGMA. https://www.isixsigma.com/voc-customer-focus/defining-ctq-outputs-key-step-design-process

Donabedian, A. (1966). Evaluating the quality of medical care. The *Milbank Memorial Fund Quarterly, 44*(3), 166–206. http://www.ncbi.nlm.nih.gov/pubmed/5338568

Dunlap, N. E., Ballard, D. J., Cherry, R. A., Dunagan, W. C., Ferniany, W., Hamilton, A. C., Owens, T. A., Rusconi, T., Safyer, S. M., Santrach, P. J., Sears, A., Waldrum, M. R., & Walsh, K. E. (2016). Observations from the field: Reporting quality metrics in health care [Discussion paper, National Academy of Medicine]. *NAM Perspectives*. https://doi.org/10.31478/201607e

Gartner, J.-B., & Lemaire, C. (2022). Dimensions of performance and related key performance indicators addressed in healthcare organisations: A literature review. *The International Journal of Health Planning and Management, 37*(4), 1941–1952. https://doi.org/10.1002/hpm.3452

Gattellari, M., Goumas, C., Jalaludin, B., & Worthington, J. (2019). The impact of disease severity adjustment on hospital standardized mortality ratios: Results from a service-wide analysis of ischaemic stroke admissions using linked pre-hospital, admissions and mortality data. *PLoS One, 14*(5), e0216325. https://doi.org/10.1371/journal.pone.0216325

Gavahi, S. S., Hosseini, S. M. H., & Arash, M. (2023). An application of quality function deployment and SERVQUAL approaches to enhance the service quality in radiology centres. *Benchmarking, 30*(5), 1649–1671. https://doi.org/10.1108/BIJ-07-2021-0411

Institute for Patient- and Family-Centered Care. (2023). *Patient- and family-centered care*. https://www.ipfcc.org/about/pfcc.html

Institute of Medicine. (1999). *To err is human*. N. A. Press. https://nap.nationalacademies.org/resource/9728/To-Err-is-Human-1999--report-brief.pdf

Kaplan, R. S., & Norton, D. P. (1992). The balanced scorecard—Measures that drive performance. *Harvard Business Review, 70*(1), 71–79. https://hbr.org/1992/01/the-balanced-scorecard-measures-that-drive-performance-2

Kaplan, R. S., & Norton, D. P. (1996). Using the balanced scorecard as a strategic management system. *Harvard Business Review, 74*(1), 75–85. https://hbr.org/2007/07/using-the-balanced-scorecard-as-a-strategic-management-system

Kaplan, R. S., & Norton, D. P. (2008). *The execution premium: Linking strategy to operations for competitive advantage*. HBS Press.

Karami, M., Safdari, R., & Rahimi, A. (2013). Effective radiology dashboards: Key research findings. *Radiology Management, 35*(2), 42–45. https://www.researchgate.net/publication/236612715_Effective_radiology_dashboards_key_research_findings

Kolata, G. (2023, June 12). When doctors use a Chatbot to improve their bedside manner. *The New York Times*. https://www.nytimes.com/2023/06/12/health/doctors-chatgpt-artificial-intelligence.html

MindTools. (2023). *Critical to quality (CTQ) trees: Translating broad needs to requirements*. https://www.mindtools.com/alif8kn/critical-to-quality-ctq-trees

National Quality Forum. (2014). *MAP families of measures—Final report*. https://www.qualityforum.org/Publications/2014/07/MAP_Families_of_Measures_-_Final_Report.aspx

Parasuraman, A., Berry, L. L., & Zeithaml, V. A. (1991). Refinement and reassessment of the SERVQUAL scale. *Journal of Retailing*, *67*(4), 420–450. https://www.proquest.com/scholarly-journals/refinement-reassessment-servqual-scale/docview/228675435/se-2

Russell, R. S., & Taylor, B. W. (2023). *Operations and supply chain management* (11th ed.). Wiley.

Saskatchewan Health Authority. (2022). *SHA Family Presence Expert Panel wins 2022 Partnership Award*. https://www.saskhealthauthority.ca/news-events/news/sha-family-presence-expert-panel-wins-2022-partnership-award

Sharifi, T., Hosseini, S., Mohammadpour, S., Javan-Noughabi, J., Ebrahimpour, H., & Hooshmand, E. (2021). Quality assessment of services provided by health centers in Mashhad, Iran: SERVQUAL versus HEALTHQUAL scales. *BMC Health Services Research*, *21*(397). https://doi.org/10.1186/s12913-021-06405-4

Tabbutt, S., Schuette, J., Zhang, W., Alten, J., Donahue, J., Gaynor, J. W., Ghanayem, N., Jacobs, J., Pasquali, S. K., Thiagarajan, R., Dimick, J. B., Banerjee, M., Cooper, D., & Gaies, M. (2019). A novel model demonstrates variation in risk adjusted mortality across pediatric cardiac intensive care units after surgery. *Pediatric Critical Care Medicine*, *20*(2), 136–142. https://doi.org/10.1097/PCC.0000000000001776

The Leapfrog Group. (2024). *Raising the bar for safer healthcare*. Author. https://www.leapfroggroup.org/about

White House. (2010). *Health care that works for Americans*. https://obamawhitehouse.archives.gov/healthreform/healthcare-overview

WHO Working Group. (2020). A minimal common outcome measure set for COVID-19 clinical research. *The Lancet Infectious Diseases*, *20*(8), e192–e197. https://doi.org/10.1016/S1473-3099(20)30483-7

Zacarias, D. (2015). *The complete guide to the Kano model*. https://foldingburritos.com/blog/kano-model

APPENDIX 4.1 BASIC CONCEPTS OF QUESTIONNAIRE DESIGN

INTRODUCTION

How easy is it to develop a "good" survey? It is extremely difficult! You must have seen and filled out many surveys in your lifetime. Do you know that many of those are poorly designed and yield useless information? Another way of saying this is that it is relatively easy to design a survey to produce the desired results which, in reality, do not convey the respondents' true opinions. Let us look at a simple example of a question in a survey of instructors teaching in a Master of Health Administration program:

- Do you consider the many healthcare administration texts adequate for most of your majors at the graduate level?

  _______ Yes _______ No

  If no, state briefly why not: ____________________________________

This question is very bad. What is meant by "many," "adequate," and "most"? All these words are very vague and may mean different things to different people. Some books may be adequate but not the others. Are they adequate in terms of type of topic coverage, breadth and/or depth of coverage, readability, or pedagogical approach? Furthermore, the response categories are too narrow; they elicit a binary response when, in fact, the level of adequacy that one associates with a particular textbook may be more nuanced. The formulation of questions and answers has an impact on data accuracy, and therefore a sloppy questionnaire can lead to a great deal of distortion in the communication of results. Questionnaire design is both an art and a science. In the next following sections, we will teach you some basic principles of questionnaire design, but in the end, practice is the best way to improve your skills. Before you start developing the questions, you should clearly identify:

- The research issues. What do you need to find out and what information do you need?
- The target respondents. Who are the people best positioned to provide the information that you need? Are they patients, administrators, clinicians, insurers, veterans, young parents, and so on? What demographics are you interested in?
- The data collection methods you will use. Ideally, multiple methods should be used (e.g., patient records and patient surveys) because this approach minimizes the risk of **common method variance** (i.e., the false appearance of a relationship between variables that is due to the common method rather than the measures themselves). For example, if executives are asked to evaluate their organization's capabilities and its financial performance in a questionnaire, they may tend to be consistent in their answers. A better approach would be to collate the survey answers on capabilities with financial records.
- The analysis you will perform. This is important because the measurement level (Chapter 7, Table 7.1) of the scale on which the answers are anchored influences the types of statistical analyses you can perform.

QUESTIONNAIRE DEVELOPMENT

Rigorous questionnaire development is time- and resource-intensive and beyond the scope of this textbook (for a scale development overview, see Boateng et al., 2018). At a minimum, designing a questionnaire will require the following steps:

STEP 1: Translate the data requirements of your project into a set of questions.

STEP 2: Check the "rough" questionnaire for form, relevance, wording, sequencing, layout, and appearance.

STEP 3: Revise and re-check.

STEP 4: Pretest the questionnaire.

TRANSLATE THE DATA REQUIREMENTS INTO A SET OF QUESTIONS

Once you have formulated your research questions and data requirements, you will need to identify the domain(s) (i.e., scope and boundaries) of the measures you want to capture. A thorough review of the literature and focus group interviews help identify the full domain(s) of your measures. For example, based on their extensive research, Parasuraman et al. (1991) determined that the domain of service quality comprises tangibles, responsiveness, reliability, assurance, and empathy. Once the domains are identified, you can start developing an initial set of questions.

CHECK THE QUESTIONNAIRE FOR FORM, RELEVANCE, WORDING, SEQUENCING, LAYOUT, AND APPEARANCE

Form

The form of a questionnaire item refers to the format of the question and response categories.

Nonstructured questions are typically open-ended. An example would be: What are the main disadvantages of your current healthcare plan? ________________. This type of question potentially yields rich answers offering valuable insights. However, it requires time and effort on the part of the respondent. As a result, the response rate on those questions is usually low. Moreover, the variety of responses make coding for analysis challenging. On the other hand, **structured questions** involve a set of two (dichotomous) or more (multiple) response categories. They are easier to answer and code than nonstructured questions. Following are examples of each type:

- Have you ever had malaria?

  _______ Yes

  _______ No

- Approximately how many times do you go to your primary care physician's office per year?

  _____ 0 to 1 time

  _____ 2 to 3 times

  _____ 4 to 5 times

  _____ More than 5 times

When there are multiple response categories involving numbers, make sure that the sequence of responses is natural. In the example given earlier, the responses should not be in random order. The response categories must be collectively exhaustive (i.e., all possible response choices are included). They must also be mutually exclusive (i.e., there may not be overlaps, e.g., 0–1, 1–2, 2–3). How many response categories are appropriate? In general, 4 to 7 response categories are recommended to provide a good balance between sufficient variability and excessive discrimination among answer options.

Relevance

A major concern in questionnaire design is parsimony. Before including a question in a survey, ask yourself the following:

- Can the research objective be met without the question? If so, do not include it. For example, if wait times are tracked electronically for each patient, it would be redundant to ask them to provide their approximate wait time in a questionnaire.
- Can the respondent answer the question? The issues covered in the questions may be too complex or technical for the respondents to be able to answer. This is why you do not see medical-type questions in patient surveys.
- Will the respondent answer the question? Some questions may be too personal or too sensitive. If they are included, respondents will tend to ignore them.

Wording

The wording of the questions should be clear, precise, and objective. This is why you should avoid the following:

- Double-barreled questions: Double-barreled questions ask two questions at the same time. For example, the question "To what extent do you feel that hospital administrators are concerned about health outcomes and efficiency?" is problematic because administrators may be concerned about health outcomes but not efficiency and vice versa. Two separate questions, one regarding quality, the other efficiency, should be asked instead.

- Biased questions and answers: The wording of a question may lead the respondent toward a positive or negative answer. Loaded questions such as "Don't you think that malpractice insurance is a major reason for high healthcare costs?" reflect the researcher's position on an issue and invite respondents, especially those who do not have a strong opinion about the issue, to adopt the same position. Similarly, unbalanced response categories introduce bias. For example, if there are five answer categories and four of them reflect a favorable opinion, whereas only one captures an unfavorable opinion, the survey results will falsely indicate that the majority of respondents have positive opinions about the issue captured in the question.
- Questions with implicit assumptions: These types of questions assume that respondents know about the topic addressed in the question. For example, the question "Does your body mass index (BMI) put you at an increased risk for heart disease?" assumes that people know what their BMI is and the ranges of values corresponding to an increased risk.
- Complex questions: Complex questions require either specialized knowledge or effort on the respondents' parts. The question, "Of the total amount you spent on insurance premiums last year, approximately what percentage was for health insurance?" involves adding up all the auto, home, life, and health insurance premiums, and then dividing the health insurance premium amount by the total. Given the amount of effort needed to answer this question and the strong probability that respondents will either ignore the question or guess an answer, it is very unlikely that results will be accurate and valuable to the researcher.

Sequencing

The order in which questions are presented and their grouping also affect the quality of the answers and the response rate.

As a general rule, demographic questions should not be placed at the beginning of a questionnaire. These questions are personal and are identifiers, potentially making the respondent uncomfortable at the onset and increasing the probability of nonresponse. Since demographics are often used for descriptive purposes in a research project, they are not as essential as the questions capturing the research issues. Consequently, placing them at the end of the questionnaire increases the chances that respondents will answer important questions before they become tired and unwilling to go further.

Have you ever taken a multiple-choice test in which the order of the questions was randomized? If so, you may remember how distracting and challenging it was for your brain to jump from the material of one chapter to that of another repeatedly. Ideally, test questions dealing with the same or related topics should be grouped together. The same applies to questionnaire items. The questions capturing responsiveness of staff or care by certain individuals should be presented as a distinct set. This will help respondents organize their thoughts around the concept and provide more reliable answers.

In paper surveys, avoid skip patterns as much as possible. In a nonnegligible number of cases, respondents who should skip forget to do so. They therefore answer questions that are not relevant to them, which complicates the interpretation of the results. These concerns do not apply to phone surveys conducted by diligent professionals and well-designed online surveys with seamlessly embedded skip patterns. An example of a skip pattern is shown here:

Question 5: Are you allergic to latex?

_________ Yes

_________ No (skip to Question 8)

Appearance and Layout

A questionnaire should look attractive, neat, and uncluttered. To create the illusion that a questionnaire is shorter than it actually is, designers are often tempted to "cram" as many questions as possible in a few pages. However, cluttered questionnaires are difficult to read, require extra effort, deter respondents, and lead to errors. A common instance of filling space with more text involves placing answer categories in a horizontal rather than vertical sequence:

- How many years have you worked in this position?

  _____ 0 to 1 year _____ 2 to 3 years _____ 4 to 5 years _____ 6 to 7 years _____ 8 or more years

As you can see from the given example, for the responses in the middle, it is difficult to determine whether the answer space is to the left or right of the stated number of years. Therefore, a respondent in her present position for 4 to 5 years might inadvertently select 6 to 7 years.

PRETEST

Once a questionnaire has been checked for form, relevance, wording, sequencing, appearance, and layout (see the checklist provided by Ekinci, 2015), it should be pretested. Pretesting involves the administration of the questionnaire draft to 5 to 15 interviewees similar to the target respondents, as well as other individuals capable of providing valuable insights. While this group fills out the questionnaire, you should observe them and solicit feedback. They might get confused, seek clarification, or find a question too sensitive to answer. This input is necessary to revise the questionnaire before it is administered.

RELIABILITY AND VALIDITY

Reliability and validity are psychometric properties that are essential in concept, or **construct**, measurement. **Reliability** denotes stability and consistency. For example, when measuring the scheduling staff's courtesy, the response to a question tapping the staff's politeness should be quite similar to the response to a question measuring the staff's willingness to accommodate your schedule. Validity, on the other hand, refers to how well questionnaire items measure the construct they are supposed to measure. You probably noticed that in CAHPS and SERVQUAL, each construct was measured using multiple survey items. This is a basic requirement to ensure reliability and validity.

RELIABILITY

Let's assume that you took the GRE test for the first time and received a quantitative reasoning score of 161. You are busy and do not have time to study before you take the test again. The second test is very similar in content to the first one, but the questions are different. This time, you get a score of 161 in quantitative reasoning. Again! This shows that the tests are very reliable because alternative forms of it generated the same score for you. The same phenomenon should occur with the measurement of attitudes and perceptions. The measurement of a given construct is reliable if independent, but comparable, measures of the construct *agree*. Let us look at an example. Assume that nurses' empathy is measured using five items or questions. On a 5-point scale, a respondent's ratings (or answers on the 5-point scale) are:

Construct	Rating
Item 1	1
Item 2	2
Item 3	3
Item 4	4
Item 5	5

You can see that the responses fluctuate widely and do not reflect any consensus on nurses' empathy. Now, contrast with the following ratings:

Construct	Rating
Item 1	4
Item 2	5
Item 3	5
Item 4	4
Item 5	5

Consistently, the respondent gave high ratings in the assessment of nurses' empathy. The measures agree. If a substantial majority of respondents also provide consistent ratings, low or high, of nurses' empathy, then the measurement of nurses' empathy will be considered reliable.

The best way to ensure reliability is to formulate questionnaire items that measure *precisely* the same construct. In other words, if you want to measure nurses' empathy, you need to avoid ambiguous terms that might not relate to empathy specifically enough.

The most popular method to measure reliability is to compute the Cronbach alpha. The Cronbach alpha reflects the extent to which the responses to questions pertaining to a given construct are internally consistent or closely related to each other. Its value is between 0 and 1. A minimum threshold for acceptable reliability in the social sciences is 0.70. Most statistical packages will generate the Cronbach alpha value for a particular set of items or measures.

The reliability of measurement does not guarantee its validity. You may think of reliability as a necessary but not sufficient condition for validity. A set of measures, also known as a measurement scale, may consistently produce the same or similar ratings (reliability), but it may not measure *accurately* the construct that the researcher is trying to examine. Whereas reliability is concerned with precision, validity deals with accuracy.

CONSTRUCT VALIDITY

Remember that we said earlier that multiple survey items were necessary to assess the reliability and validity of a construct. **Construct validity** refers to the ability of a scale to measure the construct it is supposed to measure. It subsumes content, convergent, discriminant, and criterion validity.

Content Validity. Content validity implies that the measures of a particular construct cover its entire domain. In other words, it concerns the representativeness of the content of the measures used to capture a construct under study. Consider the construct of service quality in SERVQUAL. Its domain comprises multiple facets or dimensions of service quality: tangibles, reliability, responsiveness, assurance, and empathy. Similarly, the domain of healthcare quality includes infrastructural input variables, process measures, health outcomes, and patient experience, each of which may have multiple subdimensions. A thorough review of the literature and existing scales (deductive methods), as well as focus group discussions and interviews (inductive methods), contribute to the identification of the construct's full domain.

Convergent Validity. As its name indicates, convergent validity implies the convergence of items measuring the same construct. To show convergence, the items that measure the same construct should correlate or "hang together." Let's go back to the SERVQUAL example; one would expect all the items measuring tangibles to be correlated. The same would apply to reliability, responsiveness, assurance, and empathy.

Discriminant Validity. Discriminant validity requires that the items measuring different constructs be unrelated. If the items of a measurement scale are supposed to measure Construct A, they should not measure Construct B. Using our SERVQUAL example, the items tapping responsiveness should not measure reliability, and vice versa. Why not? Because although they are dimensions of the service quality construct, they are themselves separate constructs.

Criterion Validity. Criterion validity indicates that the nature of the relationship between the measurement scale and other constructs is as expected. For example, one would expect that each dimension of SERVQUAL be positively related to customer satisfaction. On the other hand, one would expect the relationship between job satisfaction and intent to leave the organization, two separate constructs, to be negative.

By now, we think that you are convinced that designing a questionnaire with reliable and valid measurement scales is challenging. We strongly recommend that you search for existing scales with sound psychometric properties in the literature and adapt them, if necessary, rather than trying to develop measurement scales from scratch. However, sometimes, the proper scales are not available, and you should rely on professional expertise to help you develop them.

KEY TERMS

Common method variance	**Structured questions**	**Reliability**
Non-structured questions	**Construct**	**Construct validity**

REVIEW QUESTIONS

1. What is the risk of common method variance? How can you minimize it when doing your research?
2. What are the four basic steps to follow when designing a questionnaire?
3. What is the difference between a nonstructured and a structured question?
4. What wording mistakes should you avoid when designing your questionnaire?
5. What is reliability? What is a popular method to assess it?
6. What is construct validity? What other forms of validity does it subsume?

PROBLEMS

1. **For each one of the following response scales, indicate the level of measurement (nominal, ordinal, interval, ratio). Hint: Check Table 7.1 in Chapter 7.**
   a. What is your annual income before taxes? $______________
   b. During the *past 4 weeks*, how much of the time have you accomplished less than you would like *as a result of your physical health*? (Please check the appropriate category)
      All the time ______ (1)
      Most of the time ______ (2)
      Some of the time ______ (3)
      A little of the time ______ (4)
      None of the time ______ (5)
   c. Currently, what is your primary employment status (check the one that applies)?
      Self-employed ______ (1)
      Employed full-time ______ (2)
      Employed part-time ______ (3)
      Full-time student ______ (4)
      Unemployed ______ (5)
      Retired ______ (6)
   d. What is the highest level of education that you have completed?
      No formal education ______ (1)
      Some grade school ______ (2)
      Completed grade school ______ (3)
      Some high school ______ (4)
      Completed high school ______ (5)
      Some college ______ (6)
      Completed college ______ (7)
      Some graduate work ______ (8)
      Graduate degree ______ (9)
2. **Identify all potential problems for each one of the following questions. Note: These questions are not from the same questionnaire.**
   a. Approximately, how long did you wait in the exam room before seeing the doctor?
      ______ 0 to 5 minutes
      ______ 5 to 10 minutes
      ______ More than 10 minutes
   b. Does your HbA1c level put you at risk of complications from diabetes?
      ______ Yes
      ______ No

c. How often do you smoke cigarettes:
Extremely often ______ (1)
Very often ______ (2)
Often ______ (3)
Never ______ (4)

d. Our hospital has been selected by Walmart as a Center of Excellence for its employees. How much do you like the care you receive at our hospital?
____
____
____

e. During this hospital stay, how often did doctors and nurses treat you with courtesy and provide excellent care? Would you say
Never ______ (1)
Sometimes ______ (2)
Usually ______ (3)
Always ______ (4)

f. What is your religion?
Baptist ______ (1)
Catholic ______ (2)
Lutheran ______ (3)
Muslim ______ (4)

LEARNING ACTIVITIES

1. Find an empirical study dealing with burnout of healthcare staff. What instrument did the researchers use to measure burnout? Evaluate its psychometric properties as reported in the study.
2. Identify the entire knowledge domain of the course for which you are using this textbook. Select one subdomain and develop a student satisfaction survey on various forms of teaching materials in that domain.
3. Identify the customer of a particular process at work (e.g., IT training education for nurses). Develop a questionnaire to measure customer satisfaction.

REFERENCES

Boateng, G. O., Neilands, T. B., Frongillo, E. A., Melgar-Quiñonez, H. R., & Young, S. L. (2018). Best practices for developing scales for health, social, and behavioral research: A primer. *Frontiers in Public Health, 6*(Article 149). https://doi.org/10.3389/fpubh.2018.00149

Ekinci, Y. (2015). *Designing research questionnaires for business and management students*. Sage.

Parasuraman, A., Berry, L. L., & Zeithaml, V. A. (1991). Refinement and reassessment of the SERVQUAL scale. *Journal of Retailing, 67*(4), 420–450.

FOR MORE ADVANCED CONTENT ON MEASUREMENT SYSTEM ANALYSIS, SEE ECHAPTER 15: GAGE REPEATABILITY AND REPRODUCIBILITY (ONLINE STUDENT RESOURCES).

eChapter 15 is available online by visiting www.springerpub.com/courseconnect. See inside front cover and tear-out card for CourseConnect details.

CHAPTER 5

PROJECT MANAGEMENT

BRIGHT ANGEL MEDICAL CENTER 5.1

Dr. Aoki and Barbara had finished their final listening sessions with the frontline nurses, techs, and physicians to gather their input on the areas that would be most impactful to redesign the workflows in the ED. After months of critical discussions, gathering data, and garnering support from the executive team and board of directors, they were finally ready to crystalize the project and develop a plan for success. Barbara was glad to have a seasoned leader like Olina to partner with on this work.

"We need to get this formalized into a project plan," Olina shared. "This is going to be a complex project, and we need to have a comprehensive roadmap that lays out all the key elements. Just focusing on one area won't get us there."

The others nodded in agreement. "Ok," said Barbara, "where do we begin?"

Think of a project in which you have been involved. What was the hardest part for you to do well? Have you ever worked on a project that failed? Why did it fail?

LEARNING OBJECTIVES

After reading this chapter, you will be able to:

- Understand project constraints.
- Create a project charter.
- Define the roles and responsibilities of individuals involved in projects.
- Appreciate the importance of effective leadership.
- Identify the various phases of project management.
- Develop work breakdown structures (WBSs).
- Draw network diagrams.
- Schedule projects.
- Discuss the advantages and disadvantages of program evaluation and review technique (PERT)/critical path method (CPM).
- Understand the major causes of project failure.

INTRODUCTION

Chapters 3 and 4 helped us identify process improvement projects that would fulfill or even exceed customers' needs and wants. But how do you move from knowing what needs to be done to actually doing it? That is where project management comes in. Although the term *project* is often used loosely, in this chapter, a **project** denotes a set of team activities designed to produce a one-of-a-kind product or service. These types of projects are not routine or part of ongoing business operations. Examples include launching a rocket, building a bridge, implementing a hospital information system, or developing a new drug. Such endeavors involve a large number of activities and require resources (people, money, or equipment) over an extended period of time. As such, they tend to be complex and costly and must be managed carefully.

Projects require that many people from different departments and even different organizations collaborate closely. All parties concerned assume specific roles and responsibilities necessary for the successful completion of the project. Because projects have many moving parts and may be active for some time, specific tools and techniques have been developed to help you stay on track. Common tools include the work breakdown structure (WBS), the Gantt chart, and the critical path method (CPM).

WHY IS THIS MATERIAL USEFUL?

Project management ensures that the outcome of a project is what was planned and fits within an organization's strategy. Project management tools help deliver a quality product on time and within budget.

WHAT IS PROJECT MANAGEMENT?

Project management is a systematic approach to planning, implementing, monitoring, and completing the project processes to achieve the specific project goals within a particular time frame (Lippi & Mattiuzzi, 2019). Project management is difficult because it must be balanced with constraints. There is never enough time, money, or people to do everything that an organization would like to accomplish effectively. Therefore, choices need to be made to define the scope of a project so that it can meet quality standards and be completed on time and within budget. These competing constraints (scope, time, cost) are sometimes called the **triple constraint** (Hoban, 2023; Project Management for Development Organizations, 2011; Figure 5.1):

- Projects must deliver the output that is expected within specific boundaries (scope).
- Projects must be within cost (people, materials, supplies, contracts, etc.).
- Projects must be delivered on time.

If there is a change in one constraint, it affects quality and the other constraints. For example, if the project must be completed earlier than planned, more resources will be needed, and the costs will go up. If the other constraints do not change when the time is shortened, the quality may go down.

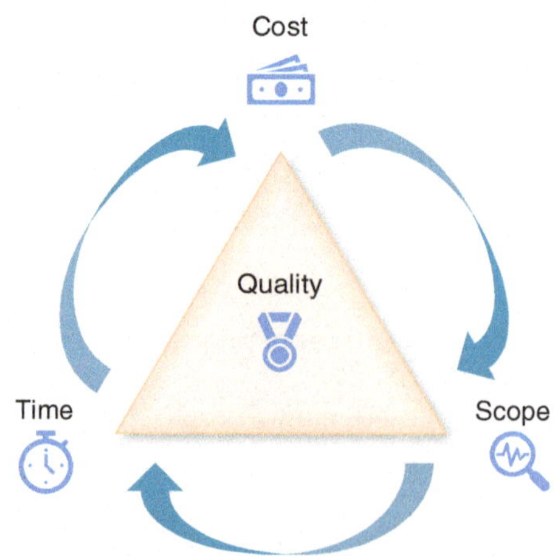

FIGURE 5.1 The triple constraint.

Source: Based on Haughey, D. (2011). Understanding the Project Management Triple Constraint. https://www.projectsmart.co.uk/role-of-the-project-manager/understanding-the-project-management-triple-constraint.php

Projects come in all sizes. For our purposes, we focus on improvement projects that require significant resources across a number of departmental units or organizations. These types of projects are usually led by a trained project manager and involve individuals working together outside their normal job roles. For example, if a hospital board decides to build a new cancer center to provide patients with cutting-edge care, a project team will be chosen from various functional areas to work on the planning and construction of the new facility and on hiring cancer research experts.

PROJECT CHARTER AND ROLES

THE PROJECT CHARTER

A **project charter** serves as a roadmap for the project. It is a document that clearly states why the project is being pursued, what the expected benefits are, who the team members are and the roles they will play, and the timeline for completion. A project leader is generally responsible for drafting the project charter with input from the other team members. This document is used as a communication tool for all members of the team. It includes:

- a business case for action—the reason for doing the project and the financial impact
- a goal statement—the desired outcome and measures of success
- project scope—the boundaries of the project (*only* the work required to complete the project successfully)
- a list of team members and their roles
- outcome measure(s)—the indicators that will show the degree of improvement delivered by the project
- milestones and deliverables—major project phases, outputs, and deadlines

As mentioned in Chapter 3, the business case for action lays the foundation for selling change to leaders and employees. It needs to clearly articulate the problem to be solved and the cost of inaction. Essentially, it justifies why the project is important for the organization to reach its strategic objectives and why it is imperative that the project be executed at a particular time. The problem should be described in terms of (a) what it is, (b) how long it has been present, and (c) the impact it has on the organization and customer(s). The group then needs to determine the desired outcomes, major actions to take, and metrics to assess performance. The roles of participants, boundaries of the project, and timelines are important to delineate because projects tend to have a way of expanding beyond what is initially intended. This situation, called "**scope creep**," can result in cost overruns and project failure.

BRIGHT ANGEL MEDICAL CENTER 5.2

Barbara was worried. Both she and Olina had full-time jobs and neither felt like they had the bandwidth to dedicate the amount of time needed to lead this complex project and do their regular jobs. They asked Dr. Paul Tibbets for some time to discuss the project plan. They knew they needed additional resources to be successful. But the hospital was under financial constraints and they weren't sure that Dr. Tibbets would approve an additional person to help out. She and Olina would have to make a persuasive argument. The three of them met to discuss the ED improvement project.

"Hello you two," Dr. Tibbets began. "How is our planning progressing for this ED improvement project?"

Olina started, "Well, that's what we need to discuss with you. We are feeling good about our progress so far in gathering preliminary data, gaining stakeholder buy-in, asking for input from the frontline, and even building a strong case for the executive team to support this work. We just need a little more help with project management. There is so much work to coordinate and organize. We really want this to be successful and both of us are so busy with our day jobs. Is there any way you could approve someone to spend part of their time for the

(continued)

BRIGHT ANGEL MEDICAL CENTER 5.2 (*CONTINUED*)

next 9 months on our team to help guide and organize this work?" Barbara held her breath, waiting for Dr. Tibbets to respond.

"This project is a big deal," he said, "and could transform our hospital's front door—the ED. If you need project management help, we would be foolish not to provide it. Let me connect with Mira and see who has the capacity to take this on. I will serve as the executive sponsor. In the meantime, how about you two start drafting a project charter to outline the key details. That will make it easier for us to communicate with other key leaders."

Barbara was thrilled at the news. "We are on it," she exclaimed.

A few days later, Dr. Tibbets told Barbara that Adeleke Mensah, a senior data scientist with a project management background, would be the project manager. Barbara and Olina inserted his name in the first draft of the following document (Exhibit 5.1).

EXHIBIT 5.1 PROJECT CHARTER FOR BAMC

Project Charter	
Improving throughput in the ED for better health outcomes and greater patient satisfaction	
Goal statement	Improve ED throughput by 30% by the end of the next calendar year.
Business case	Better ED throughput will: (a) reduce LOS and LWBS, which represent lost revenue; (b) improve health outcomes (and reimbursements) with more constructive interaction with providers and patient-friendly discharge processes; (c) improve patient satisfaction (and reimbursements) with reduced wait times; and (d) improve competitive position in the area. Inaction will result in major revenue losses and high turnover.
Scope	Staffing: Hire permanent nurses; train in LSS. Layout: Redesign processes and remodel the ED to support a more efficient workflow. Patient satisfaction: Collect data, track performance, and train for better customer service and service recovery.
Team members and roles	Dr. Paul Tibbets—executive sponsor; Adeleke Mensah—project manager; Barbara Waters—ED director; Dr. Hana Aoki—ED medical director; Olina Petrenko—director of quality and Six Sigma Master Black Belt; Loretta Romero—ED nurse manager; ad-hoc members in HR, IT, and planning design and construction.
Outcome measures	• Hand hygiene compliance rate >95% • LWBS rate <2% of arrivals • ED LOS (discharged) <150 min • ED LOS (admitted) <200 min • Door-to-doc time <45 min • Room-to-provider time <20 min, >90% time • Return to ED in <72 hr <5% • Patient satisfaction scores in top box >80% • Travel nurses FTEs <20 • Lean training >85%
Milestones and deliverables	• Staffing 4/18/25 • Layout 6/6/25 • Patient experience 4/18/25
Budget	Layout: $1,500,000 + $190,000/yr for additional staff (subsequent years) Staffing: $600,000 Patient experience: $100,000

Abbreviations: BAMC, Bright Angel Medical Center; FTE, full-time employee; HR, human resources; IT, information technology; LOS, length of stay; LSS, lean Six Sigma; LWBS, left-without-being-seen.

Why is it important to get the right people on the team? What happens if an important area is not represented? Can you recover from that oversight? How?

THE PROJECT MANAGER

The role of the **project manager** is one of great responsibility. It is the project manager's job to direct, supervise, and control the project from beginning to end. Because of the complexity of many projects and the technical skills needed to lead them successfully, certification programs have been developed to train individuals in project management. Project management software is available to help managers keep track of tasks and timelines. Organizations with multiple, simultaneous projects may require several project managers. These project managers may be located at the function unit level (e.g., human resources [HR] or finance) within the organization. However, larger organizations may pursue a pure project management organizational structure with a **project management office**, which involves a separate organizational entity with its own staff and administration dedicated to defining and maintaining project standards. It supports individual project teams within the organization to ensure that projects are aligned with organizational goals and that project management processes are efficient and standardized (Porter, 2023).

Project managers handle multiple relationships at the same time. They must be able to work with the project team, heads of functional areas within the organization, senior management, and external stakeholders. As these people are likely to hold different views, project managers must also possess leadership skills that can help them talk through their differences and come to an acceptable solution (Kerzner, 2022; Box 5.1). Project managers should not carry out project tasks because they must keep their eyes on the bigger picture. In addition to verifying that the project is defined and planned accurately and that resources are available, they must ensure that all stakeholders are kept informed, conflict is managed, and all issues are addressed. No project ever goes exactly as planned, so the project manager must be able to adapt to and manage change. Project managers get to know the organization from the ground up. This knowledge provides them with excellent opportunities to contribute in a meaningful way and prepares them for higher-level management positions. In other words, if you can get involved in a project, do not pass up the chance!

BOX 5.1 QUALITY IN PRACTICE!

Cross-Sector Collaboration for a Healthy Living Environment

Large, cross-sectional projects involve many individuals with different priorities and perspectives. From 2019 to 2022, the Dutch National Institute for Public Health and the Environment conducted a research project to determine how to facilitate collaboration among people in the public health, social, and environmental domains to develop a healthy living environment. Three different projects were examined. Semistructured interviews of project participants, quarterly updates from project leaders, and reflections on the implementation strategies by two panels yielded important insights for successful collaboration. These are noted in the following list:

1. Create trust among project participants with an independent project leader, some form of shared leadership, and investment in collaboration from the start of the project.
2. Make all stakeholders actively participate throughout the execution of the project by learning the needs and priorities of local and regional project partners, incentivizing accountability, modifying leadership style when necessary, and encouraging discussions with local residents.
3. Define roles and tasks early on and link them to societal expectations.

The research project also uncovered that trust in the project itself was as important as trust among participants. Furthermore, investments and strategies need to be clear at the onset of the project, but flexibility in adapting them during implementation maintains and reinforces cross-sector collaboration (van Vooren et al., 2023).

THE PROJECT TEAM

Essentially, the **project team** gets the necessary work done to achieve the goal. The team is a temporary organizational structure designed to harness expertise from many groups throughout the organization and to carefully define the scope and specific objectives of the project. The team is also responsible for executing tasks and producing deliverables as outlined in the project plan. However, project teams usually work with many outside contributors who have the needed expertise (e.g., information technology [IT] consultants) or are invested one way or the other in the outcome of the project. It is important that the project team reaches out to these parties who may have information or insights to contribute. This improves the chances that the overall project will be successful.

Being a project team member is a major responsibility. You must commit to the project goals and communicate honestly, particularly if you have concerns. You must also understand your work assignments and complete them on time to the best of your ability.

Characteristics of a Good Project Team

Some people are much better at working in teams than others. They tend to be constructive and positive people who are interested in giving and seeking information to solve the problem. They find areas of common ground within the group and work to build consensus. Other people can be destructive when working in teams. The negativity of these individuals can end up lengthening the time frame of the project and degrading the team's morale. But, in all fairness, many individuals who appear difficult may have valuable perspectives that are important to the quality of the project. Teams should have a balance of personality types—those who are detail-oriented and those who are more visionary. Diversity of types ensures that teams have people focusing on the specifics and the big picture simultaneously and can execute tasks while remaining creative (Wu et al., 2019).

EMPLOYEES IN FUNCTIONAL AREAS

As we mentioned earlier, the team is responsible for getting the project completed, but often this work must be done by employees in specific functional areas. Because these employees do not directly report to the project team, it may be challenging to get them to commit to the team's needs. This is why it is very important to secure the support of the employees' supervisors for the project. The team must ensure that supervisors agree with employees performing project-related tasks, that the timeline is in line with the supervisor's priorities, and that good lines of communication are maintained with the functional areas. If timelines shift or project constraints change, all involved, including supervisors, need to be informed.

EXECUTIVES

By now, you realize that project support at the highest levels of the organization is critical. Executives need to shepherd the project forward, secure the needed resources, and resolve conflicts. They have the responsibility to make effective and timely decisions to keep the project on track. Although executives may help with setting priorities and defining the project's objectives, they do not need to lead the project itself. Project sponsorship may be pushed down to middle management or committees. However, when there are differences in priorities, executives must clarify what activities take precedence.

PROJECT CHAMPIONS

It is sometimes helpful to have someone within the organization proclaim the benefits of the project and work with different stakeholder groups to explain its importance. This **project champion** is often the one who came up with the idea in the first place. Project champions can often gain support for the project more effectively than someone on the project team. As such, they should be kept apprised of progress and challenges.

IMPORTANCE OF LEADERSHIP IN PROJECT MANAGEMENT

We have discussed how a project manager must direct, supervise, and be in control of the project from beginning to end. But project managers must also be able to *lead* a group to accomplish a goal. They need to possess skills for both management and leadership. Depending on the definition of leadership, management and leadership activities have been viewed as either distinct or comparable. However, empirical evidence suggests that the activities can be placed on a continuum, with several of them overlapping both categories (Collins et al., 2023; Figure 5.2).

In healthcare today, projects often involve working with people in different disciplines (such as physicians, nurses, social workers, and financial analysts), people across different cultures (such as different ethnicities and backgrounds), and people located in different places (hospitals, clinics, nursing homes, etc.). Depending on the project, these factors make managing a project far more complex. Because different members on the project team come to the project with their own point of view, level of understanding, and intrinsic biases, the project manager must (a) ensure that everyone shares the same vision of the project's importance, (b) align people to work for a common purpose, and (c) motivate people to contribute their knowledge and expertise to assure a good outcome. In other words, the project manager must lead the group to success.

As shown in Figure 5.2, good communication is a key skill for both managers and leaders, but it is especially important with complex groups. Open and honest communication builds trust and allows everyone to share in the project's success. Continuous two-way communication helps to prevent misunderstandings and wasted effort. In order for project managers to be most effective, frequent and properly framed messages, defined communication channels, and ways to receive feedback are critical. Examples of effective compared to poor communication are shown in Table 5.1.

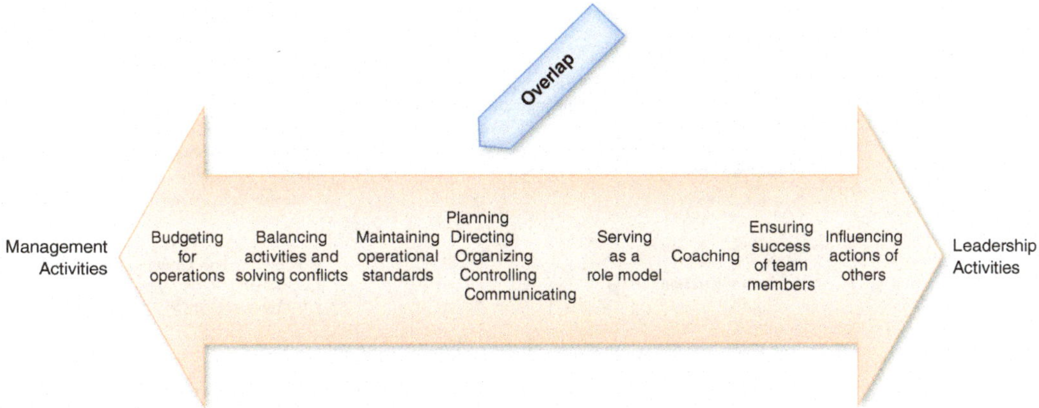

FIGURE 5.2 Types of activities related to management and leadership.

TABLE 5.1 EXAMPLES OF POOR VERSUS EFFECTIVE COMMUNICATION

Poor Communication	Effective Communication
Closed to new ideas	Open to different perspectives
Withholding information	Sharing information
Blaming and judging	Focusing on what needs to be done
Not listening	Listening to understand others' perspectives

BRIGHT ANGEL MEDICAL CENTER 5.3

On Monday morning, Olina rushed into Barbara's office at 8 a.m. sharp. "To facilitate communication within the project team, there is a simple tool that may help us get started looking at our ED workflow and care coordination with other healthcare providers. It is called a 'force field analysis'. Have you heard of it?"

Barbara replied, "Yes, in fact, it is a great way to get our ED physicians and nursing home staff working together to address a variety of problems. What do you know about it?"

Olina informed, "A **force field analysis** *helps a team examine the forces that can help improve the situation and the forces that are keeping the team from solving the problem. Once these restraining forces are identified, strategies to overcome them can be devised. It is a great way to start the brainstorming!" Barbara was smiling. "That is a great place to start!"*

Olina and Barbara were in the ED conference room with staff from the BAMC long-term care facility and several ED physicians. They had been meeting for about an hour and had a large diagram on the whiteboard in the front of the room (Exhibit 5.2).

EXHIBIT 5.2 FORCE FIELD ANALYSIS

Force Field Analysis

Each force is scored according to their "magnitude," ranging from one (weak) to five (strong)

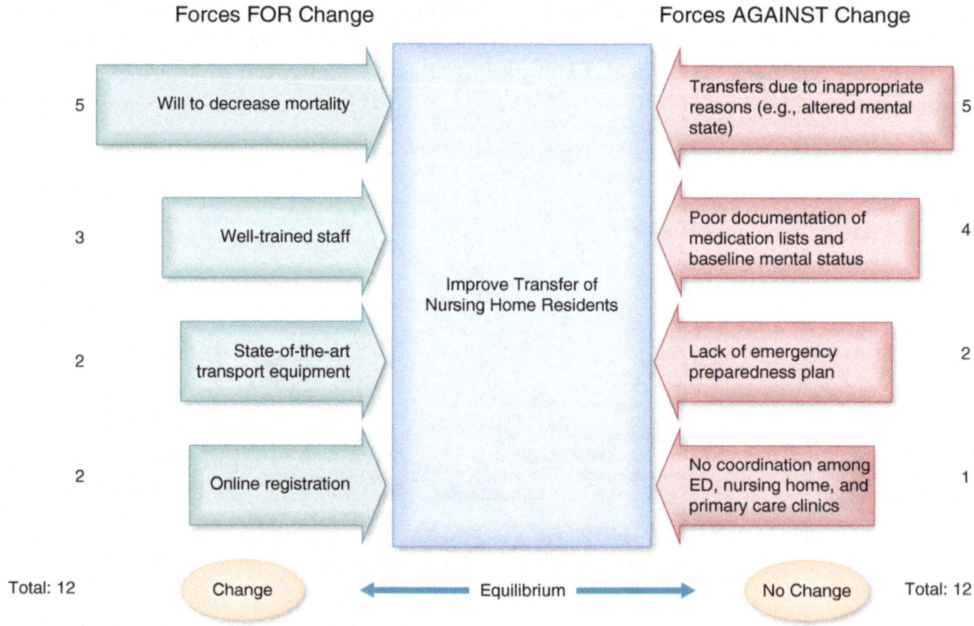

Strategies to Address Negative Forces

1. Use standardized transfer forms including patient's medical history, current medications, baseline mental status, and advance directives.
2. Establish dedicated communication channels to ensure that urgent information is relayed quickly and that follow-up care is communicated to both nursing home staff and primary care physicians to avoid errors and delays.
3. Institute joint emergency preparedness drills to help nursing home and ED staff practice their communication and coordination protocols.

Olina was standing in front of the whiteboard. "Well, I think this is a good place to start. Is everyone on board?" A hand went up. Olina recognized Dr. Patel.

(continued)

BRIGHT ANGEL MEDICAL CENTER 5.3 (*CONTINUED*)

"I did not realize that our own actions had such a bad effect on the care and safety of our nursing home patients. This discussion has been eye opening for me. I will be sure to form a task force to improve our transfer process. Thanks for getting us all together."

Olina and Barbara looked at each other. Although there was a lot more to do to improve the effective and efficient transfer of nursing home patients, this was a good start.

PHASES OF A PROJECT

Now that you understand the roles of the individuals involved in a project and the importance of effective leadership and communication, we turn to the five phases through which a project must pass: initiation, planning, execution, control, and closure (Project Management Institute, 2022; Figure 5.3).

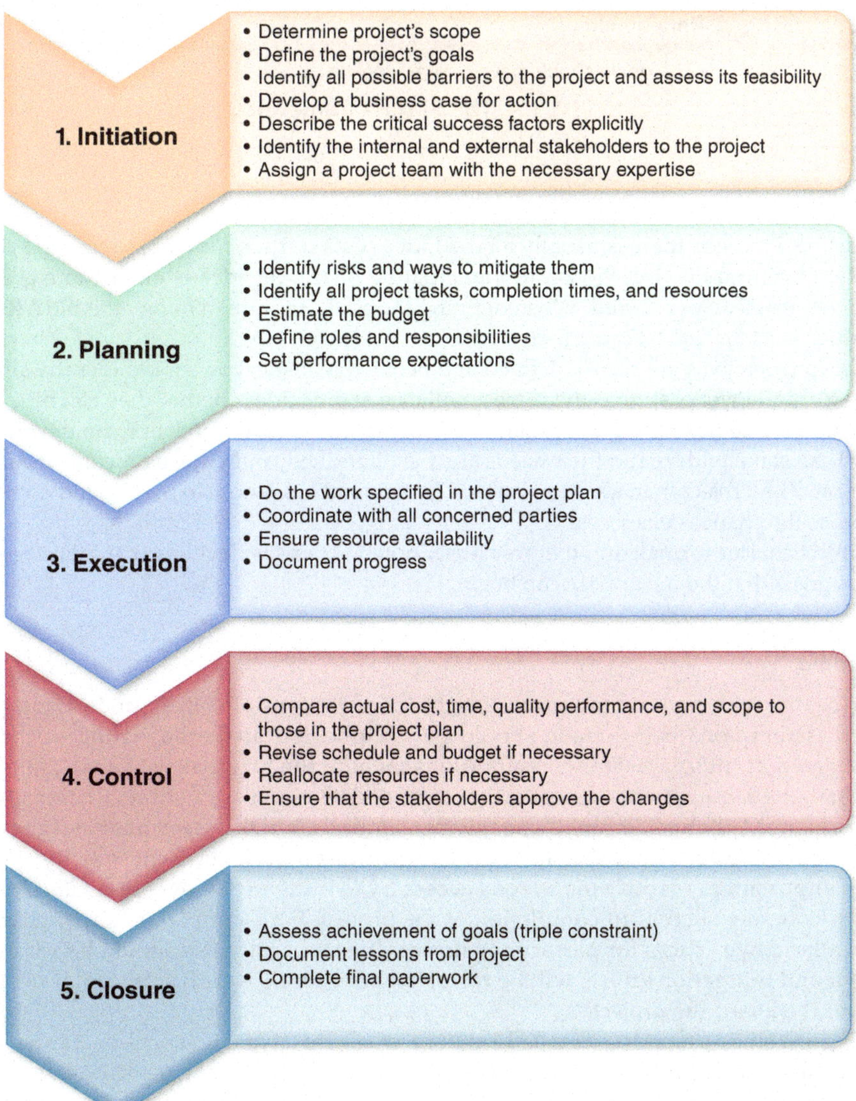

FIGURE 5.3 The five phases of project management.

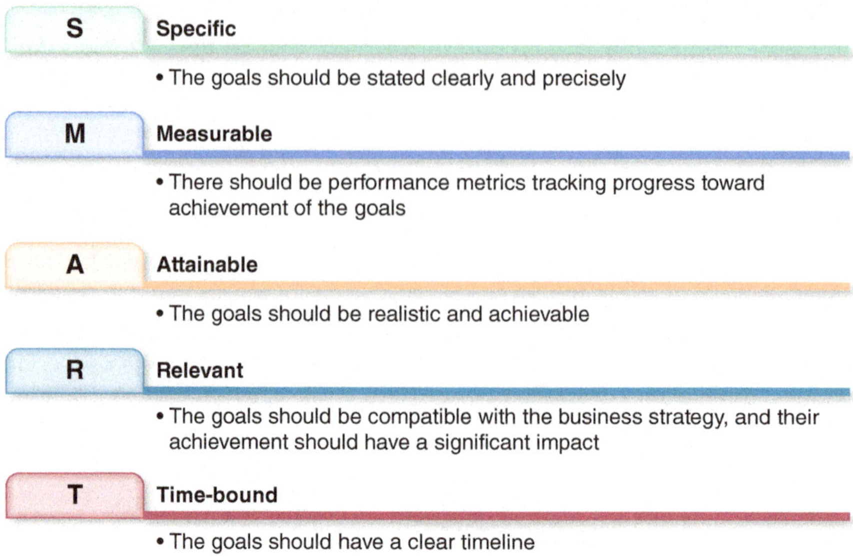

FIGURE 5.4 The SMART framework.

INITIATION

Before starting a project, there is usually a broad idea of its purpose and objectives (e.g., decrease the number of central line infections). In the initiation phase, the idea is made more precise and the objectives are clearly specified. When defining the goals, be sure to follow the **SMART framework** (Baluch & Main, 2022; Figure 5.4):

Once the project goals are clearly defined and deemed realistic, you should identify all the constraints (e.g., high-level cost) that the project will face and decide whether they can be overcome. If so, a business case describing the project's benefits and the cost of inaction are developed (see Chapter 3). All stakeholders and their needs are then identified, and critical outcome measures are agreed upon. The project manager then selects team members whose expertise and commitment will optimize the chances of success.

The project charter formalizing the previously noted actions is developed at this stage, and its approval signals that the next phase can begin.

PLANNING

Planning begins with a clear understanding of the objectives and their underlying assumptions. The assumptions being made should be documented at the beginning of the project and revalidated at intervals. These assumptions include the external risks that can affect the project, changing requirements, use of technology, and even government regulations. A SWOT analysis (Chapter 1) helps identify those threats. Similarly, a **risk assessment assignment matrix** (Figure 5.5) helps visualize the significance of various risks in terms of severity and probability. It is important to identify the actions necessary to mitigate the likelihood and/or impact of those risks on the successful completion of the project. For example, if construction delays occurred, alternative spaces for performing normal business activities should be secured. Risk assessment and mitigation efforts will be reviewed periodically—and adjusted, if necessary—throughout the life of the project.

Planning involves preparing detailed outlines of all the work that will be carried out, including people, roles, and other resource estimates. Because typical projects are large in scope, planners break down the project into identifiable, manageable parts. The **work breakdown structure (WBS)** is a hierarchical organization of a project's components at various levels of detail.

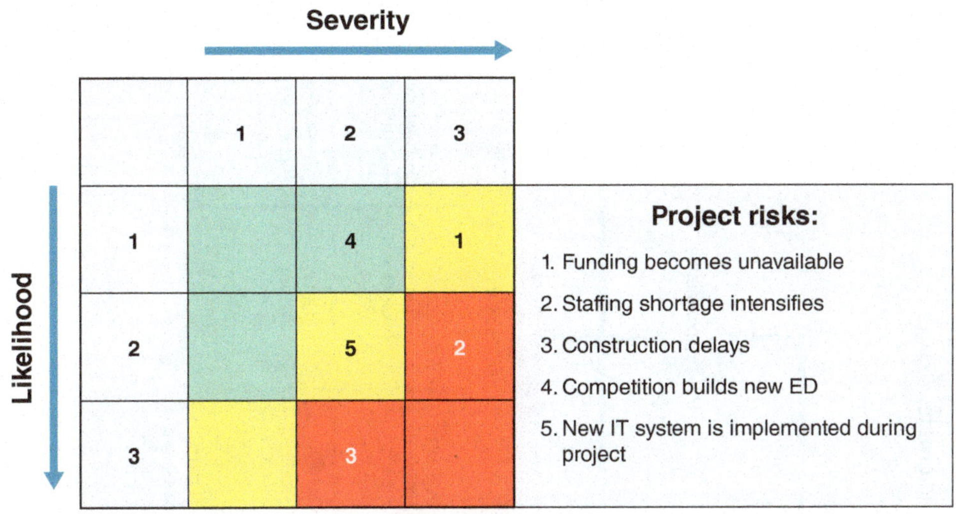

FIGURE 5.5 Risk assessment assignment matrix for BAMC's ED throughput improvement project.

Abbreviation: IT, information technology.

It helps the planner to identify all the work requirements of a project and to organize them in a logical fashion. The first step in developing a WBS is to identify the main modules of the project (Figure 5.6, Level 2). Next, these modules are divided into the major activities that need to be carried out to finish the module (Level 3). In turn, these major activities are subdivided into the activities (Level 4) required to complete them. Further breakdowns at higher levels of detail can also be performed if deemed necessary.

Once all activities have been identified, it is important to establish their sequence and estimate their individual completion times. Visual tools can be developed to chart the scheduling of activities and/or resources. One popular tool is the **Gantt chart**. A Gantt chart is a horizontal bar graph. Each bar corresponds to a specific activity, and its length indicates the duration of the activity. The Gantt chart displays important information, which includes (Russell & Taylor, 2023; Stevenson, 2021):

1. **The activities to be performed**. In the Gantt chart shown in Figure 5.7, we chose to display all Level 4 activities, but we could have elected to show a higher project view with Level 3 activities.
2. **The order in which they must be performed**. You will note that some activities must be completed sequentially, whereas others can be performed in parallel, that is, at the same time. For example, floorplan improvement opportunities can only be identified after the workflow analysis findings have been compiled and the flexibility of the floorplan has been assessed, but training for customer service can start at the same time as training for service recovery.
3. **Their expected durations**. In our example, credentialing is expected to last 6 weeks, whereas the completion of a spaghetti diagram should take 4 weeks.
4. **The estimated date of project completion**. Because certain activities can be performed in parallel (i.e., simultaneously), the project's duration is not equal to the sum of all the activity times. Rather, the project is expected to take 22 weeks or 110 work days to complete.

During the execution and control phases, project managers can use Gantt charts to monitor the progress of each activity by comparing planned progress to actual progress and react accordingly. They can incorporate "traffic light" flagging systems to keep everyone aware of what is happening and what problems may be developing: on track (green), at risk of falling behind (yellow), and behind (red) (Chapter 13, Figure 13.10).

Although appropriate for displaying simple projects with a relatively small number of activities, Gantt charts are, however, quite limited in their ability to capture the interrelationships

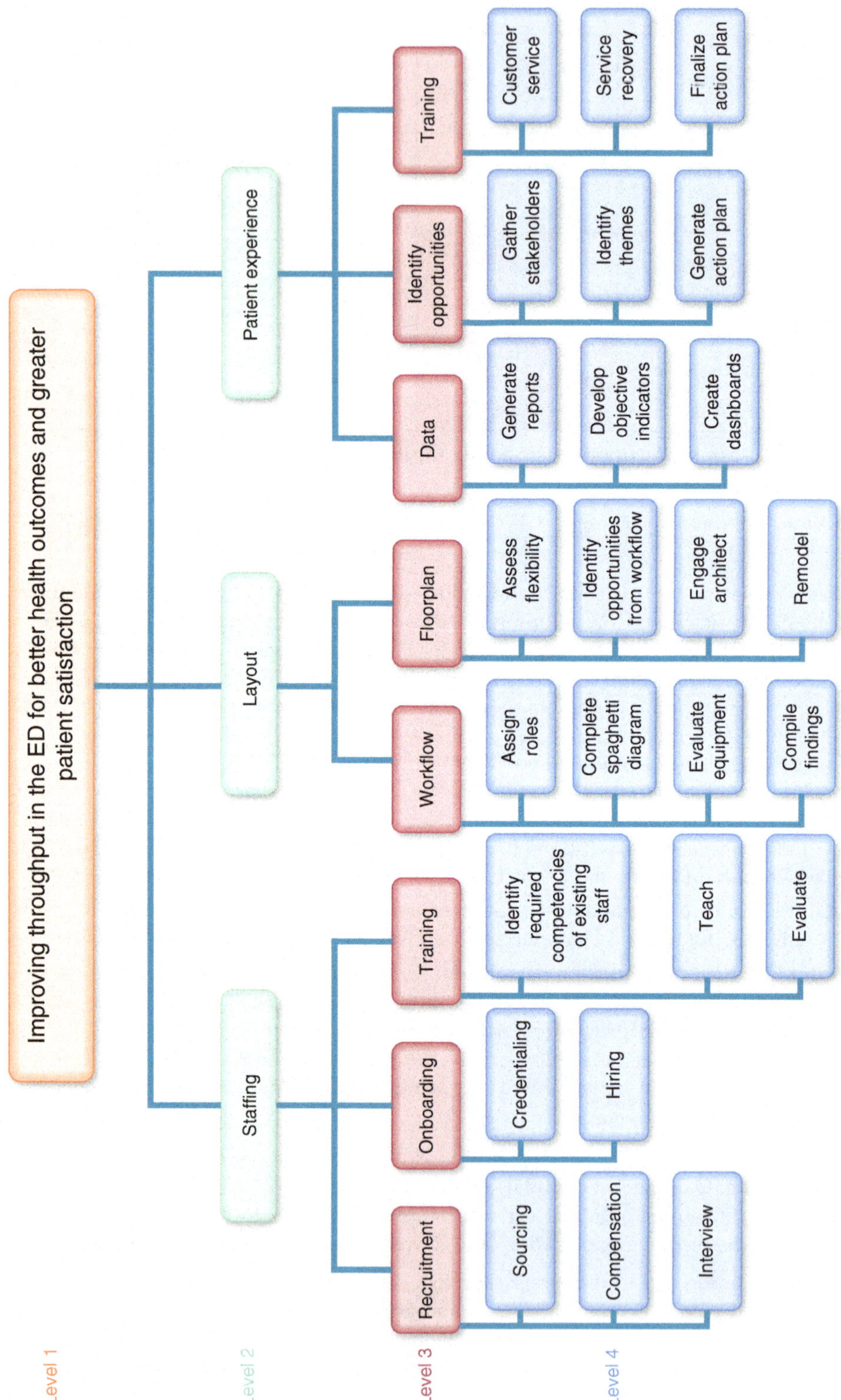

FIGURE 5.6 WBS for Bright Angel's ED throughput improvement project.

Abbreviation: WBS, work breakdown structure.

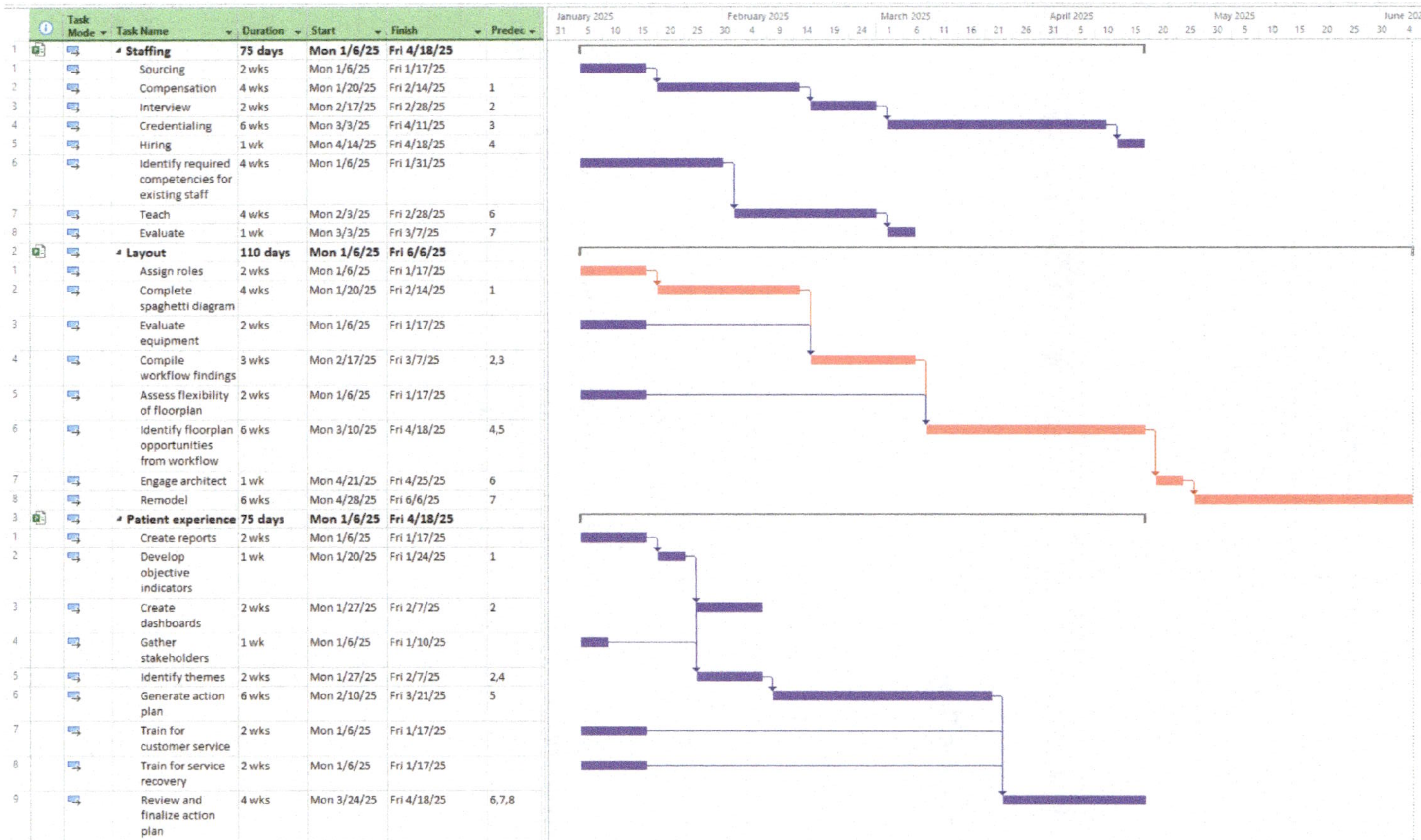

FIGURE 5.7 Gantt chart for Bright Angel Medical Center's ED throughput improvement project.

Note: Critical activities are displayed in red.

among activities that can arise in more complex projects. In such situations, more advanced project management tools are preferred.

Listing all the resources (people, materials, and supplies) needed to perform the project activities enables the development of accurate budgets, which then constitute a common frame of reference as well as a benchmark during the execution phase. The **project plan** is a roadmap intended to communicate to all concerned parties within the organization what is going to happen and when and establish performance specifications. It attempts to eliminate crises by preventing issues from falling through the cracks, and it decreases conflict by showing participants what changes need to be made. If there is disagreement regarding the project plan, it is best to settle matters before the project begins.

Planning is a rigorous process that must be systematic but flexible enough to handle unique situations. The project manager is key to creating an effective plan and ensuring that project team members thoroughly understand their responsibilities while being capable of handling inputs from diverse groups.

ON THE JOB! INTERVIEW VIDEO 5.1

Liliana Mathis
Nursing and Patient Care Manager

Creating Sustainable Change
Gantt chart
Constraints
Facilitating communication
Change management
Creating a safe space for everyone

1. Liliana shows a Gantt chart. What does she share as the most important part of her role in crafting these types of tools?
2. Scope, cost, time, and quality are typically the main variables that project managers need to juggle. According to Liliana, what are some other keys to successful project management?
3. Liliana utilizes a tool to foster conversation and create the safe space needed for an open dialogue about the project. What is it?

The interview is available online by visiting www.springerpub.com/courseconnect. See inside front cover and tear-out card for CourseConnect details.

EXECUTION

"Vision without execution is hallucination" (Thomas Edison, n.d.). The execution phase involves doing the work to deliver the product or desired outcome, and it is the hard part. One of the most common mistakes that project managers make at this stage is letting the project goals shift (i.e., scope creep). When scope creep is allowed to happen, the outputs of the initiation and planning phases are no longer relevant, and these must be reworked. Effective communication and coordination among concerned parties are crucial during execution. Resources should be made available when needed, client satisfaction should be confirmed, and progress should be documented. Unpredictable events will occur, new information will emerge, and requests for change will be made. The project manager must address and resolve these issues in a timely fashion and, if needed, revise the plan accordingly (Donato, 2022).

CONTROL

This phase runs simultaneously with the execution phase and is focused on systematic monitoring and ensuring that the project stays on track. If problems develop, troubleshooting can help determine where the project went off track. Are people not being held accountable for their tasks? Are the project's assumptions still in line? Have circumstances changed that require a change in the project plan? When assessing the triple constraint (Figure 5.1), it is important to determine whether the actual expenditures, work schedule, resource requirements, and output quality vary from the planning document. A **variance** is any deviation (schedule, technical performance, cost, etc.) from the project plan. Early identification of variances can allow the plan to get back on track through schedule revision and/or reallocation of resources.

The very act of measuring progress and communicating it to stakeholders motivates team members to focus on results. It is human nature to complete tasks when monitored. The question to be asked is, Are we on track to complete the project as planned? If not, why? What do we need to do to get back on course? (Aston, 2023)

CLOSURE

Projects must come to an end. This is the time to reflect and learn from what happened during the project. "What did we do right? What could have been done better? Did we achieve the desired quality result? Did we achieve our goal within the time frame and with the resources allocated?" In other words, did we achieve our goals within the "triple constraint"? Incorporating a process of intentional and disciplined project review will impact the success of later projects as project managers and team members will want to improve their performance in the future (Kissflow, 2023).

You must have heard of countless projects that were late and well over budget. This is often the result of poor planning, scheduling, and/or control. Fortunately, the **critical path method (CPM)** facilitates a project manager's job during those phases.

THE CRITICAL PATH METHOD

DuPont developed practices to help manage the Manhattan Project. This work was the precursor to the CPM, a powerful technique to plan and schedule project activities as well as identify those that are critical to timely project completion. In the 1950s, Morgan Walker of DuPont and James Kelley of Remington Rand started developing project scheduling algorithms at DuPont. They used plant shutdowns as pilot projects. In their first paper, they explained the need for rigorous tools to manage project complexity, which separated the functions of planning and scheduling (Kelley & Walker, 1959). Around the same time, Lockheed, the U.S. Navy, and the consulting firm of Booz, Allen, and Hamilton developed the program evaluation and review technique (PERT) to plan the complex Polaris Missile Project. Although they were developed separately for different purposes, both techniques shared a lot of common features, leading many users to "merge" the two techniques (PERT/CPM). In fact, Kelley attributed the term *critical path* to PERT's developers. Used together, the techniques provide (Heizer et al., 2023):

- a graphic display of all activities and their interrelationships
- an activity schedule
- an estimate of the duration of the project
- a list of the activities critical to the timely completion of the project
- an estimate of the time by which an activity can be delayed without delaying the entire project

THE NETWORK DIAGRAM

The graphic display of the project is known as the **network diagram** or precedence diagram. It depicts the project activities and their precedence relationships. Nodes (○) represent activities that are connected by arrows (→). Only activities take time and consume resources. Figure 5.8 illustrates common precedence relationships.

To introduce the development of a network diagram and the CPM technique, we focused solely on the longest process in the ED throughput improvement project: upgrade the layout. Based on the relationships shown in the Gantt chart (Figure 5.7) and specified more explicitly in Table 5.2, the network diagram shown in Figure 5.9 was developed. It has a Start node at the beginning and a Finish node at the end.

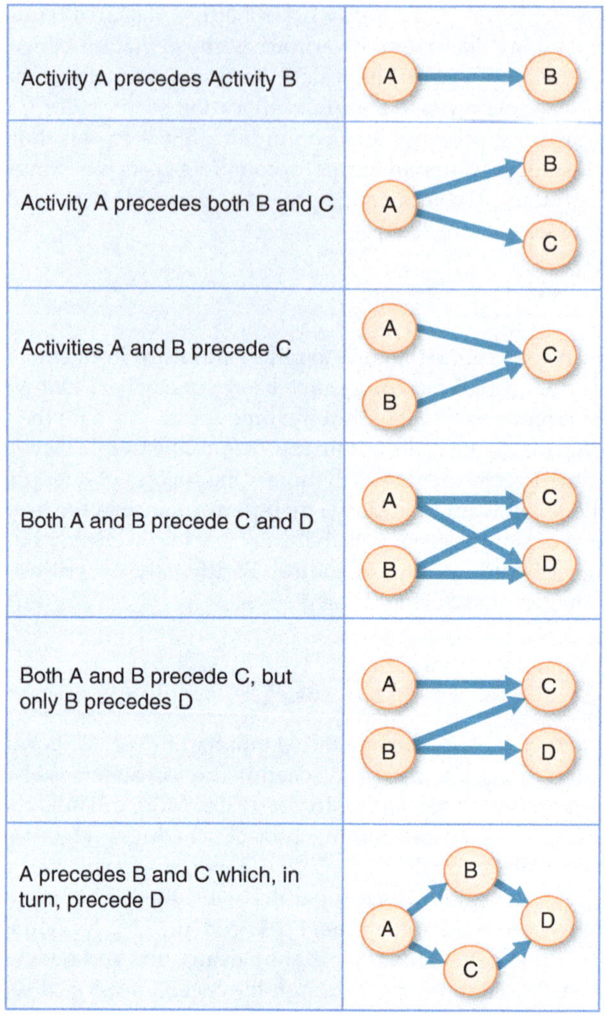

FIGURE 5.8 Examples of precedence relationships.

TABLE 5.2 PRECEDENCE RELATIONSHIPS FOR LAYOUT IMPROVEMENT IN THE ED

Activity	Description	Immediate Predecessor(s)	Estimated Duration (wks)
A	Assign roles.	-	2
B	Evaluate equipment.	-	2
C	Assess layout flexibility.	-	2
D	Complete spaghetti diagram.	A	4
E	Compile findings.	B, D	3
F	Identify opportunities from workflow.	C, E	6
G	Engage architect.	F	1
H	Remodel.	G	6

THE CRITICAL PATH

There are multiple paths in a typical network diagram. A **path** is a sequence of activities from the starting node to the ending node. In Figure 5.9, there are three paths:

1. A-D-E-F-G-H
2. B-E-F-G-H
3. C-F-G-H

The duration of a path is determined by summing the expected times of the activities on that path. Delaying one activity on a path will prolong the duration of the path. The longest path on a network is of special relevance because it determines the entire project's duration. Delays on this path would delay the entire project. Because the longest path is critical to on-time project completion, it is appropriately called the **critical path**, and the activities along the path are **critical activities**. Shorter paths can experience some delays and not affect the on-time completion of the project as long as their final completion times do not exceed that of the critical path. The amount of time by which an activity can be delayed without delaying the entire project is referred to as **slack**. Critical activities have no slack as they cannot be delayed (Box 5.2).

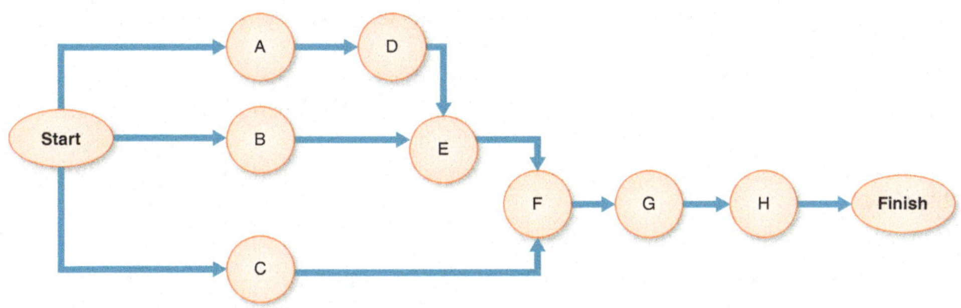

FIGURE 5.9 Network diagram of layout improvement process.

BOX 5.2 FAQs

Do critical activities have a special status?

Only the delay of the critical activities will delay the project. In complex projects with thousands of activities, limited resources make it impossible to monitor each one very closely to ensure that it does not get delayed. Focusing on the critical path is an efficient way of monitoring the project. That being said, it would be wrong to assume that complacency about the progress of noncritical activities is tolerable. When noncritical activities experience delays exceeding their slack, they delay the project as well.

- Path A-D-E-F-G-H: 2 + 4 + 3 + 6 + 1 + 6 = 22 weeks*
- Path B-E-F-G-H = 2 + 3 + 6 + 1 + 6 = 18 weeks
- Path C-F-G-H = 2 + 6 + 1 + 6 = 15 weeks

  *Critical path

At 22 weeks, path A-D-E-F-G-H is the longest and therefore the critical path. Improving the layout of the ED is expected to take 22 weeks at a minimum. Path B-E-F-G-H can be delayed by up to 4 weeks, and path C-F-G-H by up to 7 weeks, without affecting the duration of the project.

The network displayed in Figure 5.9 is quite simple and includes only eight activities. Real projects may involve dozens of paths with hundreds or even thousands of activities. In such cases, it becomes unrealistic to try to identify each path and its duration accurately. The CPM methodology offers a much more efficient way of identifying the critical path and the slack of each activity on the network. It also produces an activity schedule by indicating when an activity should start and end.

THE ACTIVITY SCHEDULE

Remember that some activities could be delayed without delaying the entire project. This means that they could start as soon as possible or later. The notion of earliest and latest start time—and, by extension, finish time—of an activity is the basic premise of the algorithm used to schedule activities. This algorithm includes two passes through the network: the forward pass and the backward pass.

The **forward pass** involves the scheduling of activities from the Start node to the Finish node. It requires the computation of the earliest start (ES) and earliest finish (EF) times of each activity on the network.

ES = earliest time an activity can start if all preceding activities have begun at their earliest possible time.

- If an activity has no immediate predecessor, its ES is 0.
- If an activity has one immediate predecessor, its ES is equal to the EF of its predecessor.
- If an activity has multiple immediate predecessors, its ES is equal to the longest of the EF times of its predecessors:

  ES = maximum (EF times of all immediate predecessors) [5.1]

  EF = earliest time an activity can finish = ES + activity time [5.2]

  In our example, A, B, and C are not preceded by any activity:

  $ES_A = 0$

  $EF_A = 0 + 2 = 2$ weeks

  $ES_B = 0$

  $EF_B = 0 + 2 = 2$ weeks

  $ES_C = 0$

  $EF_C = 0 + 2 = 2$ weeks

As soon as Activity A has been completed, Activity D can start. In other words, its ES time is equal to the EF of its predecessor, Activity A.

$ES_D = EF_A = 2$ weeks

$EF_D = 2 + 4 = 6$ weeks

Activity E is dependent on the completion of *both* Activities B and D. In other words, it cannot start until both activities are finished. Activity B will be finished in Week 2, but Activity D will only be finished in Week 6. Therefore, Activity E cannot start until Week 6.

$ES_E = \text{maximum}(EF_B, EF_D) = 6$ weeks

$EF_E = 6 + 3 = 9$ weeks

It is common to display the ES and EF times of an activity on its node (Figure 5.10).

After the forward pass (Figure 5.11), the EF time of the last activity, Activity H, connecting to the Finish node is 22 weeks. Consequently, the project of upgrading the layout of the ED is

Early start	Duration	Early finish
	Task name	
Late start	Slack	Late finish

FIGURE 5.10 Notation in nodes.

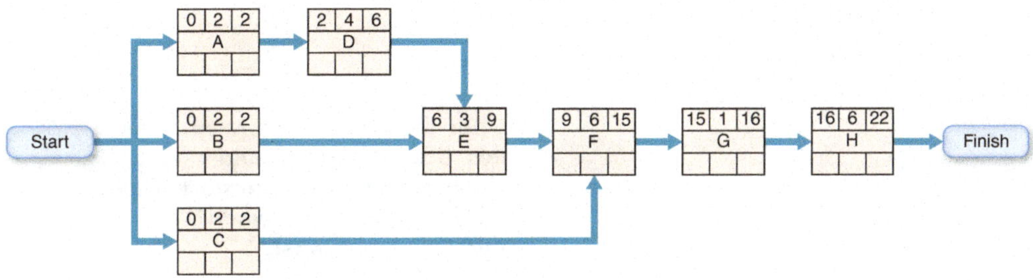

FIGURE 5.11 Earliest start and finish times.

expected to last 22 weeks. If there had been two activities converging in the Finish node, let's say Activities H and Z, and their respective EF times had been 22 and 25 weeks, respectively, the expected project completion time would have been 25 weeks because Activity Z would have had to be completed before the project could be completed. The primary output of the forward pass is the expected project completion time. However, the critical path is still unknown. To determine the activities that are critical, a backward pass through the network is necessary.

The **backward pass** through the network involves scheduling activities from the Finish node to the Start node. While performing this pass, the latest finish (LF) and latest start (LS) times of each activity are computed. Because we go "backwards," the LF time of an activity is computed before its LS time.

LF = latest time at which an activity can finish without delaying the project.

- If an activity has no immediate follower on the network, its LF is equal to the expected project completion time.
- If an activity has one immediate follower, its LF is equal to the LS of its follower.
- If an activity has multiple immediate followers, its LF is equal to the lowest of the LS times of all its followers:

LF = minimum (LS of all immediate followers) [5.3]

LS = latest time at which an activity can start without delaying the project

= LF – activity time [5.4]

In our example, only Activity H has no follower. Its LF time is therefore set equal to the expected project completion time, or 22 weeks. If there had been two activities, let's say Activity H and Activity Z, converging to the Finish node and their respective finish times had been 22 and 25, then the LF times of both Activities H and Z would have been 25 weeks. The explanation is simple: Activity H could end as early as in Week 22, but if it ends in Week 25, it will not delay the project because the project is expected to take 25 weeks to complete anyway (Box 5.3).

$LF_H = 22$ weeks

$LS_H = 22 - 6 = 16$ weeks

BOX 5.3 FAQs

Why is an activity's ES time equal to the *longest* of the EF times of its predecessors whereas the LF time is equal to the *shortest* of the successors?

Let's explain with an example.

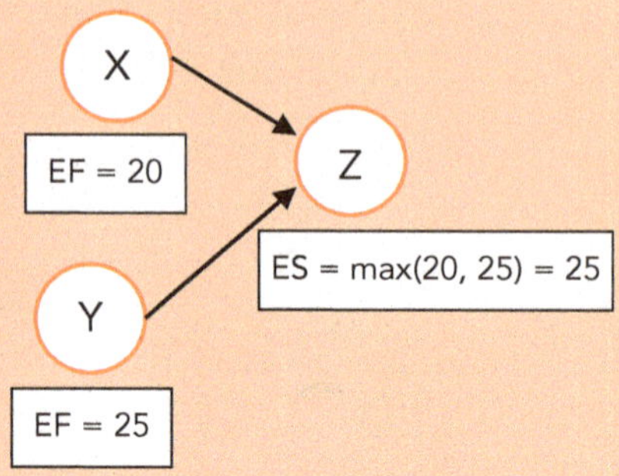

As per the precedence relationship rules, both X and Y would have to be completed before Z can start. Therefore, Z can only start when Y is finished (i.e., at 25 wks).

Now, let's look at the example that follows.

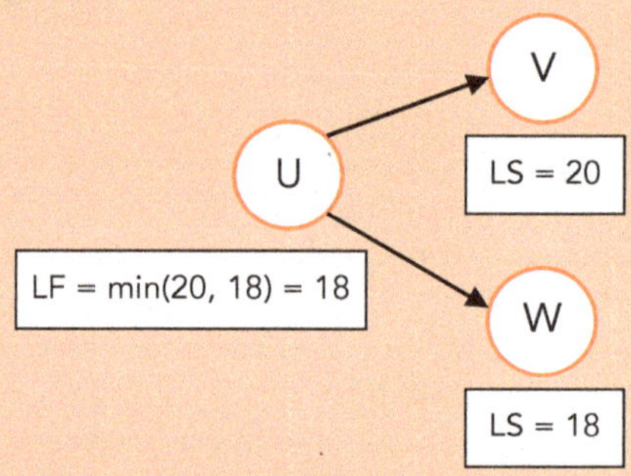

As per the precedence relationship rules, V and W could not start until U is completed. If W can start in week 18, it means that U had to be finished.

Abbreviations: EF, earliest finish; ES, earliest start; LF, latest finish; LS, latest start.

Based on the precedence rules, we know that Activity G has to be completed before Activity H can start. If Activity H has an LS at 16 weeks, it means that Activity G could have ended at that time.

$LF_G = LS_H = 16$ weeks

$LS_G = 16 - 1 = 15$ weeks

Applying the same rule to the predecessor of Activity G, we find:

$LF_F = LS_G = 15$ weeks

$LS_F = 15 - 6 = 9$ weeks

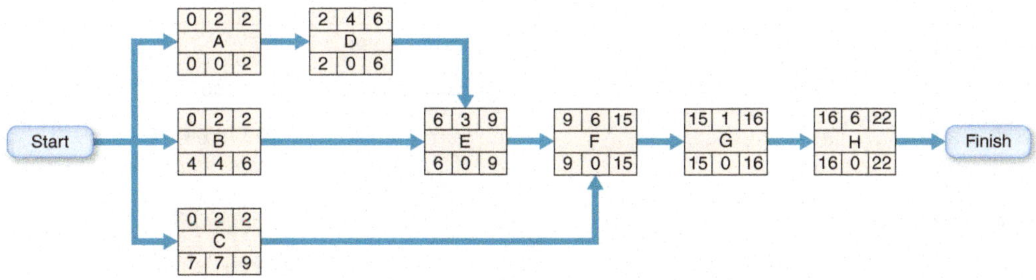

FIGURE 5.12 Latest start and finish times.

Note that Activity F follows both C and E, which means that both Activities C and E had to be completed before F could start. Because F had a late start in Week 9, the LF times of Activities C and E are 9 weeks as well.

$LF_C = LS_F = 9$ weeks

$LS_E = LS_F = 9$ weeks

After performing the backward pass, you will get a more detailed picture of how to schedule activities and monitor their progress (Figure 5.12). You will know, for example, that Activity C can start as early as Week 0, but it could start as late as Week 7 and not delay the project, assuming it does not take longer than 2 weeks to complete. In other words, Activity C has 7 weeks of slack time.

COMPUTING SLACK

What about the critical path? Remember that critical activities have zero slack. To compute slack, you need the numbers computed in the forward pass and in the backward pass:

$$S = LF - EF \quad [5.5]$$

or

$$S = LS - ES \quad [5.6]$$

Based on these computations, the Activities A-D-E-F-G-H make up the critical path, which is expected to take 22 weeks to complete. Table 5.3 displays the ES, EF, LS, LF, and S for each activity, as well as a summary of the computations.

TABLE 5.3 SUMMARY OF FORWARD AND BACKWARD PASSES

Activity	ES	t (wks)	EF	LS	LF	S
A	0	2	2	0	2	0*
B	0	2	2	4	6	4
C	0	2	2	7	9	7
D	2	4	6	2	6	0*
E	6	3	9	6	9	0*
F	9	6	15	9	15	0*
G	15	1	16	15	16	0*
H	16	6	22	16	22	0*

(continued)

TABLE 5.3 SUMMARY OF FORWARD AND BACKWARD PASSES (*CONTINUED*)

Forward pass	Backward pass
For each activity beginning from the Start node, ES = 0 For all other activities, ES = EF of immediate predecessor EF = ES + t If an activity has multiple predecessors, ES = maximum (EF times of immediate predecessors) Expected project completion time = longest EF time of activities ending at the Finish node.	For each activity ending at the Finish node, LF = expected project completion time. For all other activities, LF = LS of immediate follower LS = LF − t If an activity has multiple followers, LF = minimum (LS times of immediate followers)
Slack = LF-EF *or* LS-ES	

Abbreviations: EF, earliest finish; ES, earliest start; LF, latest finish; LS, latest start.
Note: *Critical activities.

BRIGHT ANGEL MEDICAL CENTER 5.4

Adeleke Mensah, the project manager, opened the team's first meeting by welcoming everyone and briefly explaining why he asked them to come together. "The board is on board, so to speak! And we have strong executive support for this project. Everyone feels it is a worthy effort and that the timeline and cost are reasonable. As you know, this project is three-pronged, but the timely redesign of the layout and of the processes and subprocesses patients go through is most critical to an on-time completion. Let's discuss ways to ensure that we will meet this objective. I'd like to hear everyone's input into this matter."

Barbara started, "We have a clear project plan. Let's make sure that we review it frequently and stick to it."

Dr. Aoki opined, "I agree. We should probably meet once a week and make sure we stay on track and address issues."

Adeleke added, "All good suggestions. I'll ask my assistant to set up a meeting schedule for all of us. Also, all project materials will be in a folder accessible by all of you on our team collaboration system. All our meetings will be transcribed word-for-word for proper documentation of what we discussed."

Ali Hussein, the patient experience manager, inquired, "When an activity is delayed, what shall we do?"

Adeleke replied, "Hustle and catch up. That costs money in extra resources, so let's try to avoid getting there."

The team discussed other specific issues such as accountability for complex tasks and agreed it was time to walk through the ED and follow the patient through the path.

Why is it important for the project team to review the project plan on a regular basis?

EVALUATING THE CRITICAL PATH METHOD

Before using CPM, project managers must be aware of both their pros and cons.

ADVANTAGES

1. The technique forces project managers to organize the project information in a logical fashion and quantify it.
2. The network diagram provides a graphic display of the project and its activities. It is a common point of reference for all the parties involved in the project.
3. The technique is not overly complex and can be learned easily (Note: Project management software does most of the work!).
4. Knowledge of the critical activities enables the project manager to (a) monitor closely the activities whose delay would postpone the completion of the entire project and (b) potentially allow delays for those activities that have slack. Resources can be allocated and managed accordingly.

DISADVANTAGES

1. It is sometimes impossible to identify all activities, especially in complex projects. Omissions will emerge and may require a substantial modification of the schedule.
2. Time estimates are just that: estimates. They tend to be subjective and could be quite inaccurate—fudge factor—for first-time endeavors.
3. There is a tendency to focus too much on the critical path and overlook other paths that are near critical or become critical as a result of delays.

WHY PROJECTS FAIL

Planning is never perfect, execution is difficult, and sometimes projects fail (Box 5.4). Failure can occur at any of the steps in the process. Major reasons for failure are as follows (Kerzner, 2022):

- **Goals are not understood throughout the organization.** If others within the organization do not know or understand the objectives of the project, it may be difficult to obtain the resources (people, time, money) needed to complete the project. Also, others may inadvertently interfere with the project team and may make decisions that prevent the goals from being achieved.

BOX 5.4 QUALITY IN PRACTICE!

Learning From a Failed Tech Pilot at Stanford Health Care

About 70% of hospital IT pilots are unsuccessful. Two nurse leaders from Stanford Health Care candidly discussed this topic at a conference and argued that IT project failures are bound to happen and provide opportunities to learn important lessons. They described a failed health IT pilot at Stanford that was supposed to allow inpatients to control their in-room technology at every touchpoint (e.g., call the nurse, view the menu, etc.). The rationale for providing patients with these devices was to give them the ability to contact nurses directly and bypass the inefficient steps of calling the unit secretary, who would then locate the next nurse available. Unfortunately, most devices remained unused. Patients did not know how to use them, and already overextended nurses did not have time to show them how to do so. They discontinued the pilot and realized that, in the future, similar innovations would have to be compatible with nurses' workflows and capacity (Adams, 2023).

- **There is a misalignment of the organization's strategy and the goals of the project.** If the organization is going one way and the project team is going another way, the project will fail. There needs to be a common purpose within the organization for projects to be successful.
- **Timelines are unrealistic.** If a project timeline does not take into account the realization that team members have other responsibilities, project milestones will be missed. It is discouraging for team members to be asked to do things that are impossible to do. Lack of commitment and disengagement will occur and the project will fail.
- **Resources are not available.** If team members do not have the tools (time, people, funds, expertise, etc.) to do the work, the project will fail. It is important to define what is really needed to do the work and communicate the need to the executive sponsors of the project. If resources are not available, it is better not to even start the project.
- **Planning is poor.** If the project plan is not realistic and does not have the necessary resources allocated, it will not succeed. Realistic planning is the most important step in project management.
- **Rigorous project management methodology is not followed.** If appropriate tools are not applied, it becomes more difficult to monitor tasks and predict time and cost overruns. Visual displays, such as the traffic light flagging system, make it easier for team members to see how completion of their tasks impacts completion of the overall project. If appropriate tools are not available, project managers lose sight of what needs to be done, and deadlines are missed.
- **Inadequate communication, progress tracking, and reporting.** If the project manager is not monitoring progress, communicating with their team and executive sponsors when milestones are met or unmet, and harnessing the necessary resources to be successful, the project will fail.

TEAM DYNAMICS AND COMMUNICATION

Other major reasons for failure are culture clash (Box 5.5) and poor team dynamics. Understanding what is happening within a team and being able to identify what is not working are important. In his book, *The Five Dysfunctions of a Team*, Lencioni (2002) describes how the following issues can destroy successful project management:

- absence of trust (Box 5.5)
- fear of conflict
- lack of commitment
- avoidance of accountability
- inattention to results

Effective communication is very difficult to achieve. Different people can view the same message in different ways. People tend to remember details of discussions when they are interested in the topic, but quickly forget them if they do not care about the issue. People come into discussions with preconceived notions about what will be said and do not actually listen to what the speaker is trying to communicate. Ambiguity makes us hear what we want to hear. Therefore, do not assume that the message that you are communicating always gets through to a group or that decisions made within a group will be remembered several weeks later. Taking accurate minutes of the meetings and sending them to the group within a week can help people refresh their memories and ask for clarifications. Also, meeting transcripts documenting what was actually said (word for word) are very helpful in ensuring open, honest discussions. Communication goes many ways. A project manager must communicate upward to the executives who are interested in the project; laterally to peers, groups in functional areas, and stakeholders; and downward to others in the project office or at the operational level.

In any situation in which people with different perspectives work together, conflict should be expected. Conflict is a normal and necessary part of a healthy interaction and, if handled properly,

BOX 5.5 QUALITY IN PRACTICE!

Most Mergers and Acquisitions Fail Due to a Clash of Cultures

In today's highly competitive healthcare environment, mergers and acquisitions are a fact of life. Statistics indicate that the volume of acquisitions in 2018 was up 14.4% (Lagasse, 2019). Typically, mergers and acquisitions serve one of two purposes: (1) operational efficiencies or (2) negotiating clout (Pearl, 2018). Unfortunately, the majority of the mergers and acquisitions fail to deliver the efficiencies expected, and negotiating clout results in increased prices. For example, the merger between Dignity Health and Catholic Health Initiatives in 2018 created one of the nation's largest nonprofit health systems. The combined entity, CommonSpirit, a $29 billion operation, did not consolidate any of their hospitals and posted a $582 million loss following the merger, likely resulting in increased prices (Reed, 2020). Why is it so difficult to realize operational efficiencies? The majority of merger shortfalls are due to human factors. "Culture clash" happens when two organizations' styles, values, and habits are in conflict. As Barak Richman at Duke University said, "Every place has its own flavor, and when hospitals try to integrate, you are mixing flavors. . . . Any new power structure [that] institute[s] changes in the way medicine is practiced, [causes] natural pushback. That's why it's difficult to meaningfully integrate health systems" (Ramm, 2019).

can engender energy and excitement and lead to a better outcome. Unfortunately, conflict can also be destructive and lead to hard feelings and a dysfunctional process. When conflict is mismanaged, it can harm relationships and sidetrack a project. But when handled in a respectful and positive way, conflict provides an opportunity to build trust and gain a deeper understanding of the issue as well as the person involved in the conflict. Learning to manage your emotions and to be willing to confront conflicts is addressed in *Crucial Conversations: Tools for Talking When Stakes Are High* (Grenny et al., 2021). What is a crucial conversation? According to the authors, it is a discussion between two or more people in which (a) the stakes are high, (b) opinions vary, and (c) emotions are strong. There are several concepts that are important to keep in mind when dealing with highly charged situations:

- Conflicts escalate when ignored.
- Individuals respond to conflicts based on their perceptions of the situation, not necessarily an objective review of the facts.
- Conflicts trigger strong emotions.
- Conflicts are an opportunity for growth.

Good project management is difficult. Future leaders will be those who can harness the skills of groups and solve tough problems. Good luck with your journey!

ETHICAL SCENARIO 5.1

Personal Relationships in Project Teams

Healthcare providers are people just like everyone else with feelings and emotions. Sometimes, relationships can develop between members of the healthcare team. Workplace romance can create challenges when hierarchy is involved. Managing projects that involve team members who are romantically involved can cause additional difficulties for the team.

What are the potential pitfalls to a romantic relationship developing between two members of a project team?

What can happen if a power gradient exists—for example, if one person is the project lead or at a higher level than the other? Should the couple be transparent about their relationship?

SUMMARY

In this chapter, we discussed the phases of project management: initiation, planning, execution, control, and closure. We also discussed the roles that people must play in order to have a successful project outcome. Tools, such as the WBS, Gantt charts, and CPM, that are used to help plan, schedule, and control projects were discussed in detail. You also learned why projects fail and how project managers and team members can take steps to minimize the risks of failure.

CERTIFICATION TIPS

This chapter is closely aligned with what is required for the certification exam. You need to be able to *apply* all the tools. The exam may require you to have knowledge of other tools as well (e.g., process maps in Chapter 6). Furthermore, there might be questions on project documentation beyond what is covered in this book (e.g., RACI matrix): https://www.eclipsesuite.com/project-documentation; https://www.brightwork.com/blog/a-quick-guide-to-9-essential-project-documents; RACI Chart: Definitions, Uses and Examples for Project Managers—Forbes Advisor.

KEY TERMS

Project
Project management
Triple constraint
Project charter
Scope creep
Project manager
Project management office
Project team
Project champion
Force field analysis
SMART framework
Risk assessment assignment matrix
Work breakdown structure (WBS)
Gantt chart
Project plan
Variance
Critical path method (CPM)
Network diagram
Path
Critical path
Critical activities
Slack
Forward pass
Backward pass

REVIEW QUESTIONS

1. What is a project? What are the five phases of a project, and what happens if you do not complete them all?
2. What is the triple constraint, and what does it mean?
3. What is a project charter? What does it include?
4. What are SMART goals?
5. What are the characteristics of good team members?
6. Why is communication so important when managing projects?
7. What is a WBS and what is its purpose?
8. What is a Gantt chart? Why is it used?
9. What is the CPM? Why is it useful?
10. List five reasons why projects fail.
11. Is it recommended to pilot an IT project before deciding on a full implementation? Justify your answer.

SOLVE BRIGHT ANGEL MEDICAL CENTER'S PROBLEMS

All chapter-specific data from the following problems are provided as Excel files which may be accessed via the show supplementary tab (Student Material) available online by visiting www.springerpub.com/courseconnect. See inside front cover and tear-out card for CourseConnect details.

1. The leadership team is considering building a pediatric wing. The project would be expensive, but it has the potential to bring a steady stream of revenue in the next 10 years. The project involves the following risks:

Risks	Likelihood	Severity
1. Competing hospital expands its pediatric services	3	3
2. Major employer in city closes the business	1	1
3. Donors renege on their funding promise	1	3
4. Building expenses exceed estimates	2	2
5. Inability to attract broad range of pediatric specialists	1	2

   a. Develop a risk assessment assignment matrix.
   b. What can be done to mitigate the risks?

2. A team of ICU nurses wants to improve the shift change handover between nurses. They identify the following risks:

Risks	Likelihood	Severity
1. Resistance from existing personnel	1	3
2. Lack of adherence to improved procedures	3	3
3. Staff turnover	3	2
4. Increase in patient-to-nurse ratio	2	3
5. Increase in documentation time	2	2

   a. Develop a risk assessment assignment matrix.
   b. What can be done to mitigate the risks?

3. A group of physicians wants to establish a new protocol. They have identified a list of 13 activities and their precedence relationships to design the protocol, train staff, and implement the new protocol. Draw the appropriate network diagram.

Activity	Immediate Predecessors
A	–
B	A
C	B
D	B
E	C
F	C, D
G	F
H	E, G
I	H
J	H
K	J
L	J
M	K, L

4. The Pathology Department at BAMC has planned a new project involving 18 activities. The activities and their immediate predecessors are listed in the following table. Draw the appropriate network diagram.

Activity	Immediate Predecessors
A	–
B	–
C	B
D	A, B
E	B
F	C
G	D
H	E, F
I	G
J	G
K	I, J
L	H
M	H
N	M
O	M
P	N, O
Q	L
R	K, Q

5. For problem 3, assume the following activity times:

Activity	Time (d)
A	5
B	2
C	4
D	3
E	13
F	8
G	9
H	1
I	4
J	5
K	7
L	2
M	1

Based on this information,

a. Develop a Gantt chart assuming the project starts on the first Monday of March. Assume that no work is performed on weekends.
b. Determine the ES and EF times, the LS and LF times, and slack for each activity.
c. Indicate the critical path and project duration.

6. For problem 4, assume the following activity times:

Activity	Time (wk)
A	6
B	1
C	4
D	2
E	5
F	1
G	3
H	7
I	5
J	3
K	4
L	6
M	1
N	1
O	4
P	3
Q	4
R	2

Based on this,

a. Develop a Gantt chart assuming the project starts on the last Monday of April. Assume that no work is performed on weekends.
b. What are the various paths on the project network? What is their slack?
c. Indicate the critical path(s) and project duration(s).

7. The modification of the scheduling system at BAMC's outpatient rehabilitation clinic involves the following activities and their expected durations.

Activity	Predecessor(s)	Time (d)
A	–	7
B	A	5
C	A	9
D	C	6
E	C	6
F	B	4
G	F	7
H	F	8
I	G, H, D	6
J	E	5

a. Develop a Gantt chart assuming the project starts on the first Monday of October.
b. Determine the ES and EF times, the LS and LF times, and slack for each activity.
c. Indicate the critical path and project duration.
d. If Activity C takes 4 days longer than expected, what is the impact on project scheduling and management?

8. A team of trauma surgeons is concerned about the time it takes to receive blood for transfusions. They have identified all the activities involved in the process, their precedence relationships, and their durations.
   a. Draw the network diagram.
   b. How many paths are there on the network? What is their slack?
   c. How long is this process expected to last?

Activities	Immediate Predecessors	Time (min)
A. Blood transfusion is ordered.	–	1
B. Phlebotomist draws blood sample.	A	38
C. Sample is sent to lab.	B	17
D. Nurse places blood band on patient.	B	3
E. Blood bank identifies blood type and checks for antibodies.	C	12
F. Blood bank cross-checks patient's plasma against red blood cells in blood bank.	E	28
G. Blood bank notifies nursing floor when blood is ready and sends to floor.	F	8
H. Blood is checked by two nurses to confirm patient date of birth.	D, G	21
I. Blood transfusion is performed.	H	60

9. Bright Angel Medical Center's environmental services team wants to reduce patient room turnover times without sacrificing safety and room cleanliness. Their first task involves identifying all the activities necessary to clean and disinfect a room after patient discharge and their respective durations (in minutes). Their efforts led to the following network diagram.

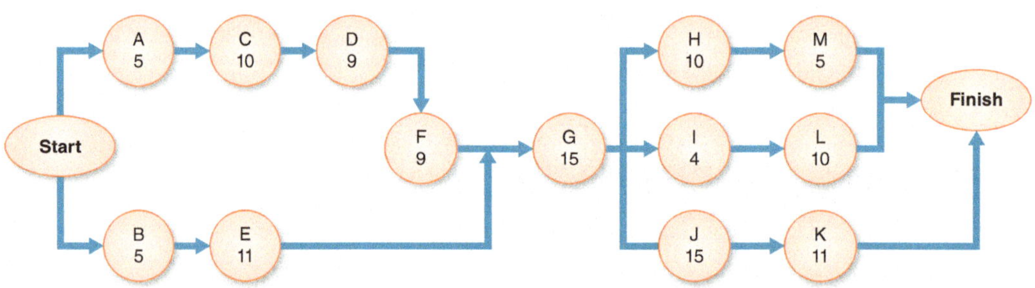

   a. Determine the ES and EF times, the LS and LF times, and slack for each activity, and identify the critical path.
   b. How long does it take to clean and disinfect a room?

LEARNING ACTIVITIES

1. Identify a failed project that is in the news. Why do you think the project failed? Point to specific factors that may have contributed to the failure.
2. What are some reasons that diverse teams may focus more on the facts and process those facts more carefully?
3. Why is it important for the project team to feel a sense of ownership in the project charter?
4. If conflicts develop into a situation where mistrust prevails, would you expect documentation of activities to increase or decrease? Why?
5. In the video, 2018 PMI Project of the Year Award Winner: Southeast Louisiana Veterans Health Care System, by PMI, October 7, 2018: https://www.youtube.com/watch?v=NjQ1Alw4xEg,

veterans and their families were involved in the design of the new healthcare system. How can patients benefit from this approach?

6. Select a potential process improvement in your organization and develop the project charter.
7. Eisenhower (1956) said: "The essence of leadership is to get others to do something because they think you want it done and because they know it is worthwhile doing." Justify this statement.

SPRINGER PUBLISHING CONNECT™ | A robust set of instructor resources designed to supplement this text is located at **http://connect.springerpub.com/content/book/978-0-8261-7976-0.** Qualifying instructors may request access by emailing **textbook@springerpub.com.**

REFERENCES

Adams, K. (2023, April 21). Here's what Stanford learned from a failed tech pilot. *MedCity News*. https://medcitynews.com/2023/04/heres-what-stanford-learned-from-a-failed-tech-pilot

Aston, B. (2023). *What is the project life cycle: The 5 main phases, explained*. The Digital Project Manager. https://thedigitalprojectmanager.com/projects/pm-methodology/project-management-life-cycle

Baluch, A., & Main, K. (2022, August 18). 5 must-know project management phases explained. *Forbes*. https://www.forbes.com/advisor/business/project-management-phases

Collins, R. T., Algaze, C., & Posner, B. Z. (2023). The Leadership/Management Concept Scale: Differentiating between actions constituting leadership and management. *Leadership & Organization Development Journal*, *44*(5), 657–677. https://www.emerald.com/insight/content/doi/10.1108/lodj-06-2022-0299/full/html

Donato, H. (2022, July 31). *5 phases of project management life cycle you need to know*. Project Management.com. https://project-management.com/project-management-phases

Eisenhower, D. D. (1956). *Quotes*. Eisenhower Presidential Library. https://www.eisenhowerlibrary.gov/eisenhowers/quotes

Grenny, J., Patterson, K., McMillan, R., Switzler, A., & Gregory, E. (2021). *Crucial conversations: Tools for talking when stakes are high* (3rd ed.). McGraw-Hill.

Heizer, J., Render, B., & Munson, C. (2023). *Operations management: Sustainability and supply chain management* (14th ed.). Pearson.

Hoban, S. (2023). *Triple constraints of project management: 3 tips & why it matters*. The Digital Project Manager. https://thedigitalprojectmanager.com/projects/scope-management/triple-constraint

Kelley, J. E., Jr., & Walker, M. R. (1959). *Critical-path planning and scheduling*. IRE-AIEE-ACM Conference, New York, NY, United States. https://doi.org/10.1145/1460299.1460318

Kerzner, H. R. (2022). *Project management: A systems approach to planning, scheduling, and controlling* (13th ed.). Wiley.

Kissflow. (2023). *5 phases of project management—A complete breakdown*. Author. https://kissflow.com/project/five-phases-of-project-management

Lagasse, J. (2019, January 28). *Healthcare mergers and acquisitions had record year in 2018, up 14.4 percent*. Healthcare Finance. https://www.healthcarefinancenews.com/news/healthcare-mergers-and-acquisitions-had-record-year-2018-144-percent

Lencioni, P. M. (2002). *The five dysfunctions of a team: A leadership fable*. Jossey-Bass.

Lippi, G., & Mattiuzzi, C. (2019). Project management in laboratory medicine. *Journal of Medical Biochemistry*, *38*(4), 401–406. https://doi.org/10.2478/jomb-2019-0021

Pearl, R. (2018, January 16). Saving America's hospitals: Why recent megamergers will fail. *Forbes*. https://www.forbes.com/sites/robertpearl/2018/01/16/hospitals/#3827d9514b03

Porter, K. (2023). Establishing a project management office. *Forbes*. https://www.forbes.com/sites/forbesbusinesscouncil/2023/03/15/establishing-a-project-management-office/?sh=7ff4b462377d

Project Management for Development Organizations. (2011). *The project constraints.* https://www.pm4dev.com/resources/docman/pm4dev-articles/14-the-project-constraints/file.html

Project Management Institute. (2022). *A guide to the project management body of knowledge (PMBOK® Guide)* (7th ed.). Author.

Ramm, M. (2019, November 25). Culture clash could be to blame for UnityPoint, Sanford Health Merger Halt. *The Gazette.* https://www.thegazette.com/health-care-medicine/culture-clash-could-be-to-blame-for-unitypoint-sanford-health-merger-halt

Reed, T. (2020, January 22). *Lloyd Dean will become the sole CEO of CommonSpirit health.* Fierce Healthcare. https://www.fiercehealthcare.com/hospitals-health-systems/lloyd-dean-will-become-sole-ceo-commonspirit-health

Russell, R. S., & Taylor, B. W. (2023). *Operations and supply chain management* (11th ed.). Wiley.

Stevenson, W. J. (2021). *Operations management* (14th ed.). McGraw-Hill.

Thomas Edison. (n.d.). *50 awesome quotes on vision.* Retrieved August 25 from http://www.ideachampions.com/weblogs/archives/2010/11/50_awesome_quot_1.shtml

van Vooren, N. J. E., Janssen, L. M. S., Drewes, H. W., Baan, C. A., & Bongers, I. M. B. (2023). How to collaborate for health throughout the project timeline—A longitudinal study reflecting on implemented strategies in three projects for a healthy living environment. *BMC Public Health, 23,* 67. https://doi.org/10.1186/s12889-022-14898-9

Wu, G., Zhao, X., Zuo, J., & Zillante, G. (2019). Effects of team diversity on project performance in construction projects. *Engineering, Construction and Architectural Management, 26*(3), 408–423. https://doi.org/10.1108/ECAM-05-2018-0220

PART III

MEASURE—Where Is the Waste and How Bad Is It?

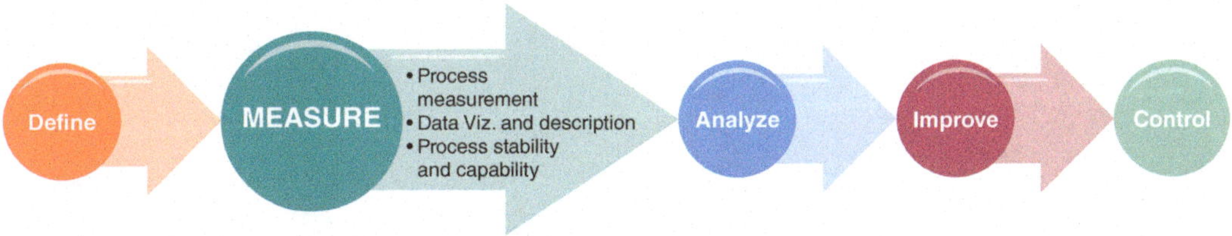

CHAPTER 6

PROCESS MEASUREMENT

BRIGHT ANGEL MEDICAL CENTER 6.1

The project team set aside 2 hours for a focused work session on the ED workflows. It was clear that ED throughput was partially impacted by unavailable hospital inpatient beds, with ED patients waiting longer than necessary to be admitted.

"Hospital throughput is outside the scope of our project. That's something the hospital leadership will have to address," Adeleke stated. "But there are several inefficiencies we can tackle in the ED itself that would shave time off the overall length of stay (LOS). We should identify where waste occurs."

Barbara liked what she was hearing. Now it seemed they were really getting down to business.

To make a real impact, shouldn't they address hospital throughput as well?

LEARNING OBJECTIVES

After reading this chapter, you will be able to:

- Develop a solid data collection plan.
- Distinguish among value-added, non–value-added, and business–value-added activities.
- Build a value stream map (VSM) to pinpoint areas that need improvement.
- Develop a process activity chart and/or a flow process chart to categorize activities and identify value-added and non–value-added steps in a process.
- Determine the efficiency of a process in delivering value.
- Understand the cumulative impact of errors or defects along a process.
- Separate facts from guesses when identifying problem areas.
- See if the facility layout supports the workflow in creating value to the customer.

INTRODUCTION

Once you have defined a dysfunctional process, it is time to identify its flaws. That means finding all the ways in which it fails to contribute value to the customer. This is precisely what you will learn in this chapter. You will view the process as a **value stream**, that is, a series of steps intended to add value for the customer from initial request to final delivery, and you will uncover all the weak links along the chain. Viewing the process from a Lean perspective is the primary objective of this chapter. This perspective will enable you to determine how efficient a process is in delivering value to the customer and to spot the areas needing improvement, namely delays, excessive movements, and errors. The process measurements will also enable you to determine the extent to which variation threatens its predictability and the quality of the outputs it should deliver. Good measurement starts with a good data collection plan.

WHY IS THIS MATERIAL USEFUL?

It is not because we "feel" that a process does not work well that we know how to fix it properly. As Lord Kelvin (2007) famously said, "if you cannot measure it, you cannot improve it." Obtaining process metrics enables us to evaluate multiple aspects of the process and pinpoint specific deficiencies, which should later become the targets of improvement efforts.

COLLECTING DATA

Data collection is the disciplined process of gathering and measuring variables of interest to answer questions, test hypotheses, monitor progress, and make informed decisions (Office of Research Integrity, 2024). In Chapter 4, we talked about capturing the voice of the customer (VOC) and voice of the process (VOP) in general terms. Now, it is time to develop a plan that everyone must follow to ensure data integrity and facilitate analysis later on. Table 6.1 provides the roadmap for this effort.

A CLOSER LOOK AT VALUE-ADDED ACTIVITIES AND WASTE

As you may recall (Chapter 1), value establishes a relationship between quality and cost; it is essentially what the customer of the process is willing to pay for. The process activities meeting or exceeding customers' expectations are therefore considered to add value. They deliver exactly what the customers want, and they do so without wasting time and resources. In Bright Angel

TABLE 6.1 DATA COLLECTION PLAN AND SEQUENCE

Objective	Define the specific purpose of the data collection effort. Identify all the research questions that will need to be answered through data analysis.
What needs to be measured?	Identify the metrics that need to be recorded. Make sure that there is a clear operational definition of each quality indicator (Chapter 4). Determine the level of measurement needed based on the type of analysis that will be conducted (e.g., interval- or ratio-level data for correlation).
Who will collect the data?	Determine who will design and administer questionnaires, observe processes, interview employees, access EHRs, and so on.
Where will the data be collected?	Identify the physical locations or sections of the process where data will be collected.
When and how often will the data be collected?	Specify when the data collection should start and when it should end. What time of day, week, or month? Establish the frequency if the data collection will be ongoing (e.g., control charts).
How will the data be collected?	Describe the methods (interview, observation, questionnaire, etc.) of data collection that will be used for each metric of interest (e.g., cameras to keep track of patients' reactions in waiting room; Chapter 4).
Sampling	Specify the sampling frame and sample size required. Provide clear instructions on sampling method (e.g., proportionate stratified random sampling; Appendix 7.1).
Analysis	Briefly list the types of analyses that will need to be performed to answer the research questions and cross-check with the level of measurement of data that will be collected. Also anticipate the types of graphs you will use to present and disseminate your findings.

Abbreviation: EHR, electronic health record.

TABLE 6.2 VALUE CATEGORIZATION OF PROCESS ACTIVITIES

Category	Description of the Steps/Activities	Example
Value-added (V)	• They are critical to meet or exceed customer expectations. • The customer thinks they are worth paying for. • They involve doing the right activities correctly and efficiently.	• Diagnosing a condition accurately • Sending a correct bill in a timely fashion • Listening attentively to a patient's concerns
Non–value-added (N)	• They are wasteful. • The customer does not want to pay for them. • They do not contribute anything positive to the care experience or to improved health outcomes.	• Waiting in line • Handoffs • Redundant activities • Redoing the work due to errors
Business–value-added (B)	• They do not benefit the customer directly, but they do so indirectly. • They involve verification, control, or inspection. • They ensure policy compliance.	• Checking x-rays for image quality • Verifying insurance information • Having each member of the surgery team (surgeon, nurses, and anesthesiologist) verify the patient's identity

Medical Center (BAMC)'s patient flow through the ED, an x-ray is certainly something the patient would value if it is performed correctly and contributes to a better diagnosis. However, the patient would not be willing to pay for delays, rework, and unnecessary transportation related to that x-ray. When we evaluate a process, we categorize each step as **value-added, non–value-added** (wasteful), or **business–value-added** (Laguna & Marklund, 2019; Table 6.2).

VALUE STREAM MAP

A value stream map (VSM) is a flowchart depicting a process flow from a Lean perspective (Chapter 2). A lean process should create optimal value for the customer with minimal or no waste. Because waste is obviously present in a dysfunctional process, all the delays, errors, unnecessary movements, redundancies, and other non–value-added steps should be identified in the current state VSM. This will facilitate their subsequent elimination and thus aid in process redesign.

Let us go back to the patient flow in the ED at BAMC. To develop the current state VSM, we will follow the steps outlined in Table 6.3 and use the basic symbols shown in Figure 6.1.

TABLE 6.3 STEPS IN VALUE STREAM MAPPING

Step	Description
1	Identify the process steps (do a Gemba walk or use a recently made flowchart).
2	Include the delays and transports required to deliver the targeted service.
3	Enter relevant process data.
4	Include the labor capacity at each process step.
5	Compute the percentage of value-added time.
6	Identify and list all areas of waste.
7	Develop a list of opportunities for improvement based on the previously noted items.

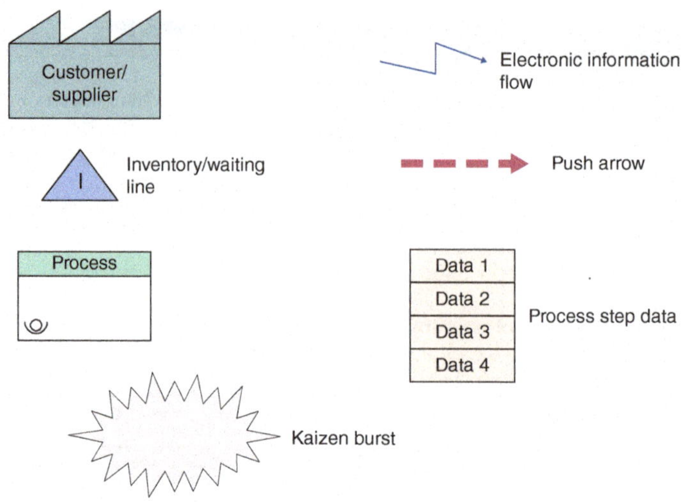

FIGURE 6.1 **Basic VSM symbols.**

Abbreviation: VSM, value stream mapping.

STEP 1: Identify the process steps.

See Figures 3.4 and 3.5.

STEP 2: Include the delays and transports involved in the process.

The triangles before each process step represent the waiting lines, and the number in each triangle refers to the average number of patients in the line.

STEP 3: Enter relevant process data.

Data such as changeover time, pace, defects, and utilization are typically entered below each process step. Here, to keep it simple, we decided to limit the data to issues of concerns, that is, long changeover time in exam rooms and defects during the discharge process.

STEP 4: Enter the capacity at each process step.

The average number of people *available* for each process step was inserted in each process box. This is different from the *required* labor capacity.

STEP 5: Compute the percentage of value-added time or process efficiency.

In order to determine **process efficiency**.

- Determine the non–value-added time. At BAMC, this time will depend on the path followed by a given patient (Table 6.4).
- For example, in the case of a patient getting both a blood test and an x-ray and being discharged after the exam, the non–value-added time would be 5 + 20 + 90 + 10 + 25 + 25 (testing of blood sample takes place during imaging) + 30 + 20 = 225 minutes.
- Determine the **total processing time**, which is the value-added time spent on all process activities.

  This time will also depend on the process path followed by a patient (Table 6.5).

  At BAMC, the total processing time for a patient who gets a blood test and is admitted is: 10 + 10 + 20 + 5 + 18 + 5 + 20 = 88 minutes.
- Divide the total processing (value-added time) by the **cycle time,** which is the time a flow unit (e.g., a patient) spends in the process from beginning to end, or the sum of the value-added and non–value-added times.

  For example, in the case of a patient getting imaging and being transferred, the percentage of value-added time is: 86/(86 + 285) = 0.2318 = 23.18%.

TABLE 6.4 NON-VALUE-ADDED TIME (MIN) FOR EACH PROCESS PATH

Process Steps	Process Paths								
	B, D	B, I, D	I, D	B, A	B, I, A	I, A	B, T	B, I, T	I, T
Registration	5	5	5	5	5	5	5	5	5
Triage	20	20	20	20	20	20	20	20	20
Initial Assessment	90	90	90	90	90	90	90	90	90
Blood Test (B)	10	10		10	10		10	10	
Imaging (I)		25	25		25	25		25	25
Treatment	35	25*	25	35	25*	25	35	25*	25
Condition Reassessment	30	30	30	30	30	30	30	30	30
Discharge (D)	20	20	20						
Admission (A)				60	60	60			
Transfer (T)							90	90	90
Total (min)	210	225	215	250	265	255	280	295	285

Abbreviations: A, admission; B, blood test; D, discharge; I, imaging; T, transfer to another facility.

*Non-value-added time before treatment is initiated is reduced to the time it takes to get imaging results; the non-value-added time to get the lab results (35 min) would be elapsed during the wait time before imaging and the imaging time itself (25 min + 15 min = 40 min).

TABLE 6.5 VALUE-ADDED TIME (MIN) FOR EACH PROCESS PATH

Process Steps	Process Paths								
	B, D	B, I, D	I, D	B, A	B, I, A	I, A	B, T	B, I, T	I, T
Registration	10	10	10	10	10	10	10	10	10
Triage	10	10	10	10	10	10	10	10	10
Initial Assessment	20	20	20	20	20	20	20	20	20
Blood Test (B)	5	5		5	5		5	5	
Imaging (I)		15	15		15	15		15	15
Treatment	18	18	18	18	18	18	18	18	18
Condition Reassessment	5	5	5	5	5	5	5	5	5
Discharge (D)	10	10	10						
Admission (A)				20	20	20			
Transfer (T)							8	8	8
Total (min)	78	93	88	88	103	98	76	91	86

Abbreviations: A, admission; B, blood test; D, discharge; I, imaging; T, transfer to another facility.

STEP 6: Identify and list all areas of waste.

- **Errors/defects**: In the VSM shown in Figure 6.2, it is clear that errors are made when vital signs are forgotten, when patients leave without being seen, and when discharge instructions are poorly understood by the patients.
- **Delays**: Major delays might occur before the initial assessment, before imaging, and before admission or transfer. Similarly, long lab turnaround times might delay treatment for patients who only get a blood test (no imaging).

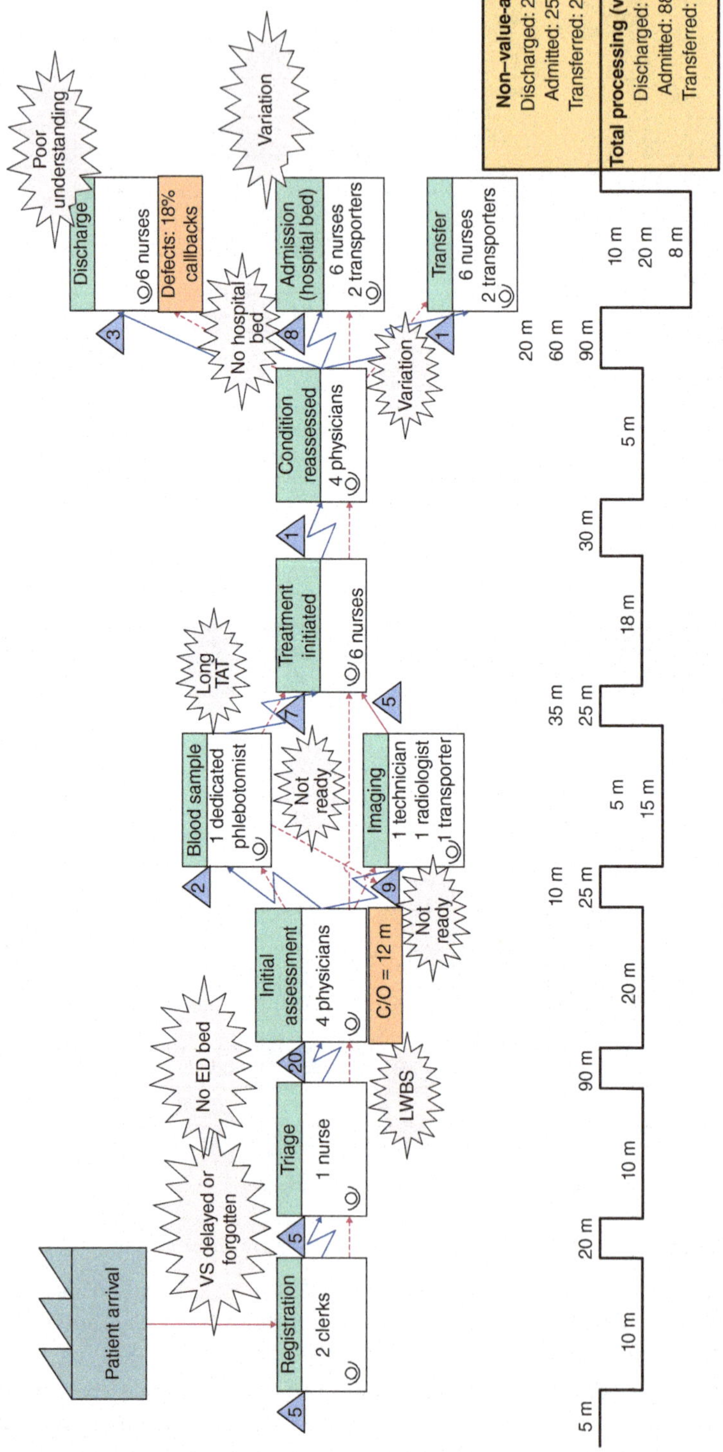

FIGURE 6.2 VSM of patient flow in the ED.

Abbreviation: LWBS, left without being seen; TAT, turnaround time; VSM, value stream map.

BOX 6.1 QUALITY IN PRACTICE!

Value Stream Mapping in an Occupational Medicine Clinic

The high demand for services at a Brazilian occupational clinic made it necessary to evaluate the patient flow and identify waste such as waiting, unnecessary displacement, and low provider productivity. Patient interarrival times and process service times were collected, and simulation of the patient flows from registration to diagnostics tests to treatment under different scenarios helped identify non–value-added steps. The study produced a proposed VSM in which patient waiting time was reduced by 37.92% and lead time by 29.86%. Furthermore, the redesigned system could accommodate a larger volume of patients with the same professional capacity (Rocha & Vasconcelos, 2021).

- **Variation**: There is also a lot of variation in wait times before transfer and in the admission step time.

  The criticality of these matters is highlighted in the map by the "kaizen burst" icons urging for the redesign of a leaner and less variable process. The cycle time for an admitted patient fluctuates between 338 and 368 min approximately, but only 88 to 103 minutes of that time is of value to the patient.

STEP 7: Develop a list of opportunities for improvement based on this list.

As each problem is being scrutinized, an intense questioning exercise (The 5 Whys; see Chapter 2) can reveal the reasons why things are not done properly, especially in processes that have been performed the same way for long periods of time. These root causes will help identify opportunities for improvement (Box 6.1). The process steps that are considered waste but cannot be eliminated should be targeted for improvement.

ON THE JOB! INTERVIEW VIDEO 6.1

Hongmey Zhen Castillo
Director of Quality Outcomes Center of Excellence and Clinical Recall Quality

Meeting Federal and State Quality Reporting Requirements

Process mapping and non–value-added work
Tracking process quality indicators
Overseeing the clinical recall program
SWOT (strengths, weaknesses, opportunities, threats), VOC, failure mode and effects analysis (FMEA).

1. Hongmey reviews the clinical recall program and highlights the value of having a detailed process map. In what ways does this tool aid in diagnosing issues?
2. What are the benefits of using a tool like FMEA in an organization with a matrixed reporting structure?
3. What are the organizational risks when different employees develop their own processes for completing a high-risk task?

The interview is available online by visiting www.springerpub.com/courseconnect. See inside front cover and tear-out card for CourseConnect details.

BRIGHT ANGEL MEDICAL CENTER 6.2

Olina shared the VSM that she and one other project team member had developed for the ED workflow.

Barbara raised her hand. "I am trying to understand what this diagram is telling us," she inquired. Olina explained, "This shows the patient's journey through the ED with all the steps

(continued)

BRIGHT ANGEL MEDICAL CENTER 6.2 (*CONTINUED*)

and wait times. Some of the steps are certainly valuable to the patient like being seen by the provider and receiving treatment. Others, such as waiting or being transported, are not valuable."

Dr. Aoki interjected excitedly, "This is exactly what I was discussing with my clinical team. If we remove some of the wasted time in the workflow, then the overall LOS and LWBS should go down." "Precisely," said Olina. The team pored over the diagram for several more minutes, discussing the process and the areas where they believed they could reduce wait times or improve efficiency. They all agreed to spend time reviewing the information and getting back together in a few days to prioritize the work ahead.

A graph is supposed to facilitate communication. If so, why would Barbara need help?

PROCESS ACTIVITY CHART

Process activity charts are also popular tools to examine the flow of activities and assess whether or not they create value. Process activity charts combine the value classification scheme with a descriptive system using symbols denoting operations; transportations, movements, or information transfers; storage; delays; and inspections (Figure 6.3). In our ED workflow, the initial assessment is an operation, going to the Imaging Department is transportation, time spent in the waiting room is a delay, and triage is an inspection/verification. Storage often implies storing physical objects—such as paper medical records in a warehouse, equipment in a stockroom, or documents in a filing cabinet—and is not explicitly captured in this example. Be aware that the classification of an activity can change depending on the process being examined. For example, when looking at the triage process alone, determining the Emergency Severity Index (ESI) classification is considered value-added. However, when looking at the entire ED care process, getting the ESI classification is downgraded to business–value-added. Moreover, the classification will vary based on the customer of the process (i.e., the recipient of its output). For example, taking the patient from imaging back to the ED exam room is a non–value-added step from the patient's perspective, but

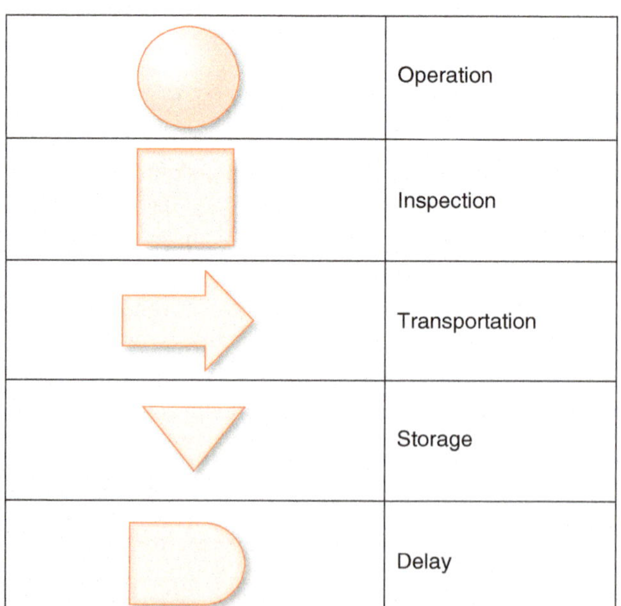

FIGURE 6.3 Symbols in process activity chart.

it is definitely a value-added one from the perspective of the employee overseeing patient transports to and from the departments.

The process activity chart for the flow of an ED patient getting a blood test and an x-ray and being admitted is depicted in Table 6.6. The symbols corresponding to the steps listed in the same row are connected to show the nature of the various steps. The time and/or distance for each step

TABLE 6.6 PROCESS ACTIVITY CHART FOR AN ED PATIENT WITH BOTH DIAGNOSTICS TESTS AND BEING ADMITTED

No.	Description	Time(Min)	Distance	Value Code (V/N/B)	Symbol
1	Patient arrives.	1	100 ft	V	○ □ ➡ D ▽
2	Patient waits.	5		N	○ □ ⇨ ◗ ▽
3	Patient is registered.	10		B	○ ■ ⇨ D ▽
4	Patient waits.	20		N	○ □ ⇨ ◗ ▽
5	Patient is triaged.	10		B	○ ■ ⇨ D ▽
6	Patient waits.	87		N	○ □ ⇨ ◗ ▽
7	Patient goes to exam room.	3	300 ft	N	○ □ ➡ D ▽
8	Patient is examined by physician.	20		V	● □ ⇨ D ▽
9	Patient waits for phlebotomist.	10		N	○ □ ⇨ ◗ ▽
10	Patient's blood is drawn.	5		V	● □ ⇨ D ▽
11	Patient goes to Imaging Department.	5	1,200 ft	N	○ □ ➡ D ▽
12	Patient waits.	20		N	○ □ ⇨ ◗ ▽
13	Patient's images are taken.	15		V	● □ ⇨ D ▽
14	Patient goes back to exam room.	5	1,200 ft	N	○ □ ➡ D ▽
15	Patient waits.	25		N	○ □ ⇨ ◗ ▽
16	Treatment is initiated.	18		V	● □ ⇨ D ▽
17	Patient waits.	30		N	○ □ ⇨ ◗ ▽
18	Patient's condition is reassessed.	5		V	○ ■ ⇨ D ▽
19	Patient waits.	60		N	○ □ ⇨ ◗ ▽
20	Patient is admitted.	20		V	● □ ⇨ D ▽

Abbreviations: B, business-value-added; N, non-value-added activities; V, value-added.

are also recorded. As can be seen from this chart, many activities do not pass the litmus test of meeting the patient's value expectations. The patient spends long periods waiting to be cared for by staff and providers and traveling distances. The situation is especially alarming for patients who undergo two diagnostics tests and wait for results while in pain.

The current process comprises 20 steps: five operations, eight delays, three inspections, and 4 transports. The total value-added time is 84 minutes, whereas the cycle time is 374 minutes. Much of the time to complete the entire process is non–value-added, signaling a need for corrective action. Computing the **efficiency of a process** helps us quantify the extent of improvement needed. The efficiency of a process expresses the proportion of time spent on value-added activities or steps in the entire process. It is computed as:

$$\text{Efficiency} = \left(\frac{\textit{Sum of the times of value-added steps in the process}}{\textit{Sum of the times of all steps in the process}}\right) \times 100 \qquad [6.1]$$

$$= \frac{84}{374} \times 100$$

$$= 22.5\%$$

An efficiency of only 22.5% is an indication that the process is cluttered with non–value-added time and must be improved. Although simple and easy to understand, the process activity chart is purely linear and does not allow for alternate paths. In our example, we would have to create another process activity chart for a patient only getting imaging and being discharged. The flow process chart circumvents this problem.

FLOW PROCESS CHART

The **flow process chart** is essentially a flowchart that also uses the symbols of the process activity chart (Figure 6.4).

Numerous handoffs in this process are clearly visible. Before each process step, there is a likely delay, and at each process step, there is an opportunity for error. These errors affect both the effectiveness and efficiency of patient care. A useful metric to see their negative impact is the yield.

YIELD

The **yield; first pass yield (FPY)**, also known as **throughput yield (TPY)**; and **rolled throughput yield (RTY)** are important Six Sigma metrics. As previously mentioned, when units flow through a process, mistakes are made, and the outcome can be a success or a failure (see BAMC 6.3).

BRIGHT ANGEL MEDICAL CENTER 6.3

The project team members reconvened to share their thinking on some of the potential errors that require rework, result in waste, and slow down throughput in the ED. Olina was taking notes and said, "Ok, here is what I have so far.

Errors can be made at each process step:

- *registration: wrong patient name or insurance information (rework);*
- *triage: inaccurate ESI classification (rework or "scrap" if this mistake proves fatal);*
- *exam: wrong diagnosis (rework or "scrap" if this mistake could also prove fatal);*
- *imaging: poor images (rework);*
- *treatment: wrong treatment (rework or "scrap" if this mistake proves fatal);*
- *reassessment: inaccurate conclusion (rework or "scrap" if this mistake proves fatal); and*
- *discharge: No or poor discharge instructions (rework later on)."*

(continued)

BRIGHT ANGEL MEDICAL CENTER 6.3 (*CONTINUED*)

"That's a great start," said Barbara. The group agreed that these were potential failure points, and that historical data had to be examined to determine the incidence of the errors made at each step.

A few days later, the team met again, and Adeleke showed the following diagram (see also Excel Video 6.1):

EXCEL VIDEO 6.1

Yield

Access the Excel video online by visiting www.springerpub.com/courseconnect. See inside front cover and tear-out card for CourseConnect details.

EXHIBIT 6.1 ERRORS MADE AT EACH PROCESS STEP FOR DISCHARGED PATIENTS

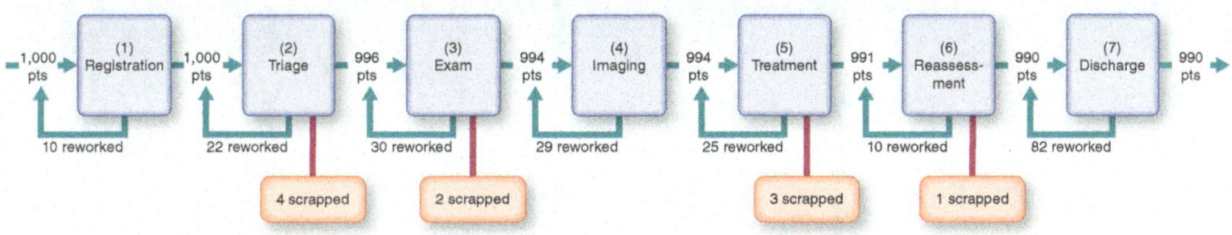

Abbreviation: Pts, patients.

Barbara frowned. "Ten patients died out of 1,000. That's unacceptable!" she lamented.

Olina replied, "It's actually a little bit more complicated. Errors compound along the way and make our system unreliable. Let me explain."

Using the BAMC case, patients flow through the steps shown in Exhibit 6.1. Out of the 1,000 patients that entered the system, deaths occurred at four different steps: triage, exam, treatment, and reassessment. When other mistakes were made, rework was necessary, using up capacity and delaying the process. For example, when x-rays were defective, new images had to be taken. There are several opportunities for defects at each stage, but let's simplify and assume that there is only one opportunity for defect per patient at each stage. For simplification, we will associate the rework at discharge with that step only. In reality, many of those might involve readmissions that would require a repeat of the entire process.

Yield measures the percentage of units (e.g., patients) that are nondefective when they exit the process. In other words, it excludes scrap but includes all the units for which rework was necessary in order to be considered acceptable and sent to the next step.

$$\text{Yield} = \frac{\textit{Number of acceptable units at end of process}}{\textit{Total number of units entering the process}} \times 100\%$$

$$= 100\% - \text{scrap rate} \qquad [6.2]$$

$$= \frac{990\,units}{1{,}000\,units} = 100\% - 1\% = 99\%$$

But rework is a wasteful activity that makes a process inefficient! First pass yield is therefore a better metric because it provides the percentage of units that passed through a process step without rework. The formula for the FPY or TPY at process step i is:

$$\text{FPY}_i = \frac{\textit{Entering units} - \textit{scrapped units} - \textit{reworked units}}{\textit{Entering units}} \times 100\% \qquad [6.3]$$

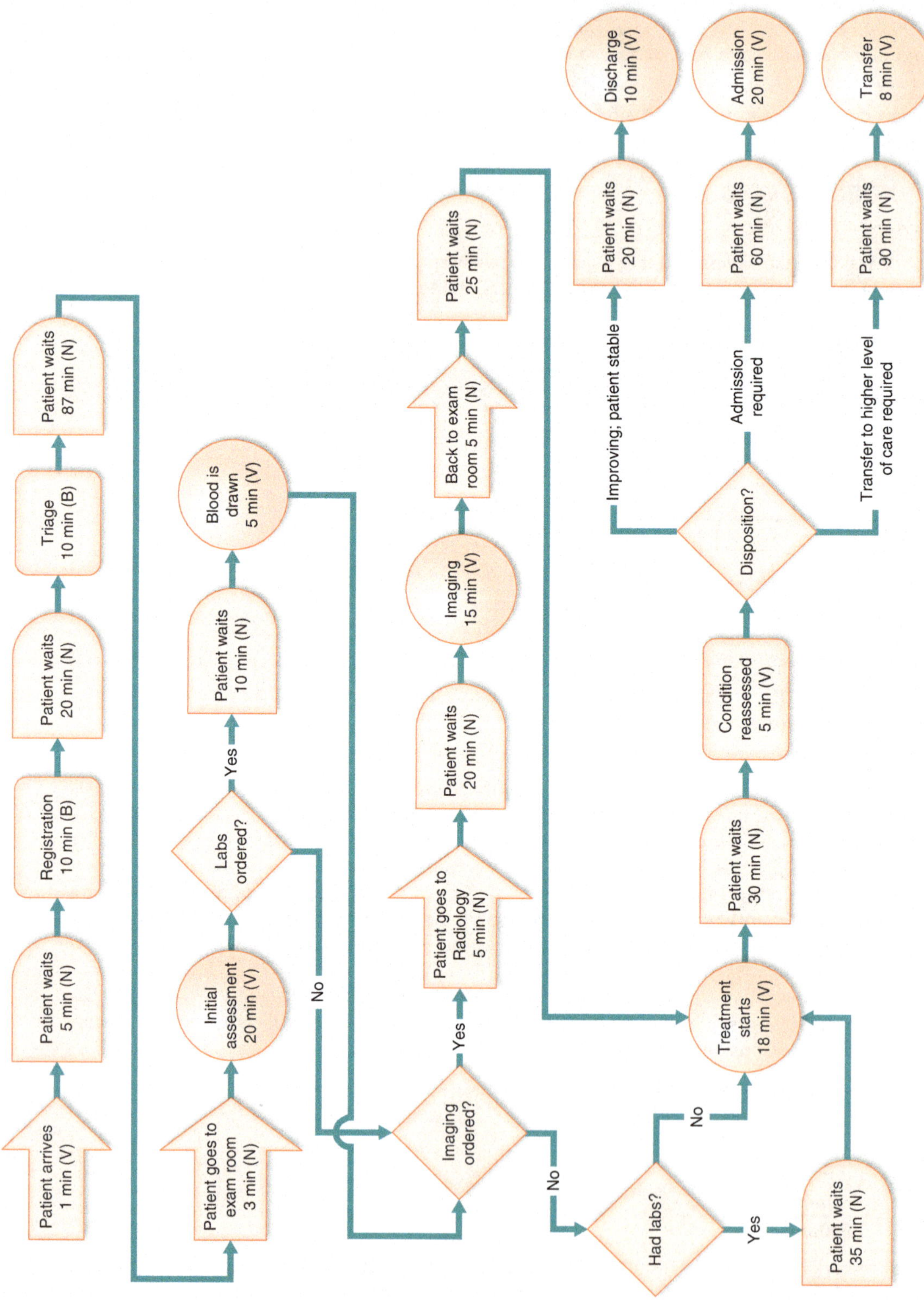

FIGURE 6.4 Flow process chart with activity chart symbols.

Abbreviations: B, business–value-added; N, non–value-added activities; V, value-added.

In our example,

$$\text{FPY}_1 = \frac{1{,}000\,units - 10\,reworked\,units}{1{,}000\,units} \times 100\% = 99.00\%$$

$$\text{FPY}_2 = \frac{1{,}000\,units - 22\,reworked\,units - 4\,scrapped}{1{,}000\,units} \times 100\% = 97.40\%$$

$$\text{FPY}_3 = \frac{996\,units - 30\,reworked\,units - 2\,scrapped}{996\,units} \times 100\% = 96.79\%$$

$$\text{FPY}_4 = \frac{994\,units - 29\,reworked\,units}{994\,units} \times 100\% = 97.08\%$$

$$\text{FPY}_5 = \frac{994\,units - 25\,reworked\,units - 3\,scrapped}{994\,units} \times 100\% = 97.18\%$$

$$\text{FPY}_6 = \frac{991\,units - 10\,reworked\,units - 1\,scrapped}{991\,units} \times 100 = 98.89\%$$

$$\text{FPY}_7 = \frac{990\,units - 82\,reworked\,units}{990\,units} \times 100 = 91.72\%$$

For the whole n-step process, the RTY is the percentage of units that passed through the entire process without ever requiring rework. Another way of defining RTY is as the probability of processing units correctly the first time. It is therefore totally consistent with the pursuit of *doing it right the first time* (Chapters 1 and 2). RTY is calculated as the product of the first pass (or throughput) yields at each process step:

$$\begin{aligned} \text{RTY} &= \text{FPY}_1 \times \text{FPY}_2 \times \text{FPY}_3 \times \ldots \times \text{FPY}_n \qquad [6.4] \\ &= (0.99 \times 0.974 \times 0.9679 \times 0.9708 \times 0.9718 \times 0.9889 \times 0.9172) \times 100\% = 79.86\% \end{aligned}$$

This means that 20.14% of the patients going through the process can expect rework or "scrap" (i.e., fatality). You can see how relatively small chances of making errors at each step of a process do add up!

In our example, the lowest FPY was at the last step, that is, discharge. Reducing fatalities at the steps where they occur should be the top priority, but the late stages of a process are also very important because costs tend to increase downstream as more resources (materials, labor, and overhead) have been utilized (Six Sigma Material, 2023). Generally speaking, improving the yield at these steps is critical.

As you can see, the more steps and handoffs in the process, the more opportunities for errors. Some can be fixed, others cannot. Combined, all these mistakes contribute to a low RTY, which impairs health outcomes, affects patient experience, and strains already scarce capacity. Many problems can occur in the ED, and staff members may feel that the problems affecting their own work are the most urgent ones that need immediate corrective action. Unfortunately, these might be *guesses* rather than *facts*. Check sheets help differentiate between serious problems and trivial issues.

CHECK SHEET

Check sheets provide an easy way to record problem occurrences and organize them by category. They are fact-finding tools that enable identification of critical concerns. Based on the check sheet presented in Table 6.7, it can be established as a fact that of all the problems plaguing the ED, *patients leaving without being seen*, with 55 occurrences during the data collection period, is the most prevalent one. To gather more data about this problem, the staff may want to develop a check sheet that organizes the occurrences per shift (day, evening, night) or even per hour (8–9 a.m., 9–10 a.m., 10–11 a.m., etc.), especially on Wednesdays. This might enable them to identify a specific pattern for these events and identify viable solutions more quickly.

All the rework arising from mistakes at each process step increases the buffers or delays, which, in turn, may cause patients to leave without being seen. The process activity chart and the flow process chart (Table 6.6 and Figure 6.4) also showed a lot of non–value-added movements. The spaghetti diagram is a simple tool that will help you identify them and evaluate their extent.

SPAGHETTI DIAGRAM

Ideally, the layout of the physical environment should facilitate the effective and efficient movement of flow units (patients, employees, materials, information, etc.) through the system. Common objectives include (Stevenson & Kull, 2024):

1. reducing errors;
2. utilizing resources and space efficiently;
3. avoiding delays and bottlenecks;
4. minimizing handoffs;
5. minimizing movements and transfers; and
6. ensuring safety.

Spaghetti diagrams depict traffic intensity and patterns within a physical area or across areas and help visualize where movements are wasted (Box 6.2). They are therefore well suited to determine whether a layout is conducive to delivering value.

In order to develop a spaghetti diagram, you need to perform the following tasks:

1. Determine what you want to observe: patients, supplies, staff, paperwork, and so on. If you want to observe several units at the same time, simply use different colors.
2. Draw the layout of the area under study.
3. Follow the unit(s) you are observing and draw the flow of their movements through the area.

TABLE 6.7 CHECK SHEET

	Number of Occurrences					
	Day					Total
Problem	Monday	Tuesday	Wednesday	Thursday	Friday	
Missing supplies in exam room	𝍸	////	𝍸 𝍸	/		20
Patients leaving without being seen	𝍸 ////	𝍸 ///	𝍸𝍸𝍸 𝍸 //	𝍸𝍸	𝍸 /	55
Soiled linen		//	//	𝍸	𝍸 /	15
Late lab results	𝍸	///	𝍸 𝍸 𝍸	///	////	30
Malfunctioning blood pressure monitors			//	//	𝍸 /	10
Inadequate discharge instructions	𝍸 //	𝍸 𝍸	𝍸 𝍸 ///	𝍸	𝍸	40

BOX 6.2 QUALITY IN PRACTICE!

Spaghetti Diagrams to Improve Flow in Neurosurgical Procedures

The number of lumbar fusion procedures has dramatically increased. Yet, with limited capacity, it is vital to improve procedural efficiency. At a U.S. university health system, intraoperative spaghetti diagrams were created to visualize surgeon motion from surgical level localization to removal of sterile drapes. The duration of component steps was measured, and in some cases the hand motion of the surgeon was videotaped. Although spaghetti diagrams were too simple to capture hand motion complexity, they helped uncover inefficiencies related to hardware placement (Liu et al., 2018).

4. Identify locations that have repeated traffic in-between, and make sure that they are located close to one another.

In Figure 6.5, you can see that:

- There is substantial patient traffic between the waiting room and the exam rooms, and between the exam rooms and the Imaging Department. Some of the exam rooms are located far away from the waiting room, resulting in traffic throughout the ED and in front of the trauma rooms.
- The trauma rooms are on the side of the ED that is opposite from the ambulance bay entrance.
- The patient restroom is located far away from the nursing station, which is inconvenient and even dangerous for patients needing assistance.
- The patient restroom is next to the supply room, creating opportunities for theft.

Although the physicians' and nurses' flows are not depicted, the layout is inefficient for them as well:

- Provider documentation is confined to only one area, far away from some patients.
- There are only two nursing stations located far away from some exam rooms.
- The simulation lab is located in the ED, taking up valuable space.
- The slit lamp is in a dedicated room, which is unnecessary.

The spaghetti diagram makes it easy to localize waste and therefore suggests opportunities to redesign the layout so that it creates flow.

BUILDING THE A3 REPORT

After measuring the process, the BAMC project team can continue to populate the A3 report and provide an overview of the current situation. In Figure 6.6, Adeleke displayed the VSM and the spaghetti diagram to shine a light on the areas where waste hinders process performance.

ETHICAL SCENARIO 6.1

Improving a process or eliminating waste can impact people and their roles within an organization. The electronic medical record (EMR) brought in sweeping changes to many healthcare organizations across the United States. Prior to using electronic records, many systems relied on paper charts and transcriptionists to type notes, operative reports, imaging results, and many other elements of the chart. Following adoption of EMR systems, most transcriptionists were no longer needed. Some were retrained to take on new tasks associated with having an EMR such as scanning in outside reports. Others obtained additional skills needed to take on new roles such as coding or insurance preauthorization. In some instances, adopting the EMR meant that jobs were eliminated, resulting in layoffs.

What is the importance of an effective change management strategy to "bring employees along" with the proposed organizational changes?

Does a healthcare organization have an obligation to its employees to offer retraining or other resources to assist them in finding new roles? What about offering other benefits such as job placement, resume writing, or other assistance?

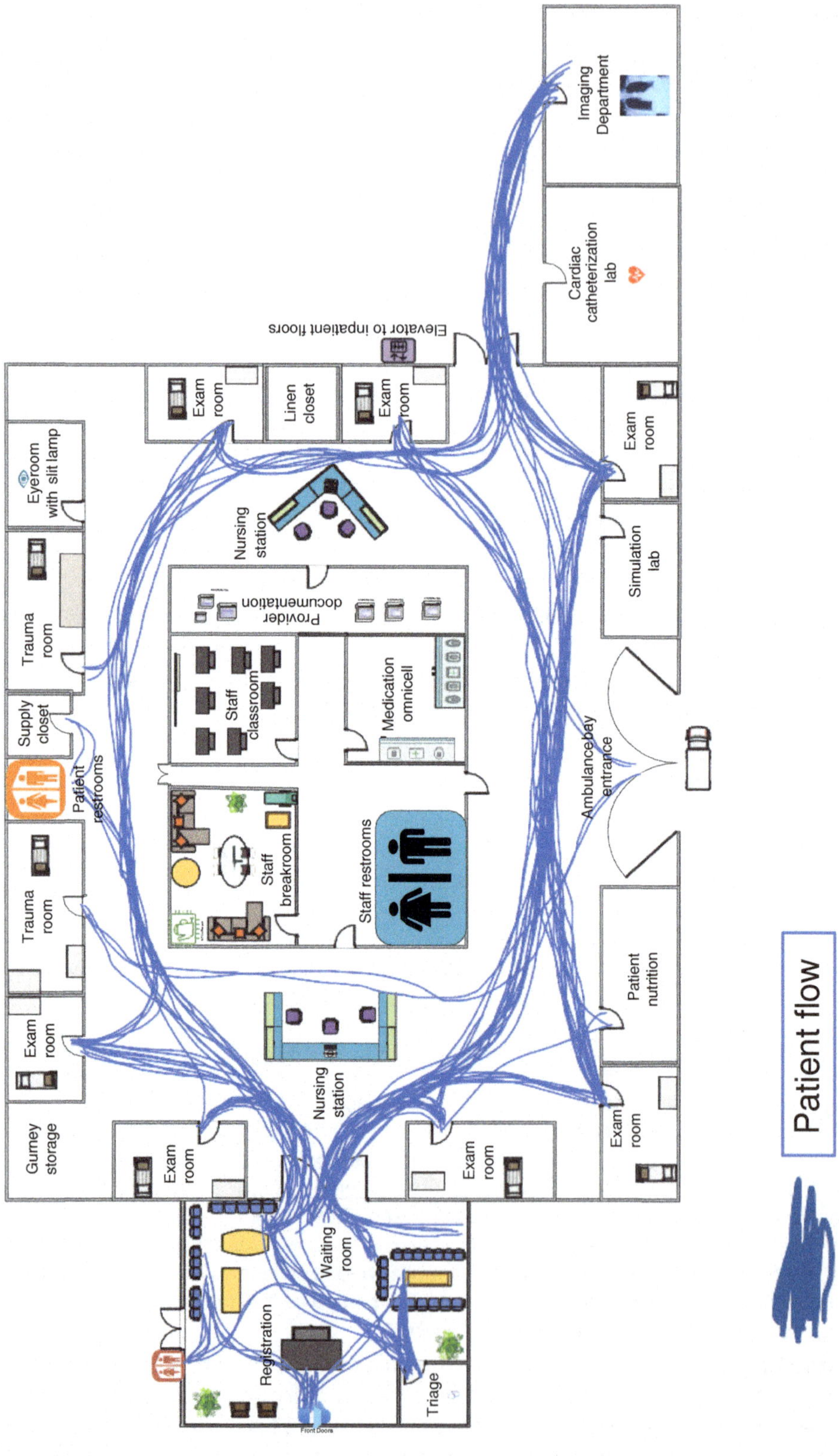

FIGURE 6.5 Spaghetti diagram at BAMC's ED.

Abbreviation: BAMC, Bright Angel Medical Center.

Prepared by Adeleke Mensah **ED throughput** **February 15, 2025**

Background

Low patient satisfaction scores and high LWBS. ALOS in the ED is over 6 hr. Average wait time in early evening exceeds 2 hr. Delays to get x-rays and lab results. High readmission rates within 72 hr. Boarding issues. Poor patient experience with providers.

Current situation

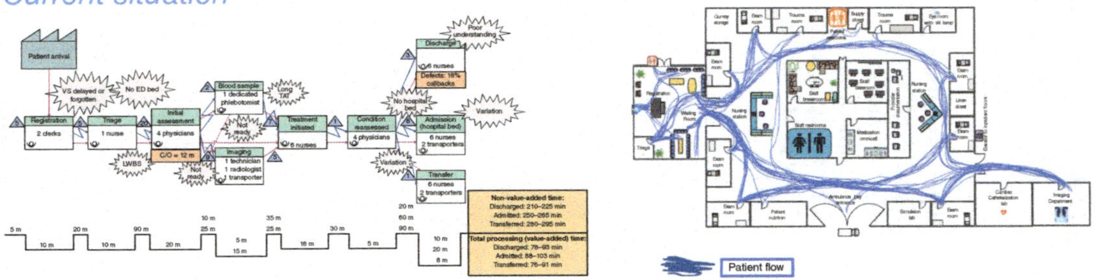

FIGURE 6.6 A3 report with *Define* and *Measure* phase findings.

Abbreviations: ALOS, average lengths of stay; LWBS, left without being seen.

SUMMARY

What is wrong with a process? Anything that does not contribute value. This chapter gives you the tools to find waste and point out errors, long delays, unnecessary movements, handoffs, excessive variation, and so forth. VSMs, process activity charts, flow process charts, and spaghetti diagrams help visualize the process flow, its handoffs and delays, and its wasted transports. Timing the process steps also helps us determine the amount of variation in the completion of an activity. Obtaining error counts at each process step and computing the RTY draw our attention to the compounding effect of errors through a process.

CERTIFICATION TIPS

You should be able to *create* process maps and flowcharts in the *measure* phase of the certification exam. Certification also requires knowledge of written procedures and work instructions that are very similar to the 5w2h framework presented in Chapter 3: What is done, by whom, why, where, when, and how. This chapter took the reader to a more granular measurement of waste (value-added, non–value-added, and business–value-added steps) with the process activity charts and flow process charts. While not required for certification, the classification (V, N, B) is a standard in process management.

KEY TERMS

Value stream
Data collection
Value-added activities
Non–value-added activities
business–value-added activities
Process efficiency
Total processing time
Cycle time
Process activity chart
Efficiency of a process
Flow process chart
Yield
First pass yield (FPY)
Throughput yield (TPY)
Rolled throughput yield (RTY)
Check sheet
Spaghetti diagram

REVIEW QUESTIONS

1. What is the purpose of the *Measure* phase?
2. Distinguish among value-added, business–value-added, and non–value-added activities.
3. Give some examples of business–value-added activities in healthcare.
4. What is a VSM? What problems can it uncover?
5. What is a process activity chart? What are the symbols used in the chart to categorize process steps?
6. Do you prefer to develop a VSM or a flow process chart? Why?
7. What is the efficiency of a process from a value standpoint?
8. What is the purpose of a spaghetti diagram?
9. When would you use a check sheet?
10. Distinguish among yield, FPY, and RTY.

SOLVE BRIGHT ANGEL MEDICAL CENTER'S PROBLEMS

All chapter-specific data from the following problems are provided as Excel files which may be accessed via the show supplementary tab (Student Material) available online by visiting www.springerpub.com/courseconnect. See inside front cover and tear-out card for CourseConnect details.

1. The following is a VSM for medication ordering and administration. Compute the efficiency of this process and recommend areas that need improvement.

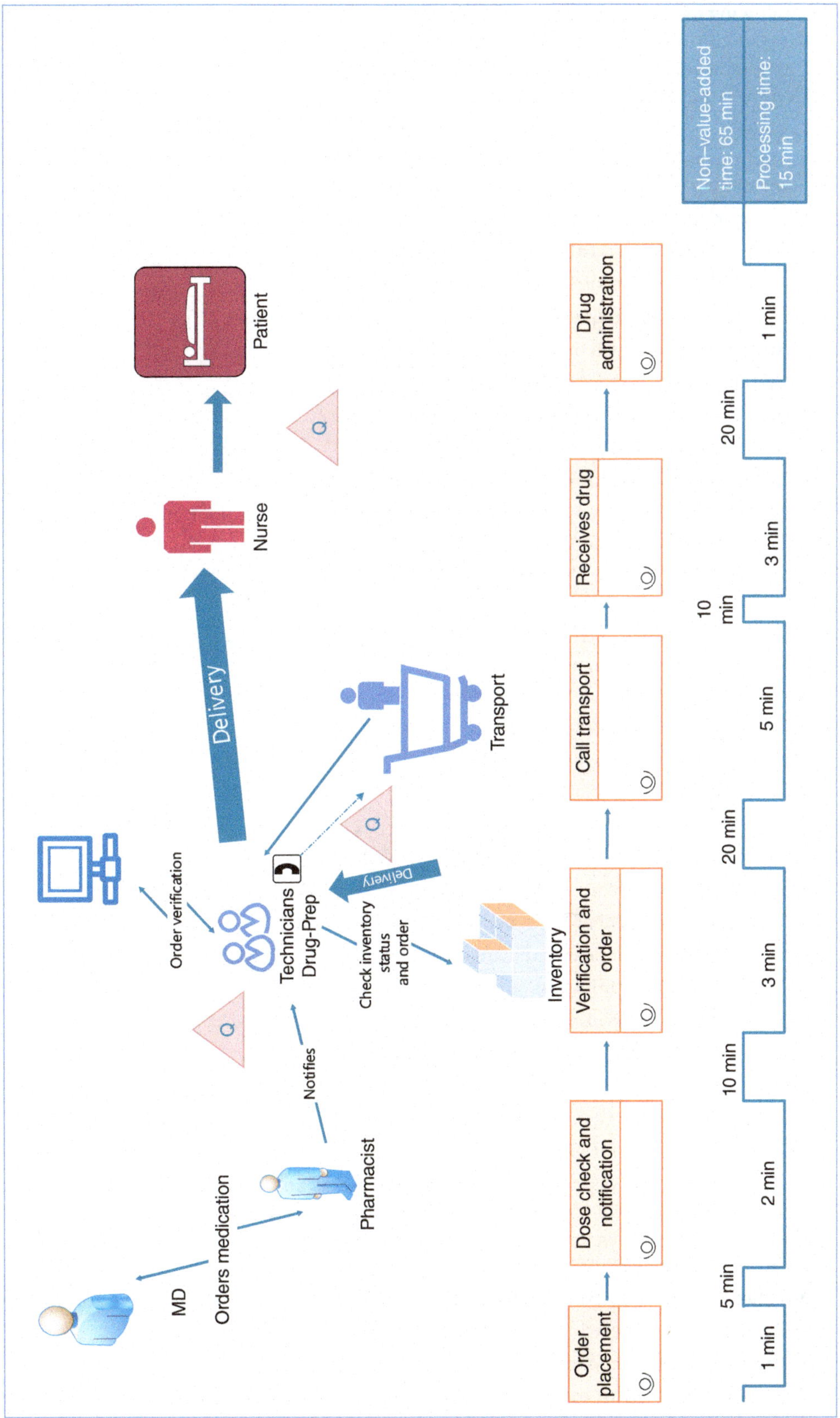

MD
Orders medication
Pharmacist
Notifies
Technicians Drug-Prep
Order verification
Check inventory status and order
Inventory
Delivery
Transport
Delivery
Nurse
Patient
Q
Q
Q
Order placement
Dose check and notification
Verification and order
Call transport
Receives drug
Drug administration
1 min
5 min
2 min
10 min
3 min
20 min
5 min
10 min
3 min
20 min
1 min
Non–value-added time: 65 min
Processing time: 15 min

2. The following are the steps for patients' paper record requests and recovery at one of BAMC's clinics. Develop a process activity chart and identify areas for improvement.
   a. Categorize activities as value-added, non–value-added, and business–value-added.
   b. Compute the efficiency of this process.
      - Staff member pulls list of patients with appointments to pick up their records (1 min).
      - Staff member requests paper medical records from file clerk through email, call, instant messaging, or paper note (10 minutes).
      - File clerk checks all communication methods (10 minutes).
      - File clerk finds the location of each requested file (5 minutes).
      - File clerk goes to record storage location (5 minutes).
      - File clerk places a request to have records pulled (2 minutes).
      - Storage clerk reviews the request (2 minutes).
      - File clerk collects the records (3 minutes).
      - Staff member makes copies (19 minutes).
      - Staff member gives copies to patient (1 minute).
      - File clerk returns records to storage location (5 minutes).
3. The following are the steps for a patient to receive an echocardiogram. Develop a process activity chart and identify areas for improvement.
   a. Categorize activities as value-added, non–value-added, and business–value-added.
   b. Compute the efficiency of this process.
      - Patient checks in (1 minute).
      - Patient sits in waiting area (1 minute).
      - Patient is registered (3 minutes).
      - Patient is sent to third floor for exam (3 minutes).
      - Patient sits in waiting area (11 minutes).
      - Echo staff checks paperwork (1 minute).
      - Echo staff enters order (2 minutes).
      - Echo staff goes to procedure room (2 minutes).
      - Echo staff enters demographic patient data into machine (1 minute).
      - Echo staff takes patient to procedure room (1 minute).
      - Echo staff gets a blanket and brings it to the room (1 minute).
      - Patient changes (2 minutes).
      - Echo staff performs exam (23 minutes).
      - Patient changes and is dismissed (2 minutes).
      - Echo staff writes down exam information (3 minutes).
      - Echo staff moves to control area (1 minute).
      - Echo staff charges for exam (2 minutes).
4. The following are the steps of the check-in process at an outpatient therapy department. Develop a process activity chart and identify areas for improvement.
   a. Categorize activities as value-added, non–value-added, and business–value-added.
   b. Compute the efficiency of this process.
      - Patient checks in at front desk (1 minute).
      - Patient fills in paperwork (4 minutes).
      - Patient is given arm band (1 minute).
      - Patient is escorted to the second floor where outpatient physical therapy clinic is located (1.5 minutes).

- Paperwork is given to registration staff in the physical therapy clinic (1 minute).
- Registration staff determines what papers should be kept, thrown away, or duplicated (1 min).
- Registration staff checks patient in on electronic health record (EHR) system (0.3 min).
- Registration staff pages therapist (0.5 minute).
- Patient waits for therapist (2 minutes).
- Therapist escorts patient back to a physical therapy evaluation room (1.5 minutes).
- Patient fills out a questionnaire as part of the evaluation (5 minutes).
- Patient waits for therapist to enter questionnaire data into the system (3 minutes).
- Therapist performs evaluation (10 minutes).

5. Compute the yield and the RTY for each one of the two processes that follow. In each case, state the meaning of these performance metrics.

a.

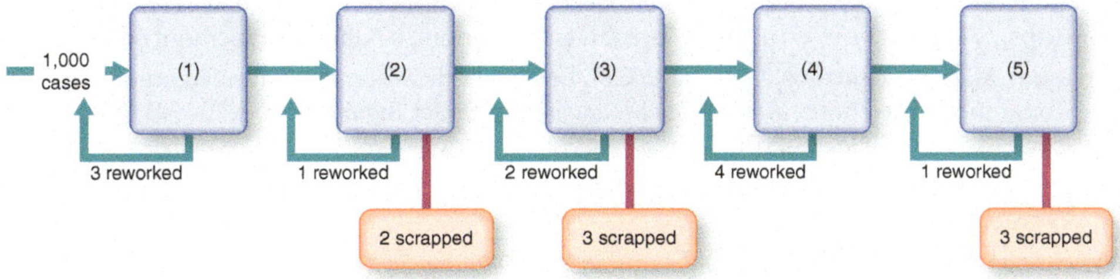

b.

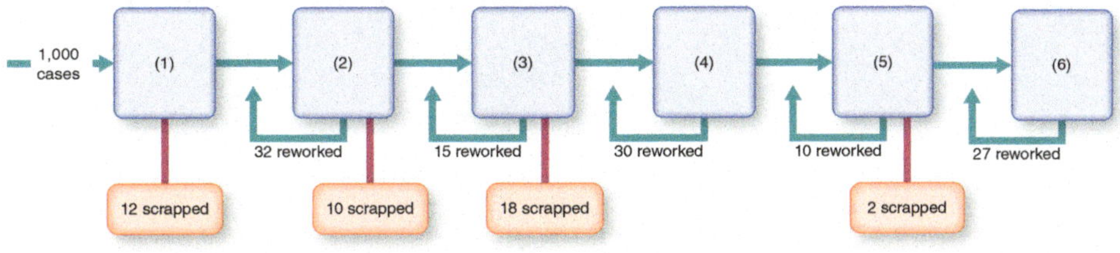

LEARNING ACTIVITIES

1. In a healthcare organization, what are the roadblocks to measurement? What can be done to overcome them?
2. Imagine that you are the billing supervisor at a large clinic. You want to redesign the process to make it more efficient. As you explain the measurement process to your staff, you meet strong resistance immediately. They feel that they do a great job, work as fast as they can, and that the process cannot be improved. Prepare a speech that will convince them that your idea is a good one.
3. In your work environment, select a process that is dysfunctional.
   a. Identify all the steps (including waits, transports, etc.).
   b. Select 10 flow units going through the steps and time each step for each one of the 10 flow units.
   c. Develop a process activity chart.
   d. Suggest improvements.
4. Draw the layout of a high traffic area at your workplace. Observe staff or customers going through the area for about 1 hour while developing a spaghetti diagram. What are your findings?

SPRINGER PUBLISHING CONNECT™ A robust set of instructor resources designed to supplement this text is located at **http://connect.springerpub.com/content/book/978-0-8261-7976-0.** Qualifying instructors may request access by emailing **textbook@springerpub.com.**

REFERENCES

Laguna, M., & Marklund, J. (2019). *Business process, modeling, simulation, and design* (3rd ed.). Routledge.

Liu, J. J., Raskin, J. S., Hardaway, F., Holste, K., Brown, S., & Raslan, A. M. (2018). Application of Lean principles to neurosurgical procedures: The case of lumbar spinal fusion surgery, a literature review and pilot series. *Operative Neurosurgery*, *15*(3), 332–340. https://doi.org/10.1093/ons/opx289

Lord Kelvin. (2007). *In praise of Lord Kelvin*. Physics World. https://physicsworld.com/a/in-praise-of-lord-kelvin

Office of Research Integrity. (2024). *Data collection*. Department of Health & Human Services. https://ori.hhs.gov/education/products/n_illinois_u/datamanagement/dctopic.html

Rocha, Í. J. A., & Vasconcelos, C. R. d. (2021). Lean healthcare implications in an occupational medicine clinic. *International Journal of Lean Six Sigma*, *12*(5), 973–991. https://doi.org/10.1108/IJLSS-05-2020-0056

Six Sigma Material. (2023). *Rolled throughput yield*. https://www.six-sigma-material.com/Rolled-Throughput-Yield.html

Stevenson, W. J., & Kull, T. J. (2024). *Operations and supply chain management*. McGraw-Hill.

CHAPTER 7

DATA VISUALIZATION AND DESCRIPTION

BRIGHT ANGEL MEDICAL CENTER 7.1

Adeleke, Olina, and Barbara were reviewing ED patient arrival data gathered by the analytics team. Just then, the CFO, Joe García, popped his head in the conference room. "I wanted to swing by and better understand the request for additional staff," Joe stated. "We are trying to sort that out ourselves," said Barbara. Olina interjected, "it might be more about matching our staffing with patient arrivals. It looks like we have times when our staff is overwhelmed, and other times when it's slow, we have too many people on shift. If we adjust the shifts to better align with the busy times, I bet we could pull this off and stay budget neutral." That was music to Joe's ears. Staffing was their largest expense, and he knew they needed to try to save money, not spend more.

How can data help make better decisions? What about experience?

LEARNING OBJECTIVES

After reading this chapter, you will be able to:

- Understand the purposes of the various types of data analytics.
- Determine the level of measurement of the data in a data set.
- Produce graphs that are appropriate for each level of measurement.
- Understand how probabilities and distributions are related.
- Recognize the importance of the law of large numbers (LoLN) and the central limit theorem (CLT) in statistics.
- Identify the discrete (binomial, Poisson) and continuous (normal, standard normal) distributions of your data.
- Compute measures of central tendency and dispersion.

INTRODUCTION

Let the data tell the story! Healthcare collects massive amounts of data every day on patients' demographics, experience, diagnoses, procedures, screenings, family history, and outcomes. This is in addition to financial, process, supply chain, workforce, and other data generated by delivering care to those patients. These raw data have very little use unless they are processed to generate meaningful insights. Always important, the role of data analytics has taken a special significance in the 21st century as data science has emerged as an independent discipline, and the mining of large data sets has become commonplace in private and public organizations. What are data analytics? **Data analytics** are the processing of data using information technology, statistics, mathematical models, simulation, and computer-based models to get a deeper understanding of clinical and business conditions and make better decisions based on facts rather than gut feelings. There are several types of data analytics. In this chapter, we focus on descriptive analytics so that you can get an initial "feel" for the data and see where further analysis is warranted. We also stress the importance of data visualization to facilitate understanding and interpretation.

WHY IS THIS MATERIAL USEFUL?

Measurement enables us to describe the data in a graphical or numeric format. This description helps us summarize the data and understand their behavior. In turn, this knowledge guides further analysis.

ON THE JOB! INTERVIEW VIDEO 7.1

Paula Lewis
Director for Clinical Learning

Using Data to Optimize Learning
Barriers to education
Working with leaders
Curriculum redesign

1. Paula uses a line chart to show new nurse employee attendance in specific training sessions and retention over a 3-year period. Is this the best way to display the data? Why or why not?
2. Why would a health system want to focus time and resources on nurse retention? What are the benefits of retaining seasoned nurses versus continually hiring new graduates? What value do new graduates bring to the workforce?
3. How did collecting and analyzing these data result in changes to the processes for new nurses? Would this have been possible without this information?

The interview is available online by visiting www.springerpub.com/courseconnect. See inside front cover and tear-out card for CourseConnect details.

TYPES OF DATA ANALYTICS

There are three types of data analytics: descriptive, predictive, and prescriptive.

1. **Descriptive analytics** is the categorization or summarization of historical data to understand what is or has been happening. It is the simplest and most widely used type of data analytics and lends itself very well to visualization with charts, graphs, maps, and dashboards. It presents data in a way that is easy to comprehend and often serves as a first step toward further data analysis. Questions that can be answered with descriptive analytics include: Which payer takes the longest time to reimburse the hospital? At what time of the day do we have the biggest bottlenecks in the ED? Which doctors account for the majority of malpractice settlements? How many patients live more than 20 miles from our facility? The descriptive analytics covered in this book include dashboards, basic charts and quality tools, frequency distributions, probability distributions, descriptive statistics, measures of association, and hypothesis tests.
2. **Predictive analytics** help predict the future based on patterns and relationships in historical data. The underlying assumption is that the same "behavior" in the data will continue in the future. Examples of questions that can be answered with predictive analytics include: How many outpatient visits can we expect during each quarter of the next year? Which patients will be most likely to miss their appointments? What will our monthly supply expenses be next year?

Which departments will be the most understaffed in the next 2 years? How long will patients have to wait in the ED given our current capacity levels? By giving managers a picture of what can be expected in the future, predictive analytics are very helpful in formulating strategies (Chapter 1) and developing effective plans. The predictive analytics technique covered in this book is regression (Chapter 9); the benefits of another, simulation, are noted in Chapter 11.

3. **Prescriptive analytics** rely on optimization models to determine the course of action that will maximize (e.g., profit) or minimize (e.g., cost) an objective. Typically, the problems that are solved using prescriptive analytics are so complex that the decision-maker alone cannot identify all possible alternatives and select the best one. Typical questions that can be answered with prescriptive analytics are: What is the best patient appointment schedule that will minimize wait time? To which project activities should we allocate more resources in order to complete the project earlier while minimizing the extra expenses? What is the nursing schedule that will provide the necessary nurse-to-patient ratio while accommodating their preferences for days off?

Please note that many decisions will require all three types of data analytics. For example, to improve the flow of patients in the ED, hospital staff and/or consultants would collect data on patient arrivals and times at each process step to develop probability distributions (descriptive analytics). Given those distributions, simulation models would be run to predict wait times at various stages in the process and for various levels of capacity (predictive analytics). Then, staff schedules that minimize the cost of providing care with fewer bottlenecks would be developed (prescriptive analytics).

DATA SETS

The data are usually organized in a data set. A **data set** is a collection of data that are organized in rows and columns, with each column representing a variable, and each row representing a record. For example, in the data set shown in Figure 7.1, the variables are patient ID, age, race, and so forth. Each row shows the values of these variables for a given patient with a unique identifier.

Coding:

Race: (1) Native American/Alaska Native; (2) Asian; (3) Black or African American; (4) Native Hawaiian or Other Pacific Islander; (5) White

Education: (1) 8th grade or less; (2) Some high school; (3) High school graduate or GED; (4) Some college or 2-year degree; (5) 4-year college graduate; (6) More than 4-year college degree

Insurance status: (1) Insured; (2) uninsured

Health rating: (1) Excellent; (2) Very good; (3) Good; (4) Fair; (5) Poor

You will notice that all the data are in a numerical rather than textual format. For example, Patient 126381's race is coded "1" for "Native American." This facilitates analysis using statistical software.

	A	B	C	D	E	F	G	H
1	Patient ID	Age	Race	Education	Insurance status	Resting Heart rate	BMI	Overall health rating
2	126381	18	1	3	1	50	20	1
3	138019	56	5	4	2	68	23	2
4	226582	32	5	5	1	98	28	5
5	156609	51	2	4	1	103	30.5	4
6	196648	69	3	6	1	70	19	2
7	326512	22	4	5	1	61	21	1
8	546010	81	3	3	1	91	26	5
9	663273	46	2	6	1	63	20.5	1
10	189071	52	5	4	2	92	29.5	4
11	272008	18	5	2	1	63	18.5	1
12								

FIGURE 7.1 Data set.

MEASUREMENT LEVELS

The level of measurement of the collected data influences the range of analyses that can be performed. Table 7.1 shows the various levels of measurement, their meanings, and some examples. In the data set shown in Figure 7.1, the numbers representing patient ID, race, and insurance status convey no meaning at all; they are mere labels. For example, "uninsured," which is coded "2," is not higher in value than "insured," which is coded "1." These are **nominal or categorical data**. This is different from the numbers representing education. Notice that the numbers 1, 2, 3,

TABLE 7.1 LEVELS OF MEASUREMENT

Level of Measurement	Explanation	Example	Appropriate Measures of Central Tendency (see later section in chapter)
Nominal	The numbers associated with the answers have no meaning. They are mere labels like the numbers on NBA players' jerseys.	What is your marital status? 1. Single, never married 2. Married or domestic partnership 3. Separated 4. Divorced 5. Widowed	Mode
Ordinal	The ordering or rank of the numbers associated with the answers has meaning. There is an actual progression: 1 < 2 < 3 < 4 < 5 < 6 < 7.	What is your age? 1. 20 years old and under 2. 21–34 years old 3. 35–44 years old 4. 45–54 years old 5. 55–64 years old 6. 65–74 years old 7. 75 years or older	Mode, median
Interval	Not only do the numbers reflect an actual progression, but we can assume that the distances between the answer categories are equal. For example, the semantic difference between a "1" and a "2" is the same as between a "4" and a "5."	Indicate the extent to which you agree or disagree with the following statements (not shown here) on the scale below: 1. Strongly disagree 2. Disagree 3. Neither agree nor disagree 4. Agree 5. Strongly agree	Mode, median, mean
Ratio	The numbers associated with the answer categories have the same properties as interval-scaled data, but additionally, they have a true zero. Therefore, we can compare the numbers and say, for example, that $50,000 is twice as much as $25,000 or that 60 years old is three times as old as 20 years old.	How old are you? __________ years old.	Mode, median, mean

4, 5 show a progression in the highest level of education attained. Their order or rank matters, and they are referred to as **ordinal data. Interval data** are very similar to ordinal data, but we can reasonably assume that the distances between the numbers of the scale used to measure the data, for example, 1 to 2 and 4 to 5, are equal. In the data shown in Figure 7.1, the difference between "fair" and "poor" for health rating is very similar to the difference between "fair" and "good." That was not the case with ordinal data since the difference between, let's say "8th grade or less" and "some high school" is dissimilar to the difference between "some college or a 2-year degree" and "4-year college graduate." Interval data may have a zero point as a reference, but it is not a "meaningful" zero. For example, the pH level of a solution is its level of acidity or alkalinity, measured on a scale of 0 to 14. The level "0" is the most acidic state and does not mean the "absence" of anything. The final and fourth measurement level, **ratio data**, is the richest because it has a true zero or origin, allowing us to make several meaningful comparisons between variables. For example, a 40-year-old person is twice as old as a 20-year-old (Table 7.1).

More powerful analyses can be performed with interval and ratio data. Therefore, you should always try to collect such data even if you decide to categorize them later for simplicity. For example, you could measure patients' exact heights (ratio data) and later decide to categorize the patients as short, average, and tall.

DATA VISUALIZATION EXAMPLES FOR DIFFERENT MEASUREMENT LEVELS

"**Data visualization** is the graphical representation of information and data" (Tableau Software, 2024). As you know, a picture is worth a thousand words. It displays complex information in a way that everyone can understand, helps uncover patterns and relationships, and facilitates collaboration and decision-making. Data tell their own story through graphs, maps, and charts. It is important to use the most appropriate type of visualization for your data. The text that follows features some of the charts appropriate for different measurement levels.

NOMINAL AND ORDINAL DATA

Let us assume that we want to show the number of ED patients discharged, admitted, or transferred in a given month. Figure 7.2 displays the absolute frequency distribution of patients with disposition 1, 2, and 3. **Absolute frequencies** refer to the number of times a certain value, or group of values, occurs in a data set. A **frequency distribution** shows the frequencies for all possible outcomes in a data set in a tabular or graphical format.

Bar Chart

Bar charts are frequently used to represent the frequency of nominal data. As shown in the text that follows, the variable labels can be displayed on the horizontal axis (Figure 7.3A) or the

	A	B	C
1	Disposition	Number of Patients	
2	1	3972	
3	2	616	
4	3	113	
5			
6	1 = discharge; 2 = admission; 3 = transfer		

FIGURE 7.2 Absolute frequencies for each disposition in tabular format.

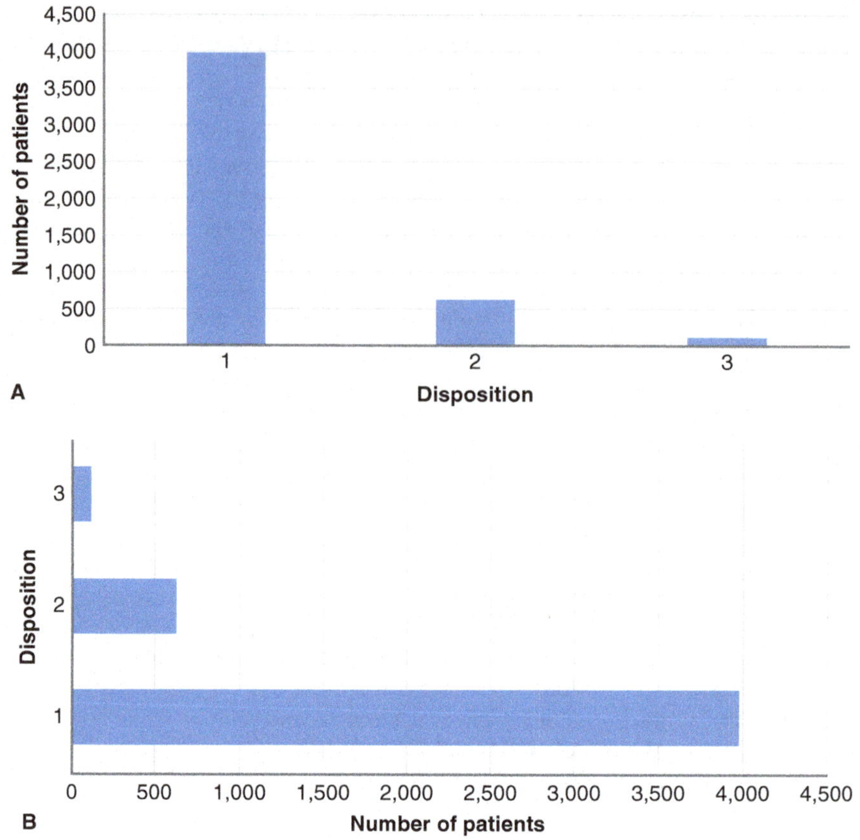

FIGURE 7.3 Frequency distribution on vertical (A) and horizontal (B) bar charts.

Note: In Excel, the numbers 1, 2, and 3 were formatted as text to indicate that they had no numerical value.

vertical axis (Figure 7.3B; see also Excel Video 7.1). The numbers used to designate the variable "disposition"—that is, 1, 2, and 3—are simple labels. The length of the bars indicates the absolute frequencies of the data, that is, 3,972 discharged, 616 admitted, and 113 transferred patients. Bar charts can also display **relative frequencies**, that is, frequencies expressed as percentages of the total number of values.

EXCEL VIDEO 7.1

Bar Chart

Access the Excel video online by visiting www.springerpub.com/courseconnect. See inside front cover and tear-out card for CourseConnect details.

Pie and Doughnut Charts

Nominal data can also be summarized and depicted with pie charts. **Pie charts** are typically a preferred graph to display relative frequencies or percentages. Figure 7.4 (see also Excel Video 7.2) indicates that 85%, 13%, and 2% of the ED's patients were discharged, admitted, and transferred, respectively.

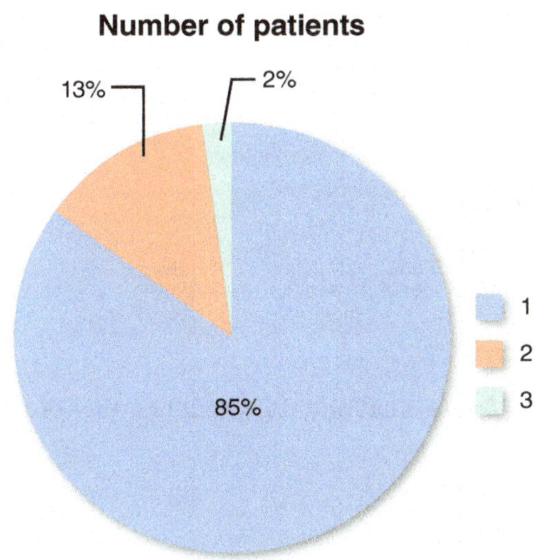

FIGURE 7.4 Pie chart.

EXCEL VIDEO 7.2

Pie Chart

Access the Excel video online by visiting www.springerpub.com/courseconnect. See inside front cover and tear-out card for CourseConnect details.

Tables, bar charts, and pie charts can be used with ordinal data as well. Figure 7.5 features an example for education levels in a set of 228 patient surveys. The bar chart and **doughnut chart** (a type of pie chart) shown in Figure 7.6 depict summaries of ordinal data.

The previous charts can also be used to describe interval and ratio data. However, other charts are often used to depict data with higher levels of measurement, as shown in the text that follows.

	A	B
1	Years of Formal Education	Number of Patients
2	0-8	2
3	9-11	6
4	12-13	120
5	14-15	58
6	16-17	37
7	18-19	5
8	20 and more	2

FIGURE 7.5 Absolute frequencies for years of formal education.

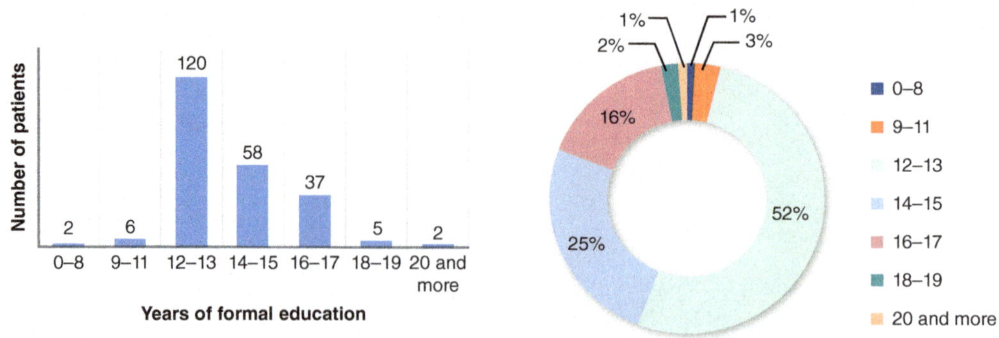

FIGURE 7.6 Bar chart and doughnut chart for ordinal data.

INTERVAL AND RATIO DATA

Interval and ratio variables are not associated with specific categories and provide meaningful information about the difference between values.

Histogram

Histograms display the frequencies for each value or each equal range of values (i.e., bin) of interval or ratio data in a set. Because the distances between two consecutive values are equal in interval and ratio data, we use histograms rather than bar charts to represent them. For example, if instead of grouping age into intervals, we considered every value, let's say from 20 to 30 (Figure 7.7; Box 7.1), we would depict the number of patients for each age with a histogram. The histogram looks like a bar chart, but there are no gaps between the bars (Figure 7.8).

	A	B
1	Age	Number of Patients
2	20	6
3	21	26
4	22	39
5	23	55
6	24	62
7	25	120
8	26	66
9	27	57
10	28	36
11	29	12
12	30	7

FIGURE 7.7 Absolute frequency distribution for patients' ages.

BOX 7.1 FAQs

In Figure 7.5, the education groups are equal: 12–13; 14–15; 16–17; and so on. Why can't we assume they are interval data?

In order to capture all possible education groups, some of the intervals will be larger. For example, the first interval, 0–8, and especially the last one, 20 or more, are substantially larger than the other intervals.

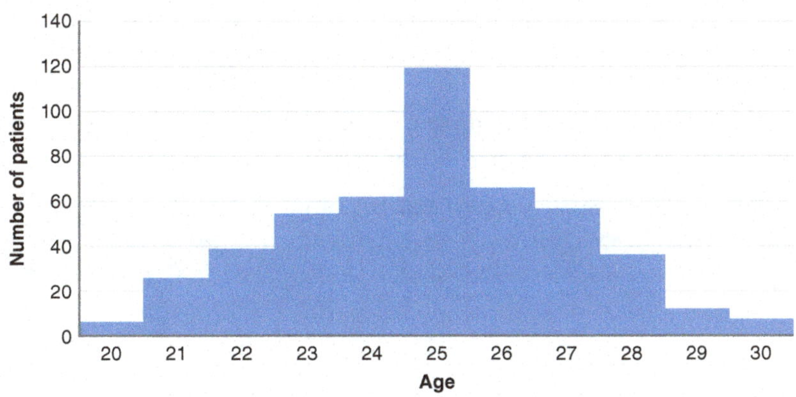

FIGURE 7.8 Histogram and absolute frequency distribution for age.

Line Chart

Line charts are useful to display changes in interval or ratio data over time. Data are taken at fixed time intervals and are connected by a line. Time is on the horizontal or ***x*-axis**, whereas the metric being tracked is on the vertical or ***y*-axis**. For example, let us assume that a diabetic patient has been on a diet for 10 months. Her doctor has been charting her weight as shown in the text that follows to show her progress (Figure 7.9; see also Excel Video 7.3).

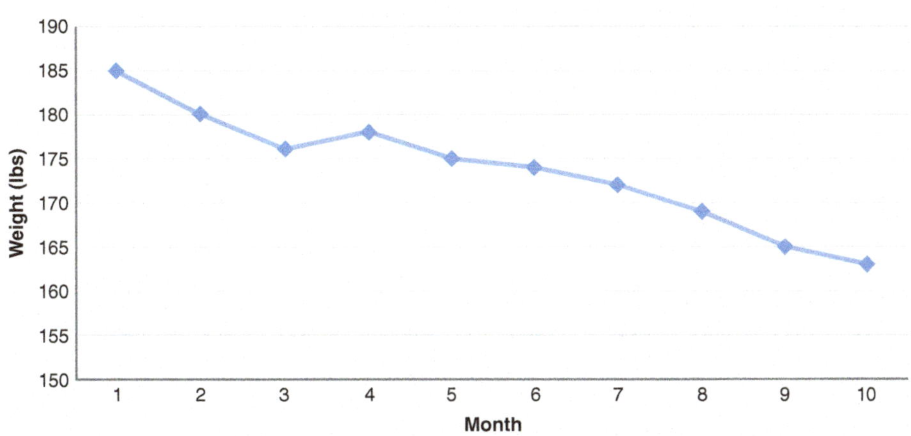

FIGURE 7.9 Line chart for weight.

EXCEL VIDEO 7.3

Line Chart

Access the Excel video online by visiting www.springerpub.com/courseconnect. See inside front cover and tear-out card for CourseConnect details.

The intent in this chapter is not to show all available charts, but just to give an overview of the most common ones. The text that follows features a list of other, common charts that you can develop using Excel (Table 7.2).

BRIGHT ANGEL MEDICAL CENTER 7.2

Adeleke and Olina were still pondering how to reschedule the ED staff based on the following graphs (Exhibit 7.1). Olina said, "It took us longer than expected to get these data because of miscommunication. We talked about waits, and our analytics team first started gathering data on the times in the waiting room. We had to clarify the operational definition of our indicator of interest: door-to-doc time."

Adeleke nodded. "I should have been more clear at the beginning. It's on me. I'll upload the precise definitions of our indicators on the shared drive."

EXHIBIT 7.1 LINE CHART FOR DOOR-TO-DOC TIMES AND BAR GRAPH FOR NUMBER OF DAILY VISITS

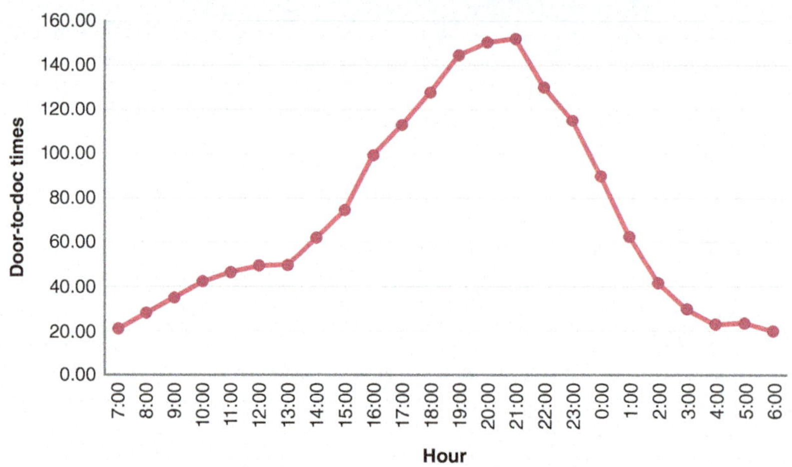

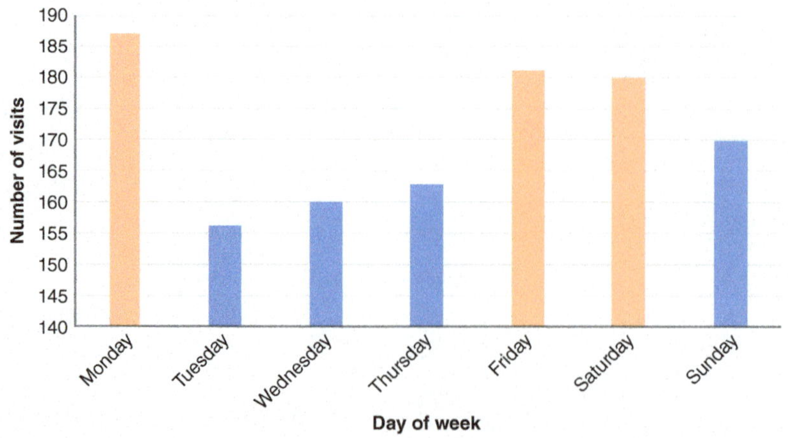

(continued)

BRIGHT ANGEL MEDICAL CENTER 7.2 (*CONTINUED*)

Olina said, "No worries. We need to schedule more staff in the evening and fewer people in the morning. We also need more people on weekends than during the week. As simple as that."

Adeleke frowned. "Good luck getting our staff to agree to less desirable shifts!" he pouted.

"Hmm, you've got a point," Olina agreed. "The leadership will have to make that option somewhat attractive; otherwise, we might lose people, which is the last thing we want. Let's call Barbara."

Could Olina and Adeleke get a better idea of staffing needs by plotting the data at a more granular level? Explain.

How could they persuade staff to give up a convenient shift for another, less attractive one?

TABLE 7.2 COMMON CHARTS IN EXCEL

Chart	Purpose
Area	Show the change in one or more quantities over time
XY (scatter plot)	Display the relationships between two metric variables (Chapter 5)
Map	Compare values for different categories in different geographic regions
Surface	Show relationship between two metric, independent variables and a dependent variable and help identify optimal combinations
Radar	Compare entities/categories across multiple metric variables in a two-dimensional format
Treemap	Display hierarchical data using nested shapes (e.g., rectangles)
Sunburst	Display hierarchical data in a circular format, with each ring representing a hierarchy level
Box and whisker	Depict the center (median) and spread (minimum, maximum, interquartile range) of a metric variable
Waterfall	Visualize the impact of sequential increases and decreases in data with a running total
Funnel	Display the progressive reduction of data from one stage to the other (e.g., number of job candidates after each interview stage)

Dashboard

Dashboards (Chapter 4) track performance on key metrics and are automatically updated as soon as new data become available. Conceptually, they are identical to the dashboard in your car with at-a-glance visual displays of the odometer, speedometer, fuel gauge, and so forth. Dashboards can be in a tabular or graphical format (Box 7.2). Specialized software can be used to develop sophisticated dashboards, but even simple tools like PivotChart in Excel help you visualize performance over time. The text that follows shows an example for mortality index and hospital-acquired conditions per 1,000 discharges (Figure 7.10). You can also create interactive Excel dashboards with slicers and timelines (see Quality Dashboard data set in online student resources; https://support.microsoft.com/en-ie/office/create-and-share-a-dashboard-with-excel-and-microsoft-groups-ad92a34d-38d0-4fdd-b8b1-58379aae746e).

BOX 7.2 QUALITY IN PRACTICE!

What Types of Charts Do Patients Prefer?

Patients facing different options of carotid stenosis treatment must understand their risks of stroke or death over time. Graphical representations of these risks may enhance risk perceptions, but it is unclear which type of graphical format patients prefer. Patients at the Dartmouth Vascular Clinic were presented with icon arrays, bar charts, line charts, and pie charts. Patients overwhelmingly preferred the pie charts over the other types of graphs. They also preferred the quantification of risk as probability of major stroke or death over the proportion of time lived without major stroke or death. These visualizations of risk facilitated patients' and providers' shared decision-making regarding treatment options (Scalia et al., 2019).

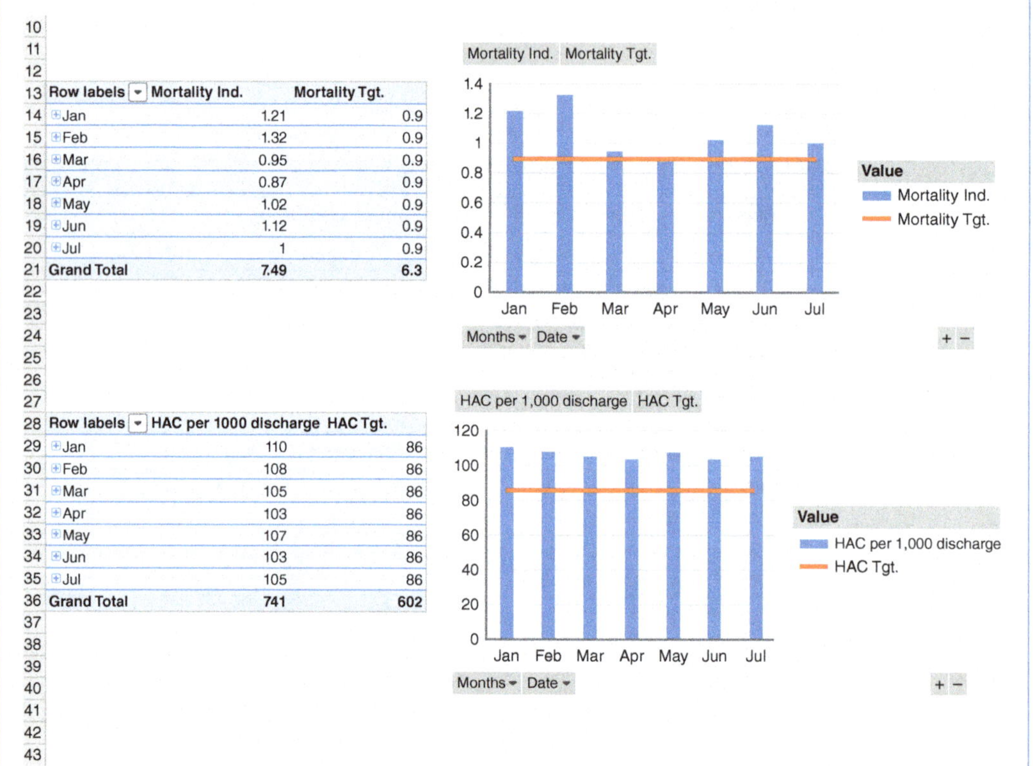

Row labels	Mortality Ind.	Mortality Tgt.
Jan	1.21	0.9
Feb	1.32	0.9
Mar	0.95	0.9
Apr	0.87	0.9
May	1.02	0.9
Jun	1.12	0.9
Jul	1	0.9
Grand Total	**7.49**	**6.3**

Row labels	HAC per 1000 discharge	HAC Tgt.
Jan	110	86
Feb	108	86
Mar	105	86
Apr	103	86
May	107	86
Jun	103	86
Jul	105	86
Grand Total	**741**	**602**

FIGURE 7.10 Simple dashboard with PivotChart.

POPULATION AND SAMPLE

In statistics, the target **population** represents a complete group of similar units of interest in a study. For example, if you were interested in patient satisfaction with the ED care provided at a particular hospital, the satisfaction scores of *all* the patients having presented to the ED at that hospital would be the population of interest. However, only a random **sample** of patients having visited the ED will receive the invitation to participate in the survey. The sample is therefore a subset of the target population. The **sampling frame** is a listing of all the patients in the population. The total number of the units in the population, or **population size**, is denoted by N. The total number of units in a sample, or **sample size**, is denoted by n.

PROBABILITIES

A **probability** is a chance of occurrence determined by the ratio of favorable outcomes to the total number of possible outcomes. It has a value between 0 and 1. The **outcomes** of an experiment are the results that we observe. Let us define $P(O_i)$ as the probability that outcome *i* occurs (Evans, 2013).

There are several types of probability:

1. **Theoretical probability**: It is a known chance of occurrence. There is no need to conduct an experiment, make observations, or collect data. For example, when rolling a die, theoretically you would expect any of the following outcomes: 1, 2, 3, 4, 5, and 6. Each outcome has a chance (or probability) of 1/6 of being selected.
2. **Experimental probability**: It is not based on a known fact. Rather, it pertains to actual observations. For example, if you roll a die six times, it is possible that you will get "1" 6 times. In that particular experiment, the probability of getting "1" would not be 1/6. Let's use another example. Assume that there are 10 students in one class, and their ages, in ascending order, are 23, 25, 25, 26, 26, 26, 28, 30, 35, 51. The probability of randomly selecting a student who is 26 is 3/10. This probability is specific to this data set.
3. **Subjective probability**. It is based on judgment. For example, based on your family history, you may think that you have at least a 50% chance of developing breast cancer. (Let's hope not!)

As you may have already noticed, frequencies are related to probabilities. In the die example, there is one chance of getting a "3" out of the six possible outcomes. Therefore, the probability of getting a "3" is 1/6. In the student age example, the age value 26 is observed three times (absolute frequency) out of 10, yielding a 0.3 probability of selecting a 26-year-old student out of that set.

For a given data set, the sum of the probabilities of occurrence for each value or groups of values is 1. Let's illustrate this fact with the die example. The probability of getting a 1, 2, 3, 4, 5, OR 6 is 1/6. The sum of probabilities for all possible outcomes is $P(1) + P(2) + P(3) + P(4) + P(5) + P(6) = 1/6 + 1/6 + 1/6 + 1/6 + 1/6 + 1/6 = 6/6 = 1$.

More advanced probability concepts are explained in the online Student Resources, eChapter 14 (eChapter 14 is available online by visiting www.springerpub.com/courseconnect. See inside front cover and tear-out card for CourseConnect details).

THEORETICAL AND EMPIRICAL DISTRIBUTIONS

Theoretical distributions are based on mathematical formulas, not collected data. Their shapes and other characteristics are firmly established. **Empirical distributions** start with collecting data and then building a frequency distribution. The distribution depicted in Figure 7.8 is an empirical distribution. There are both frequency and probability distributions. A frequency distribution shows the number of times each value occurs in a data set. A **probability distribution** indicates the likelihood that each possible value will occur. Obtaining a probability distribution for all possible values of, let's say, the ages of U.S. patients who died of a heart attack, would be rather complex. Fortunately, theoretical distributions help us make predictions about the likelihood of an event occurring without a huge data collection effort.

Although we could develop an empirical distribution based on a small sample, let's say 10 patients' ages, we can all agree that we would get a better estimate of the average age if we collected the data in many other samples or in a very large sample. This is where the **law of large numbers (LoLN)** and the **central limit theorem (CLT)** come into play.

The *LoLN* tells us that the average of the results obtained from a large number of independent samples of a random variable (here, the random variable is age) will approach the average of the variable in the population. Remember that the population would involve the ages of ALL the patients. The metrics used to summarize population data are called **parameters**; those used to describe sample data are called **statistics**.

LoLN: As the sample size increases, the probability that the sample mean approaches the true mean gets closer to 1.

What does that mean? Let's go back to our original example of rolling a die. If we roll the die 10 times, we may never get a "5". However, if we repeat this action 1,000 times, the results will probably show that we get a "5" about 166 times out of 1,000 or 1/6th of the time. The implication is important! It says that ***as our sample size increases, our empirical distribution starts resembling a theoretical distribution.***

The CLT tells us that the distribution of the averages of many, sufficiently large samples (Box 7.3) of a random variable is approximately normal. In other words, irrespective of the original population distribution, the distribution of the sample means will be approximately normal.

CLT: As the sample size increases, the distribution of the sample means approaches the normal distribution.

What does that mean? It means that as we draw larger, independent samples from a population that is not normally distributed, the distribution of the sample averages will resemble the normal distribution. By extension, ***when we have a large enough random sample, we can assume normality when doing various types of statistical analysis.***

Look at Figure 7.11. It displays the **sampling distribution**—the distribution of a sample statistic across many random samples taken from a population—of heads in 250 trials of 50 coin tosses. Note that in 50 coin tosses, 13H and 35H were obtained very few times. On the other hand, about 25H (50/2) were obtained most often, which is what you would expect if you tossed the coin 50 times since the theoretical probability of getting a head is ½. This is the illustration of the LoLN. Moreover, the distribution of this collection of large sample results approximates the normal distribution (look at the bell curve that has been superimposed over the empirical distribution) even though coin tosses have binary outcomes (H or T) and therefore follow the binomial distribution. This is the illustration of the CLT. Note: The normal distribution is a *theoretical* distribution.

BOX 7.3 FAQs

What do you mean by "large enough" sample size?

In most cases, it means that $n \geq 30$

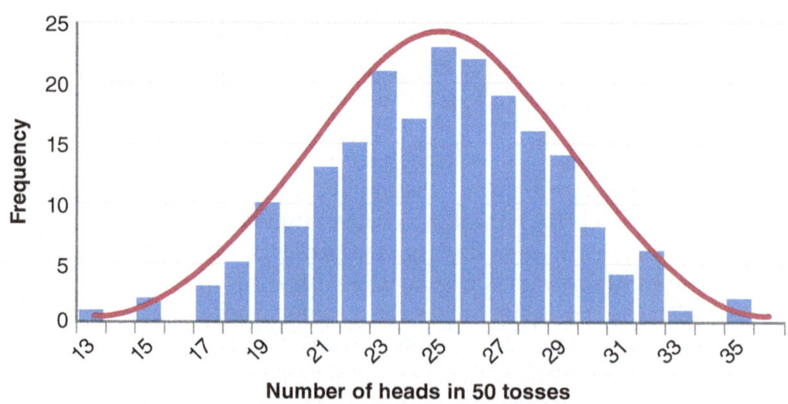

FIGURE 7.11 Illustration of LoLN and CLT with 250 experiments of 50 coin tosses.

Abbreviations: CLT, central limit theorem; LoLN, law of large numbers.

BRIGHT ANGEL MEDICAL CENTER 7.3

The proposal to reschedule staff right away had not convinced Barbara Waters. She felt that process improvements should be done before changing capacity. These improvements would streamline processes and improve flow. She wanted Dr. Aoki's perspective on the issue.

A week later, Barbara called Philip Robinson, the chief pharmacy officer. "Hi, Phil. Do you have a few minutes? Adeleke and I would like to discuss something with you."

Phil said: "Sure, my next meeting is 2 hours from now. Come on over."

In Phil's office, Barbara said, "We reviewed multiple components of the length of stay in the ED. It appears that long delays can occur when waiting for medications to come from central pharmacy. The high-usage drugs are often simple ones that could be stored securely in the ED if the medications we don't use often were removed. What do you think?"

Barbara showed Phil the usage distribution of blood thinners, insulin, lidocaine, epinephrine, nitroglycerin, and antibiotics. "This idea came from our frontline clinical team," Barbara continued. "Dr. Aoki, our ED medical director, asked the providers for ideas to improve our throughput. They suspected that the medications we keep in the ED had not been reviewed in years. After pulling data and reviewing what we stored versus what we use, it became clear we need to make changes."

Philip nodded, "I am all for it. It would also save time for our inpatient pharmacy team, so they don't have to spend time pulling medications and sending them to the ED." "Sounds like a win-win!" Adeleke agreed.

Why is it important to review drug usage on a regular basis?

SOME IMPORTANT THEORETICAL DISTRIBUTIONS

Discrete Distributions

Discrete data produce discrete probability distributions. **Discrete data** represent whole units that are *counted*. For example, you count the number of people who arrive at McDonald's from 12 to 1 p.m., the number of readmissions within 30 days during the month of April, the number of postoperative deaths per 1,000 surgeries, the number of food trays returned in a given week, and so forth. These counts involve whole numbers: 1, 2, 3, 4, 5, and so forth. Of course, if you compute an average, you will get fractional amounts. That's where the 1.94 children per family come into play!

Popular theoretical discrete probability distributions include the binomial distribution and the Poisson distribution. We will specify the parameter(s)—or population characteristic(s)—for each distribution.

Binomial Distribution

A **binomial distribution** displays the probability of obtaining binary (success or failure) outcomes in n trials. For example, the number of "yes" in yes–no questions, the number of tails in coin tosses, the number of defective (as opposed to nondefective) items in a production lot, the number of incorrect (as opposed to correct) insurance claims sent by a clinic, and so on. Depending on the sample size, it may be the underlying distribution of the proportion defective in p-charts (Chapter 8). A few interesting points about the binomial distribution:

- It is applicable when the population size, N, is greater than 50 and when the sample size $n < 0.10N$.

- For smaller values of p, the probability of success, the distribution is skewed to the right; for higher values of p, the distribution is skewed to the left (Figure 7.12). For $p = 0.5$, it is symmetric.
- It is described by two parameters: the number of trials (n) and p.
  - The mean, $\mu = np$ [7.1]
  - The *SD*, $\sigma = \sqrt{np(1-p)}$ [7.2]
- As n increases, the binomial distribution approximates the normal distribution (CLT; Figure 7.11). As a general rule, the normal approximation applies if $np \geq 10$ and $n(1-p) \geq 10$. (Note: some say that a value of 5 is sufficient.)

If you need to determine the probability of getting a certain number of defective items in a sample taken from a population with a known percent defective, you will use the Excel function BINOM.DIST(*number_s, trials, probability_s, cumulative*)

where: *number_s* is the number of defective items, the probability of which we are trying to determine;

trials is the sample size;

probability_s is the known proportion of defectives in the population; and

cumulative is the option to obtain cumulative probabilities; type TRUE for cumulative probabilities, FALSE otherwise.

	A	B	C
1	n	10	
2	p	0.12	
3			Probability
4	x	1	0.37977
5		2	0.23304
6		3	0.08474
7		4	0.02022
8		5	0.00331
9		6	0.00038
10		7	0.00003
11		8	0.00000
12		9	0.00000
13		10	0.00000
14			
15			
16			
17			
18	n	10	
19	p	0.88	
20			Probability
21	x	1	0.00000
22		2	0.00000
23		3	0.00003
24		4	0.00038
25		5	0.00331
26		6	0.02022
27		7	0.08474
28		8	0.23304
29		9	0.37977
30		10	0.27850
31			
32			

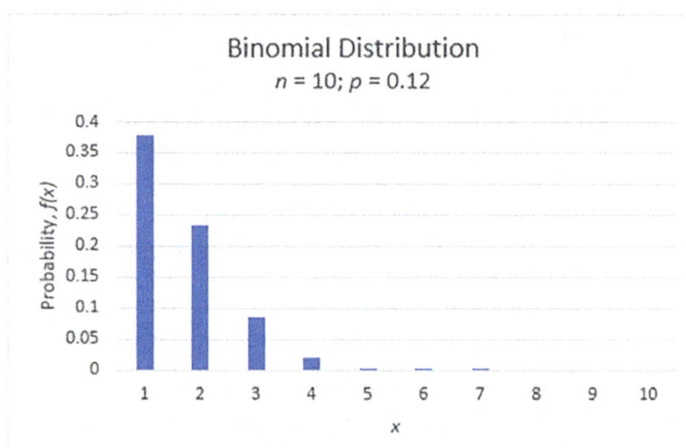

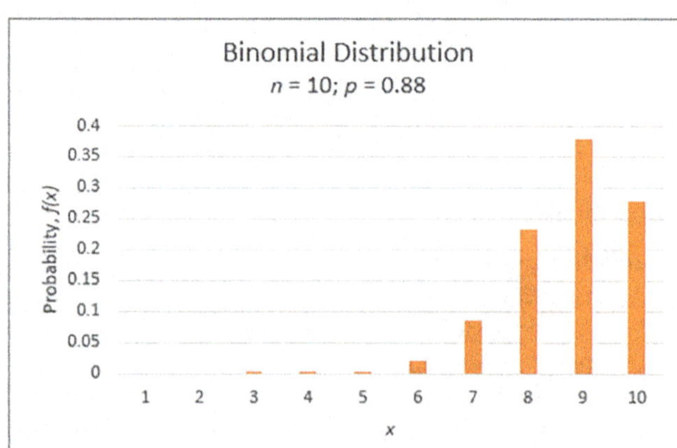

FIGURE 7.12 Binomial distributions with $p = 0.12$ and $p = 0.88$.

For example, the probability of having one complication in a sample of 10 surgeries with a known complication rate of 12% is BINOM.DIST(1, 10, 0.12, FALSE) = 0.380. Probabilities for different numbers of complications out of 10 surgeries for $p = 0.12$ and $p = 0.88$ are shown in Figure 7.12.

Poisson Distribution

The **Poisson distribution** models the number of events per unit (e.g., number of patient arrivals per hour, number of errors per claim, number of incorrect entries per patient record, etc.). It is the underlying distribution for *c*-charts (Chapter 8). A few interesting points about the Poisson distribution:

- It is defined by a parameter, λ, which is the mean number of events per unit.
- The variance, σ^2, is equal to the mean, λ.
- As λ increases, the distribution starts to resemble a normal curve (Figure 7.13).

If you need to find the number of defects per unit in a Poisson process known to have λ defects, you can use the Excel function POISSON.DIST(*x*, *mean*, *cumulative*)

where: *x* is the number of defects specified in the quesstion;

mean is λ; and

cumulative is the option to obtain cumulative probabilities; type TRUE for cumulative probabilities, FALSE otherwise.

Assume that the number of incorrect entries in a clinic's patient records is described by the Poisson distribution with a mean of 3. The probability of finding 2 incorrect entries in a patient record is POISSON.DIST(2, 3, FALSE) = 0.224.

Continuous Distributions

Continuous distributions are based on continuous data. **Continuous data** are *measured, not* counted. They are measured with an instrument (e.g., temperature, weight, height, length, blood pressure, blood sugar level, time in the waiting room, etc.). Since they are measured on a continuous scale, values with decimals are frequent (e.g., 1.3 meters, 3.67 minutes). A continuous distribution has an infinity of possible outcomes. The probabilities of continuous random variables only apply to intervals [$P(a \leq X \leq b)$], not specific values. Examples of continuous distributions include the normal, Student's *t*, chi-square, and *F* distributions. In this chapter, we will only discuss the normal and standard normal distributions, but the other continuous distributions mentioned here are discussed in the online Student Resources, eChapter 14.

Normal Distribution

The **normal distribution** is the bell curve; it is the most widely used continuous distribution in statistics and is also known as the Gaussian distribution. It is often used to:

- Compare means and proportions between two or more groups (see online Student Resources).

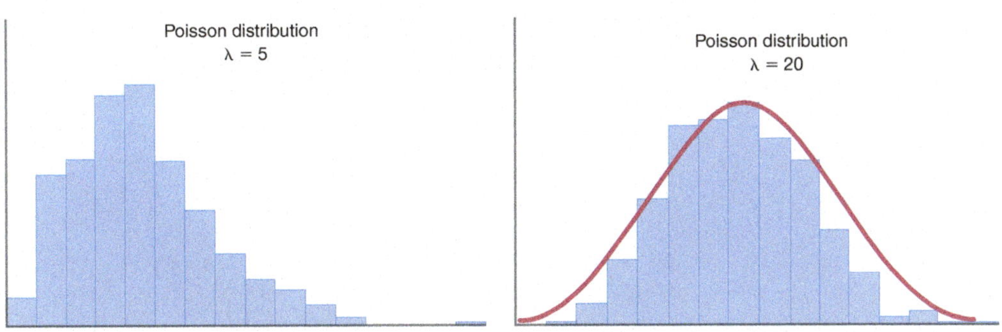

FIGURE 7.13 Example of Poisson distribution with $\lambda = 5$ and $\lambda = 20$.

- Develop confidence intervals (see online Student Resources, eChapter 16).
- Develop and analyze statistical process control charts (Chapter 8).

There are several interesting facts about the normal distribution:

- Its two parameters are its mean (μ) and its *SD* (σ).
  - The mean, $\mu = \frac{\sum_{i=1}^{N} X_i}{N}$ [7.3]
  - The *SD*, $\sigma = \sqrt{\frac{\sum_{i=1}^{n} (X_i - \mu)^2}{N}}$ [7.4]
- It is symmetric around its mean (Figure 7.14), with 99.7% of the data comprised within ±3 *SD* from the mean (total = 6 *SD*). In other words, almost *all* the data are within 6 *SD*. The 6 *SD* represent the natural width of the distribution. Any value outside the limits set by ± 3 *SD* is possible, but unexpected and inconsistent with the distribution; it would be considered an anomaly.
- The mean, median, and mode are equal.
- The tails of the normal distribution do not end. *Any* value is therefore possible. However, practically, we know that 99.7% or *nearly all* values are within ± 3 *SD* from the mean.

To compute the probability of a given random variable being less than equal to a certain value, we can use the Excel function NORM.DIST(*x, mean, standard_deviation, cumulative*)

where *x* is the value that the random variable cannot exceed;

cumulative is the option to obtain cumulative probabilities, which is the case here; therefore, type TRUE.

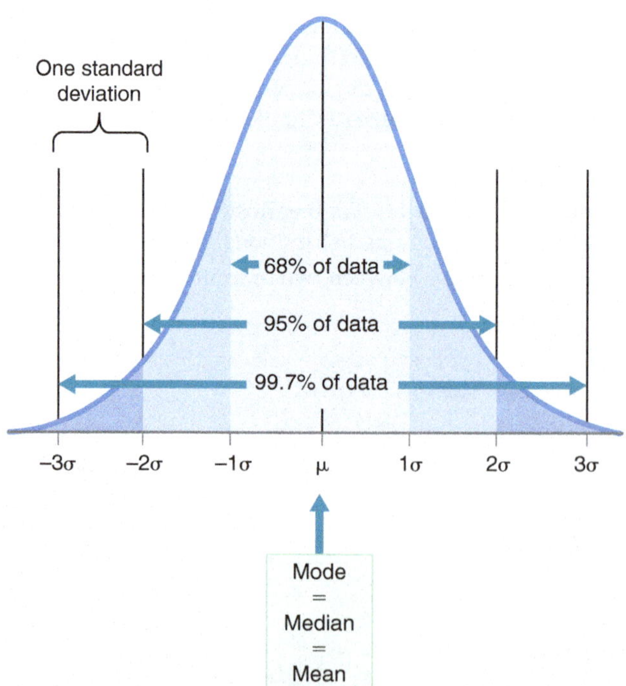

FIGURE 7.14 Normal distribution.

Let's assume that the door-to-doc times in the ED are normally distributed with $\mu = 120$ min and $\sigma = 20$ min. The probability that the door-to-doc time would not exceed 100 min is $P(X \leq 100)$ = NORM.DIST(100, 120, 20, TRUE) = 0.159. $P(X > 100)$ is simply $1 - P(X \leq 100) = 1 - 0.159 = 0.841$.

Standard Normal Distribution

Although probabilities for normal distributions with different values for μ and σ can be easily obtained with Excel (see the previous discussion), most reference manuals provide probability tables for the standard normal distribution (Appendix A). The **standard normal distribution** is a special case of the normal distribution:

- $\mu = 0$, and $\sigma = 1$
- The values for which cumulative probabilities are given (see Appendix A) are known as *z*-values
- Random *x* variables with a given μ and σ can be standardized to *z*-values on the standard normal distribution, using the formula:

$$z = \frac{X - \mu}{\sigma} \qquad [7.5]$$

For example, if *x* is normally distributed with a mean of 63 and an *SD* of 4.83, $P(X \leq 60)$ can be found with NORM.DIST(60, 63, 4. 84, TRUE) = 0.2676. Alternatively, *x* can be standardized to $z = \frac{60-63}{4.84} = -0.62$. $P(z \leq -0.62) = 0.2676$ (Figures 7.15 and 7.16). Conversely, $P(X > 60) = P(z > -0.62) = 1 - P(z \leq -0.62) = 1 - 0.2676 = 0.7324$.

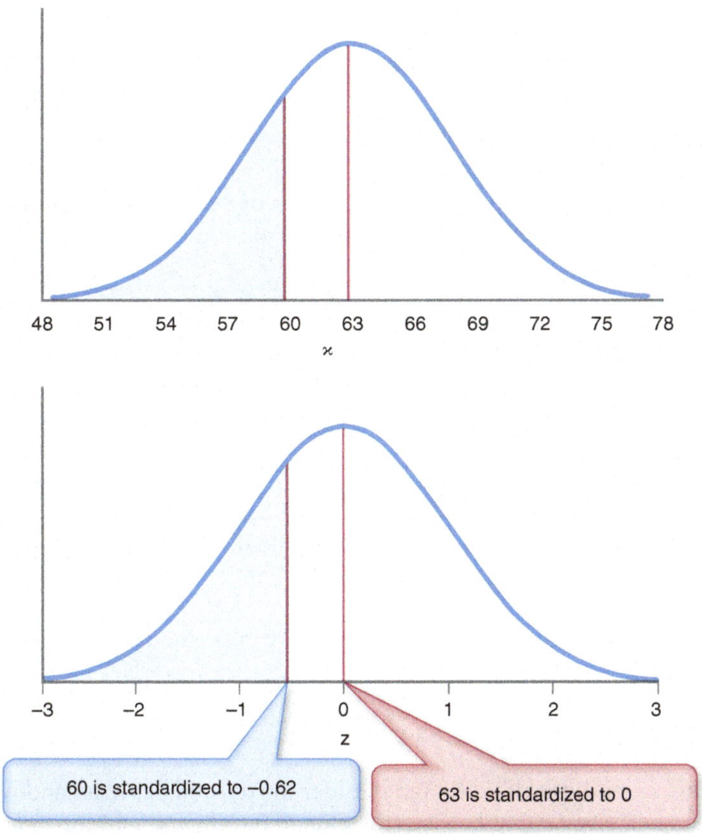

FIGURE 7.15 Standardizing the normal distribution.

Table

Z	0.00	0.01	0.02	0.03	0.04
−0.0	0.5000	0.4960	0.4920	0.4880	0.4840
−0.1	0.4602	0.4562	0.4522	0.4483	0.4443
−0.2	0.4207	0.4168	0.4129	0.4090	0.4052
−0.3	0.3821	0.3783	0.3745	0.3707	0.3669
−0.4	0.3446	0.3409	0.3372	0.3336	0.3299
−0.5	0.3085	0.3050	0.3015	0.2981	0.2946
−0.6	0.2743	0.2709	0.2676	0.2643	0.2610
−0.7	0.2417	0.2385	0.2354	0.2323	0.2291

FIGURE 7.16 $P(z \le -0.62)$ in negative standard normal distribution.

In statistics, we often try to find the center of the frequency distribution and the extent to which the data vary. The former refers to central tendency, and the latter to dispersion.

MEASURES OF CENTRAL TENDENCY

Central tendency refers to the center of the distribution of a particular variable. The measures of central tendency are the mode, the median, and the mean.

THE MODE

The **mode** is the value that occurs most frequently in the data set. As a result, its frequency is the peak of a distribution. For example, at Bright Angel Medical Center (BAMC)'s ED, the percentages of top box scores for "Understanding care after leaving the hospital" from January to November were the following (Chapter 4):

86	85	80	68	70	71	76	78	63	62	70

The mode is 70 because it occurred more often than any other number in the data set (Figure 7.17). In Excel, the function to obtain the mode in a data set is: MODE.SNGL(number1, [number2], …).

In the normal distribution, there is only one mode; it is unimodal. But in other distributions, there could be multiple modes (Figure 7.18).

THE MEDIAN

The **median** is the center of the data. To find it, order the data values in ascending or descending order. The median is the value that has half the data to its left, and half the data to its right. The position of the median is given by the following formula:

Position of the median = $(n+1)/2$ where n is the total number of data points or values [7.6]

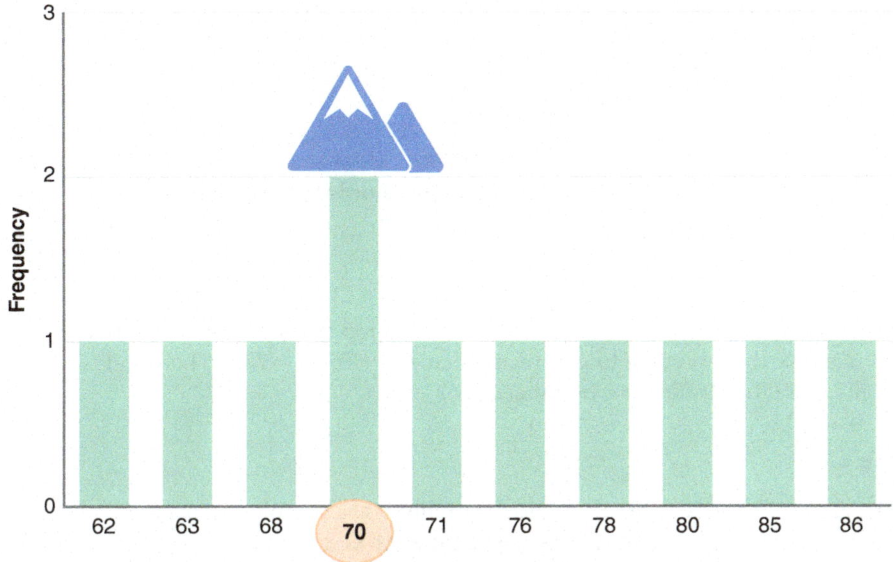

FIGURE 7.17 Mode = peak frequency.

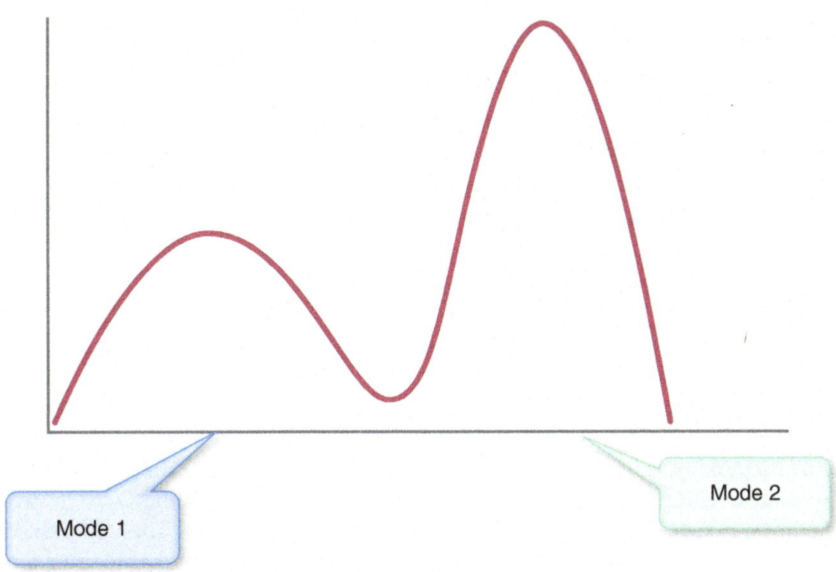

FIGURE 7.18 Bimodal distribution.

To find the median of BAMC's ED top box scores for "Understanding care after leaving the hospital" from January to November, you will follow these steps:

STEP 1: Reorganize the data in ascending order: 62, 63, 68, 70, 70, 71, 76, 78, 80, 85, 86.

STEP 2: Find the position of the median. There are 11 scores. Therefore, the position of the median is the $(11 + 1)/2 = 6$th top box score.

STEP 3: State the median: The median is 71 (Figure 7.19)

What if the number of data points is even? Let's find out by adding one more top box score: 62, 63, 68, 70, 70, 71, 76, 78, 80, 85, 86, 88

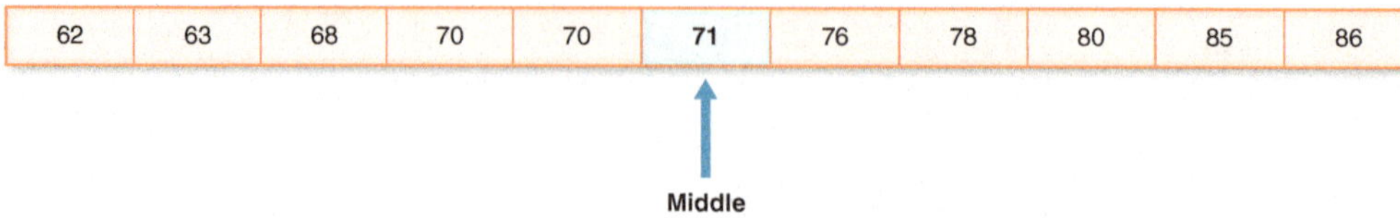

FIGURE 7.19 Median = middle of ordered data values.

Now, the position of the median is (11 + 1)/2 = 6.5th top box score. This is between the 6th and 7th score. We take their average to get the median: (71 + 76)/2 = 73.5. The Excel function to find the median is MEDIAN(number1, [number2], ...)

THE MEAN

The **mean** is simply the average of all the data points. The population mean or parameter is referred to as μ; the sample mean or statistic is referred to as $\bar{X}$. It is found with the following formula:

$$\bar{X} = \frac{\sum_{i=1}^{n} X_i}{n} \quad [7.7]$$

where $\bar{X}$ is the sample mean;

X_i is the value of variable X for the ith observation; and

n is the number of observations in the sample or sample size.

The numerator is the sum of all the data points. In the example used to determine the median, x_i is an individual top box score expressed as a percentage.

$$\bar{X} = \frac{86+85+80+68+70+71+76+78+63+62+70}{11} = 73.5\%$$

The sample mean is 73.5%. The Excel function to get the mean is: AVERAGE (number1, [number2], ...)

MEASURES OF DISPERSION

Variability or dispersion refers to the spread of the data distribution. The wider the spread, the more variety and uncertainty there is. Take the example of swings in the Dow Jones Industrial Index. Sometimes, it keeps going up and up, with hardly any decrease. Then all of a sudden, we see a 500-point drop followed the next day by an 1,100-point drop. At the same time, the volatility index which measures uncertainty starts going up. It is therefore important for us to measure the dispersion in the distribution of our data. The measures of dispersion or variability are the range, the variance, and the *SD* (and *SE*).

If there was no variability, all the data points would be the same!

THE RANGE

The **range** is the simplest measure of dispersion. It is computed by subtracting the smallest value in our data from the largest value.

$$R = \text{Maximum} - \text{Minimum} \quad [7.8]$$

Using the top box scores as an example, we find that the minimum value is 62, and the maximum value is 86.

86, 85, 80, 68, 70, 71, 76, 78, 63, 62, 70

The range, R, is 86% − 62% = 24%.

As mentioned in Table 7.2, the boxplot helps visualize the spread of the data by displaying the range and the **interquartile range**—the difference between the third and first quartiles—of the data. Using Excel, the boxplot (see box and whisker plot in Table 7.2) for the top box scores shown earlier is displayed in Figure 7.20. The Excel function to obtain the range is MAX(number1, [number2], …) – MIN(number1, [number2], …).

THE VARIANCE

The **variance** is simply an average of squared deviations from the mean. In other words, the extent to which a data point deviates from the average is a measure of variability. The population variance is referred to as σ^2; the sample variance is referred to as S^2. They are computed using the following formulas:

$$\sigma^2 = \frac{\sum_{i=1}^{N}(X_i - \mu)^2}{N} \quad [7.9]$$

$$S^2 = \frac{\sum_{i=1}^{n}\left(X_i - \bar{X}\right)^2}{n-1} \quad [7.10]$$

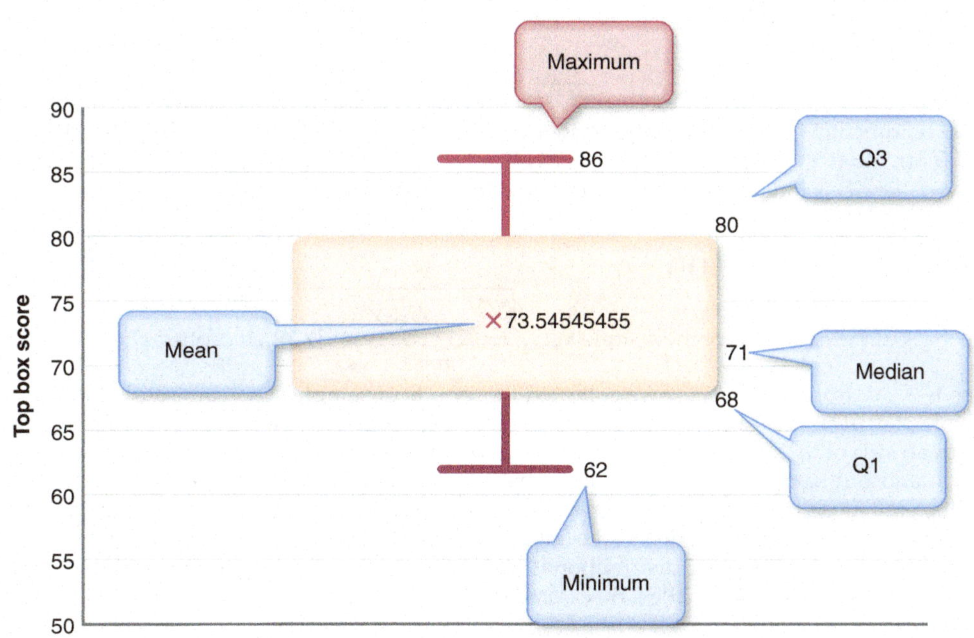

FIGURE 7.20 Boxplot for top box scores.

where X_i is the value of variable X for the ith observation;

μ is the population mean;
N is the population size; and
n is the sample size.

Note that to determine the population variance, we sum up the squared deviations of each data point from the mean and divide the sum by the population size, N. If we want to find the sample variance, we divide the sum of squared deviations by the sample size, n, minus 1. Why? Because we lose one **degree of freedom,** the number of independent values that can vary, for the estimation of the statistic $\bar{X}$.

Using the sample of top box scores as an example, let's find the variance.

$$S^2 = \frac{(86-73.55)^2 + (85-73.55)^2 + \ldots + (70-73.55)^2}{11-1} = 66.07$$

The Excel functions for the population and sample variances are VAR.P(number1, [number2], ...) and VAR.S(number1, [number2], ...), respectively. The problem with the variance is that it gives us a value in units squared. Squared percentages in the top box? We would all prefer a measure in terms of top box scores because it is easier to interpret! Therefore, let's get rid of the squares and compute the *SD*.

THE STANDARD DEVIATION

The **standard deviation (*SD*)** is the square root of the variance. The population *SD* is referred to as σ; the sample *SD* is referred to as *S*. The formulas are:

$$\sigma = \sqrt{\frac{\sum_{i=1}^{N}(X_i - \mu)^2}{N}} \qquad [7.11]$$

$$S = \sqrt{\frac{\sum_{i=1}^{n}(X_i - \bar{X})^2}{n-1}} \qquad [7.12]$$

In our example of exam scores, $S = \sqrt{66.07} = 8.13\%$. (Note that now we have meaningful units!) The Excel functions for the population and sample *SD* are STDEV.P(number1, [number2], ...) and STDEV.S(number1, [number2], ...), respectively.

A smaller *SD* is indicative of less variation, which is good since variation denotes uncertainty.

THE STANDARD ERROR

Look back at the equation for the sample *SD*, $\sqrt{\frac{\sum_{i=1}^{n}(X_i - \bar{X})^2}{n-1}}$ [7.12]. It captures how far a given value is away from the mean. If we collected thousands of samples and computed the mean for each one, the *SD* of the sample means, also known as the **standard error (SE)** of the mean, would give us an idea of the spread of the sample means around μ. If the SE is large, the means are widely spread, and our sample may not be representative of the population. If it is small, the means are clustered close to the population mean, and our sample is likely to be representative of the population. But we did not collect thousands of samples! Fortunately, as samples get larger, the CLT tells us that the sampling distribution is normal with a mean equal to the population mean, μ, and an *SD* of $\sigma / \sqrt{n}$ (Field, 2013). By extension, if we collect a large enough sample ($n \geq 30$), the *SE* $\hat{\sigma}_{\bar{x}}$, is equal to

$$\hat{\sigma}_{\bar{x}} = S / \sqrt{n} \qquad [7.13]$$

where *S* is the sample *SD*.

BRIGHT ANGEL MEDICAL CENTER 7.4

Kimberly Mitchell, CEO of the health system, was on a Gemba walk in the ED and ran into Barbara and Olina looking at their performance management board.

"Impressive," said Michael Chen, the chief nursing officer who was accompanying Kimberly.

"The data tell the story," said Olina. The team had decided to look at the variation in their key performance indicators from month to month and throughout the day.

"Sharing the data like this helps everyone to see our deviations in performance and where we need to go. Well done!" complimented Kimberly. Barbara smiled, knowing they still had a long way to go.

Why is variation in performance relevant to improvement?

ETHICAL SCENARIO 7.1

Reporting Quality Data

The Agency for Healthcare Research and Quality has promoted the public reporting of healthcare data for many years to improve transparency and to help patients make informed decisions. Several rating agencies such as the Leapfrog Group give out grades or scores based on these reported data. Patients can then use this information to assess their care options and, hopefully, make better provider selection when given the opportunity. However, some hospitals choose not to report their data or to opt out of certain data sets. This may be due to poor performance or a lack of resources to collect the data. In the end, patients may not have access to all relevant information.

What are the advantages and disadvantages of sharing healthcare data with the public? Should it be mandatory or optional?

Can you think of information that would influence your decision to seek care with a specific physician or at a certain facility?

SUMMARY

In the measurement phase, you describe the process quantitatively. The numbers tell the story of what works and what does not. In this chapter, you learned the four levels of measurement: nominal, ordinal, interval, and ratio. These levels determine how you may describe the data and analyze them. Describing the data graphically helps you identify certain data patterns or behaviors that can reveal issues that might be overlooked in a tabular display. You also learned about various probability distributions and their parameters. More importantly, the LoLN and the CLT underscored the importance of drawing larger samples (Appendix 7.1). Measures of central tendency (mode, median, and mean) and dispersion (range, variance, and *SD*) summarize the data succinctly. They will also be very useful once you start analyzing your data.

CERTIFICATION TIPS

In this chapter, it was difficult to strike a balance between the needs of a traditional Healthcare Quality course and certification requirements. Just a few differences:

The American Society for Quality certification materials provide the probability mass functions of the discrete distributions and the probability density functions of the continuous distributions. These tend to be complicated, and we do not think that their omissions in the chapter affect understanding. Yet, be reminded that they may appear on the certification test.

Rules of probability and other distributions are also beyond the scope of this book, but are available in the online Student Resources, eChapter 14 for students seeking certification.

In this chapter, we distinguished between the LoLN and the CLT. The LoLN is not explicitly mentioned in some certification guides. However, the CLT is covered in depth.

When data are collected from different sources or situations (e.g., patients with different Emergency Severity Index (ESI) levels, different shifts, different methods, etc.), you may want to stratify or sort your data. Stratification will enable a more meaningful description and interpretation of the data. A good source for the stratification procedure is:

American Society for Quality. (2024). *What is stratification?* https://asq.org/quality-resources/stratification

KEY TERMS

Data analytics
Descriptive analytics
Predictive analytics
Prescriptive analytics
Data set
Nominal (or categorical) data
Ordinal data
Interval data
Ratio data
Data visualization
Absolute frequency
Frequency distribution
Bar chart
Relative frequency
Pie chart
Doughnut chart
Histogram
Line chart
***x*-axis**
***y*-axis**
Population
Sample
Sampling frame
Population size, *N*
Sample size, *n*
Probability
Outcome
Theoretical probability
Experimental probability
Subjective probability
Theoretical distribution
Empirical distribution
Probability distribution
Law of large numbers (LoLN)
Central limit theorem (CLT)
Parameter
Statistic
Sampling distribution
Discrete data
Binomial distribution
Poisson distribution
Continuous data
Normal distribution
Standard normal distribution
Central tendency
Mode
Median
Mean
Variability or dispersion
Range
Interquartile range
Variance
Degrees of freedom
Standard deviation (*SD*)
Standard error (*SE*)

REVIEW QUESTIONS

1. What are the three types of data analytics? Briefly describe each one.
2. What are the different measurement levels? Explain and provide an example for each one.
3. What is the difference between absolute and relative frequencies?
4. What is a histogram?
5. What is the difference between a bar chart and a pie chart?
6. Differentiate among theoretical, experimental, and subjective probabilities.
7. What is the law of large numbers?
8. What is the central limit theorem?
9. What is the difference between discrete and continuous data?
10. Give an example of a discrete distribution and specify its parameters.
11. What are the three measures of central tendency?
12. What are the three primary measures of dispersion?
13. List three characteristics of the normal distribution.

SOLVE BRIGHT ANGEL MEDICAL CENTER'S PROBLEMS

1. The following are examples of questions in a patient survey. For each question, determine the level of measurement and the appropriate measure(s) of central tendency.
   a. Which one of our facility's providers is your primary care physician?
      1. Dr. Banville
      2. Dr. Ponce
      3. Dr. Sethuraman
      4. Katia Serafimov, NP
   b. What is your age?
      1. 18 to 25 years old
      2. 26 to 35 years old
      3. 36 to 45 years old
      4. 46 to 55 years old
      5. 56 to 64 years old
      6. 65 years old and over
   c. What is your race?
      1. White
      2. Black or African American
      3. Asian
      4. Native Hawaiian or other Pacific Islander
      5. Native American or Alaska Native
      6. Other
   d. Approximately, how long does it take to drive from your home to our clinic? ___________ minutes.
   e. Please indicate the extent to which you agree or disagree with the following statements on the scale that follows.

Statement	Strongly Disagree 1	Disagree 2	Neither Agree nor Disagree 3	Agree 4	Strongly Agree 5
The provider listened to my concerns carefully.					
The provider explained my condition in a way I could easily understand.					
The provider was courteous.					

2. Dr. Mitra is a primary care physician. Last month, the types of visits billed by her office fell into the following categories:

Type of Visit	Frequency
Establish care (new patient)	4
Consultation (new patient)	19
Annual physical examination	33
Follow-up visits	130

(continued)

Type of Visit	Frequency
Non-urgent problem visits	97
Urgent/Same-day appointments	65
Medicare annual wellness visits	26
Total	374

a. What type(s) of chart is(are) appropriate to display these data? Explain.
b. Use an appropriate chart to display the problem data.

3. Dr. Mitra's practice cares for over 500 patients who fall into the following age groups:

Age (years)	Frequency
0–5	22
6–12	68
13–18	86
19–25	71
26–35	55
36–45	69
46–55	51
56–64	56
65 and over	40
Total	518

a. What is the level of measurement of these data? Explain.
b. Develop a bar graph to display the age distribution of Dr. Mitra's patients. What do you observe?

4. A nurse in Dr. Mitra's office has been tracking the average time patients spend in the waiting room over the past year.

Month	Jan	Feb	March	April	May	Jun	Jul	Aug	Sep	Oct	Nov	Dec
Time (min)	6.2	6.5	5.9	6	6.7	6.9	7.1	7	7.3	7.5	7.7	8

a. What is the level of measurement of these data? Explain.
b. What type of graph would you recommend to display these data? Why?
c. Create the graph you selected in part (b) and determine the average wait time over the last 12 months.
d. Should Dr. Mitra be concerned? Why or why not?

5. The fall rate (falls per 1,000 occupied bed days) at a nursing home has been fluctuating over the past year.
a. What is the level of measurement of these data?
b. What type of graph would you recommend to display these data? Why?
c. Create the graph you selected in part (b) to display the fall rate over the last 12 months.
d. Should providers and administrators be concerned? Why or why not?
e. Compute the mode, median, and mean.
f. What is the range?

Month	Jan	Feb	March	April	May	Jun	Jul	Aug	Sep	Oct	Nov	Dec
Fall rate	25	28	29	30	28	31	33	34	34	36	37	39

6. There are 20 patients who have a 50-50 chance to survive a certain illness. What is the probability that all 20 will survive?

7. The age of the patients in the ED is normally distributed with a mean of 42 and an *SD* of 10. What is the probability that the next patient entering the ED will be younger than 50 years old?

8. A sample of 20 patients is drawn randomly from a population of 300. There is a 20% chance that a patient will be a smoker. Which probability distribution is appropriate for modeling the smoker status in this sample?

9. The following are the blood pressure readings of 30 patients.

Patient	Systolic Blood Pressure	Diastolic Blood Pressure
1	107	68
2	145	91
3	139	87
4	125	79
5	141	89
6	140	88
7	130	82
8	107	68
9	146	92
10	146	92
11	124	78
12	146	92
13	134	84
14	137	86
15	121	76
16	130	82
17	129	81
18	157	98
19	140	88
20	131	83
21	134	85
22	125	79
23	140	88
24	124	79
25	134	84
26	142	89
27	117	74
28	138	87
29	139	87
30	144	91

a. What are the mode, median, and mean systolic blood pressure?
b. What are the mode, median, and mean diastolic blood pressure?
c. What are the ranges and *SD* of the systolic and diastolic blood pressure?

10. Develop the boxplot for the systolic blood pressure readings shown in the table. At first sight, does it look like the data could be described by the normal distribution? Why or why not?

11. The problem is based on the supplemental medical tourism data set available in the online Student Resources. The coding for each variable is explained in the first worksheet. For the problem that follows, copy the data that you need and paste them on a new worksheet.

a. Develop a bar graph showing the absolute frequencies of the three gender categories. (Hint: Develop a table on the side of the worksheet with the Gender category in one column and the frequencies obtained with the COUNTIF Excel function in a second column.)
b. Develop a pie chart showing the relative frequencies of the three gender categories.

LEARNING ACTIVITIES

1. Mock interview with two students, the interviewer and the interviewee. The interviewee is Steven Jobs. The topic is: "How to make data tell a story?" Hint: Research Steven Jobs's biography and contribution to design before the interview.
2. Do a Pecha Kucha (20 slides, 20 seconds each) on the special role of the normal distribution in statistics.
3. Data scientist has been labeled by many as the "sexiest job of the 21st century." Search the literature and determine if you agree.
4. Get a copy of the Hospital Consumer Assessment of Healthcare Providers and Systems (HCAHPS) survey. Identify the level of measurement of the answers to each question.
5. Find a data set that interests you and determine the levels of measurement of at least five variables. Display the frequency distribution of these variables.

SPRINGER PUBLISHING CONNECT™ | A robust set of instructor resources designed to supplement this text is located at **http://connect.springerpub.com/content/book/978-0-8261-7976-0.** Qualifying instructors may request access by emailing **textbook@springerpub.com.**

REFERENCES

Evans, J. R. (2013). *Statistics, data analysis, and decision making* (5th ed.). Pearson.

Field, A. (2013). *Discovering statistics using IBM SPSS statistics* (4th ed.). Sage.

Scalia, P., O'Malley, A. J., Duranda, A.-M., Goodney, P. P., & Elwyn, G. (2019). Presenting time-based risks of stroke and death for patients facing carotid stenosis treatment options: Patients prefer pie charts over icon arrays. *Patient Education and Counseling, 102*(10), 1939–1944. https://doi.org/10.1016/j.pec.2019.05.004

Tableau Software. (2024). *What is data visualization? Definitions, examples, and learning resources.* Salesforce. https://www.tableau.com/learn/articles/data-visualization

FOR MORE ADVANCED CONTENT ON PROBABILITIES AND DISTRIBUTIONS SEE ECHAPTER 14: EXPANDED COVERAGE OF PROBABILITIES AND DISTRIBUTIONS

eChapter 14 is available online by visiting www.springerpub.com/courseconnect. See inside front cover and tear-out card for CourseConnect details.

APPENDIX 7.1 PROBABILITY AND NONPROBABILITY SAMPLING

BRIGHT ANGEL MEDICAL CENTER A.7.1.1

Adeleke knocked on Barbara's office door. "Come in," replied Barbara in a tired voice. Adeleke walked in and fell into the chair across from Barbara's desk.

"I know it has been a long day," Adeleke said, "but we need to get ready for the next step. We have been collecting some preliminary data. Unfortunately, our busy employees essentially collect what they can when they can. I'm not sure we can place too much confidence in what these data tell us. There should be a more rigorous data collection and sampling process."

Barbara did not reply right away. She seemed to absorb this information slowly. Finally, she looked up from her laptop and smiled. "We never thought about it seriously," she said. "We just assumed it was straightforward. It's not just in the ED. Last week, the HR director sent a satisfaction survey to the new nurses that had just completed orientation, and all they received were a few, very negative responses. Only 10% of the nurses had replied .... Were they the only angry ones? Carol, the preceptor, had never seen anything like that. She was wondering what to do in the next class."

Adeleke sighed, "Knowing Carol, she did a great job. Just bad luck with the sample of respondents." Barbara stood up, "OK, I don't know anything about sampling, but it is obviously important. Let's bring in Olina. She can teach us how it should be done."

LEARNING OBJECTIVES

After reading this appendix, you will be able to:

- Draw simple random samples, proportionate stratified random samples, systematic samples, and cluster samples.
- Know the precautions required to select convenience samples and judgment samples.

INTRODUCTION

In the previous chapter, we distinguished between a target population and a sample. Because a sample is used to make inferences about the population, you might wonder why sample at all and not take the whole population? The answer is simple: because it is easier, faster, and cheaper to sample. For example, collecting data on the entire ED patient population in the city where you live would be extremely difficult to organize and implement. It would also be time-consuming and costly. Obtaining data from a sample of patients who visited the ED at one of the major hospitals would be more practical and, if the sample is representative of the population, it will yield valid findings. Representativeness is the key! Although a sample will never yield the exact same results as the population, it can come close. In this chapter, we review **probability and nonprobability sampling** methods. With probability sampling methods, each unit in the target population has an objective, known probability or chance of being selected through a random process, irrespective of the personal preferences or biases of the person collecting the data. For example, a nurse keeping track of wait times could not arbitrarily (and conveniently!) select patients who show up during the first hour of her shift so that she can be "done with it" early! Nonprobability sampling involves the subjective or nonrandom selection of units that have no known chance of being selected. Depending on the approach and care taken, nonprobability samples can be representative as well.

PROBABILITY SAMPLING

Probability sampling is preferred when we need to make inferences about the population with great accuracy. An obvious case is medical research where generalizing sample results to the population has important repercussions. There are several types of sound, probability-based sampling plans. The most common are simple random sampling, proportionate stratified random sampling, systematic sampling, and cluster sampling.

SIMPLE RANDOM SAMPLING

As its name indicates, **simple random sampling** is simple and requires only minimum knowledge of the target population! Just think of drawing a name from a hat. It means that every sample of a certain size within a population has a known and equal probability of being selected. By extension, it also means that any person in the population would have the same chance of being selected.

Let us demonstrate this principle. A total of 100 patients visited the ED on September 1 (Table A.7.1.1). The average wait time in the waiting room was 75.64 minutes. If you were going to pick a sample of 10 patients, there would be 17,310,309,456,440 possible samples of size 10! You could write them all out on 17,310,309,456,440 pieces of paper, put them in a hat, and draw one of them. Each sample of 10 patients would have a 1/17,310,309,456,440 chance of being selected.

TABLE A.7.1.1 WAIT TIMES DATA—FEBRUARY 1

Patient	Arrival Time	Wait Time (min)	
1	02-01 00:04:34	124	
2	02-01 00:21:00	194	
3	02-01 00:52:00	17	
4	02-01 01:01:00	170	
5	02-01 02:05:00	36	
6	02-01 02:24:24	4	
7	02-01 02:50:00	15	
8	02-01 05:02:10	3	**Night shift: midnight to 8:00 a.m.**
9	02-01 05:14:00	16	
10	02-01 05:43:00	9	15 patients
11	02-01 06:05:00	14	
12	02-01 07:09:00	12	Average wait time: 44 min
13	02-01 07:28:00	17	
14	02-01 07:44:41	20	
15	02-01 07:50:00	3	
16	02-01 08:14:00	34	
17	02-01 08:23:00	8	
18	02-01 08:24:02	0	
19	02-01 08:36:00	10	
20	02-01 08:37:00	2	
21	02-01 08:42:00	13	
22	02-01 08:47:50	5	

(continued)

TABLE A.7.1.1 WAIT TIMES DATA—FEBRUARY 1 (*CONTINUED*)

Patient	Arrival Time	Wait Time (min)	
23	02-01 09:16:15	14	
24	02-01 09:36:00	18	
25	02-01 09:38:00	21	
26	02-01 09:41:00	29	
27	02-01 09:42:00	10	
28	02-01 09:42:00	10	
29	02-01 09:48:00	33	
30	02-01 09:52:00	20	Day shift: 8 a.m. to 4 p.m.
31	02-01 10:04:00	23	
32	02-01 10:11:00	0	48 patients
33	02-01 10:12:00	88	
34	02-01 10:14:00	102	Average wait time: 64.31 min
35	02-01 10:31:26	62	
36	02-01 10:32:00	76	
37	02-01 10:38:36	112	
38	02-01 10:51:00	20	
39	02-01 10:52:00	119	
40	02-01 11:27:00	215	
41	02-01 11:33:00	142	
42	02-01 11:40:47	252	
43	02-01 11:49:00	16	
44	02-01 11:55:00	59	
45	02-01 12:14:00	119	
46	02-01 12:46:00	92	
47	02-01 12:53:00	9	
48	02-01 12:57:10	62	
49	02-01 13:04:00	32	
50	02-01 13:05:00	5	
51	02-01 13:22:00	148	
52	02-01 13:47:00	152	
53	02-01 13:58:00	197	
54	02-01 14:10:58	213	
55	02-01 14:24:37	102	
56	02-01 14:31:00	4	
57	02-01 14:37:08	13	
58	02-01 14:49:00	18	
59	02-01 14:56:00	131	
60	02-01 15:20:00	19	
61	02-01 15:29:00	245	

(*continued*)

TABLE A.7.1.1 WAIT TIMES DATA—FEBRUARY 1 (*CONTINUED*)

Patient	Arrival Time	Wait Time (min)	
62	02-01 15:42:00	2	
63	02-01 15:46:00	11	
64	02-01 16:00:25	134	
65	02-01 16:07:21	162	
66	02-01 16:14:00	225	
67	02-01 16:44:00	281	Evening shift: 4 p.m. to midnight
68	02-01 16:54:00	248	
69	02-01 16:57:00	7	37 patients
70	02-01 16:59:45	5	
71	02-01 17:06:00	11	Average wait time: 103.32 min
72	02-01 17:06:16	217	
73	02-01 17:24:00	220	
74	02-01 17:35:59	1	
75	02-01 17:36:53	22	
76	02-01 17:46:00	11	
77	02-01 17:56:00	0	
78	02-01 18:37:00	168	
79	02-01 18:40:00	171	
80	02-01 18:51:00	166	
81	02-01 18:54:00	112	
82	02-01 18:59:00	6	
83	02-01 19:07:00	13	
84	02-01 19:33:00	221	
85	02-01 20:09:00	93	
86	02-01 20:10:29	139	
87	02-01 20:29:00	72	
88	02-01 20:36:00	183	
89	02-01 20:39:00	82	
90	02-01 21:11:10	70	
91	02-01 21:26:00	168	
92	02-01 21:39:00	129	
93	02-01 21:49:00	57	
94	02-01 21:54:00	37	
95	02-01 21:58:00	77	
96	02-01 22:31:00	78	
97	02-01 22:36:00	108	
98	02-01 22:54:00	35	
99	02-01 23:24:00	12	
100	02-01 23:27:00	82	
	Average	75.64	

TABLE A.7.1.2 SIMPLE RANDOM SAMPLE OF 10 PATIENTS

Patient	Arrival Time	Shift	Wait Time (min)
93	02-01 21:49:00	Evening	57
69	02-01 16:57:00	Evening	7
5	02-01 02:05:00	Night	36
78	02-01 18:37:00	Evening	168
57	02-01 14:37:08	Day	13
24	02-01 09:36:00	Day	18
64	02-01 16:00:25	Evening	134
40	02-01 11:27:00	Day	215
97	02-01 22:36:00	Evening	108
85	02-01 20:09:00	Evening	93
Average			84.90

Fortunately, this was just a demonstration of the concept. Nobody would actually do it this way. Instead, we could just put our finger on the list of patients and their associated wait times, close our eyes, pick one patient, write down the wait time for that patient, and repeat the process 10 times. Or we could use the sampling tool in Excel to select 10 patients and their wait times. When using this procedure, we obtain the sample shown in Table A.7.1.2. For this sample, the average wait time is 84.9 min. Why is it so much higher than the average of 75.64 minutes found for the population of patients seen in the ED on February 1? Note that the sample included three patients from the day shift, six from the evening shift, and one from the night shift. However, the percentages of patients in the population seen during the day, evening, and night shifts were 48, 37, and 15, respectively. In other words, patients who arrived during the evening shift are overrepresented, whereas patients who arrived during the other two shifts are underrepresented in our sample. As wait times tend to be longer during the evening shift, it is therefore no surprise that the average wait time for our sample of patients is substantially longer than that of the population. To overcome this problem, we can use a sampling procedure called "proportionate stratified random sampling."

Simple Random Sampling Using Excel

It is quite simple to use Excel to generate samples. Next is the series of steps you need to follow to draw simple random samples (see Figures A.7.1.1–A.7.1.5; see also Excel Video A.7.1). Note that Figure A.7.1.1 was truncated; in reality, the 100th patient's arrival and wait data are on the 103rd row.

STEP 1: Click on the *Data* Tab, and select *Data Analysis* in the *Analyze* group (Figure A.7.1.2).

STEP 2: Select *Sampling* and click *OK* (Figure A.7.1.3).

STEP 3: In the *Input Range* box (Figure A.7.1.4), specify the numbers from which the sample is going to be drawn. Here, it is patients 1 through 100. Click on *Labels* to indicate that the first cell corresponds to a column title. Select the number of units to be sampled (*Number of Samples*), and click on the cell where you want the sample to be displayed (e.g., K4).

Ten patients were selected using this tool (Figure A.7.1.5, column K). Note that the procedure involves sampling with replacement. If you see that a patient was selected more than once, you will need to select another patient. Use the VLOOKUP function to extract the patients' wait times. For example, the formula in cell L4 is VLOOKUP(K4,$A$4:$C$103,3). This formula looks for the sampling unit (or patient number) value "11" in the data set including the Patient Number, Arrival Time, and Wait Time (Figure A.7.1.1) and retrieves the corresponding wait time in column C.

TABLE A.7.1 – Wait Times Data — February 1st

Patient	Arrival Time	Wait Time (min)	
1	02-01 00:04:34	124	
2	02-01 00:21:00	194	
3	02-01 00:52:00	17	Night Shift
4	02-01 01:01:00	170	12:00 a.m. - 8:00 a.m.
5	02-01 02:05:00	36	
6	02-01 02:24:24	4	
-	-	-	
-	-	-	
42	02-01 11:40:47	252	
43	02-01 11:49:00	16	
44	02-01 11:55:00	59	Day Shift
45	02-01 12:14:00	119	8:00 a.m. - 4:00 p.m.
46	02-01 12:46:00	92	
47	02-01 12:53:00	9	
48	02-01 12:57:10	62	
-	-	-	
-	-	-	
95	02-01 21:58:00	77	
96	02-01 22:31:00	78	
97	02-01 22:36:00	108	Evening Shift
98	02-01 22:54:00	35	4:00 p.m. - 12:00 a.m.
99	02-01 23:24:00	12	
100	02-01 23:27:00	82	

FIGURE A.7.1.1 Selection of waiting times data in Excel spreadsheet.

Note: Microsoft Excel 2019 application interface is used with permission of Microsoft.

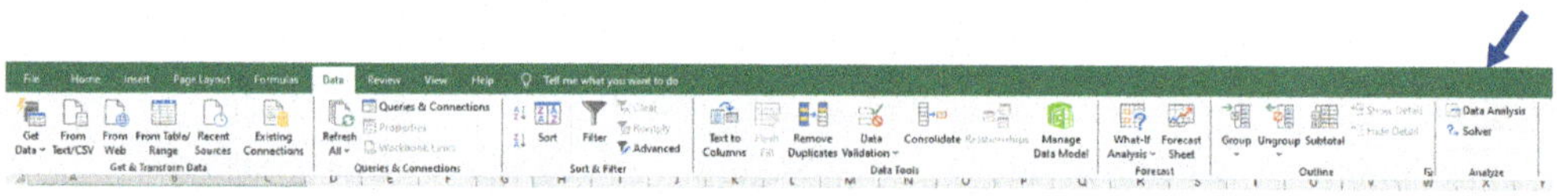

FIGURE A.7.1.2 Tool bar.

Note: Microsoft Excel application interface is used with permission of Microsoft.

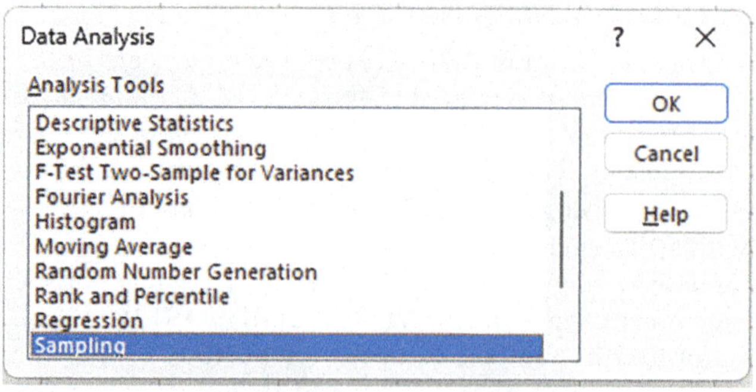

FIGURE A.7.1.3 Data analysis menu.

Note: Microsoft Excel 2019 application interface is used with permission of Microsoft.

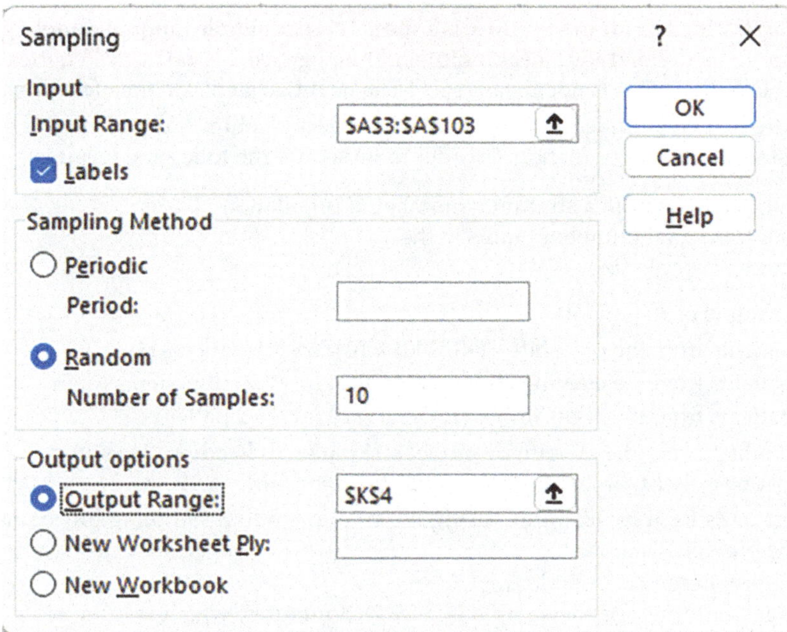

FIGURE A.7.1.4 Sampling dialog box for simple random sampling.

Note: Microsoft Excel 2019 application interface is used with permission of Microsoft.

	K	L
1		
2	Sampling Unit	Wait Time
3		
4	11	14
5	80	166
6	50	5
7	34	102
8	79	171
9	14	20
10	19	10
11	97	108
12	39	119
13	4	170
14		

FIGURE A.7.1.5 Simple random sample generated in Excel.

Note: Microsoft Excel 2019 application interface is used with permission of Microsoft.

EXCEL VIDEO A.7.1

Simple Random Sampling

Access the Excel video online by visiting www.springerpub.com/courseconnect. See inside front cover and tear-out card for CourseConnect details.

PROPORTIONATE STRATIFIED RANDOM SAMPLING

Proportionate stratified random sampling is a special case of simple random sampling. It requires the population to be divided into meaningful and homogeneous strata or categories (e.g., shift), such as in Table A.7.1.1. This is not always easy! The next two steps are then followed:

STEP 1: Ensure that the number of sample units from each stratum is proportionate to the size of the stratum in the population. In order to do so, use the following formula:

Number of sample units from a stratum = (number of population units in the stratum/total number of units in the population) × total sample size. [A.7.1.1]

For BAMC's sample of 10 patients:

Number of patients from the day shift = $(48/100) \times 10 = 4.8 \approx 5$ patients.

Number of patients from the evening shift = $(37/100) \times 10 = 3.7 \approx 4$ patients.

Number of patients from the night shift = $(15/100) \times 10 = 1.5 \approx 2$ patients.

Due to rounding, we came up with a sample of 11 patients. To adjust, we will make a judgment call and select one rather than two patients from the night shift.

STEP 2: Select units from each stratum using the simple random sampling procedure described in the previous section.

The results are presented in Table A.7.1.3.

The average wait time for the sample is now 78.3 minutes, which is quite close to the population average. When the strata are homogeneous, proportionate stratified random sampling yields very representative samples. Another popular sampling technique is systematic (or periodic) sampling.

SYSTEMATIC SAMPLING

Systematic (or periodic) sampling is a rather simple procedure, which involves selecting units from the population according to a fixed interval. The requirement is that the population units must be assigned the numbers 1 to *N* (population size). For BAMC, that would be patients 1 to 100. These steps are then followed.

TABLE A.7.1.3 PROPORTIONATE STRATIFIED RANDOM SAMPLE OF 10 PATIENTS

Patient	Arrival Time	Shift	Wait Time (min)
13	02-01 7:28:00	Night	17
21	02-01 8:42:00	Day	13
58	02-01 4:49:00	Day	18
26	02-01 9:41:00	Day	29
39	02-01 0:52:00	Day	119
56	02-01 4:31:00	Day	4
80	02-01 8:51:00	Evening	166
68	02-01 6:54:00	Evening	248
81	02-01 8:54:00	Evening	112
93	02-01 21:49:00	Evening	57
Average			78.3

TABLE A.7.1.4 SYSTEMATIC RANDOM SAMPLE OF 10 PATIENTS

Patient	Arrival Time	Shift	Wait Time (min)
6	02-01 02:24:24	Night	4
16	02-01 08:14:00	Day	34
26	02-01 09:41:00	Day	29
36	02-01 10:32:00	Day	76
46	02-01 12:46:00	Day	92
56	02-01 14:31:00	Day	4
66	02-01 16:14:00	Evening	225
76	02-01 17:46:00	Evening	11
86	02-01 20:10:29	Evening	139
96	02-01 22:31:00	Evening	78
Average			69.2

STEP 1: To sample n units, compute the sampling interval $k = N/n$. If you obtain a fractional amount, round k to the closest integer.

For BAMC, $k = 100/10 = 10$.

STEP 2: Randomly select a number from 1 to k. This will be the first unit sampled from the population.

For BAMC, let us assume that this number is 6. Patient #6 will be the first unit sampled.

STEP 3: The selected unit and every kth unit thereafter will be included in the sample until the desired sample size is obtained.

In BAMC's case, the sampled patients would therefore be:

[1] 6
[2] $6 + 10 = 16$
[3] $16 + 10 = 26$
⋮
[10] $86 + 10 = 96$

The resulting sample and wait times are shown in Table A.7.1.4.

Systematic sampling can produce representative samples, especially when the data are organized in strata. Although practical, it can also be problematic when the periodicity coincides with another phenomenon. For example, if the room temperature in the ED was recorded every hour over a period of 10 days, selecting a sample of 10 room temperatures would result in $k = 240/10 = 24$. This means that the sample data would all correspond to room temperatures recorded at the same time each day, let us say 5 a.m. Because room temperature is likely to fluctuate during the day due to sun exposure and volume of patients, it is likely that the average room temperature in our sample would be quite lower than the population's.

To use the systematic sampling method with $k = 10$ in Excel, start your Input range with the 6th patient which you selected randomly, select "Periodic", and enter "10" for "period" in the *Sampling Method* box, as shown in Figure A.7.1.6.

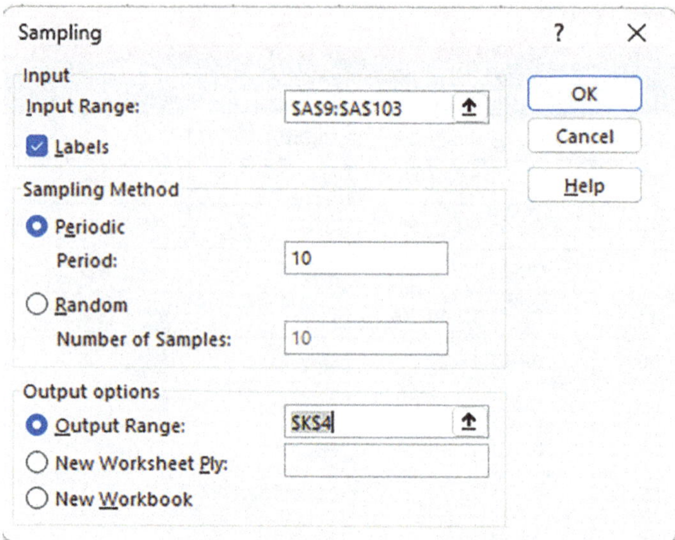

FIGURE A.7.1.6 **Sampling dialog box for systematic sampling.**

CLUSTER SAMPLING

Cluster sampling requires dividing the population into "mini-populations" or clusters that are essentially alike. For example, a researcher wanting to examine the use of antidepressants among high school students in Springfield, Missouri, could consider each high school as a cluster (Figure A.7.1.7). The researcher could then randomly select one cluster/high school and select every student in that cluster for participation in the study, assuming of course that informed consent was obtained. Alternatively, the researcher could randomly select students from that cluster.

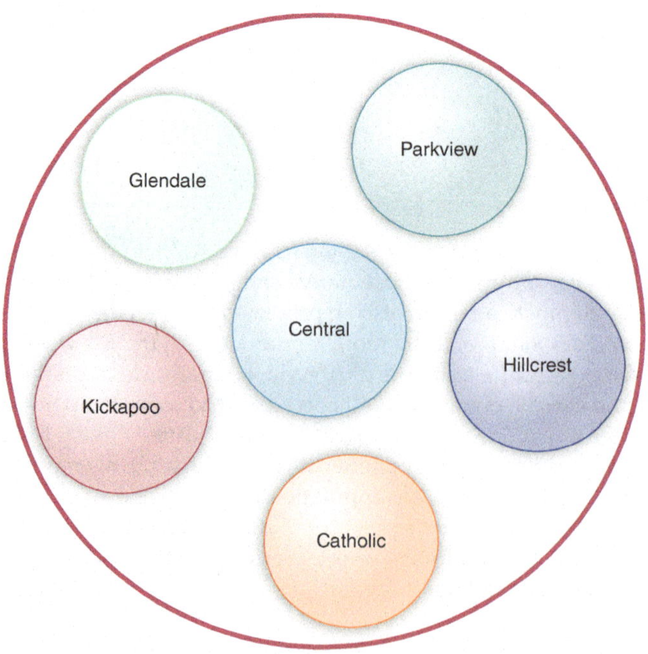

FIGURE A.7.1.7 **High schools in Springfield, Missouri.**

Unlike the previous three sampling methods, cluster sampling does not require a complete sampling frame, only the cluster(s) of interest. This is a simple method, but we must acknowledge the difficulty in forming equivalent clusters. In our example, the social determinants of health may vary significantly in the districts where students live and the high schools they attend. Therefore, clusters might not be interchangeable for a study on mental health.

BRIGHT ANGEL MEDICAL CENTER A.7.1.2

Olina was looking at the small group of nurses, technicians, and clerical staff in front of her.

She was not sure how the two lectures on sampling had been received. Some had grasped the material right away, whereas others appeared to be overwhelmed. Peter, the most outspoken student in the class, said, "Honestly, this material is too abstract. It would make more sense if we actually used these sampling techniques in the field." Several heads nodded in agreement. "Excellent idea," Olina admitted. "Let me ask the lab manager if we can get access to some data, and if he agrees, we will meet at the lab conference room for our final class."

Two days later, they all met in the lab. "Here are the lab turnaround times for orders placed by ED providers over the past week," Olina said. "We have removed all patient identifiers so that you could have access to these data on your laptops. Your objective is to examine whether turnaround times may have something to do with the long lengths of stay in the ED. Draw a sample of 1,000 turnaround times. Get together in teams of 2 or 3 and go to work!"

NONPROBABILITY SAMPLING

Nonprobability sampling is subjective and may not be as rigorous, but it may be the best you can achieve, and sometimes, it is actually more useful. In this section, we will describe convenience and judgment sampling.

CONVENIENCE SAMPLING

It may come to you as a surprise that, in a field as demanding and meticulous as healthcare, convenience sampling is quite common. **Convenience sampling** is involved when participation is voluntary or when the researcher personally selects the participants (e.g., a pharmacist's record of prescriptions for diabetic patients). In that case, there is no way to ascertain that a representative sample is drawn. The HCAHPS survey results are also the product of data obtained through a convenience sample because only the patients who agree to respond will be included (Figure A.7.1.8). Their opinions and experiences could be very different from those who chose not to respond.

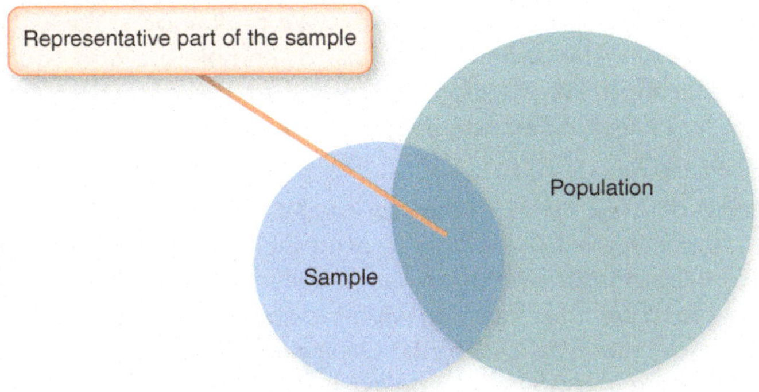

FIGURE A.7.1.8 **Representativeness of convenience sample.**

To determine whether there is a difference between the respondents and the nonrespondents, known as **nonresponse bias**, it is common to compare some demographic characteristics of the population with those of the respondents. If significant differences exist, it is best to exert efforts to entice nonrespondents to participate. This is precisely why you get frequent reminders when you don't respond to a survey!

JUDGMENT SAMPLING

Judgment sampling involves selecting respondents based on the researcher's assessment that they are very relevant to what is being studied. For example, nurses working in the ED or the ICU would be ideal participants in a study on nurses' burnout. Similarly, patients in assisted-living facilities might be good candidates to participate in a study on the effects of strength training and yoga on fall rates. Judgment samples do not represent the entire population of interest (Figure A.7.1.9). Therefore, caution should be taken in generalizing the results.

This concludes this chapter appendix on sampling. Always check the data you have collected. Computing minimum, maximum, and averages can tell you a lot about the quality of your sample and its representativeness.

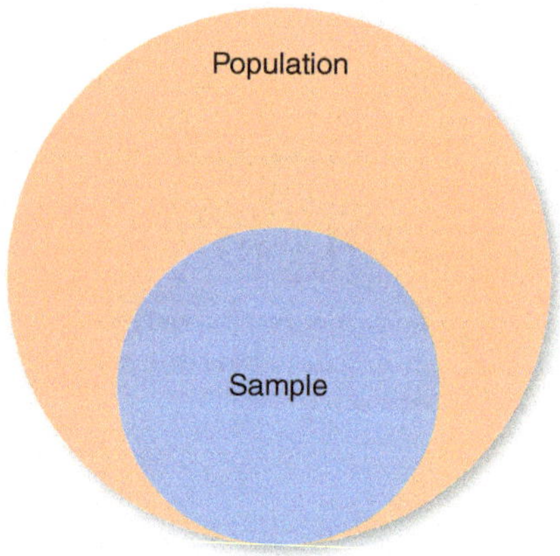

FIGURE A.7.1.9 Judgment sample.

BRIGHT ANGEL MEDICAL CENTER A.7.1.3

Olina was watching the groups hard at work on the sampling exercise. After about 30 min, she asked, "Anyone want to share their results?"

"Yes," said Rajiv. "First, Tania and I did a simple random sample of turnaround times. We took the sample average and realized it was rather low. We took another look at our sample and realized that it included mostly turnaround times for complete blood count (CBC)-d tests, which tend to be rather short. We therefore grouped the types of tests on the sampling frame and then used proportional stratified sampling. Our average turnaround time went from a few minutes to almost 2 hours!"

Jordan raised her hand. "Hey, I work in the lab, and I can tell you that we work as fast as we can. Sometimes, people in the ED are slow to send their orders. Once we get an order, we have to dispatch a phlebotomist who often has to collect multiple samples in the ED. By the time we get all the blood samples in, a considerable amount of time may have elapsed. The lab gets a bad rap, and it's unfair." "All right," Olina said. "This is a good starting point. Now we need to find out where and why all the delays occur. That's the next step!"

SUMMARY

This chapter supplement covered sampling basics. Table A.7.1.5 provides a summary of the probability and nonprobability sampling techniques as well as their advantages and disadvantages.

TABLE A.7.1.5 SUMMARY OF SAMPLING TECHNIQUES

Type	Technique	Advantages	Disadvantages
Probability Sampling Objective; probability of selection is known in advance	Simple random sampling • Draw randomly from the sampling frame • Same probability of selection for every sample of a given size	• Simple • Minimum knowledge of population	• May not be representative
	Proportionate stratified random sampling • Divide population into homogeneous strata • Randomly draw a number of units proportionate to size of stratum	• Representative	• Higher knowledge of population • May be difficult to get homogeneous strata
	Systematic sampling • Compute sampling interval, *k* • Select a unit randomly between 1 and *k* and add *k* units thereafter until desired sample size is obtained	• Simple • Can be representative	• Periodicity may create bias
	Cluster sampling • Divide population into mini-populations or clusters • Select a cluster randomly	• Simple • Can be representative	• Difficult to form comparable clusters
Nonprobability Sampling Subjective; probability of selection cannot be determined in advance	Convenience sampling • Based on personal convenience and/or availability	• All that one can get	• Only partially representative
	Judgment sampling • Units are sampled because of their special relevance to study	• Purposeful	• Only partially representative

CERTIFICATION TIPS

The material on sampling is quite sparse and general in certification materials. It only includes random, sequential (destruction of testing units), and stratified sampling. The emphasis is more on data collection methods than the specifics of sampling techniques. Yet, you should be able to *apply* the material presented in this appendix.

KEY TERMS

Probability sampling
Nonprobability sampling
Simple random sampling
Proportionate stratified random sampling
Systematic (or periodic) sampling
Cluster sampling
Convenience sampling
Nonresponse bias
Judgment sampling

REVIEW QUESTIONS

1. What is the difference between probability and nonprobability sampling?
2. Differentiate among simple random sampling, proportionate stratified random sampling, and systematic sampling.
3. When would you use judgment sampling?
4. What are the advantages and disadvantages of proportionate stratified random sampling?
5. What are the advantages and disadvantages of simple random sampling?
6. What circumstances justify the use of convenience sampling?

SOLVE BRIGHT ANGEL MEDICAL CENTER'S PROBLEMS

All chapter-specific data from the following problems are provided as Excel files which may be accessed via the show supplementary tab (Student Material) available online by visiting www.springerpub.com/courseconnect. See inside front cover and tear-out card for CourseConnect details.

1. Your objective is to draw a sample of 600 patients. Using proportionate stratified random sampling, determine how many sample units there will be for each stratum.

Marital Status	*N* (population)	*n* (sample)?
Single (never married)	4,000	
Married	7,000	
Widowed	2,750	
Divorced	4,250	
Total	**18,000**	

2. Your objective is to obtain feedback on BAMC's diversity policies from 500 staff members. Using proportionate stratified random sampling, determine how many sample units there will be for each stratum.

Race/Ethnicity	*N* (population)	*n* (sample)?
White	4,250	
Black or African American	680	
Native American or Alaska Native	25	
Asian	1,024	
Native Hawaiian or Other Pacific Islander	26	
Hispanic, Latino, Spanish origin	1,350	
Other race	145	
Total	7,500	

3. Use the BAMC ED data set (CBC stats); filter to obtain the data on the urine pregnancy tests (Column A) for the month of October. Select a simple random sample of five total lab turnaround times (Column J).
4. Use the BAMC ED data set (CBC stats); filter to obtain the data on acetaminophen level tests (Column A) for October. Form a sample of 10 total lab turnaround times (Column J) using systematic sampling.
5. Use the BAMC ED data set (left-without-being-seen [LWBS] and left without being treated [LWBT]) for the month of November 2024:
   a. Create a sample of 10 average lengths of stay (Column AO) using simple random sampling.
   b. Create a sample of 10 average lengths of stay (Column AO) using systematic sampling.

LEARNING ACTIVITY

1. There are many online reviews (e.g., Google reviews) for every type of medical provider. Do you trust the validity of these reviews? Explain.

CHAPTER 8

PROCESS STABILITY AND CAPABILITY

BRIGHT ANGEL MEDICAL CENTER 8.1

Barbara booted up her computer early Monday morning. As soon as she logged in, an instant message appeared on her screen from the ED nursing shift supervisor. "ED on divert due to lack of capacity and 24 patients in the waiting room. Please advise." Barbara groaned. Every time it felt like they were making a little progress, she was painfully reminded of how slow they were moving. Thankfully, the process improvement team had been pulling and organizing the data on ED throughput, left without being seen (LWBS), and ED length of stay (LOS). Barbara picked up her cell phone and called Olina Petrenko, director of quality and Six Sigma Black Belt. They agreed to get together later that morning to see what else could be done in the short term to address the growing concern that the ED just could not handle the volume of patients presenting every day.

Why is it valuable to use supporting data when evaluating workflows? Will this make the change management effort harder or easier?

LEARNING OBJECTIVES

After reading this chapter, you will be able to:

- Understand the concept of variation, which affects all processes.
- Develop process control charts to track attributes (*p*-chart, *np*-chart, *c*-chart, and *u*-chart) over time.
- Develop process control charts to track variables (*IX* and moving ranges [*MR*] charts; $\overline{X}$ and *R* charts; $\overline{X}$ and *s* charts; cumulative sum [CUSUM] charts) over time.
- Evaluate a process control chart and determine whether the process being monitored is behaving as expected or becoming unstable.
- Decide whether a process is capable of meeting predetermined quality requirements.

INTRODUCTION

In Chapter 4, you learned how to translate customer requirements into objective quality indicators. In Chapter 7, you were introduced to basic statistics concepts. You are therefore ready to determine from those quality indicators whether the processes are stable and generating output in a reliable fashion. But, even if a process is behaving the way you expected, it may still not be good enough to meet specific targets and will need to be improved.

Do you like numbers? If the answer is "yes," great! If the answer is "no," no problem! You are like millions of other highly educated individuals who may not like numbers because they are a little "intimidated" by math. As a result, we try to introduce you to this material in a step-by-step, nonthreatening way.

WHY IS THIS MATERIAL USEFUL?

Statistical process control (SPC) charts are great tools to manage quality because:

- They help you visualize the performance of a process indicator.
- They help you identify variation due to specific causes.
- They signal potential changes in the process and help you be proactive in addressing them and formulating improvement plans.
- They show you whether an improvement initiative has had positive results (Chapter 11).

VARIATION

As suggested in Box 8.1, it is impossible to determine exactly how long it takes to drive from your house to your best friend's. It depends on the time of day, the traffic, whether you hit every red light, whether a cop is right behind you, and so on. Even if you drove at the exact same time of day, got green lights all the way, and tried to drive consistently at the same speed, it might take you a little less time on some days and a little more time on others. This is the phenomenon of variation, and it exists in everything we do.

Process variation reflects the deviations of process output values from the mean or expected value for that process. When process output values deviate significantly from the mean, they create uncertainty about the ability of the process to produce quality output. For example, at a university health center, patients may usually wait 5 to 15 minutes before going to the exam room. However, it is possible that some will have to wait much longer than 15 minutes, in which case they will likely get irritated and dissatisfied with the responsiveness of the service. Why do some patients wait for 5 minutes, whereas others wait for 10, or even 30 minutes? There are many possible reasons, but they fall into two major categories, as explained in the text that follows.

ASSIGNABLE CAUSES OF VARIATION

Assignable or **special causes of variation** occur for reasons that are external to the process. They reflect unusual faults arising from temporary situations. In the preceding health center example, the

BOX 8.1 FAQs

How long does it take you to drive from your house to your best friend's?

About 20 minutes.

About 20 minutes? Do you mean 17, 18, 19, 20, 21, 22, or 23 minutes?

??? Are you serious? ... It depends!

x-ray machine may have malfunctioned intermittently, resulting in the increased utilization of exam rooms by patients waiting for their x-ray results. Another possibility is that the clinical information system became uncharacteristically slow when various scheduled reports were printed. These sources of variation do not indicate a "bad" process per se; they signal atypical disturbances that can be identified and eliminated because they cause the process to be "out of control" and therefore unstable or unpredictable. In the previous examples, repairing the x-ray machine and scheduling the printing of reports at nonpeak times in the clinic will resolve a majority of the delays.

COMMON OR RANDOM CAUSES OF VARIATION

Common or **random causes of variation** are inherent to the process. They reflect the faults of the system and result from the combined influences of many regular, ordinary causes that occur randomly. Each one of these causes is insignificant by itself. Even if we could isolate and eliminate one, the impact on process variability would be negligible (Stevenson & Kull, 2024). As mentioned before, you may have to wait between 5 and 15 minutes before seeing a physician at the university health center. This would be expected given the number of doctors and nurses usually on duty, the number of exam rooms, and so on, to accommodate the existing patient population. Why do patients sometimes wait 6 minutes and at other times 14 minutes? Because some patients arrive early for their appointments, whereas others arrive late; because some exams last longer than expected, whereas others are finished promptly. All these little variations add up, creating variation in wait times. Minimizing wait times and keeping them low for all patients would require changing the process itself (e.g., building new facilities with additional exam rooms and increasing staff). In other words, an investment in process redesign would be necessary.

The type of variation that is intrinsic to the process is also referred to as the *natural* variation of the process because it determines the *natural* statistical variation, or width, in the distribution of the process output. The *SD* is a measure of this type of variation. When the normal distribution can be assumed, most of the process values (99.7%) fall within ±3 *SD*s from the mean or expected process value (Chapter 7). Because this variation is expected, it does not impair the stability and predictability of the process. In fact, it provides the "control settings" for the **statistical process control (SPC)** charts, which are covered in depth in this chapter. This does not mean that random variation is desirable (Figure 8.1). For example, infection rates in a hospital could remain predictably high over time. This would of course be a stable but unacceptable situation. Continued surveillance and institution of sound infection control procedures would need to be implemented in order to change the process and, therefore, shift the average infection rate downward as well as reduce its variability.

ON THE JOB! INTERVIEW VIDEO 8.1

John Barnes
Director of Systems Integration and Planning for Supply Chain

Visualizing Progress Toward Standardization
Dashboards
Tracking variability

1. John first displays a dashboard with key performance indicators (KPIs) relating to supply chain and overall spending. What are the benefits, especially for leaders, of having access to this type of dashboard?
2. What are some of the most useful dashboard features used to display the performance for the Supply Chain Department? Hint: Focus especially on the second example.
3. Brainstorm on the various ways that supply use variation can negatively impact the bottom line. How could supply standardization backfire?

The interview is available online by visiting www.springerpub.com/courseconnect. See inside front cover and tear-out card for CourseConnect details.

At BAMC, data were collected on waiting times in the ED for the past year. The frequencies of those times were plotted to obtain the process distribution. If you were Barbara Waters, which one of the following normal distributions of the process would you prefer to see?

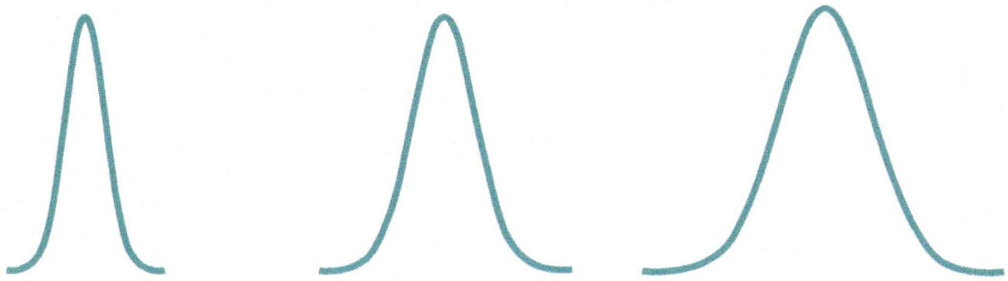

Process A	**Process B**	**Process C**
Mean wait time: 82 min	Mean wait time: 82 min	Mean wait time: 82 min

A? B? C? Not sure? Here is a little hint. As you recall, the *SD* is a measure of random variation. Let's assume that the *SD*s in processes A, B, and C are 5, 10, and 15, respectively. Now, which one of the process distributions do you find more desirable?

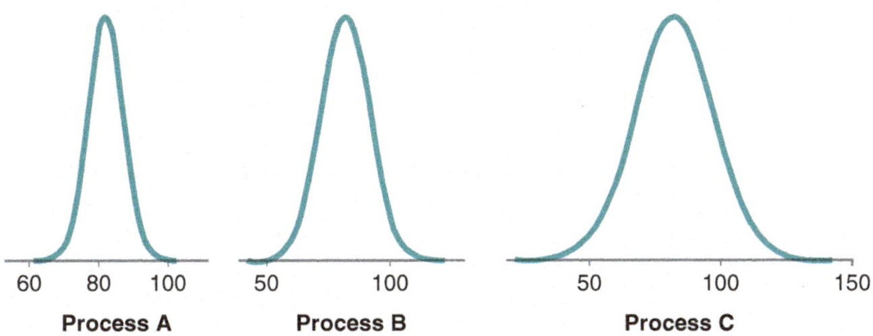

A! The more compact distribution (82 min ± 3*5 min) has less variation, giving the decision-maker more certainty about the process output. On the other hand, process output values that are all over the place (82 min ± 3*15 min) make it very difficult to determine adequate staffing levels.

FIGURE 8.1 **Let us explore variability.**

FUNDAMENTALS OF STATISTICAL PROCESS CONTROL

SPC involves the use of statistical methods to determine whether a process is stable and therefore performing as expected. **Control charts** illustrate the voice of the process! These SPC tools depict the consistency of process performance indicators over time. They are line graphs with a centerline representing the overall process average and control limits set by the random variation of the process (Ransom et al., 2022). They serve three primary purposes: (1) to help you detect special causes of variation, (2) signal potential changes in the process, and (3) gauge the effectiveness of a process improvement (Chapter 11). A process is considered "in control" if (Russell & Taylor, 2023; Figure 8.2):

1. There are no points outside the control limits.
2. The majority of the points are close to the centerline, that is, the process average, and only a few points approach the control limits.
3. The points are approximately equally distributed above and below the centerline.
4. The points are randomly distributed around the centerline with no visible pattern.

To build control charts, we have to draw samples or select subgroups. As indicated in Chapter 7, a sample is a subset of observations taken from a population that it is supposed to represent. If you

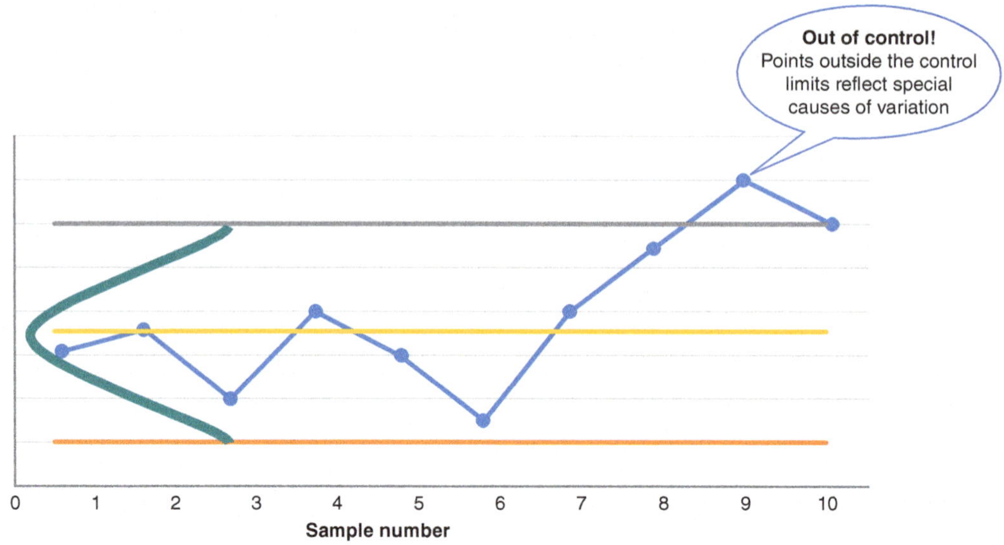

FIGURE 8.2 Process control chart.

select a sample that is not representative, it will produce results that will be either better or worse than those obtained by using the entire population of observations. In the Bright Angel Medical Center (BAMC) example shown in Appendix 7.1, the average wait time for *all* patients seen in the ED on February 1 was 76 minutes. If we took a sample of 30 patients that is perfectly representative of the population, the sample average wait time would also be 76 minutes. Realistically, close to 75 minutes would be good enough! The choice of the sampling technique has a significant impact on the representativeness of the sample.

A **subgroup** is similar in concept to a sample, but the units in the subgroup are created under the same conditions. For example, all the surgeries on a given day of the week would be a subgroup, whereas a group of surgeries comprising surgeries randomly selected over several days would be a sample. Unless the selected subgroup is taken on an atypical day, the difference between sample and subgroup is subtle and does not affect our analysis and its interpretation.

THE CENTERLINE

According to the law of large numbers (LoLN; Chapter 7), the probability that the sample mean approaches the true mean gets closer to 1 as the sample size increases. Therefore, if we take many samples and compute the average for each sample, the average of these statistics is a good approximation of the true process average. This approximation is the centerline on a control chart.

THE CONTROL LIMITS

The central limit theorem (Chapter 7) specifies that the distribution of the averages of many, sufficiently large samples of a random variable is approximately normal even if the population from which the samples are drawn is not normal. We also know that 99.7% of the values are within ± 3 *SD* from the mean. As you recall, the *SD* of the sampling distribution of a statistic (e.g., mean) is known as the *SE*. The three *SE*s on each side of the average represent the extent to which sample statistics can vary randomly. These boundaries are the **control limits** of a control chart. The process distribution displays the probabilities of occurrence for all values of process output. It is essentially the population. As you can see in Figure 8.3, the process distribution is wider than the sampling distribution.

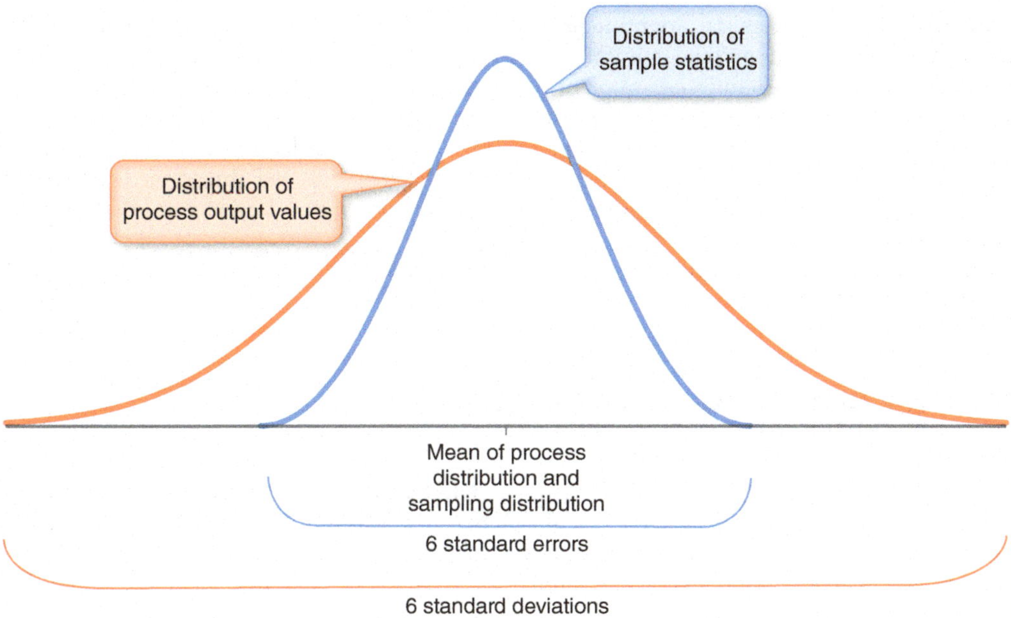

FIGURE 8.3 **Process distribution and sampling distributions of means.**

ON THE JOB! INTERVIEW VIDEO 8.2

Mandy Studebaker
Performance Improvement Specialist and Physician Assistant

Making the Right Thing to Do the Easy Thing to Do

Training leaders
Facilitating process improvement work
Tracking opioid prescriptions with SPC charts
Process capability
Using data to make changes
Change in SPC chart after improvement

1. Mandy describes a project focused on patient safety and opioid prescriptions in acute care. What tools does she use to display the data? Are these tools appropriate? Explain.
2. Outside of education, what else did the project team do to help surgeons meet the target of prescribing 10 pills or less? Why was this support important?
3. What elements can SPC charts help differentiate in the data? Why is it important?
4. On the Outcomes and Conclusions: Overall slide, the control chart displays a sudden change in centerline and control limits. Is it good or bad? Explain.

The interview is available online by visiting www.springerpub.com/courseconnect. See inside front cover and tear-out card for CourseConnect details.

PROCESS CONTROL CHARTS

There are several types of process control charts, and one challenge is knowing which one to use. This decision partly hinges upon whether the quality indicators (Chapter 4) you are monitoring are attributes or variables.

ATTRIBUTE OR VARIABLE

Attributes refer to discrete (i.e., identifiable, separate) units that are *counted* and can be classified as defective units in a sample (e.g., number of postoperative deaths in a sample of surgeries), or as number of defects per unit (e.g., number of medical errors per 1,000 patient-days). Attributes are counted with minimal effort. Was the outcome good or bad? Was an error made or not? How many patient falls occurred last month? On the other hand, **variables** are *measured* on a continuous scale using some type of instrument, such as a balance (e.g., weight), ruler (e.g., length), or timer (e.g., wait time). They therefore yield a more informative and precise assessment of the quality indicator.

The control charts used to monitor attributes are *p*-charts, *np*-charts, *c*-charts, and *u*-charts. The charts used to monitor variables are *IX* and *MR* charts, $\bar{X}$ and *R* charts, $\bar{X}$ and *s* charts, and CUSUM charts.

CONTROL CHARTS FOR ATTRIBUTES

p-Charts

When the attribute data consist of two categories (defective versus nondefective; nonconforming versus conforming), it is appropriate to use the *p*-chart to assess process stability. ***p*-charts** display the proportion of defective items in each sample. The theoretical basis for a *p*-chart is the binomial distribution (Chapter 7), and it is recommended to use large sample sizes ($50 \leq n \leq 200$) to obtain good statistical results.

To construct the *p*-chart for BAMC, Olina Petrenko followed these steps (see also Excel Video 8.1):

EXCEL VIDEO 8.1

p-Chart

Access the Excel video online by visiting www.springerpub.com/courseconnect. See inside front cover and tear-out card for CourseConnect details.

BRIGHT ANGEL MEDICAL CENTER 8.2

Olina and Barbara reviewed last month's data (Exhibit 8.1) outlining patient arrivals and the rate of patients who left without being seen (LWBS). Olina recommended plotting these numbers into a control chart to get a better understanding of the variation (Figure 8.4).

EXHIBIT 8.1 PROPORTION OF LWBS PATIENTS IN JANUARY

These are the numbers that will be plotted.

Weekday	Day	Number of Visits (*n*)	LWBS ("Defective Visits")	Proportion (*p*) (LWBS/*n*)
Saturday	1	176	18	0.1023
Sunday	2	170	14	0.0824
Monday	3	188	20	0.1064
Tuesday	4	160	7	0.0438
Wednesday	5	155	3	0.0194

(*continued*)

EXHIBIT 8.1 PROPORTION OF LWBS PATIENTS IN JANUARY (*CONTINUED*)

Thursday	6	160	6	0.0375
Friday	7	192	23	0.1198
Saturday	8	182	20	0.1099
Sunday	9	160	9	0.0563
Monday	10	190	19	0.1000
Tuesday	11	146	10	0.0685
Wednesday	12	150	2	0.0133
Thursday	13	104	0	0.0000
Friday	14	175	16	0.0914
Saturday	15	178	18	0.1011
Sunday	16	159	9	0.0566
Monday	17	185	19	0.1027
Tuesday	18	158	6	0.0380
Wednesday	19	150	5	0.0333
Thursday	20	172	6	0.0349
Friday	21	185	21	0.1135
Saturday	22	186	19	0.1022
Sunday	23	179	16	0.0894
Monday	24	187	19	0.1016
Tuesday	25	156	7	0.0449
Wednesday	26	160	5	0.0313
Thursday	27	163	1	0.0061
Friday	28	181	25	0.1381
Saturday	29	180	16	0.0889
Sunday	30	170	12	0.0706
Monday	31	212	26	0.1226
	Total	5,269	397	

Abbreviation: LWBS, left without being seen.

STEP 1: Compute the mean proportion of LWBS patients, $\overline{p}$.

This is the estimate of the population proportion (π) and the centerline of the control chart.

$$\overline{p} = \frac{\textit{Total number (sum) of nonconforming items}}{\textit{Total number (sum) of items inspected}}$$

$$= \frac{\textit{Total number (sum) of patients who LWBS}}{\textit{Total number (sum) of patients who visited the ED}} \quad [8.1]$$

$$= \frac{397}{5,269} = 0.0753$$

STEP 2: Compute each sample *SD* of the proportion, S_p.

This reflects the variation or spread in the sample data.

$$S_p = \sqrt{\frac{\overline{p}(1-\overline{p})}{\textit{Number of items inspected in each sample or subgroup}}} \quad [8.2]$$

Note: As the subgroup size changes every day, S_p will also change daily.

On January 1 (day 1),

$$S_p = \sqrt{\frac{0.0753(1-0.0753)}{176}} = 0.0199.$$

STEP 3: Determine the control limits or upper and lower bands of the chart (±3 *SD* from the centerline), UCL_p and LCL_p.

$$\text{Upper control limit } (UCL_p) = \bar{p} + 3\,S_p \qquad [8.3]$$

$$\text{Lower control limit } (LCL_p) = \bar{p} - 3\,S_p \qquad [8.4]$$

On January 1 (day 1),

$UCL_p = 0.0753 + (3 \times 0.0199) = 0.1350.$

$LCL_p = 0.0753 - (3 \times 0.0199) = 0.0156$ (Box 8.2).

BOX 8.2 FAQs

Is it possible to get a negative value when computing the *LCL*?

Yes! In fact, it happens on day 13. The *LCL* is –0.0023.

It doesn't make sense! How could a proportion of patients who left without being seen be negative?

You're right. It's impossible. That's why we have to round it up to 0. Anything else?

Yes. Why add and subtract 3 *SD* to and from the average proportion?

Because the control chart essentially depicts the distribution of the process. Three *SD* or *SE* below and above the mean represent most of its natural width, that is, its random variation (see Figure 8.3).

STEP 4: Draw the control limits (Figure 8.4).

Note that the control limits change for every subgroup point. This is because the number of observations or patient visits to the ED (the denominator in the *SD* formula used to determine control limits) changes each day. In Table 8.1, the subgroup sizes vary between 104 and 212. If they had been rather stable, let us say between 154 and 162, Olina Petrenko could have taken the average subgroup size and developed an *np*-chart (see next section). If she had decided to sample 50 visits each day and determine the number of LWBS patients in each sample, the control limits would have been straight lines, and she could have used either a *p*- or an *np*-chart.

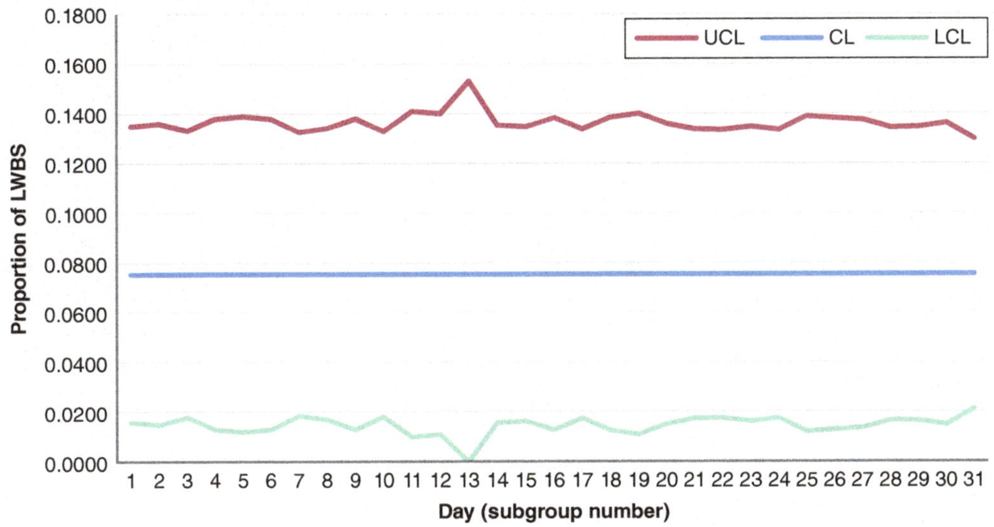

FIGURE 8.4 Centerline and control limits of *p*-chart.

Abbreviations: CL, centerline; LCL, lower control limit; LWBS, left without being seen; UCL, upper control limit.

TABLE 8.1 NUMBER OF LWBS PATIENTS IN JANUARY

These are the numbers that will be plotted.

Day	Number of Visits (*n*)	LWBS ("Defective Visits")
1	154	16
2	161	13
3	159	17
4	155	7
5	160	3
6	159	6
7	156	19
8	154	18
9	161	9
10	161	16
11	155	11
12	161	2
13	158	0
14	159	15
15	155	16

(continued)

TABLE 8.1 NUMBER OF LWBS PATIENTS IN JANUARY (*CONTINUED*)

Day	Number of Visits (*n*)	LWBS ("Defective Visits")
16	156	9
17	156	16
18	162	6
19	160	5
20	157	6
21	158	18
22	155	16
23	160	14
24	155	16
25	158	7
26	160	5
27	154	1
28	159	22
29	159	14
30	161	11
31	155	20
Total	4,893	354
Average	157.8 ≈ 158	11.42

Abbreviation: LWBS, left without being seen.

STEP 5: Plot the proportion defective (proportion of LWBS patients) for each day (column 5, Exhibit 8.1), *p*.

$$p = \frac{Number\ of\ nonconforming\ items\ in\ a\ sample\ or\ subgroup}{Number\ of\ items\ in\ the\ sample\ or\ subgroup\ (i.e., sample\ or\ subgroup\ size)} \quad [8.5]$$

On day 1, $\frac{18}{176} = 0.1023$ (Figure 8.5).

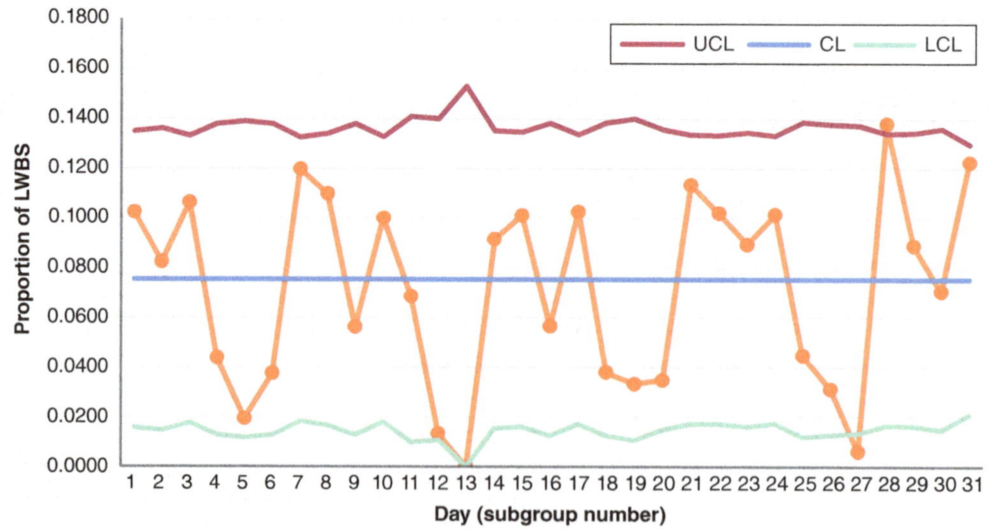

FIGURE 8.5 *p*-chart.

Abbreviations: CL, centerline; LCL, lower control limit; LWBS, left without being seen; UCL, upper control limit.

STEP 6: Determine whether the process is in control.

The process is out of control. The proportion of LWBS patients was outside the control limits on days 27 and 28. On day 28, the special cause(s) of variation that led to a larger-than-expected proportion of LWBS patients should be investigated and eliminated. As for day 27 (same for day 13), the percentage of LWBS patients was lower than expected, which is a good thing! Again, the cause(s) should be investigated so that the favorable conditions that led to these outcomes can be reproduced. Finally, there was a cyclical pattern in the data. You will notice that on Fridays, Saturdays, and Mondays, the proportion of LWBS is above average, and during the middle of the week, it tends to be lower. This is consistent with the visit pattern shown in Chapter 7, BAMC story 7.2.

np-Charts

As indicated previously, ***np*-charts** are used when subgroup or sample sizes are not substantially different. Let us illustrate with the following data set (Table 8.1; see also Excel Video 8.2). The lowest subgroup is 154 and the largest is 162. With a difference of only eight visits, we can assume that the subgroups are roughly equal, take the average subgroup size of 158 for our calculations of constant LCLs and UCLs, and create an *np*-chart.

EXCEL VIDEO 8.2

np-Chart

Access the Excel video online by visiting www.springerpub.com/courseconnect. See inside front cover and tear-out card for CourseConnect details.

To develop the *np*-chart, follow these steps:

STEP 1: Compute the average number of defective items, or, in this case, the daily average of LWBS patients, $n\bar{p}$.

$$n\bar{p} = \frac{\textit{Total number (sum) of nonconforming items}}{\textit{Number of subgroups}} \qquad [8.6]$$

This is the centerline of the control chart

$$= \frac{\textit{Total number (sum) of patients who LWBS}}{\textit{Number of days}}$$

$$= \frac{354}{31} = 11.42 \text{ patients}$$

Note that the denominator is no longer the total number of items inspected but the number of subgroups. Likewise, the centerline is no longer a proportion but a number of nonconforming items, that is, LWBS.

STEP 2: Determine the UCL and LCL of the *np*-chart, UCL_{np} and LCL_{np}.

$$UCL_{np} = n\bar{p} + 3\sqrt{n\bar{p}\left(1 - \frac{n\bar{p}}{n}\right)} \qquad [8.7]$$

$$= 11.42 + 3\sqrt{11.42\left(1 - \frac{11.42}{158}\right)}$$

$$= 11.42 + 3(3.255)$$

$$= 21.18 \text{ patients}$$

$$LCL_{np} = n\bar{p} - 3\sqrt{n\bar{p}\left(1-\frac{n\bar{p}}{n}\right)} \qquad [8.8]$$

$$= 11.42 - 3\sqrt{11.42\left(1-\frac{11.42}{158}\right)}$$

$$= 11.42 - 3(3.255)$$

$$= 1.65 \text{ patients}$$

STEP 3: Draw the centerline, UCL, and LCL of the *np*-chart.
STEP 4: Plot the daily number of LWBS patients (column 3 in Table 8.1; Figure 8.6).
STEP 5: Determine whether the process is in control.

The results are similar to those observed on the *p*-chart. The daily number of LWBS patients is unstable, that is, out of control, with the number of LWBS patients on days 13, 27, and 28 outside the control limits.

c-Charts

***c*-charts** are used to plot the number of defects per unit over time. The **area of opportunity**, or the number of units inspected, for the defect to occur must be constant (e.g., number of falls per 1,000 occupied bed days in a long-term care facility, number of occurrences of system downtime per 1,000 hours, number of sharps injuries per 100 full-time equivalents (FTEs) per year). The number of defects per unit (or fixed set of units) follows the Poisson distribution. One important distinction between these attributes and those in *p*-charts is that *multiple* defects can be found in each unit or area of opportunity, whereas an item in a *p*-chart is determined to be defective or nondefective only once. In other words, a patient may fall multiple times, and the system could be down several times in a month. In contrast, LWBS patients leave or they do not (*p*-chart); they do not leave multiple times (Box 8.3).

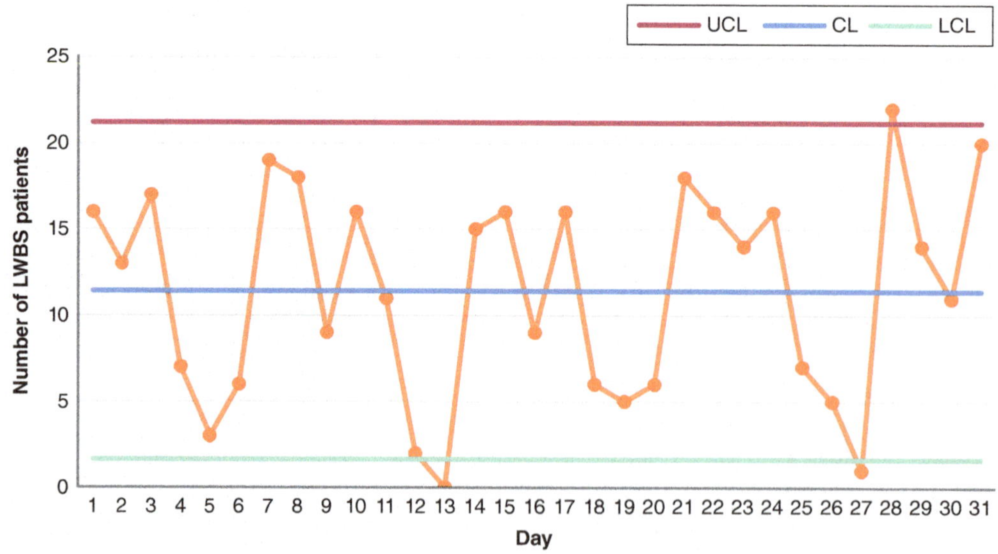

FIGURE 8.6 *np*-chart.

Abbreviations: CL, centerline; LCL, lower control limit; LWBS, left without being seen; UCL, upper control limit.

BOX 8.3 FAQs

I still don't understand the difference between *p*- and *c*-charts. How can you tell which one to use?

The *p*-chart focuses on inspecting a sample of items and putting the defective ones in a "separate pile." You end up with two piles: a pile of defective items and a pile of non-defective ones. Keep in mind that a defective item could have multiple defects, but that is not your concern with the *p*-chart.

On the other hand, the number of defects in each item that you inspect is the focus of the *c*-chart. Each unit inspected could have multiple defects, but the nonoccurrence of defects cannot be counted.

Can you give an example?

Sure. If you take a sample of 100 patients and identify those who fell during a week, you are distinguishing between those who fell ("defective") and those who did not fall ("non-defective"). You have two groups and could determine the proportion of patients who fell in a given week. This proportion would be tracked each week on a *p*-chart.

A single patient could have fallen multiple times during a week. If you record the number of falls ("defects") per week in a set of 100 patients, you could track that number on a *c*-chart. But there is no way you could count the number of "non-falls"!

BRIGHT ANGEL MEDICAL CENTER 8.3

Barbara had heard anecdotal reports of exam rooms lacking the needed supplies and shared her concerns with Adeleke. Adeleke said, "I heard that too. The staff has to go on a treasure hunt to find what they need to care for patients. That wastes time and slows everything down. This is why we had been focused on this issue for a month. The nurses documented every shortage, and I personally organized the data in a table (Exhibit 8.2; see also Excel Video 8.3). One shortage is one too many, but I wonder if we have a pattern here. I have already asked Olina to help us sort this out."

(continued)

BRIGHT ANGEL MEDICAL CENTER 8.3 (*CONTINUED*)

EXCEL VIDEO 8.3

c-Chart

Access the Excel video online by visiting www.springerpub.com/courseconnect. See inside front cover and tear-out card for CourseConnect details.

EXHIBIT 8.2 NUMBER OF SHORTAGES IN EXAM ROOMS

These are the numbers that will be plotted.

Day	Number of Shortages, *c*
1	5
2	4
3	6
4	6
5	5
6	6
7	7
8	9
9	8
10	8
11	7
12	8
13	10
14	11
15	9
16	11
17	10
18	11
19	12
20	14
21	11
22	12
23	13
24	15
25	13
26	12
27	14
28	16
29	15
30	16
31	18
Total	322

(*continued*)

BRIGHT ANGEL MEDICAL CENTER 8.3 (*CONTINUED*)

Olina determined that shortages were actually defects. She verified that the number of patients treated in the exam rooms did not fluctuate much from day to day and decided that the c-chart was appropriate.

To construct the c-chart, Olina used the following steps.

STEP 1: Compute the average number of defects per unit, $\bar{c}$.

$$\bar{c} = \frac{\textit{Total number of defects}}{\textit{Total number of units inspected}} \quad [8.9]$$

$$= \frac{\textit{Total number of shortages}}{\textit{Total number of exam room floors inspected 31 days}}$$

All exam rooms are on the same floor (constant)

$$= \frac{322}{31} = 10.39 \text{ shortages.}$$

STEP 2: Compute the *SD* of the number of defects, S_c. With the Poisson distribution, the *SD* is the square root of the mean (Chapter 7).

$$S_c = \sqrt{\bar{c}} \quad [8.10]$$

$$= \sqrt{10.39} = 3.22 \text{ shortages.}$$

STEP 3: Determine the control limits, UCL_c and LCL_c.

$$UCL_c = \bar{c} + 3S_c \quad [8.11]$$

$$= 10.39 + (3 \times 3.22) = 20.05 \text{ shortages}$$

$$LCL_c = \bar{c} - 3S_c \quad [8.12]$$

$$= 10.39 - (3 \times 3.22) = 0.73 \text{ shortages}$$

STEP 4: Draw the centerline and control limits.

STEP 5: Plot the number of defects, that is, shortages, *c* (Exhibit 8.3).

EXHIBIT 8.3 *c*-CHART

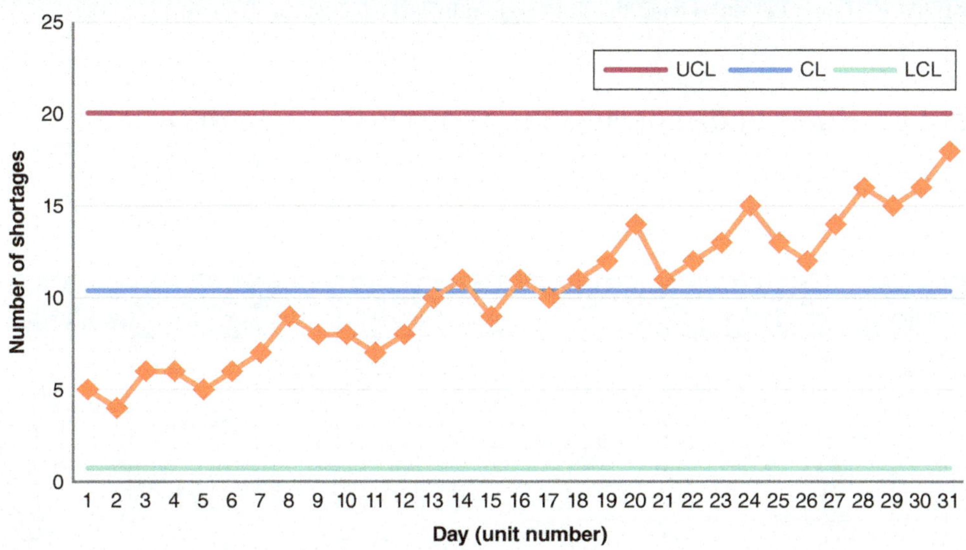

Abbreviations: CL, centerline; LCL, lower control limit; UCL, upper control limit.

(*continued*)

BRIGHT ANGEL MEDICAL CENTER 8.3 (*CONTINUED*)

STEP 6: *Determine whether the process is in control.*

There are no points outside the control limits, but there is a clear, upward trend, which indicates that the process is out of control.

"Well," Adeleke said, "The staff had a reason to complain, and the situation is getting worse. Clearly, the daily number of shortages is increasing over time. How are the rooms being stocked? Whatever is being done, it's not working!"

"What are you thinking?" questioned Olina. She empathized with Adeleke and how difficult his job to turn around the ED on a short timeline seemed.

"I am thinking this job is really tough," said Adeleke, appearing a little bit dejected.

"This is hard work, and we believe that you and Barbara are the right people to make things happen. Besides, you're not alone. It's a team effort," encouraged Olina. Adeleke flashed a brief smile.

"Well, let's move on and review the data on patient complaints. Might as well just rip the whole band-aid off!"

u-Charts

***u*-charts** are similar to *c*-charts. They are used to plot defects per unit (or set of inspected units) when the area of opportunity fluctuates. Each day the number of patients visiting the ED varies. When there are more patients, one would expect more complaints about wait times and vice versa. Therefore, the set of inspected units, that is, the number of patients seen on a given day, is not constant; there is not an equal area of opportunity for defects to occur. Other examples include the number of needle-stick injuries in a hospital per month (the number of occupied beds fluctuates), or the number of discrepancies in surgery patient charts per week (the number of weekly surgeries fluctuates). In the absence of an equal area of opportunity for the defects to occur, we need to unitize, that is, make the set of inspected units constant, so that comparable values can be plotted on the *u*-chart.

At BAMC, Olina Petrenko used the data shown in Table 8.2 (see also Excel Video 8.4).

TABLE 8.2 NUMBER OF COMPLAINTS ABOUT WAIT TIMES IN THE ED

These are the numbers that will be plotted.

Day	Visits	*c* Complaints	*n* Visits ÷ Predetermined Set Size (100)	*u* *c*/*n*
1	176	13	1.76	7.39
2	170	10	1.7	5.88
3	188	16	1.88	8.51
4	160	10	1.6	6.25
5	155	7	1.55	4.52
6	160	12	1.6	7.50

(continued)

TABLE 8.2 NUMBER OF COMPLAINTS ABOUT WAIT TIMES IN THE ED (*CONTINUED*)

Day	Visits	*c* Complaints	*n* Visits ÷ Predetermined Set Size (100)	*u* *c*/*n*
7	192	17	1.92	8.85
8	182	14	1.82	7.69
9	160	10	1.6	6.25
10	190	18	1.9	9.47
11	146	5	1.46	3.42
12	150	12	1.5	8.00
13	104	9	1.04	8.65
14	175	13	1.75	7.43
15	178	13	1.78	7.30
16	159	15	1.59	9.43
17	185	18	1.85	9.73
18	158	10	1.58	6.33
19	150	12	1.5	8.00
20	172	12	1.72	6.98
21	185	15	1.85	8.11
22	186	18	1.86	9.68
23	179	19	1.79	10.61
24	187	17	1.87	9.09
25	156	15	1.56	9.62
26	160	16	1.6	10.00
27	163	16	1.63	9.82
28	181	28	1.81	15.47
29	180	20	1.8	11.11
30	170	17	1.7	10.00
31	212	24	2.12	11.32
Total		451	52.69	

EXCEL VIDEO 8.4

u-Chart

Access the Excel video online by visiting www.springerpub.com/courseconnect. See inside front cover and tear-out card for CourseConnect details.

To construct the *u*-chart, Olina followed the following steps.

STEP 1: Compute the number of sets of inspected units in each area of opportunity, n (column 4 in Table 8.2). For the data in Table 8.2, Olina had decided to use a set of 100 visits to unitize.

$$n = \frac{\textit{Number of observations in the original area of opportunity}}{\textit{Number of observations in the agreed–upon set of inspected units}} \quad [8.13]$$

For day 1, $n = \dfrac{176}{100} = 1.76.$

STEP 2: Convert c (column 3 in Table 8.2), the number of defects, to u (column 5 in Table 8.2), the unitized number of defects.

$$u = \frac{\textit{Number of defects in the original area of opportunity}}{\textit{Number of sets of inspected units}} \quad [8.14]$$

$$= \frac{\textit{Number of complaints}}{\textit{Number of sets of 100 visits}}$$

For day 1, $u = \frac{13}{1.76} = 7.39$ complaints.

STEP 3: Compute the average unitized number of defects, $\bar{u}$.

This is the centerline value of the u-chart

$$\bar{u} = \frac{\textit{Total number (sum) of defects}}{\textit{Total number (sum) of sets of inspected units}} \quad [8.15]$$

$$= \frac{\textit{Total number (sum) of complaints about wait times in January}}{\textit{Total number (sum) of sets of 100 visits in January}}$$

$$= \frac{451}{52.69} = 8.56 \text{ complaints.}$$

STEP 4: Compute the *SD* of the unitized number of defects, S_u.

$$S_u = \sqrt{\frac{\bar{u}}{n}} \quad [8.16]$$

For day 1, $S_u = \sqrt{\frac{8.56}{1.76}} = 2.21.$

STEP 5: Determine the control limits, UCL_u and LCL_u.

$$UCL_u = \bar{u} + 3S_u \quad [8.17]$$

For day 1, $UCL_u = 8.56 + (3 \times 2.21) = 15.19$ complaints.

$$LCL_u = \bar{u} - 3S_u \quad [8.18]$$

For day 1, $LCL_u = 8.56 - (3 \times 2.21) = 1.93$ complaints.

STEP 6: Draw the centerline and control limits.
STEP 7: Plot the unitized number of defects, u (column 5 in Table 8.2; Figure 8.7).
STEP 8: Determine whether the process is in control.

Data Point #28 is outside the control limits. Furthermore, two other phenomena are worth discussing. It seems that in the first half of the month, a large number of values were below average, whereas the opposite is true for the later part of the month. It seems that the average has shifted to a higher value. Further supporting this observation is the presence of nine consecutive data points above the average for the last days of January. The points, therefore, do not appear to be randomly distributed around the mean. The process is out of control.

BRIGHT ANGEL MEDICAL CENTER 8.4

Adeleke stared at these results. Why were patients complaining about wait times? Was it true? Did they actually spend too much time in the waiting room? Waiting to see the doctor? Or was the entire experience too long? He read another article on the use of SPC charts in hospitals (Box 8.4) and decided to examine the ED LOS first.

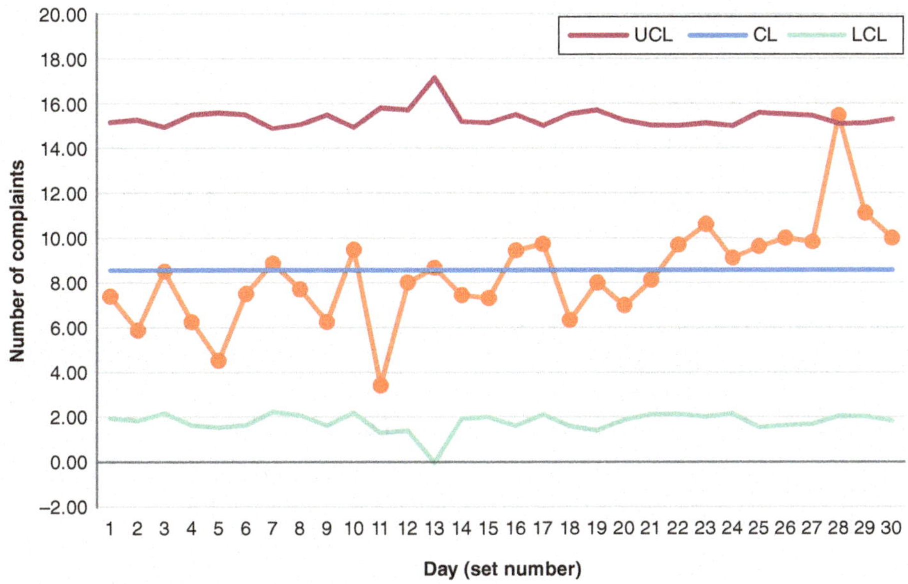

FIGURE 8.7 *u*-chart.

Abbreviations: CL, centerline; LCL, lower control limit; UCL, upper control limit.

BOX 8.4 QUALITY IN PRACTICE!

Using Statistical Process Control Charts for Surveillance of Surgical Site Infections

Researchers in the southeast United States monitored 29 community hospitals for the incidence of surgical site infection (SSI) outbreaks. By implementing new weekly analysis using SPC charts, there was a greater recognition of outbreaks or "clusters" of SSIs. This led to the identification of various deficiencies in adopting infection prevention best practices. Unfortunately, there was no overall improvement in SSI rates despite the increased identification of noncompliance. The reasons for the discrepancy between detection and prevention were a lack of direct communication with the surgeons and insufficient implementation of the recommendations provided to decrease SSI risk (Baker et al., 2022).

CONTROL CHARTS FOR VARIABLES

Unlike the number of LWBS patients or the number of complaints, time is a continuous variable. Other examples of variables include weight, height, temperature, and blood pressure. Variables are not counted; they are measured precisely on a continuous scale, using an instrument. The control charts for variables are (a) *IX* and *MR* charts, (b) $\bar{X}$ and *R* charts, (c) $\bar{X}$ and *s*-charts, and (d) CUSUM charts. The principles for constructing control charts for variables are the same as for attributes: Draw a centerline and establish the control limits three SEs (based on sampling distribution of means) from the centerline. However, there are always two charts for variables: one to track the process central tendency (*IX* or $\bar{X}$) and the other to track its variability or dispersion (*MR*, *R*, or *s*).

IX and *MR* Charts

IX and *MR* charts are used when evaluating the consistency of an individual data point ($n = 1$) over time. This is typically the case when the data or indicators are collected individually and not in subgroups, reported infrequently (e.g., monthly or even yearly), and are independent of one another. Examples include yearly healthcare expenditures, monthly revenue, and average length of stay (ALOS). The ***IX* chart** displays the individual data points. The ***MR* chart** depicts the *MR*s or the absolute differences between two consecutive, individual measures or *IX*s.

The following steps were used to construct the *MR* chart:

STEP 1: Compute the *MR* for each data point.

$$MR = |IX_n - IX_{n-1.}| \quad [8.19]$$

Since there is no data point before month 1, the first *MR* is computed for the second month. For month 2, *MR* = |275 min – 210 min| = 65 minutes. This value shows the spread between the first two ALOS.

BRIGHT ANGEL MEDICAL CENTER 8.5

Olina pulled the ALOS data for discharged patients over the past 24 months from the ED dashboard (Exhibit 8.4; see also Excel Video 8.5) and developed the IX and MR charts.

EXCEL VIDEO 8.5

IX and *MR* Charts

Access the Excel video online by visiting www.springerpub.com/courseconnect. See inside front cover and tear-out card for CourseConnect details.

EXHIBIT 8.4 ALOS IN THE ED

These values will be plotted on the *IX* chart

These values will be plotted on the *MR* chart

Month	ALOS (min)	*MR*
1	210	–
2	275	65
3	209	66
4	279	70
5	332	53
6	249	83
7	299	50
8	251	48
9	341	90
10	237	104
11	270	33
12	215	55
13	155	60
14	185	30
15	257	72
16	265	8
17	285	20
18	275	10
19	285	10

(continued)

EXHIBIT 8.4 ALOS IN THE ED (*CONTINUED*)

Month	ALOS (min)	*MR*
20	330	45
21	325	5
22	345	20
23	385	40
24	365	20
Sum	6,624	1,057

Abbreviations: ALOS, average length of stay; IX, individual X; *MR*, moving range.

STEP 2: Compute the mean moving range, $\overline{MR}$.

This is the centerline value of the *MR* chart

$$\overline{MR} = \frac{\Sigma MR}{k-1} = \frac{\textit{Sum of moving ranges across all individual data points}}{\textit{Number of subgroups included in analysis} - 1} \quad [8.20]$$

$$= \frac{\textit{Sum of ALOS moving ranges}}{\textit{Number of months} - 1}$$

$$= \frac{1{,}057}{23} = 45.96 \text{ minutes}$$

STEP 3: Determine the control limits, UCL_{MR} and LCL_{MR}.

Table values (see Appendix 8.1; $n = 1$) have been developed to determine the lower (D_3) and upper (D_4) control limits for the range charts based on different sample sizes. These values enable you to produce control limits that are similar to three SEs away from the mean.

$$UCL_{MR} = D_4\,\overline{MR} \quad [8.21]$$

$$= (3.267) \times (45.96)$$

0 and 3.267 are the D_3 and D_4 values for $n = 1$

$$= 150.15 \text{ minutes.}$$

$$LCL_{MR} = D_3\,\overline{MR} \quad [8.22]$$

$$= (0) \times (45.96)$$

$$= 0 \text{ minute.}$$

STEP 4: Draw the centerline and control limits.
STEP 5: Plot all moving ranges, *MR* (Figure 8.8).
STEP 6: Determine whether the process is in control.

The process dispersion does not appear to be in control. There are no points outside the control limits, there is an approximately equal number of data points above and below the centerline, but there has been a decrease in variability over the last 12 months. Lower variability is good, but it does not mean that it has reduced ALOS as we will see shortly. Note that the D_3 value of 0 has caused a lack of symmetry around the average *MR*.

The next steps were followed to develop the *IX* chart.

STEP 1: Compute the mean of the individual *X* values.

$$\overline{IX} = \frac{\Sigma IX}{k} \quad [8.23]$$

$$= \frac{\textit{Sum of the individual IX values}}{\textit{Number of subgroups included in analysis}}$$

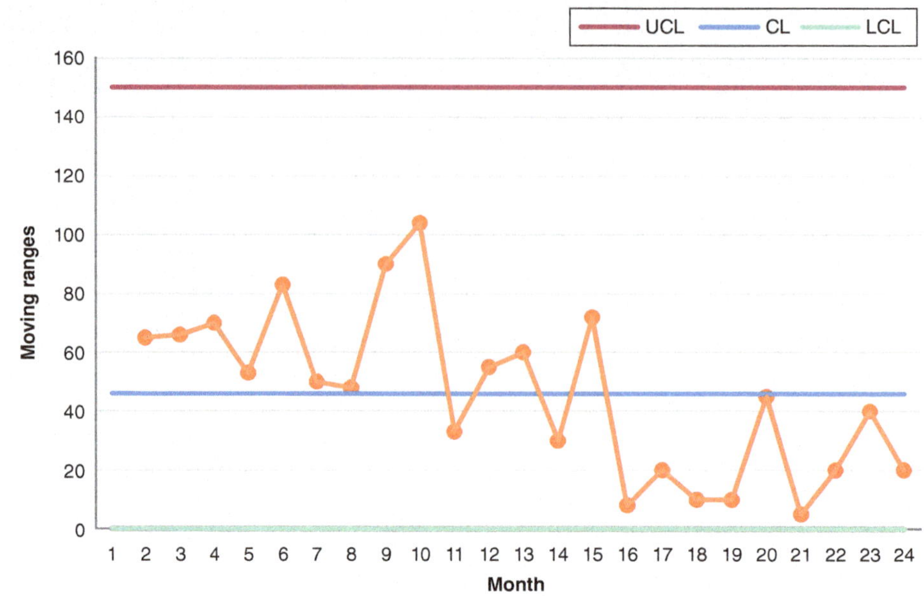

FIGURE 8.8 **Moving range (*MR*) chart.**

Abbreviations: CL, centerline; LCL, lower control limit; UCL, upper control limit.

$$= \frac{\textit{Sum of the ALOS values}}{\textit{Number of months considered}}$$

$$= \frac{6{,}624}{24} = 276 \text{ minutes.}$$

This is the centerline value of the *IX* chart

STEP 2: Determine the control limits, UCL_{IX} and LCL_{IX}.

Table values (A_2) have been developed to determine the LCLs and UCLs for the *IX* chart (see Appendix 8.1). These values enable you to produce control limits that are similar to three SEs away from the mean.

$$UCL_{IX} = \overline{IX} + A_2\overline{MR} \quad [8.24]$$

$$= 276 + (2.660) \times (45.96)$$

2.66 is the A_2 value for $n = 1$

$$= 398.25 \text{ minutes.}$$

$$LCL_{IX} = \overline{IX} - A_2\overline{MR}$$

$$= 276 - (2.660) \times (45.96)$$

$$= 153.75 \text{ minutes.} \quad [8.25]$$

STEP 3: Draw the centerline and control limits.
STEP 4: Plot all individual *X* values, *IX* (Figure 8.9).
STEP 5: Determine whether the process is in control.

The chart with ALOS times is not in control. The ALOS in month 13 is rather low, yet still above the LCL. However, after a brief stabilization around the mean, there is an upward shift in ALOS.

For variables, both the charts for central tendency and dispersion must be in control for the process to be in control. It is not the case here, with the sudden and sustained decrease in variability (Figure 8.8) corresponding to a steady increase in ALOS (Figure 8.9). Both the *MR* and *IX* charts are out of control. Therefore, the process is not in control.

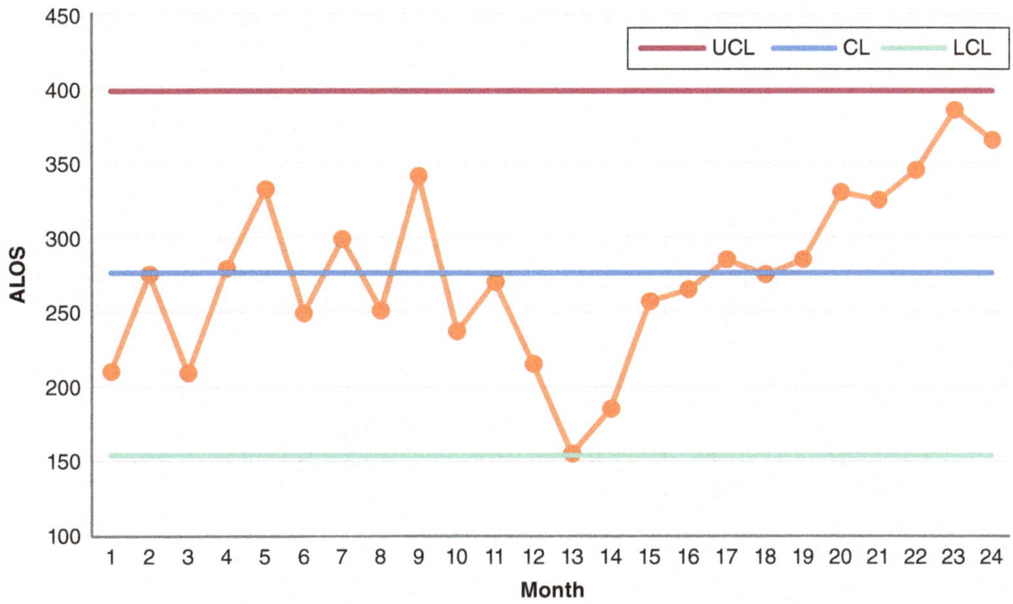

FIGURE 8.9 Individual *X* (*IX*) chart.

Abbreviations: ALOS, average length of stay; CL, centerline; LCL, lower control limit; UCL, upper control limit.

BRIGHT ANGEL MEDICAL CENTER 8.6

Adeleke and Olina were in Barbara's office. There was an uncomfortable silence before Barbara, visibly flustered, pointed to the IX and MR charts on her screen and said, "We are so far from our target length of stay . . . I just don't see how we could improve this situation dramatically in a short amount of time."

After a long sigh, Adeleke suggested, "Well, let's see if most of this time is actually door-to-doc time. That would give us a preliminary idea of how this length of stay is distributed and where the bottleneck might be."

Barbara pondered. "Shall we start reviewing the door-to-doc times for each patient seen in the month of January? What do you think, Olina?"

Olina smiled. "That's a good idea, but given the large volume of patients, let's take random samples of five patients each day and their associated door-to-doc time. We will then develop $\bar{X}$ and R charts."

The next day, she showed Adeleke the times shown in Exhibit 8.5 (see also Excel Video 8.6).

EXCEL VIDEO 8.6

$\bar{X}$ and *R* Charts

Access the Excel video online by visiting www.springerpub.com/courseconnect. See inside front cover and tear-out card for CourseConnect details.

(*continued*)

EXHIBIT 8.5 DOOR-TO-DOC TIMES (MIN) IN JANUARY

These values will be plotted on the $\bar{X}$ chart

These values will be plotted on the R chart

Day	Patient 1	Patient 2	Patient 3	Patient 4	Patient 5	$\bar{X}$	R
1	118	145	65	140	131	119.8	80
2	194	118	147	121	142	144.4	76
3	117	151	113	145	162	137.6	49
4	178	164	161	107	165	155.0	71
5	75	118	176	122	137	125.6	101
6	164	84	141	126	113	125.6	80
7	121	133	158	127	164	140.6	43
8	134	136	117	157	123	133.4	40
9	133	112	143	121	126	127.0	31
10	107	169	119	141	117	130.6	62
11	112	163	99	67	144	117.0	96
12	198	139	102	151	88	135.6	110
13	97	101	115	158	144	123.0	61
14	112	157	121	130	116	127.2	45
15	94	125	106	97	78	100.0	47
16	170	167	185	123	154	159.8	62
17	157	78	195	162	124	143.2	117
18	134	181	158	158	115	149.2	66
19	131	124	124	111	169	131.8	58
20	132	89	145	122	163	130.2	74
21	127	151	135	167	135	143.0	40
22	108	193	179	141	117	147.6	85
23	73	67	153	109	144	109.2	86
24	92	148	144	151	146	136.2	59
25	107	138	99	135	155	126.8	56
26	84	136	36	124	119	99.8	100
27	100	161	150	119	148	135.6	61
28	157	160	134	180	98	145.8	82
29	164	145	151	148	160	153.6	19
30	138	102	89	123	150	120.4	61
31	96	141	120	149	57	112.6	92
Total						4,087.2	2,110.0

$\bar{X}$ and *R* Charts

Mean ($\bar{X}$) and range (R) charts are used when the sample size is small ($2 \le n \le 9$). The **$\bar{X}$ chart** displays the sample means; the ***R* chart** displays the sample ranges. The range helps track the amount of variability or dispersion in the process. The range is the simplest measure of variability and is therefore easy and practical to use.

The following steps were used to construct the R chart.

STEP 1: Compute the range for each sample, R.

$$R = \text{largest value in the sample} - \text{lowest value in the sample} \quad [8.26]$$

$$= \text{longest door-to-doc time in sample} - \text{shortest door-to-doc time in sample.}$$

For day 1, $R = 145$ minutes $- 65$ minutes

$= 80$ minutes.

This value shows the spread in the sample data.

STEP 2: Compute the mean range, $\bar{R}$.

$$\bar{R} = \frac{\sum R}{k} = \frac{\textit{Sum of the ranges across all samples}}{\textit{Number of samples taken}} \quad [8.27]$$

$$= \frac{\textit{Sum of the door-to-doc time ranges}}{\textit{Number of samples of five patients taken}}$$

$$= \frac{2{,}110}{31} = 68.06 \text{ minutes}$$

STEP 3: Determine the control limits, UCL_R and LCL_R.

Table values (see Appendix 8.1) have been developed to determine the LCL (D_3) and UCL (D_4) for the range charts based on different sample sizes. These values enable you to produce control limits that are similar to three SEs away from the mean.

$$UCL_R = D_4\bar{R} \quad [8.28]$$

$$= (2.114) \times (68.06)$$

$$= 143.89 \text{ minutes}$$

0 and 2.114 are the D_3 and D_4 values for a sample size of 5 (Box 8.3)

$$LCL_R = D_3\bar{R} \quad [8.29]$$

$$= (0) \times (68.06)$$

$$= 0 \text{ minute}$$

STEP 4: Draw the control limits.
STEP 5: Plot all sample ranges, R (Figure 8.10).
STEP 6: Determine whether the process is in control.

With no points outside the control limits, no visible pattern, the majority of the points near the centerline, and points equally distributed above and below the mean, the process dispersion appears to be in control.

The following steps are needed to construct an $\bar{X}$ chart.

STEP 1: Compute the mean for each sample, $\bar{X}$.

$$\bar{X} = \frac{\sum X}{n} = \frac{\textit{Sum of sample values}}{\textit{Number of units in sample (sample size)}} \quad [8.30]$$

$$= \frac{\textit{Sum of door-to-doc times}}{\textit{Number of patients in sample}}$$

For day 1, $\bar{X} = \dfrac{118 + 145 + 65 + 140 + 131}{5} = 119.8$ minutes.

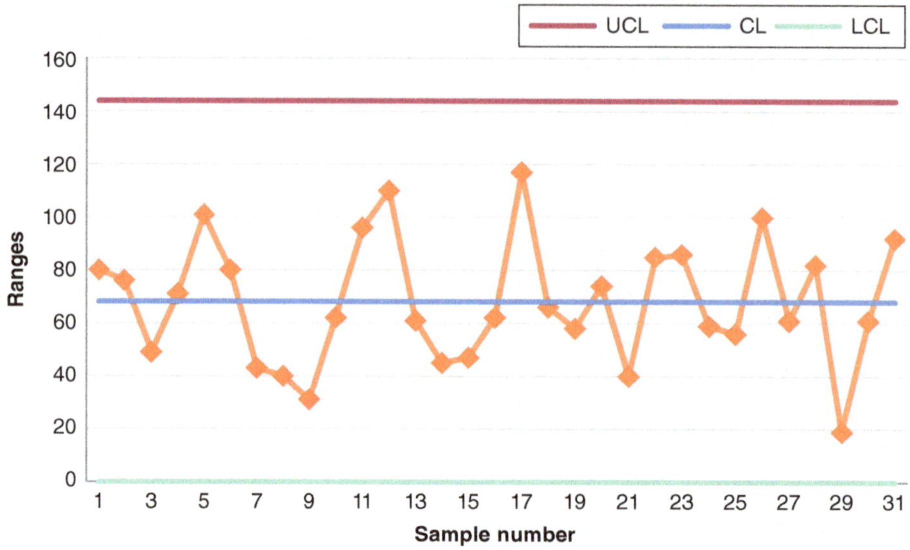

FIGURE 8.10 ***R* chart.**

Abbreviations: CL, centerline; LCL, lower control limit; UCL, upper control limit.

STEP 2: Compute the average of the sample means or grand mean, $\bar{X}$.

$$\bar{\bar{X}} = \frac{\sum \bar{X}}{k} = \frac{\textit{Sum of the sample means}}{\textit{Number of samples taken}} \quad [8.31]$$

$$= \frac{\textit{Sum of the average door-to-doc times for each sample of five patients}}{\textit{Number of samples of five patients taken}}$$

$$= \frac{4{,}087.2}{31} = 131.85 \text{ minutes.}$$

STEP 3: Compute the control limits, $UCL_{\bar{X}}$ and $LCL_{\bar{X}}$.

Just like for the R chart, table values (A_2) have been developed to determine the LCL and UCL for the $\bar{X}$ charts based on different sample sizes. These values enable you to produce control limits that are similar to three SEs away from the mean.

$$UCL_{\bar{X}} = \bar{\bar{X}} + A_2\bar{R} \quad [8.32]$$

The A_2 value for a sample size of 5 is 0.577

$$= 131.85 + (0.577) \times (68.06)$$

$$= 171.12 \text{ minutes}$$

$$LCL_{\bar{X}} = \bar{\bar{X}} - A_2\bar{R} \quad [8.33]$$

$$= 131.85 - (0.577) \times (68.06)$$

$$= 92.58 \text{ minutes}$$

STEP 4: Draw the control limits.

STEP 5: Plot the sample means, $\bar{X}$ (Figure 8.11).

STEP 6: Determine whether the process is in control.

Although a few larger sample averages emerged in the last days of January, the process appears to be in control. Because both central tendency and dispersion are in control, the process is in control.

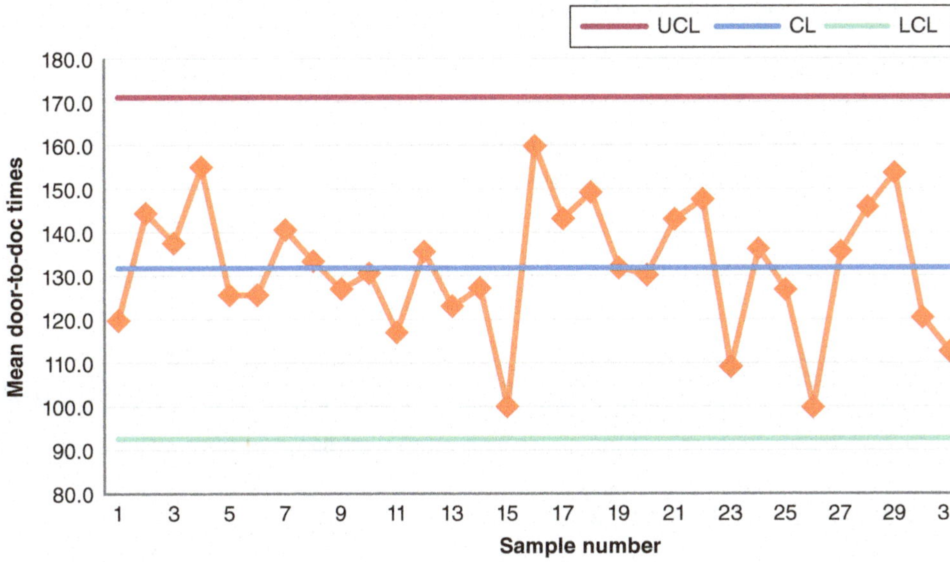

FIGURE 8.11 $\bar{X}$ **chart.**

Abbreviations: CL, centerline; LCL, lower control limit; UCL, upper control limit.

Just like *IX* and *MR* charts, $\bar{X}$ and *R* charts are used together. Because variables are evaluated both in terms of central tendency and dispersion, both the process average and its variability must be in control for the process to be in control. This makes sense. After all, the ranges could be consistently small, suggesting little variability, but the averages could be out of control. For example, if the control limits of the $\bar{X}$ chart were 5 and 10 minutes, and those of the *R* chart were 3 and 4 minutes, sample values of 9, 10, and 12.5 minutes would yield a range of 3.5 (within limits), but the sample mean of 10.5 minutes would be outside the limits. On the other hand, sample values of 1, 5, and 10 minutes would yield a mean of 5.33 minutes (within limits), but the sample range would be 9, a value clearly outside of the UCL.

BRIGHT ANGEL MEDICAL CENTER 8.7

Barbara and Adeleke were somewhat puzzled. Adeleke started, "At about 132 minutes, the average door-to-doc time is high. However, it is not the only concern. It looks like the increasingly long stays are due to delays in other areas."

Barbara agreed and added, "Something else that sticks out in the ED is the turnaround time for blood work and imaging tests. Physicians and nurses often complain that once they have ordered tests, it takes way too long to get the results. The patients are occupying exam rooms, causing a 'log jam.' Everyone is waiting, and the system is at a standstill." Adeleke nodded.

The health information system was used to pull the data on lab turnaround time. Again, Olina was called in to help. She drew daily samples of 10 patients and tracked the turnaround times for a complete blood count (CBC), one of the most common lab tests (Exhibit 8.6; see also Excel Video 8.7).

(continued)

EXHIBIT 8.6 CBC TURNAROUND TIMES IN JANUARY

EXCEL VIDEO 8.7

$\bar{X}$ and *s* Charts

Access the Excel video online by visiting www.springerpub.com/courseconnect. See inside front cover and tear-out card for CourseConnect details.

These numbers will be plotted on the $\bar{X}$ chart

These numbers will be plotted on the *s* chart

Day	Patient											
	1	2	3	4	5	6	7	8	9	10	$\bar{X}$	*s*
1	23.55	19.33	3.93	29	22.88	19.73	27.21	26.84	19.73	18.13	21.03	7.09
2	14.3	18.66	22.67	18.42	25.27	18.56	17.99	13.63	15.19	13.97	17.87	3.83
3	9.87	55.06	34.53	208	16.4	55.06	21.85	19.95	92.55	12.8	52.61	60.38
4	10.84	18.12	47.05	38.8	27.46	64.45	47.05	70.83	85.77	34.22	44.46	23.72
5	21.06	27.38	22.59	67.93	19.85	38.57	27.38	38.57	19.85	13.97	29.72	15.62
6	27.84	35.58	16.45	37.11	26.41	24.2	16.45	26.41	35.58	14.47	26.05	8.36
7	13.99	16.19	27.24	18.13	22.98	10.84	46.22	67.00	17.63	16.87	25.71	17.59
8	96.74	16.27	43.64	15.37	24.31	20.26	15.37	11.05	17.33	18.83	27.92	25.79
9	18.99	18.09	14.41	24.1	28.64	18.09	50.65	16.16	15.63	44.19	24.90	12.69
10	15.52	11.83	39.11	15.69	14.84	22.91	10.87	15.52	29.29	14.3	18.99	8.93
11	37.39	13.7	18.9	51.29	47.95	51.29	18.9	51.29	55.6	18.66	36.50	17.03
12	142.96	30.43	29.86	23.35	22.17	15.56	24.64	23.35	30.1	22.67	36.51	37.68
13	18.13	13.97	12.8	34.22	13.97	14.47	16.87	18.83	44.19	18.42	20.59	10.31
14	17.98	17.98	6.89	52.98	137.14	14.66	16.2	20.06	21.78	25.27	33.09	38.51
15	10.61	21.12	73.04	56.27	27.48	43.79	13.3	12.8	52.41	18.56	32.94	21.90
16	11.55	23.02	93.52	11.55	11.11	28.2	17.62	18.69	17.77	17.99	25.10	24.63
17	20.56	96.45	33.63	19.88	28.46	10.75	19.88	29.21	20.45	13.63	29.29	24.61
18	21.74	66.14	44.14	36.99	5.01	32.06	39.64	5.01	19.85	15.19	28.58	19.07
19	53.95	26.2	9.27	70.81	27.34	9.15	27.71	25.07	27.93	17.49	29.49	19.19
20	14.16	14.51	18.76	40.86	23.78	28.13	13.91	203.23	16.7	18.06	39.21	58.23
21	8.54	15.77	5.58	17.47	13.63	16.59	109.92	20.19	7.48	6.51	22.17	31.26
22	20.91	7.82	22.55	35.06	7.82	22.55	23.17	13.41	127.66	10.04	29.10	35.67
23	13.41	13.33	16.55	18.63	162.66	44.36	16.55	30.29	22.06	28.93	36.68	45.30
24	39.35	79.98	17.4	9.34	24.31	19.41	14.49	19.16	19.92	15.04	25.84	20.62
25	40.57	14.4	15.62	79.32	30.89	17.62	40.57	13.56	19.19	18.42	29.02	20.47
26	17.23	57.77	25.24	72.74	23.34	18.16	195.77	72.74	23.34	18.69	52.50	55.16
27	30.03	20.63	44.79	26.35	94.98	20.63	63.85	17.23	25.13	32.93	37.66	24.46
28	17.49	18.06	6.51	10.04	28.93	15.04	18.42	18.69	32.93	19.73	18.58	7.80
29	22.81	8.84	19.69	22.81	16.77	19.69	19.69	19.76	21.38	27.21	19.87	4.77
30	17.96	14.51	52.97	70.87	30.75	27.86	29.37	26.56	5.49	26.84	30.32	18.89
31	18.7	32	29.4	18.5	20.2	31.7	33.9	21.3	20.8	11.7	23.82	7.39
Total											926.08	726.94

Note: Totals are based without rounding.

$\bar{X}$ and s-Charts

Mean ($\bar{X}$) and *SD* (*s*) charts are used when the sample size is larger than 9. These are the most powerful control charts, but compared to the *R* chart, constructing the **s-chart**, which displays the sample *SD*s, is more computationally demanding.

To develop the *s*-chart, Olina used the following steps.

STEP 1: Compute the *SD* for each sample, *s*.

$$s = \sqrt{\frac{\sum_{i=1}^{n}(X_i - \bar{X})^2}{n-1}} \quad [8.34]$$

$$= \sqrt{\frac{\textit{Sum of (each sample value} - \textit{the sample mean})^2}{\textit{Sample size} - 1}}$$

On day 1, $s = \sqrt{\frac{(23.55-21.03)^2 + (19.33-21.03)^2 + \ldots + (18.13-21.03)^2}{10-1}}$

$= 7.09$ minutes.

STEP 2: Compute the average sample *SD*, $\bar{s}$.

$$\bar{s} = \frac{\Sigma s}{k} \quad [8.35]$$

$$= \frac{\textit{Sum of sample SD}}{\textit{Number of samples taken}}$$

$= \frac{726.94}{31} = 23.45$ minutes.

The B_3 and B_4 values for a sample size of 10 are 0.284 and 1.716, respectively (Appendix 8.1)

STEP 3: Determine the control limits, UCL_s and LCL_s.

$$UCL_s = B_4\bar{s} \quad [8.36]$$

$= (1.716) \times (23.45) = 40.24$ minutes.

$$LCL_s = B_3\bar{s} \quad [8.37]$$

$= (0.284) \times (23.45) = 6.66$ minutes.

STEP 4: Graph the control limits.
STEP 5: Plot the *SD*s for each sample, *s* (Figure 8.12).
STEP 6: Determine whether the process is in control.

Several *SD*s (samples #2, #3, #20, #23, #26, and #29) are outside the control limits, indicating unstable variability. The process is out of control.

To build the $\bar{X}$ chart, the next steps were followed.

STEP 1: Compute the mean for each sample $\bar{X}$.

$$\bar{X} = \frac{\Sigma X}{n} \quad [8.38]$$

$$= \frac{\textit{Sum of sample values}}{\textit{Number of units in sample (sample size)}}$$

$$= \frac{\textit{Sum of turnaround times in a sample}}{\textit{Number of patients in sample}}$$

For day 1,

$$\bar{X} = \frac{23.55 + 19.33 + 3.93 + 29 + 22.88 + 19.73 + 27.21 + 26.84 + 19.73 + 18.13}{10}$$

$= 21.03$ minutes.

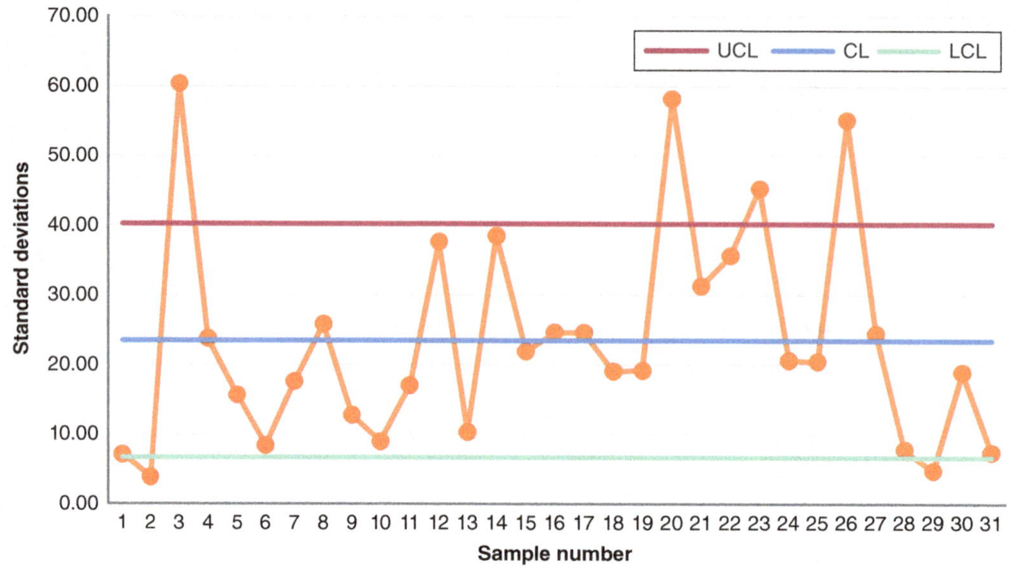

FIGURE 8.12 ***s*-chart.**

Abbreviations: CL, centerline; LCL, lower control limit; UCL, upper control limit.

STEP 2: Compute the average of the sample means or grand mean, $\bar{X}$.

$$\bar{\bar{X}} = \frac{\Sigma \bar{X}}{k} \tag{8.39}$$

$$= \frac{\textit{Sum of sample means}}{\textit{Number of samples taken}}$$

$$= \frac{\textit{Sum of the average turnaround times for each sample of 10 patients}}{\textit{Number of samples of 10 patients taken}}$$

$$= \frac{926.08}{31} = 29.87 \text{ minutes.}$$

STEP 3: Compute the control limits, $UCL_{\bar{X}}$ and $LCL_{\bar{X}}$.

$$UCL_{\bar{X}} = \bar{\bar{X}} + A_3 \bar{s} \tag{8.40}$$

$$= 29.87 + (0.975) \times (23.45)$$

$$= 52.73 \text{ minutes.}$$

The A_3 value for a sample size of 10 is 0.975 (Appendix 8.1)

$$LCL_{\bar{X}} = \bar{\bar{X}} - A_3 \bar{s} \tag{8.41}$$

$$= 29.87 - (0.975) \times (23.45)$$

$$= 7.01 \text{ minutes.}$$

STEP 4: Graph the control limits.

STEP 5: Plot the $\bar{X}$ values for each sample (Figure 8.13).

STEP 6: Determine whether the process is in control.

All sample values are within the control limits, and there does not seem to be a pattern. The two values close to the *UCL*, with none close to the *LCL*, suggest some skewness. More data points would be needed to see if this is a valid concern, but given that the dispersion of the process (*s*-chart) is out of control, the process is unstable overall and therefore out of control.

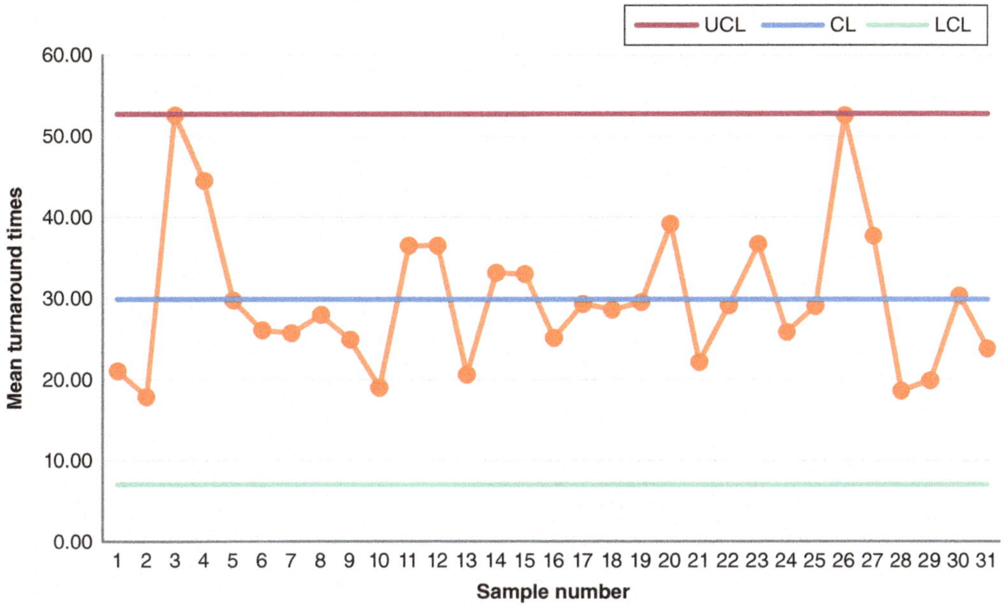

FIGURE 8.13 $\bar{X}$ chart.

Abbreviations: CL, centerline; LCL, lower control limit; UCL, upper control limit.

When using both charts together, you can see that for samples #2 and #29, the *SD*s are very low, indicating low variability. The average turnaround times for these two samples are also relatively low. This is a desirable situation that we would want to reproduce in the future! Identifying the conditions that led to these situations would be time well spent. On the other hand, the *SD*s for samples #3, #20, #23, and #26 are high because of the unusually high turnaround times for some patients.

BRIGHT ANGEL MEDICAL CENTER 8.8

It was late, and Adeleke wanted to go home. This week, he had spent long hours in the office and had missed his sons' football games. He was feeling down. To make matters worse, the SPC charts for lab turnaround times were discouraging. With the current technology, CBC test results should be available within minutes! What was taking so long and why was there so much variability? And time was also wasted when patients were sent to Imaging. Everything in the ED was a mess! He sent an invite to Dr. Aoki, the ED medical director. He needed to find out why all these problems were occurring.

So many charts to remember! Figure 8.14 helps you determine which SPC chart is to be used based on the characteristics of the data.

CONTROL CHART PATTERNS

As previously mentioned, a sample value could be inside the control limits and yet the process could be deemed unstable or out of control. A consistent pattern, even inside the limits, would suggest the presence of assignable causes of variation, not the random variation that we normally expect in a process. In most cases, patterns—that are, by definition, nonrandom—would warrant efforts to identify the causes of variation and eliminate them to get the process back in control. Three examples of patterns are shown in Figure 8.15. Note that if Figure 8.15B represented the

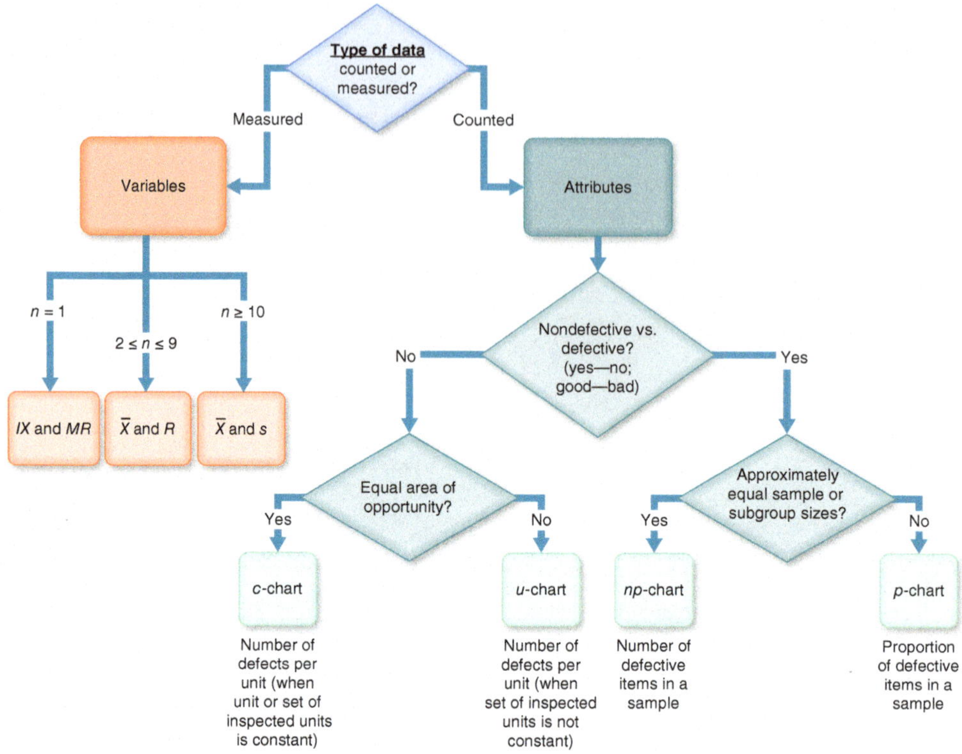

FIGURE 8.14 Control chart decision tree.

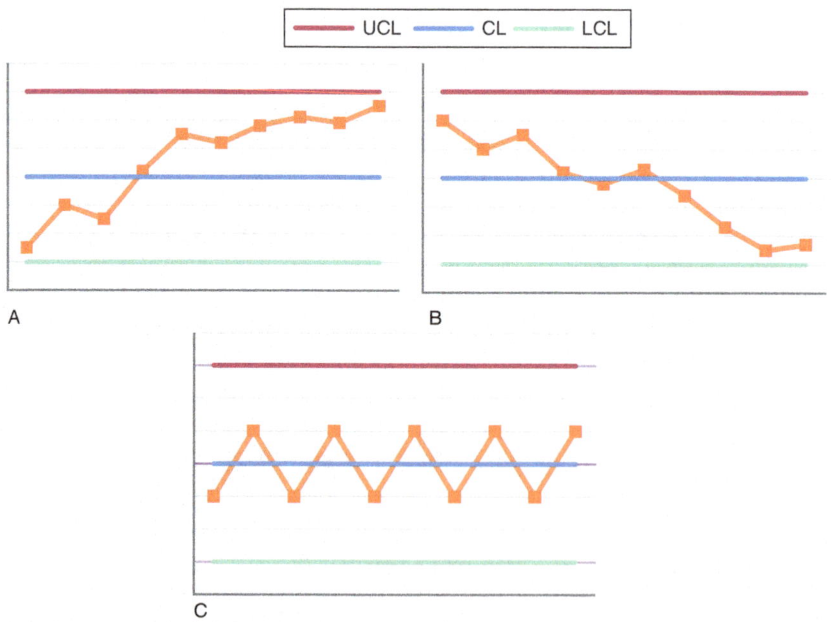

FIGURE 8.15 Examples of patterns.

Note: (A) Sample values consistently increasing. (B) Sample values consistently decreasing. (C) Points alternating above and below the centerline.

Abbreviations: CL, centerline; LCL, lower control limit; UCL, upper control limit.

proportion of defective items (p-chart) or the number of defects (c- or u-chart), the consistent decrease would be desirable! In this situation, just like for any out-of-control process, you would want to identify the causes of assignable variation. However, instead of eliminating the causes that led to a better outcome, you would ensure that they become permanent elements of a new, improved process.

PATTERN TESTS

Sometimes, the patterns are not as obvious as those shown in Figure 8.15, and we need to do a **pattern test** to detect their presence (Lighter & Fair, 2004). To conduct a pattern test, we divide the control chart into three zones above and below the centerline. Zone A includes values between two and three *SD*s from the mean. Zone B contains values between one and two *SD*s from the mean. Zone C contains values that are less than one *SD* from the mean. Remember that to reflect a process that is in control, sample value points should be *randomly* distributed around the mean, with most of the values close to the mean and only a few values close to the control limits. Figure 8.16 shows several deviations from this rule.

CUMULATIVE SUM CONTROL CHARTS

The control charts we discussed so far are known as "Shewhart charts," so named for the man who invented them. As you know by now, they are meant to determine whether a process is stable, that is, operates as expected over time, or to display the results of an improvement (Chapter 11). Data points outside the 3-sigma control limits are the clearest sign of an out-of-control situation, but sometimes, 2-sigma limits can be treated as early warnings (Box 8.5). Building on this tightened scrutiny of a process, the **CUSUM chart** is a control chart intended to detect sudden and small (<2 *SD*s) shifts from a target value quickly. As such, its purpose is to keep a process on target. To accomplish this, the CUSUM chart displays the CUSUM of the deviations from the target value. To illustrate this

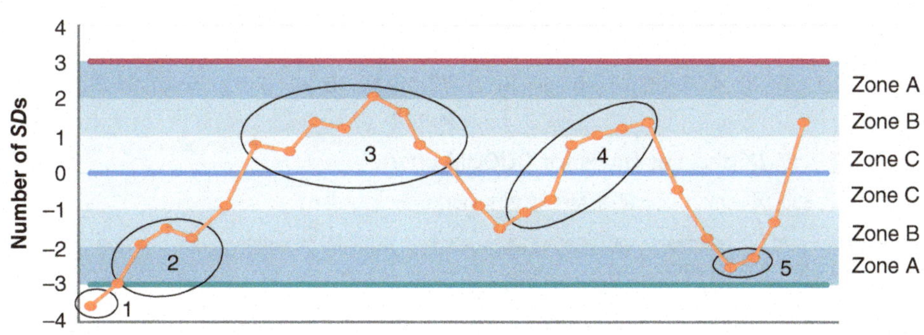

Pattern	Characteristics
1	Point outside the band determined by the control limits
2	Four of five consecutive points in Zones A or B
3	More than seven consecutive points either above or below the centerline
4	More than five points with consistently increasing or decreasing values
5	Two of three consecutive points in Zone A

FIGURE 8.16 Zones and patterns.

BOX 8.5 QUALITY IN PRACTICE!

Use of Statistical Process Control Charts for Monitoring *Staphylococcus aureus* Bloodstream Infections

In Australia, *Staphylococcus aureus bloodstream* (SAB) rates are reported as healthcare performance indicators. In a study of 155 healthcare facilities, researchers relied on *u*-charts to track SAB rates over time and signal higher-than-expected rates. Facility data were therefore plotted on those charts, using 2-sigma limits for warning and 3-sigma limits for control. Because of very high variability in rates at several facilities, some distribution adjustments were made. Nevertheless, the *u*-chart proved to be an effective, easily understood, and proactive tool to detect problematic SAB rates over a 2-year period (Imam et al., 2019).

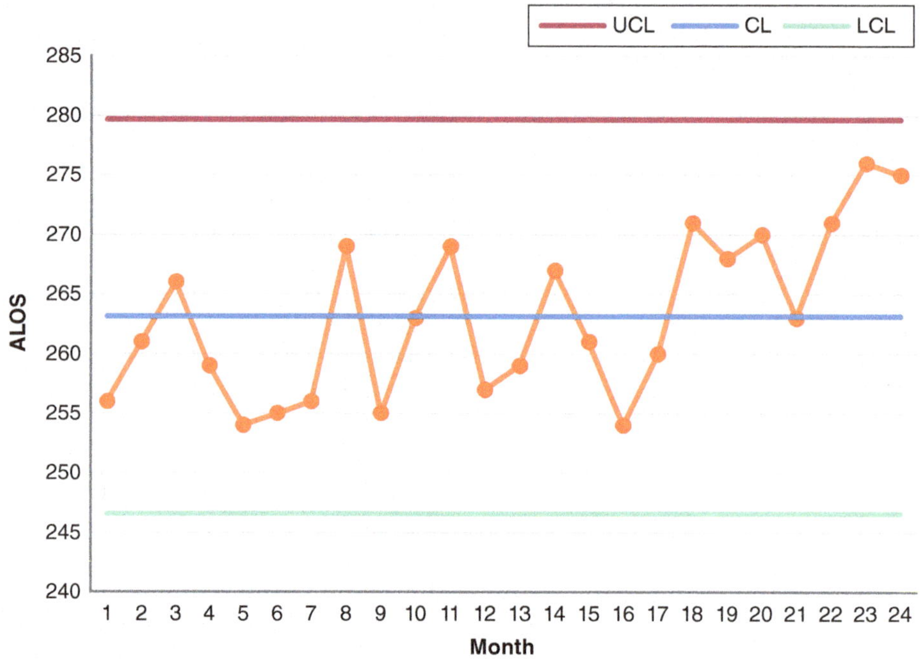

FIGURE 8.17 ***IX*** **chart as basis for CUSUM chart.**

$n = 1$; $A_2 = 2.660$; $\overline{IX} = 263.13$ minutes; $\overline{MR} = 6.22$ minutes.

Abbreviations: ALOS, average length of stay; CL, centerline; CUSUM, cumulative sum; LCL, lower control limit; UCL, upper control limit.

point, let us look at the *IX* chart in Figure 8.17. At first sight, the process appears to be in control, but we notice that six of the last seven points are above the centerline. Are they indicative of an upward shift in ALOS? Let us also assume that an average target of 260 minutes for ALOS in the ED has been set, and that any noticeable upward deviations from this target value would be causes for concern and corrective action. To develop the CUSUM chart, these steps should be followed:

STEP 1: Determine the *SD* of the process.

If the dispersion in the sample data is measured by the *SD*, the process *SD* is approximated by the following formula:

$$\hat{\sigma} = \frac{\bar{s}}{c_4} \qquad [8.42]$$

where: $\hat{\sigma}$ is the estimate of the process *SD*,
$\bar{s}$ is the average of all sample *SD*s in the data set, and
c_4 is a factor obtained from Appendix 8.1.

If the range measures the dispersion in the sample data, the process *SD* is approximated by the following formula:

$$\hat{\sigma} = \frac{\overline{R}}{d_2} \quad [8.43]$$

where: $\hat{\sigma}$ is the estimate of the process *SD*,
$\overline{R}$ is the average of all sample ranges in the data set, and
d_2 is a factor obtained from Appendix 8.1.

In the example shown in Figure 8.17, the *MR* was used to measure dispersion (Table 8.3; see also Excel Video 8.8). Therefore, the estimate of the process *SD* is

$$\hat{\sigma} = \frac{\overline{MR}}{d_2}$$

The d_2 value when $n = 1$ is 1.128

This is the small change or shift mentioned earlier

$$= \frac{6.22}{1.128} = 5.51 \text{ minutes (rounded).}$$

STEP 2: Determine the allowable deviation from the target value, *k*. Typically, this value is 0.5 to 1 *SD*.

$k = 0.5 \times (5.51) = 2.755.$

TABLE 8.3 POSITIVE AND NEGATIVE CUMULATIVE DEVIATIONS

Month	ALOS	*MR*	*SP*	*SN*
1	256	–	0	–1.244
2	261	5	0	0
3	266	5	3.244	0
4	259	7	0	0
5	254	5	0	–3.244
6	255	1	0	–5.488
7	256	1	0	–6.732
8	269	13	6.244	0
9	255	14	0	–2.244
10	263	8	0.244	0
11	269	6	6.488	0
12	257	12	0.732	–0.244
13	259	2	0	0
14	267	8	4.244	0
15	261	6	2.488	0
16	254	7	0	–3.244
17	260	6	0	–0.488
18	271	11	8.244	0
19	268	3	13.488	0
20	270	2	20.732	0
21	263	7	20.976	0
22	271	8	29.220	0
23	276	5	42.464	0
24	275	1	54.708	0

Abbreviations: ALOS, average length of stay; *MR*, moving range; *SP*, cumulative sum on the positive side; *SN*, cumulative sum on the negative side.
Note: The computations of *SP* and *SN* were done in Excel with a lower level of rounding error than shown in Step 4.

STEP 3: Determine the UCL and LCL for the CUSUM chart, usually, ±4 *SD*s.

$UCL_{CUSUM} = +(4) \times (5.51) = 22.04$

$LCL_{CUSUM} = -(4) \times (5.51) = -22.04.$

STEP 4: Compute the CUSUMs on the positive side, *SP*, and on the negative side, *SN*, using the following formulas (see Box 8.6):

$$SP_i = \max[0, SP_{i-1} + X_i - \text{Target} - k] \quad [8.44]$$

$$SN_i = \min[0, SN_{i-1} + X_i - \text{Target} + k]. \quad [8.45]$$

In Period 1, SP_{i-1} and SN_{i-1} are equal to 0

In month 1 of the ED ALOS data set (Table 8.3),

$SP_1 = \max[0, 0 + X_1 - 260 - 2.755] = [0, 256 - 260 - 2.755] = [0, -6.755] = 0$

$SN_1 = \min[0, 0 + X_1 - 260 + 2.755] = [0, 256 - 260 + 2.755] = [0, -1.245] = -1.245.$

In month 2,

$SP_2 = \max[0, SP_1 + X_2 - 260 - 2.755] = [0, 0 + 261 - 260 - 2.755] = [0, -1.755] = 0$

$SN_2 = \min[0, SN_1 + X_2 - 260 + 2.755] = [0, -1.245 + 261 - 260 + 2.755] = [0, 2.510] = 0.$

In month 3,

$SP_3 = \max[0, SP_2 + X_3 - 260 - 2.755] = [0, 0 + 266 - 260 - 2.755] = [0, 3.245] = 3.245$

$SN_3 = \min[0, SN_2 + X_3 - 260 + 2.755] = [0, 0 + 266 - 260 + 2.755] = [0, 8.755] = 0.$

BOX 8.6 FAQs

The formulas for the positive and negative cumulative sums are quite convoluted. They don't make much sense to me.

A deviation is essentially the difference between a data point and the target value. Because we allow some "slack" or tolerate a small change, we incorporate *k* into the computations. A deviation of zero from the target value is ideal.

On the positive or high side, if the value of the data point exceeds the target value, the deviation is positive. Yet, a small shift, *k*, is allowed. Therefore, we subtract *k* from the deviation. If the result is positive (>0), it is added to the previous deviation, which explains the term *cumulative deviation.*

On the negative or low side, if the value of the data point is lower than that of the target, the deviation is negative. Again, we tolerate a small shift, *k*. We therefore add it to the negative deviation. If the result is still negative (<0), it is accumulated with the previous deviation.

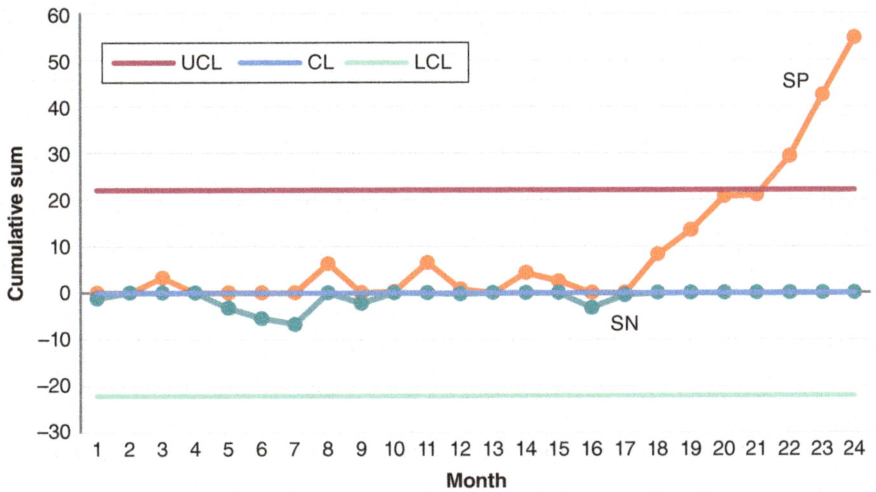

FIGURE 8.18 CUSUM chart.

Abbreviations: CL, centerline; CUSUM, cumulative sum; LCL, lower control limit; *SP*, cumulative sum on the positive side; *SN*, cumulative sum on the negative side; UCL, upper control limit.

EXCEL VIDEO 8.8

CUSUM Chart

Access the Excel video online by visiting www.springerpub.com/courseconnect. See inside front cover and tear-out card for CourseConnect details.

All *SP* and *SN* values are shown in Table 8.3.
STEP 5: Draw the centerline (it is 0), UCL, and LCL.
STEP 6: Plot the SP_i and SN_i values (Figure 8.18).
STEP 7: Determine whether the process is on target.

The process is not on target. The CUSUMs start increasing in month 18 and continue to do so until the CUSUMs on the positive side for months 22, 23, and 24 are outside the UCL.

At this point, you may think that once a process is in control, everything is fine, right? Not really! A process in control is not necessarily a "good" process in that it may not be capable of meeting established requirements.

BRIGHT ANGEL MEDICAL CENTER 8.9

Dr. Paul Tibbets, the chief medical officer (CMO), emailed Barbara asking for an update on what she and the quality team had uncovered. As the CMO and clinical sponsor for the ED improvement project, Dr. Tibbets felt accountable for ensuring the team was on the right track and had the resources they needed to be successful. Barbara emailed back and suggested they meet in person.

Dr. Tibbets welcomed Barbara into the conference room, noting that she looked a little fatigued. "Hana Aoki shared with me that you're all trying hard to find out why our length of stay keeps going up," he said.

"We are getting there," said Barbara. "We don't know yet the reasons for the sustained increase in ALOS over the past year. However, we noticed several issues that might delay treatment and disposition. They frequently run out of supplies in the exam rooms, and the nurses waste precious time retrieving them from the supply room. Another problem is the

(continued)

BRIGHT ANGEL MEDICAL CENTER 8.9 (*CONTINUED*)

ridiculously long lab turnaround times for simple CBC tests. They are so highly variable that I wonder what is going on at the lab. As for our door-to-doc times in the ED, the good news is that they are in control. The bad news is that they average more than 2 hours. No wonder that patients complain about wait times and leave without being seen! That being said, sometimes they leave when wait times are relatively short. Go figure!" Barbara smiled. "But there has been one improvement. We talked to Philip Robinson, and he agreed to let some of the high-usage drugs be stored in the ED. Too much time was wasted waiting for them to be delivered from central pharmacy."

"Well, that is good news," Dr. Tibbets exclaimed. "I hope this is just the beginning of our turnaround. I'm a little puzzled, though. If the door-to-doc times are in control, as you said, how badly are they off from what our patients really want and deserve?"

Barbara nodded. "That's a great question. We need to find out. I'll ask Olina to talk to Ali Hussein, our patient experience manager. He is quite involved in helping revamp the training for customer service and service recovery, but I'm sure he'll give us some insights into the door-to-doc time issue. He knows that all the parts of this project must come together in the end."

"There we go!" said Dr. Tibbets enthusiastically. "Let's get rolling."

Although average door-to-doc times were within the control limits and did not follow a particular pattern, they did not meet patients' expectations. Why not?

How would you explain that on some days, patients leave without being seen even though wait times are not particularly high?

PROCESS CAPABILITY

Process capability indicates the ability of a process to produce outputs within **specification or tolerance limits.** These limits are the boundaries within which process output values must fall to be considered acceptable. The lower specification limit (*LSL*) and upper specification limit (*USL*) may be imposed by the customer of the process, evidence-based guidelines, regulations, competition, and so on (Figure 8.19). They are *not* related to the control limits of the sampling distribution of a statistic or to the process variation (Figure 8.3). Only control limits and process variation are related because they depend on the variability of the process output from which samples are drawn.

If a process is out of control, it is too unpredictable to ever be capable of meeting preestablished requirements. In other words, being in control is a *necessary* but not *sufficient* condition for a process to be capable. Process capability involves the comparison of the natural variability of a process with the variation between specification limits (Stevenson & Kull, 2024).

Let us revisit BAMC's door-to-doc times (see $\overline{X}$ chart in section on $\overline{X}$ and R charts). The process was found to be in control with no signs of assignable or nonrandom variation. The $LCLX_{\overline{X}}$ and $UCLX_{\overline{X}}$ were equal to 92.58 minutes and 171.12 minutes, respectively. The samples were drawn from process output. The distribution of process output values is $\mu \pm 3\sigma$. The process *SD*, σ, is usually unknown, but it can be estimated (see equations 8.41 and 8.42). In the BAMC example,

$$\hat{\sigma} = \frac{\overline{R}}{d_2}$$

$$= \frac{68.06}{2.326} = 29.26 \text{ minutes.}$$

The LoLN allows us to assume that $\overline{\overline{X}}$ is a good approximation of μ. Therefore, an average door-to-doc time of 131.85 minutes will be considered as the average of the process distribution.

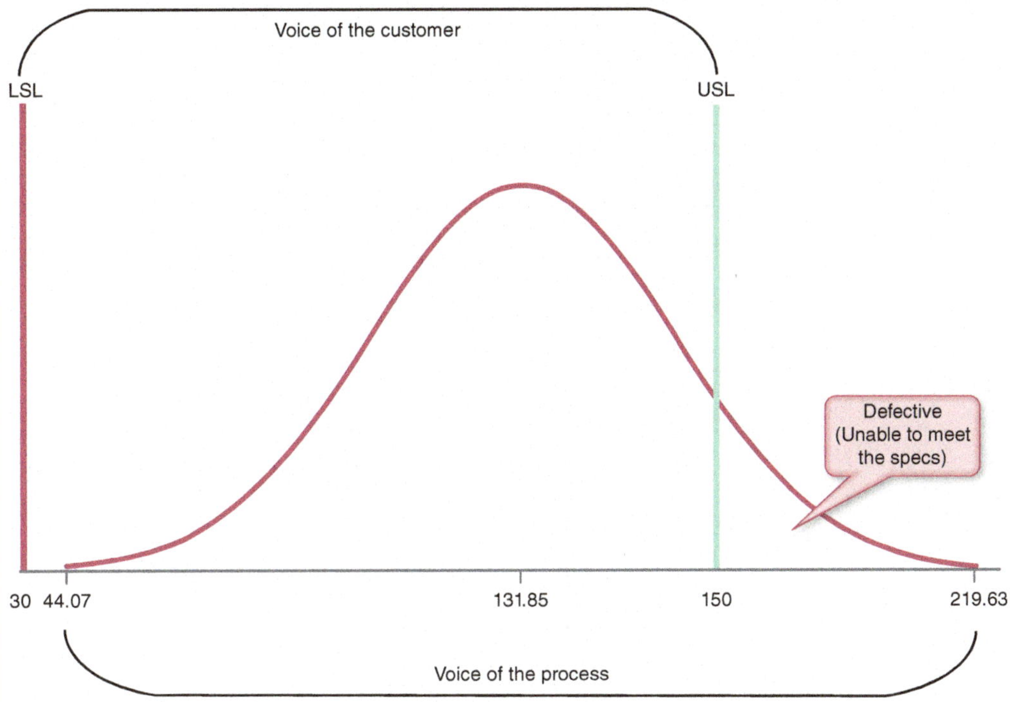

FIGURE 8.19 Process distribution and specification limits.

Abbreviations: LSL, lower specification limit; USL, upper specification limit.

What if surveys of low-acuity patients indicated that they would tolerate a time of 90 ± 60 minutes, but would leave the ED after spending 2.5 hours (150 minutes) before seeing a doctor? In that case, the process, which is in control, would not be capable of meeting patient requirements (Figure 8.19).

There are two reasons why a process that is in control may not be capable of meeting the specifications: (1) its natural distribution is too wide and/or (2) its distribution is not properly centered.

IS THE PROCESS DISTRIBUTION TOO WIDE?

Look at Figure 8.19. You can see that the natural or random variation in the process is too "spread out" to fit between the *LSL* and *USL*. You do not have to plot the distribution to determine whether a process distribution will fit within the band established by the *LSL* and *USL*. All you have to do is compute C_p, the **process capability ratio**, which compares the width of the process distribution with the width or range of the specifications:

$$C_p = \frac{VOC}{VOP}$$

$$= \frac{USL - LSL}{6\sigma} \qquad [8.46]$$

(Width of specs: $USL - LSL$; Width of process: 6σ)

In our BAMC example, the process capability ratio is:

$$C_p = \frac{150 - 30}{6 \times 29.26} = 0.68$$

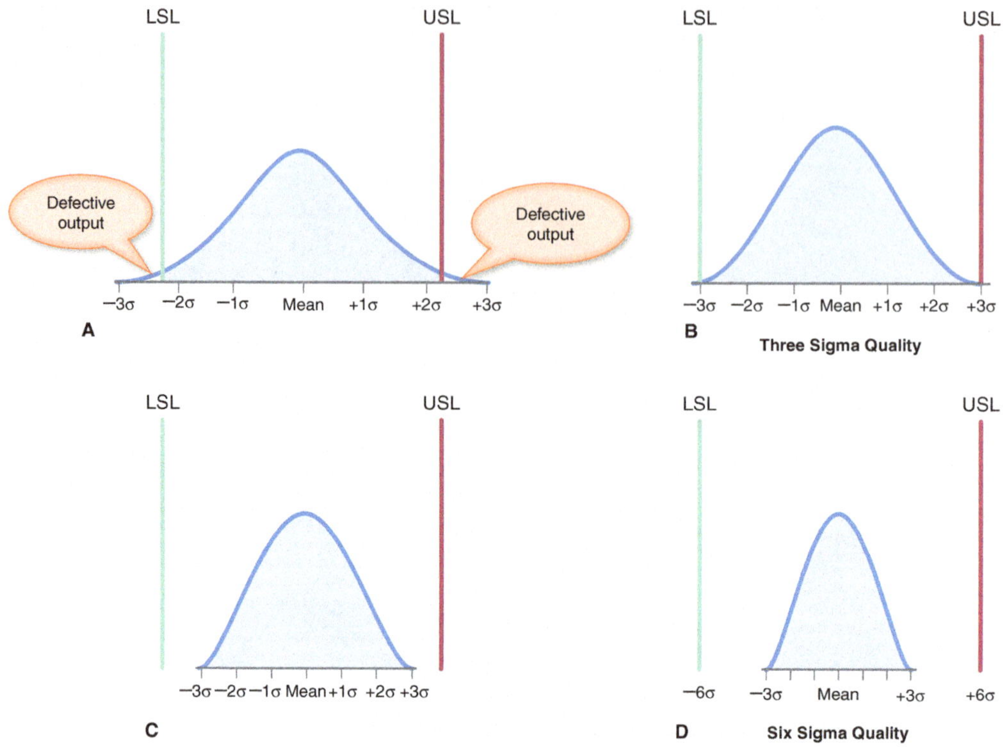

FIGURE 8.20 Process capability ratio scenarios.

Note: (A) Process variability exceeds the specification limits: *Cp* <1; (B) process variability corresponds to the specification limits: *Cp* = 1; (C) process variability is well within the specification limits: *Cp* ≥ 1.33; (D) the specification limits are six *SD*s away from process mean: *Cp* = 2.

Abbreviations: LSL, lower specification limit; USL, upper specification limit.

This value indicates that the denominator, or process variation, is larger than the tolerable range of specifications. The process, or random variation, is too large for the process to be capable. At a minimum, C_p should be equal to 1, which means that the width of the process and the range of the specifications are exactly the same (Figure 8.20[B]). The larger the C_p, the tighter the process distribution compared to the spread of the specification limits, and therefore the greater is the ability of the process to meet specifications. Table 8.4 and Figure 8.20 provide insights into the interpretation of C_p values. In all four scenarios depicted in Figure 8.20, the specification limits are identical *and* the process is perfectly centered; what changes is the process variability. When process variability is half the spread between the specification limits, that is, $C_p = 2$, the process is highly capable and extremely unlikely to produce defective output. It is associated with Six Sigma quality and 3.4 defects per million opportunities.

TABLE 8.4 INTERPRETATION OF C_p AND C_{pk} VALUES

C_p , C_{pk} Values*	Interpretation
<1	Process is not capable.
=1	Process is theoretically (but not practically) capable.
>1.33	Process is capable (good).
>2.0	Process is capable (excellent).

Note: * Unless the process mean is centered between the specification limits, C_{pk} will be smaller than C_p

IS THE PROCESS WELL CENTERED?

In our example, because the process distribution is too wide, it is obvious that the process is generating unacceptable output. However, sometimes, even if the process distribution is narrower than the range of the specification limits, the process may not be capable of meeting the specifications because it is poorly centered, that is, the process mean is not equidistant from the *LSL* and *USL*. In those cases, C_p may overstate the process capability (Figure 8.21). Note that sometimes the **target value** or desired value for the process output is simply a minimum or maximum (e.g., wait time < 40 minutes). In those cases, the process mean will likely not be centered between the specification limits, and C_{pk}, the **process capability index**, is preferable to C_p. Using BAMC's wait times data,

$$C_{pk} = \text{minimum}\left(\frac{USL - Process\ mean}{3\sigma}, \frac{Process\ mean - LSL}{3\sigma}\right) \tag{8.47}$$

$$= \text{minimum}\left(\frac{150-131.85}{(3\times 29.26)}, \frac{131.85-30}{(3\times 29.26)}\right)$$

$$= \text{minimum}\ (0.21, 1.16) = 0.21.$$

The larger the C_{pk} value, the better it is; our concern is about the ability of the lower of the two computed values to meet process capability criteria. Based on Table 8.4, the C_{pk} value of 0.21 is unacceptable. This value is associated with the first term, that is, $\frac{USL - \text{Process mean}}{3\sigma}$. It shows that the process mean is less than three *SD*s away from the *USL* and is therefore too close to it. Not only is our process distribution too wide, but it is also poorly centered, which was clearly depicted in Figure 8.19. You must have noticed that both C_p and C_{pk} are ratios with a numerator and a denominator. They are also indices because they are measures or signs of capability. In this chapter, we differentiated between the two by labeling C_p a ratio and C_{pk} an index.

A useful analogy to C_p and C_{pk} is driving your car into a garage (Figure 8.22). The garage door provides the specification limits. The car's width is the distribution of the process output. If the car is wider than the garage, it does not matter whether you have it centered or not; it will not fit at all (Figure 8.22A). If the car is only a little bit narrower than the garage, you must park it right in the middle of the garage, or it will not fit (Figure 8.22B); good luck opening the door! If the car is significantly smaller than the garage, there is plenty of room on either side, and it will fit whether or not you center it (Figure 8.22[C]). In a Six Sigma situation, think of the ease of parking one car in a two-car garage! C_p gives you the relationship between the size of the car and the size of the garage. C_{pk} tells you how far away from the middle of the garage you parked the car.

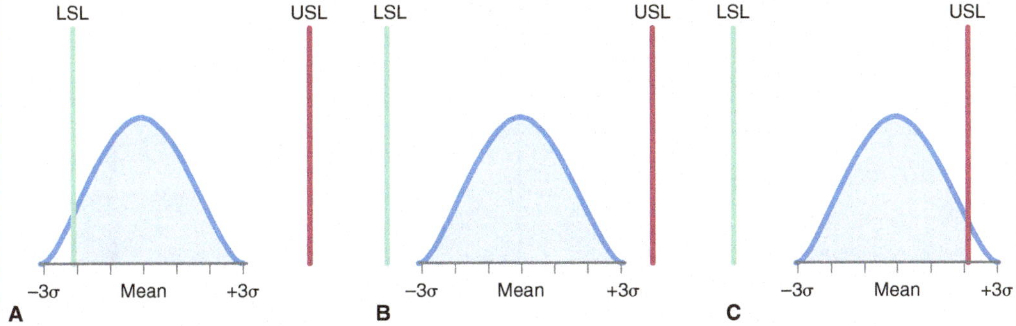

FIGURE 8.21 Process centering.

Note: (A) Process mean is too close to the LSL; (B) process is well centered; (C) process mean is too close to the USL.

Abbreviations: LSL, lower specification limit; USL, upper specification limit.

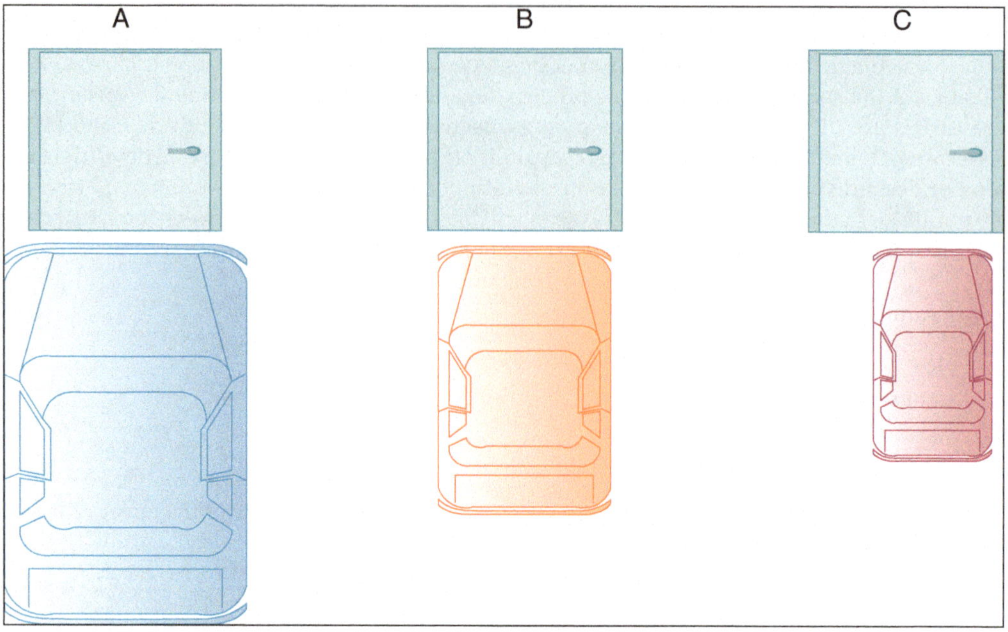

FIGURE 8.22 Process capability analogy. (A) Car is wider than the garage; (B) car is only a little bit narrower than the garage and must be perfectly centered; (C) car fits nicely within the garage and does not have to be centered.

Why is it so important for the process distribution to be much narrower than the range between the specification limits? Because things change! Over the long term, a process will usually shift by 1.5 *SD*s (Figure 8.23).

So, if the process is in control but incapable of meeting the specifications, what should be done? We are no longer talking about assignable causes of variation here. Instead, we are looking at the natural variation of the process and realize that it must change. This means that the process must be changed or redesigned, which is the topic of Chapters 10 and 11.

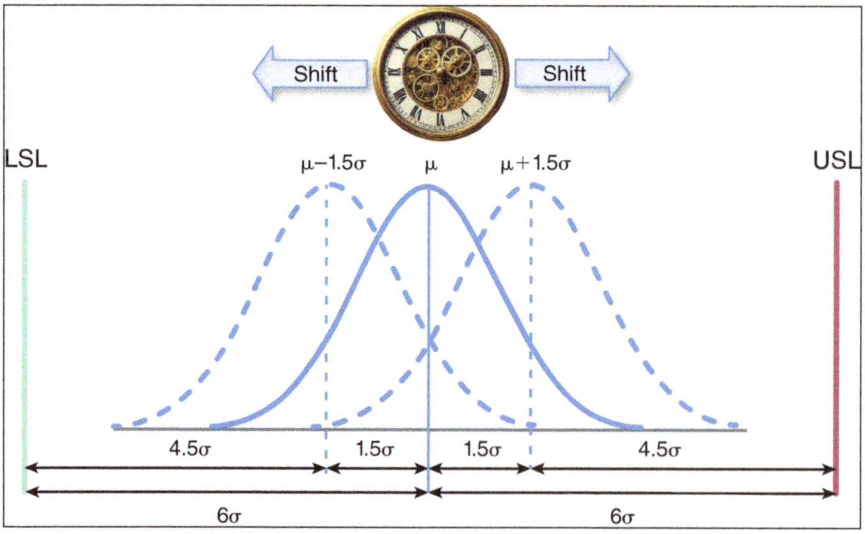

FIGURE 8.23 Shifts in performance over time.

Abbreviations: LSL, lower specification limit; USL, upper specification limit.

ETHICAL SCENARIO 8.1

"Quiet Quitting" and Output Variation

Following the COVID-19 pandemic, a workplace trend called "quiet quitting" occurred. Employees who followed this trend essentially decided they would just do the bare minimum to not get fired and simply do the very basic requirements of their jobs. They would not put forth any discretionary effort beyond the very minimal. This trend gained popularity as many people were reevaluating their priorities and putting less emphasis on the importance of work in their lives.

What type of variation in work output would you expect to see from those who ascribed to quiet quitting compared with others?

Are there strategies that leaders can employ (besides termination) to deal with employees who are doing the bare minimum?

What impact would this have on the morale of those who are giving their very best?

SUMMARY

In this chapter, you were introduced to the concept of variation: assignable or random. Processes must be stable and predictable. In order to monitor their behavior, we use a multitude of SPC charts. For attributes, common charts are *p*-, *np*-, *c*-, and *u*-charts. For variables, we use *IX* and *MR*, $\bar{X}$ and *R*, or $\bar{X}$ and *s*-charts, depending on the sample or subgroup size. If some of the process output values are not randomly distributed around the mean and/or are not within the control limits, the process is deemed out of control. This means that assignable causes of variation are present and, in most cases, need to be eliminated. However, even if a process is in control, it may be incapable of meeting target specifications. The process capability ratio and the process capability index help you determine whether the process is capable. If it is not capable, it needs to be redesigned (Chapters 10 and 11).

CERTIFICATION TIPS

Chapter 8 covers a great deal of material required for Green Belt Six Sigma certification. Nevertheless, a few concepts not considered paramount to a deep understanding of SPC and process capability in healthcare were omitted. They include:

- The operating characteristic (OC) curve, which displays information about the probability that a sample statistic will fall within the control limits: https://www.6sigma.us/six-sigma-in-focus/operating-characteristic-curve
- Median control charts which plot the median rather than the sample average: https://www.spcforexcel.com/knowledge/variable-control-charts/medians-individuals-control-chart
- Process performance indices that, unlike capability indices, focus on the short term. The formulas for P_p and P_{pk} are the same as those for C_p and C_{pk}, respectively, but a sample *SD* (*S*) is used rather than the process *SD* (σ): https://www.6sigma.us/process-improvement/ppk-process-performance-index

During the certification exam, be prepared to do computations and interpret your results. This chapter gives you ample opportunities to test your understanding of the material and apply it.

KEY TERMS

Process variation
Assignable/Special causes of variation
Common/Random causes of variation
Statistical process control (SPC)
Control charts
Subgroup
Control limits

Attributes
Variables
***p*-chart**
***np*-chart**
***c*-chart**
Area of opportunity
***u*-chart**
***IX* chart**
***MR* chart**
$\bar{X}$ chart
***R* chart**
***s*-chart**
Pattern test
Cumulative sum (CUSUM) chart
Process capability
Specification (or tolerance) limits
Process capability ratio, C_p
Target value
Process capability index, C_{pk}

REVIEW QUESTIONS

1. What are the two major causes of variation? Explain each one.
2. What is SPC? What is the purpose of control charts?
3. How do you determine whether a process is in control?
4. Differentiate between attributes and variables.
5. How do you know when to use a *p*-chart versus a *c*-chart? A *c*-chart versus a *u*-chart?
6. What are the differences and similarities between a *p*-chart and an *np*-chart?
7. When do you use *IX* and *MR* charts, $\bar{X}$ and *R* charts, and $\bar{X}$ and *s*-charts?
8. Distinguish between "sample size" and "number of samples taken." Use examples to illustrate your answer.
9. What are examples of patterns in a control chart?
10. What is a CUSUM chart? What is its purpose?
11. What is process capability? What is the purpose of C_p? What is the purpose of C_{pk}?

SOLVE BRIGHT ANGEL MEDICAL CENTER'S PROBLEMS

All chapter-specific data from the following problems are provided as Excel files which may be accessed via the show supplementary tab (Student Material) available online by visiting www.springerpub.com/courseconnect. See inside front cover and tear-out card for CourseConnect details.

1. At BAMC, door-to-doc times seemed to be in control (Figures 8.10 and 8.11). Does it mean that the situation is satisfactory? Explain why or why not.
2. Samples of 100 medication orders placed in the ED are checked each day against five potential types of errors. The following table shows the number of orders that were found to include errors during the past 16 days. Develop the appropriate control chart(s). Is the process in control? Why or why not?

Day	Number of Orders Containing Errors
1	4
2	12
3	8
4	14
5	0
6	8
7	16
8	6

Day	Number of Orders Containing Errors
9	10
10	2
11	12
12	14
13	8
14	6
15	8
16	6

(continued)

3. For each sample of 100 medication orders described in problem 2, the number of medication errors is also recorded. Develop the appropriate control chart(s). Is the process in control? Why or why not?

Day	Number of Errors
1	3
2	14
3	8
4	10
5	0
6	12
7	22
8	4

Day	Number of Errors
9	14
10	4
11	4
12	8
13	12
14	6
15	2
16	8

(continued)

4. The manager of a nursing home wants to keep track of the number of falls per 150 patients on a weekly basis. Data were recorded over a period of 20 weeks.
   a. Develop the appropriate chart(s).
   b. Is the process in control? Why or why not?
   c. Why do the LCLs appear to be closer to the CL than do the UCLs?

Week	Falls	Number of Patients at Nursing Home
1	7	217
2	4	210
3	6	156
4	2	182
5	3	165
6	8	179
7	2	182
8	6	160
9	6	150
10	6	142
11	4	144
12	7	120
13	1	132
14	5	88
15	6	132
16	3	112
17	4	110
18	1	115
19	5	138
20	5	105

5. One of the accountants at BAMC has tracked the monthly savings achieved from outsourcing transcription services to a new vendor over the past 2 years. The data are shown in the following table. Develop the appropriate chart(s) and determine whether the process is in control.

Month	Savings ($)	Month	Savings ($)
1	8,000	13	6,600
2	8,200	14	8,200
3	5,700	15	6,500
4	6,800	16	4,200
5	4,300	17	6,900
6	6,800	18	8,100
7	7,750	19	6,900
8	6,500	20	5,900
9	7,100	21	7,100
10	6,900	22	6,500
11	4,800	23	8,000
12	6,800	24	7,100

6. The head of the Surgery Department is concerned about the incidence of patient readmissions after being discharged from the hospital. In several cases, a patient had to be readmitted multiple times. The following data are available for the past 18 months. Develop the appropriate control chart and help the head of surgery determine whether the process involving readmissions per 500 discharges is stable. Based on your findings, does he have a reason to be concerned?

Month	Number of Discharges	Number of Readmissions
January	748	121
February	708	108
March	528	98
April	587	91
May	700	127
June	770	119
July	728	119
August	678	89
September	736	97
October	715	110
November	757	122
December	778	135
January	712	120
February	607	107
March	590	88
April	698	122
May	766	141
June	670	127

7. Dr. Giri wants to reduce the wait times in his office. Eight random observations of times spent between arrival and exam were made over a period of 20 days.
   a. Develop the appropriate chart(s) and determine whether the process is in control.
   b. If patient surveys indicate that they are willing to wait between 5 and 20 minutes before seeing Dr. Giri, is the process capable? Assume a process mean of 17 minutes and an *SD* of 1.5 minutes.

Day	1	2	3	4	5	6	7	8
1	13	19	18	15	18	18	16	15
2	13	19	19	15	19	17	17	16
3	15	16	16	20	18	16	17	16
4	16	18	15	17	18	14	17	20
5	18	18	15	15	18	16	17	18
6	16	17	20	19	15	17	19	16
7	19	18	16	16	16	15	16	19
8	15	16	16	16	19	16	18	16
9	16	15	17	17	17	18	16	17
10	16	17	17	17	17	18	14	16
11	19	20	19	16	17	16	16	19
12	15	17	18	17	16	17	17	16
13	16	18	18	18	18	18	17	17
14	16	17	16	19	20	16	17	16
15	16	18	16	18	14	18	19	16
16	17	18	16	15	17	17	20	16
17	19	18	15	16	14	16	18	16
18	18	18	17	17	17	15	17	15
19	19	17	17	19	17	17	17	16
20	16	17	16	16	18	17	20	20

8. You have been asked to determine whether the sound level at night is acceptable in cancer patient rooms. Using a digital sound–pressure-level meter, you collect data in 12 patient rooms, every night, for 21 days. Recommended sound levels are 27.5 ± 7.5 dB. Is the process in control? Why or why not? If the process mean and *SD* are 29 and 1.8 dB, respectively:
   a. Is the process capable of meeting recommended sound levels? Why or why not?
   b. Based on your answer in part (a), what actions should be taken?

Day	1	2	3	4	5	6	7	8	9	10	11	12
1	20.5	28.6	33.8	24.6	29.5	27.6	30.6	27.5	25.6	22.9	26.5	28.8
2	29.4	25.7	33	22.4	28	28.5	28.8	30.8	30.8	25.6	27.8	29.7
3	26.6	21.7	29.3	32.9	26.1	24.9	25.8	29.5	27.6	28.7	26.4	30
4	31.4	22.4	26	27.3	26.9	34.1	28.1	26.6	33.4	30.9	36.2	32
5	29.6	28.1	28.7	27.3	28.5	30.3	31.7	31	27.4	30.4	28.7	31.7
6	28.9	29.2	27	29.6	31.4	26.1	23.9	31.8	27.8	29.3	37.1	29.9
7	27.9	29.5	32.1	30.4	29.1	32.3	29.1	28.3	26	24.9	25.4	30.6
8	32.5	29.7	26.7	31.8	35.5	31.6	30.2	29	30.7	28.6	29.9	29.5
9	31.6	29.8	31.2	30.7	30.9	29.6	28.5	32.4	31.7	26.7	25.3	28.1
10	30.9	26.3	31.8	28.9	27.9	26.6	25.5	23.6	30.5	30.4	28.6	26.5
11	26.4	30.2	36.6	26.7	26.3	26.4	33.6	36.1	29.7	27.5	33.2	30.8
12	32	28.7	38.6	30.8	30.1	31.5	33	29.5	30.9	28.6	24.4	29.4
13	30.6	27.9	29.8	28.8	28.9	28.8	29.3	24.4	27.1	27	32.5	32.7
14	29.1	24.6	28.2	28.7	24.7	26.2	27.9	29.2	26	29.6	27.5	27
15	27.6	29.8	27.3	33.6	30.5	29	28.8	26.6	20.8	29.2	26.9	26.5
16	22.9	31.2	27.5	30.8	29	30.7	28.1	31.8	24.7	29.9	31.1	29.7

(continued)

Day	1	2	3	4	5	6	7	8	9	10	11	12
17	25.3	31.4	31.8	25.5	26.1	28.3	31.9	29.9	31.4	26.2	28.4	30.5
18	28	29.1	23.5	29.7	33.6	27.4	27.7	30.1	31.9	29	26.7	29.6
19	26.1	27.5	28.1	28.2	26	29.5	28.7	26.6	26.7	34	29.9	27.9
20	26.3	32.2	25.3	30.8	32.7	30.3	27.3	31.8	25.6	30.4	29.7	29
21	35.4	30.7	30.3	29.8	30.4	30.9	34.9	25.8	29.4	33	28.7	25.1

9. To reduce patient arrivals and wait times at the ED, BAMC has implemented a Nurse Hotline to give around-the-clock medical information and advice. A nurse can recommend if the patient must see a doctor, go to an urgent care clinic, or rush to the ED. Because of heavy call volume during certain times of the day, patients are often put on hold. Management has determined that a wait of 1 to 2 minutes is reasonable. Times on hold (in minutes) for samples of 10 callers over 20 days are shown in the following table.
   a. Develop the appropriate control chart(s).
   b. Is the process in control? Why or why not?
   c. If the process mean is 1.46 minutes with an *SD* of 0.17, is the process capable of meeting management's expectations?

	Callers									
Day	1	2	3	4	5	6	7	8	9	10
1	1.9	2.2	1.8	2	1.8	1.9	1.6	1.7	1.8	1.7
2	1.9	1	1.6	1.5	1.2	1.8	1.6	1.7	1.8	2.2
3	1.8	1.5	1.7	1.5	2.3	1.6	1.3	1.5	1.6	1.5
4	1.9	1.8	1.6	1.4	2.5	1.7	1.3	1.2	1.7	1.9
5	1.9	2.2	1.9	1.5	1.5	1.1	1.6	1.7	2	1.6
6	1.7	2.1	1.5	1.7	1.5	1.6	1.9	1.9	1.7	1.7
7	1.9	1.9	1.7	2	1.2	1.6	1.8	2.2	2.2	1.3
8	1.9	1.4	1.8	1.5	1.5	1.4	1.6	1.8	1.7	1.7
9	1.9	1.9	2	1.2	1.7	1.5	1.9	1	1.4	2.3
10	2.5	2.2	1.7	1.9	1.5	1.8	2.1	2.3	1.8	1.1
11	1.8	1.2	1.6	1.4	1.8	1.9	1.9	2	1.4	1.7
12	2.1	1.9	1.8	1.9	1.6	1.9	1.6	1.8	1.2	2.3
13	2.1	1.9	1.6	2.1	2.4	2	1.7	1.8	1.7	1.7
14	2.2	1.9	1.7	1.8	1.9	1.9	2.1	1.9	2.5	1.9
15	2	2	1.7	2.4	2.1	2.1	1.7	1.7	2.3	1.8
16	2.3	2.2	2	2.2	2	2	2	2.3	2	2
17	1.7	2.3	2.2	1.7	1.9	1.9	2.3	1.8	2.3	2.3
18	1.8	2.2	2	2.2	2.5	1.9	2.6	2.2	2	2
19	1.8	1.9	2.1	2.3	2.1	2.5	2.5	1.9	1.7	2.2
20	1.7	2.2	2.1	2.1	2.2	2.1	2.5	2.5	2.1	2.2

10. You are not sure whether a process is in control or not. You decide to do a pattern test. The values shown in the following table will help you develop the appropriate chart. Divide the chart into Zones A, B, and C and identify ALL patterns being displayed. Briefly explain each pattern and determine whether the process is in control or not.

−3 *SD*	−2 *SD*	−1 *SD*	CL	+1 *SD*	+2 *SD*	+3 *SD*	Sample Values
1	2	3	4	5	6	7	1.5
1	2	3	4	5	6	7	1.8

(continued)

−3 *SD*	−2 *SD*	−1 *SD*	CL	+1 *SD*	+2 *SD*	+3 *SD*	Sample Values
1	2	3	4	5	6	7	3.8
1	2	3	4	5	6	7	4.4
1	2	3	4	5	6	7	4.6
1	2	3	4	5	6	7	4.8
1	2	3	4	5	6	7	5
1	2	3	4	5	6	7	5.2
1	2	3	4	5	6	7	4
1	2	3	4	5	6	7	3.8
1	2	3	4	5	6	7	3.6
1	2	3	4	5	6	7	3.7
1	2	3	4	5	6	7	2.8
1	2	3	4	5	6	7	2.2
1	2	3	4	5	6	7	3
1	2	3	4	5	6	7	3.1
1	2	3	4	5	6	7	3.3
1	2	3	4	5	6	7	5
1	2	3	4	5	6	7	4.8

11. In problem 5, the accountant thinks that the transcription savings have been getting higher lately. Develop a CUSUM chart to determine whether there has been a shift in savings from a target value of $6,500. Use $k = 0.5$ *SD* and set the control limits at ±4 *SD*s from the centerline. Explain your findings.
12. Based on the following scenarios, determine the type of data (attribute vs. variable) involved and identify the appropriate control chart.

Type of Data	Scenario	Chart(s)
	In the patient surveys received by BAMC, the number of responses that are not in the "top boxes" is recorded.	
	Complaints about room cleanliness from 100 inpatients are recorded each day.	
	At a clinic, the number of no-shows (patients who had an appointment but failed to show up for it) is recorded each day.	
	Each day, the registration clerk of a clinic records the time at which a patient checks in and the time when they are called by the nurse to see the doctor. The difference between these two times is the wait time. The registration clerk reports the number of patients who had to wait more than 20 minutes.	
	Hospital staff records the number of Medicare patient rehospitalizations within 30 days following surgery.	
	Each week, the director of financial services determines the number of bills that contained errors.	
	Each week, the director of financial services reports the number of billing errors identified by her staff.	
	When billing Medicare outpatients, claims must be filed within 72 hours of service. Each week, a hospital administrator selects a sample of 20 late claims and records for each claim the time by which the 72-hour deadline was exceeded.	

(continued)

Type of Data	Scenario	Chart(s)
	To track financial performance, the CFO requests to see monthly revenue for the past 2 years.	
	A new hospital information system has just been implemented. This implementation required extensive training of the nursing staff. To assess the quality of the training program, the education specialist requests to see the daily log of calls (seeking assistance with the new system) to the information technology help desk. The number of staff interactions with the system varies daily.	
	To better assess the quality of the discharge process, the time it takes to explain discharge instructions to each patient is recorded. Each day, 7 discharge times are randomly sampled.	

13. Use the supplemental BAMC ED data set (LWBS and LWBT; ALOS) for May. The proportion of LWBS + LWBT patients relative to the total number of visits is provided for each day (Column Q). Construct the appropriate *p*-chart. Is the process in control? Why or why not? Hint: Convert percentages (LWBS + LWBT rate) to decimals.
14. Use the BAMC ED data set (CBC-Stats) for October. Filter the data to extract the tests for CBC-d (Column A). For tests ordered from October 10 to October 29, randomly select samples of four total lab turnaround times (Column J) *each day*. Using the 20 samples (one sample of four times each day), track sample means and conduct a pattern test. Is there any reason for concern? Hint: Use $\frac{1}{3} A_2 \bar{R}$ for the width of each zone.

LEARNING ACTIVITIES

1. Why do A_2 values decrease as sample size increases?
2. Explain how SPC benefits patients.
3. Formulate an SPC training plan (content and schedule) for new hires with no prior knowledge in the unit where you work.
4. Mock interview: one interviewer and one interviewee. The interviewee is Dr. Atul Gawande, the author of *The Checklist Manifesto*. The topic of the interview will be: How does process variation affect health outcomes and revenue? Hint: Research Dr. Gawande's biography before the interview.
5. SPC knowledge by itself is insufficient to bring about quality. Inability to apply this knowledge is a major obstacle to quality achievement and is the result of numerical illiteracy.

   > "Numerical illiteracy is not a failure with arithmetic, but it is instead a failure to know how to use the basic tools of arithmetic to understand data. Numerical illiteracy is not addressed by traditional courses in elementary or secondary schools, nor is it addressed in advanced courses in mathematics. This is why even highly educated individuals can be numerically illiterate" (Wheeler, 1993, vi).

   Explain why and how numerical illiteracy can be a serious problem in healthcare management. What can be done to overcome this obstacle?
6. From a statistical standpoint, why are CUSUM charts especially relevant for individual values?
7. What is an EWMA chart? What purpose does it serve?

REFERENCES

Baker, A. W., Ilies, J., Benneyan, J. C., Lokhnygina, Y., Foy, K. R., & Lewis, S. S. (2022). Early recognition and response to increases in surgical site infections using optimised statistical process control charts—The early 2RIS trial: A multicentre stepped wedge cluster randomised controlled trial. *eClinicalMedicine*, 54, 101698. https://doi.org/10.1016/j.eclinm.2022.101698

Imam, N., Spelman, T., Johnson, S. A., & Worth, L. J. (2019). Statistical process control charts for monitoring *Staphylococcus aureus* bloodstream infections in Australian health care facilities. *Quality Management in Health Care*, 28(1), 39–44. https://doi.org/10.1097/QMH.0000000000000201

Lighter, D. E., & Fair, D. C. (2004). *Quality management in health care* (2nd ed.). Jones & Bartlett Publishers.

Ransom, E. R., Joshi, M. S., Ransom, S. B., & Nash, D. B. (2022). *The healthcare quality book: Vision, strategy, and tools* (5th ed.). AUPHA/HAP Book.

Russell, R. S., & Taylor, B. W. (2023). *Operations and supply chain management* (11th ed.). Wiley.

Stevenson, W. J., & Kull, T. J. (2024). *Operations and supply chain management*. McGraw-Hill.

Wheeler, D. (1993). *Understanding variation: The key to managing chaos*. SPC Press.

FOR MORE ADVANCED CONTENT ON MEASUREMENT SYSTEM ANALYSIS, SEE ECHAPTER 15: GAGE REPEATABILITY AND REPRODUCIBILITY

eChapter 15 is available online by visiting www.springerpub.com/courseconnect. See inside front cover and tear-out card for CourseConnect details.

APPENDIX 8.1 FACTORS FOR CONTROL CHARTS

Sample Size (n)	Chart for Averages		Chart for SDs			Chart for Ranges		
	Factors for Control Limits		Factors for:			Factors for:		
			Centerline	Control Limits		Centerline	Control Limits	
	A_2	A_3	c_4	B_3	B_4	d_2	D_3	D_4
1	2.660	–	–	–	–	1.128	0	3.267
2	1.880	2.659	0.7979	0.000	3.267	1.128	0.000	3.267
3	1.023	1.954	0.8862	0.000	2.568	1.693	0.000	2.575
4	0.729	1.628	0.9213	0.000	2.266	2.059	0.000	2.282
5	0.577	1.427	0.9400	0.000	2.089	2.326	0.000	2.114
6	0.483	1.287	0.9515	0.030	1.970	2.534	0.000	2.004
7	0.419	1.182	0.9594	0.118	1.882	2.704	0.076	1.924
8	0.373	1.099	0.9650	0.185	1.815	2.847	0.136	1.864
9	0.337	1.032	0.9693	0.239	1.761	2.970	0.184	1.816
10	0.308	0.975	0.9727	0.284	1.716	3.078	0.223	1.777
11	0.285	0.927	0.9754	0.321	1.679	3.173	0.256	1.744
12	0.266	0.886	0.9776	0.354	1.646	3.258	0.283	1.717
13	0.249	0.850	0.9794	0.382	1.618	3.336	0.307	1.693
14	0.235	0.817	0.9810	0.406	1.594	3.407	0.328	1.672
15	0.223	0.789	0.9823	0.428	1.572	3.472	0.347	1.653
16	0.212	0.763	0.9835	0.448	1.552	3.532	0.363	1.637
17	0.203	0.739	0.9845	0.466	1.534	3.588	0.378	1.622
18	0.194	0.718	0.9854	0.482	1.518	3.640	0.391	1.609
19	0.187	0.698	0.9862	0.497	1.503	3.689	0.404	1.596
20	0.180	0.680	0.9869	0.510	1.490	3.735	0.415	1.585
21	0.173	0.663	0.9876	0.523	1.477	3.778	0.425	1.575
22	0.167	0.647	0.9882	0.534	1.466	3.819	0.435	1.565
23	0.162	0.633	0.9887	0.545	1.455	3.858	0.443	1.557
24	0.157	0.619	0.9892	0.555	1.445	3.895	0.452	1.548
25	0.153	0.606	0.9896	0.565	1.435	3.931	0.459	1.541
Over 25	$\frac{3}{\sqrt{n}}$	–		$1-\frac{3}{\sqrt{2n}}$	$1+\frac{3}{\sqrt{2n}}$			

PART IV

ANALYZE—Why Is There Waste in the Process?

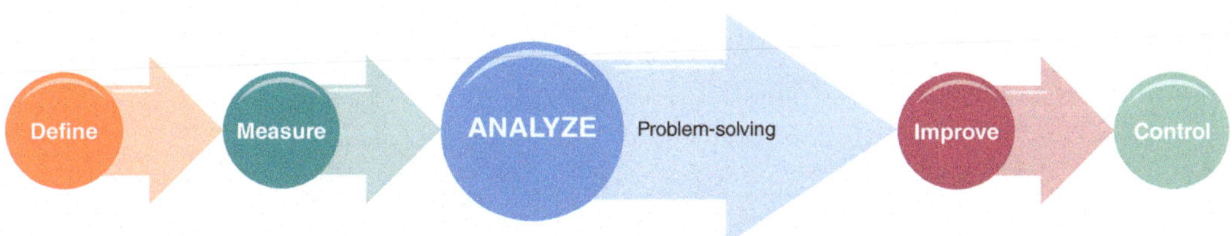

CHAPTER 9

PROBLEM-SOLVING

BRIGHT ANGEL MEDICAL CENTER 9.1

Adeleke sat at his desk, which was covered with tables and statistical process control (SPC) charts. After carefully reviewing all the information, he was convinced that all the possible reasons for a long ED length of stay (LOS) had to be investigated. "That is the whole ballgame," Adeleke whispered to himself. The patient complaint data mostly focused on the long amount of time spent in the ED waiting room. The backed up waiting room resulted in some patients leaving to seek care at other sites. Once in an exam room, the long ED LOS resulted in patients becoming frustrated at their perceived lack of attention. It was all starting to come together. Yet, he was unsettled by the ***gap analysis*** *produced by the team. Before sharing it with the leadership team, he wanted to discuss it with Barbara and Dr. Aoki. He scheduled a meeting for the next day.*

Barbara and Dr. Aoki were looking at the gap analysis report.

"What's this?" asked Barbara.

Adeleke replied, "It's a comparison between the actual and desired process performance. I don't want to sound pessimistic, but we may not be able to accomplish our objectives on time."

Dr. Aoki smiled. "Let's take a deep breath here. Let's uncover what is really causing these long LOS. Then, we'll have a better idea of what needs to be done and whether it is realistic."

Besides increased cost, what impact does inefficiency have on healthcare teams and patients?

LEARNING OBJECTIVES

After reading this chapter, you will be able to:

- Organize the ideas formulated during a team brainstorming session.
- Classify the primary causes of a problem into various categories and drill down to the root causes.
- Establish with confidence that a proposed "cause" is a real one and not a guess.
- Show the effect of causes on problems.
- Prioritize the causes that need immediate remedial action.

INTRODUCTION

Once you know what went wrong and to what extent, you need to find out *why* it went wrong. This is precisely the purpose of the *Analyze* phase of a Lean Six Sigma (LSS) project. It is important to remember that this is a team exercise that requires the collaboration of different individuals with different perspectives. In other words, it can be a messy and confrontational exercise because we all tend to blame others for mistakes. At this stage, the project manager must stress that the emphasis is on problem-solving and not on playing the "blame game." Creating a positive mindset, as opposed to finger pointing, will generate more valuable ideas and enthusiasm for identifying sources of dysfunction.

Several LSS tools can help you detect the root causes of the problems identified in the *Measure* phase. We invite you to see how these tools can be used together to explain how certain "ways of doing things" lead to errors, delays, and higher costs. Who suffers the most? The patients that you are trying to help.

WHY IS THIS MATERIAL USEFUL?

The tools presented in this chapter assist healthcare professionals to set the stage for targeted improvements. They help teams organize brainstorming sessions into meaningful themes, uncover and verify cause-and-effect relationships, and prioritize efforts for optimal effectiveness and efficiency.

BASIC TOOLS

The "seven basic quality tools" are shown in the text that follows because they require minimal training (Figure 9.1). You are already familiar with several of them. The flowchart was introduced in the *Define* phase; the check sheet, histogram, and control chart were presented in the *Measure* phase. The cause-and-effect diagram, scatter plot, and Pareto chart will be presented in this chapter. In addition to these simple tools, we include the **failure mode and effects analysis (FMEA)** tool, a proactive methodology designed to identify potential failure points in the process and assess the relative impact of these failures, because it complements some of the basic tools. We present the tools in a logical order of purpose:

1. organizing the team's thoughts
2. verifying the association between cause and effect
3. predicting the effects of causes
4. prioritizing the causes that contribute to the problem/waste

ORGANIZING THE TEAM'S THOUGHTS

CAUSE-AND-EFFECT DIAGRAM

Cause-and-effect diagrams, also called fishbone (see shape) or Ishikawa diagrams, are commonly used in **root cause analysis (RCA)**, a systematic search for the root causes of a problem. In the fishbone diagram, the quality problems are the "effects" of the causes and are depicted by the "head of the fish." The potential causes are represented by the "bones" and typically fall into six major categories:

1. **people:** the people involved in the process
2. **materials:** the raw materials, parts, and supplies needed to produce the good or provide the service
3. **methods:** the methods, approaches, practices, systems, and procedures used to perform the process
4. **measurement:** the data collected to assess process quality

5. **environment:** the nature of the surroundings (e.g., temperature, humidity, noise levels, and lighting) in which the process is performed
6. **equipment:** the machines, computers, tools, devices, and instruments used to perform the process

When developing a cause-and-effect diagram, all the individuals involved in various stages of the process should voice their opinions about the potential causes of a given problem. This plurality

Flowchart

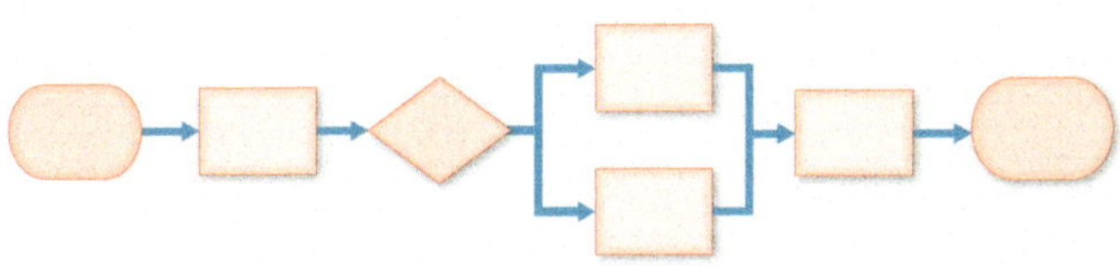

Graphic representation of process steps

Check sheet

Defect Type	Day					TOTAL
	Monday	Tuesday	Wednesday	Thursday	Friday	
A	///		///	///	//	11
B	/	//	//	//		7
C	~~////~~	///	//	////	/	15
D		/	///	//		6

Fact-finding tool to record problems and occurrences

Cause-and-effect diagram

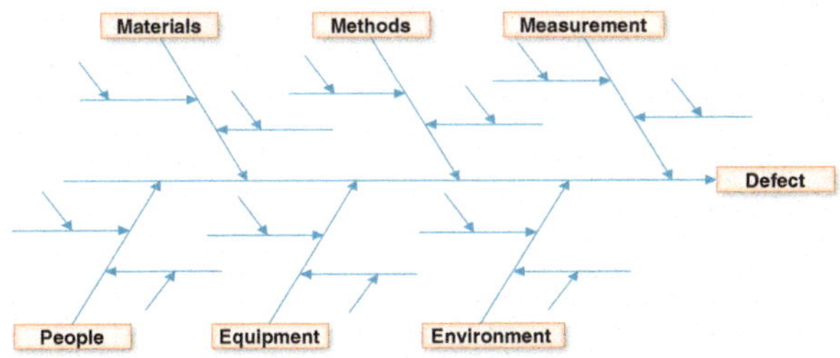

Diagram to identify and organize the potential causes of quality problems

Histogram

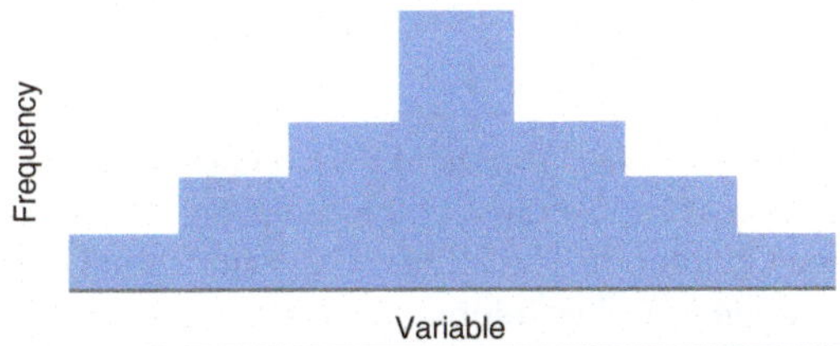

Chart to display frequency distributions

FIGURE 9.1 The seven basic quality tools.

(continued)

Pareto chart

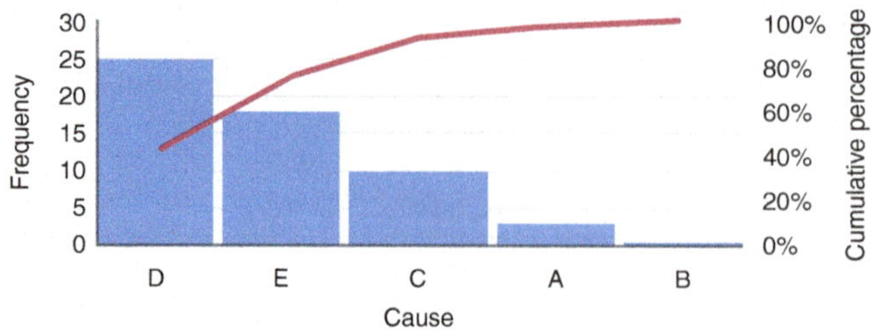

Chart displaying the frequencies of causes or problems in descending order to identify the most significant

Scatter diagram

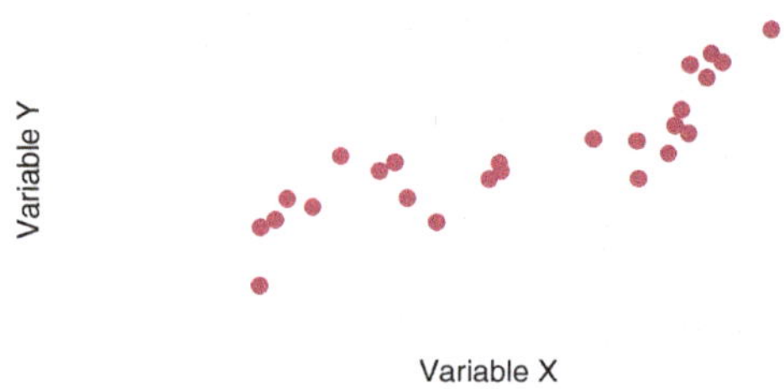

Diagram showing the type, strength, and direction of the relationship between two variables

Control chart

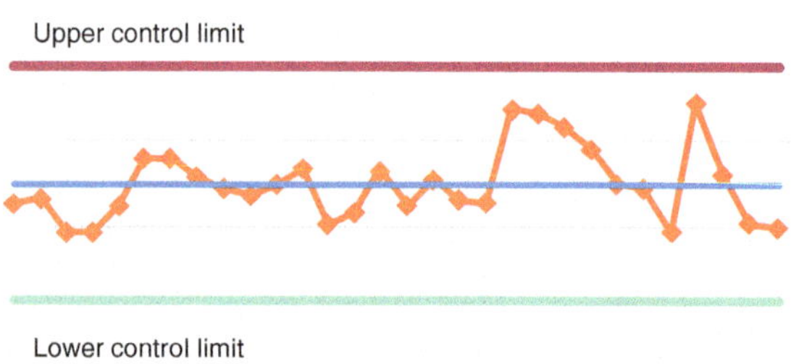

Chart depicting the behavior of a process over time

FIGURE 9.1 ***(continued)***

of opinions is instrumental in effective problem-solving. The development of the diagram involves multiple phases:

- Identify the problem clearly.
- List the causes that have the most influence on the problem.
- Brainstorm to identify the "causes of the causes," that is, the secondary branches on the diagram. Two useful supplemental tools that can be used at this stage are the affinity diagram (see Chapter 4) and the "5 Whys (see Chapter 2). The affinity diagram fosters creative thinking and facilitates the organization of ideas and opinions into logical groups. The 5 Whys is a Lean technique that drills down to the root causes. Why was the staff unfriendly? Because they are too busy. Why are they too busy? Because there is not enough capacity. Why is there insufficient capacity? Because of vaccination requirements and a labor shortage, and so forth.

BRIGHT ANGEL MEDICAL CENTER 9.2

Adeleke, Olina, and Dr. Aoki were reviewing the project team's findings about the potential reasons for long ED LOS (Exhibit 9.1).

Adeleke said: "As you can see on the fishbone diagram, one cause that keeps on surfacing is a layout that does not support our workflow."

EXHIBIT 9.1 CAUSE-AND-EFFECT OR FISHBONE DIAGRAM

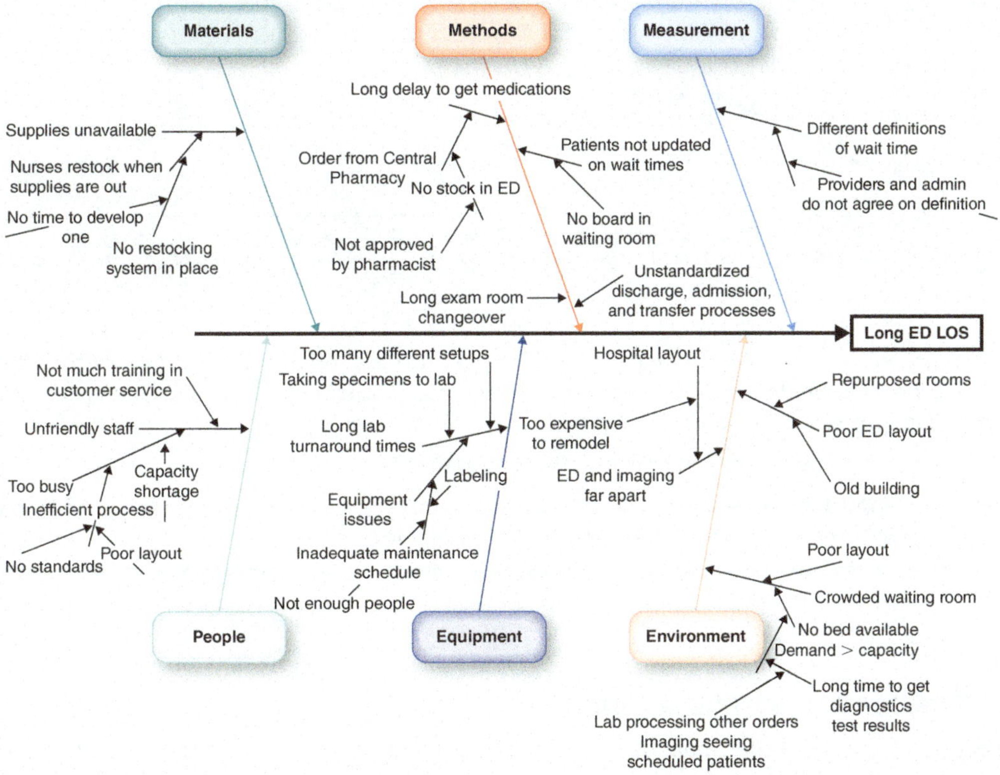

Dr. Aoki chuckled, "We have known that for a long time, but there is nothing we can do about it. So, what's next?" Olina suggested: "Look at this line chart (Exhibit 9.2) we had developed some time ago. The door-to-doc times were the longest between 5 and 10 p.m. That's also when both the LOS and left without being seen (LWBS) rates shoot up. Of course, we get more patients during that time. The outpatient clinics are closed, and the local urgent cares only stay open until 8, but is there anything else going on?"

Dr. Aoki pondered for a second and said: "At those times, we tend to get kids who were injured during sports practice. We also get patients who fell after a prolonged Happy Hour." They all laughed. Dr. Aoki added: "What's the common thread? More diagnostic tests!" Adeleke mumbled: "A double whammy on our capacity."

EXHIBIT 9.2 DOOR-TO-DOC TIMES THROUGHOUT THE DAY

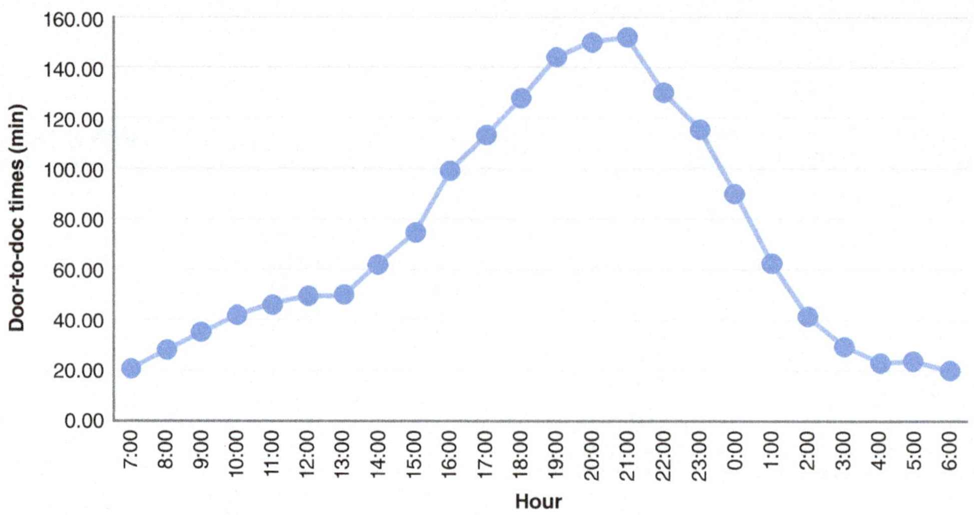

Olina urged caution. "We are making really good progress. Now, we should verify that the causes identified in the fishbone diagram have an actual impact on the long LOS. Adeleke, can your team get started on this? I'll help whenever you need me."

What are the benefits of using several tools together?

Why is it important to analyze the data prior to starting an improvement project? What can happen if reliable data are ignored or not available?

INTERRELATIONSHIP DIAGRAM

In Bright Angel Medical Center (BAMC) 9.2, Adeleke correctly says that the poor ED layout emerges multiple times as a cause for the long LOS. He is right. The multiple occurrences of causes suggest interrelationships. After creating an affinity or fishbone diagram, it is therefore a good practice to explore connections among causes. **Interrelationship diagrams (or diagraphs or digraphs)** depict the links among different aspects of a complex situation. In doing so, they help identify improvement areas that will have the greatest impact (American Society for Quality [ASQ], 2024). To develop an interrelationship diagram, consider the following steps.

STEP 1: Select the factors for possible relationships.

STEP 2: Place these factors on a wall or whiteboard in a circular shape.

STEP 3: For each factor, determine which other factors it influences and draw arrows to represent these relationships.

STEP 4: For each factor, write down the number of incoming and outgoing arrows.

STEP 5: The factors with mostly outgoing arrows are primary causes; the factors with mostly incoming arrows are the final effects of the causes.

In Figure 9.2, the factor with the largest number of outgoing arrows and no incoming arrow is the poor ED layout. This confirms Adeleke's suspicions. Another interesting fact is that contrary to expectations, insufficient exam room capacity is not a primary cause of long LOS; rather, it is the result of multiple inefficiencies in other areas!

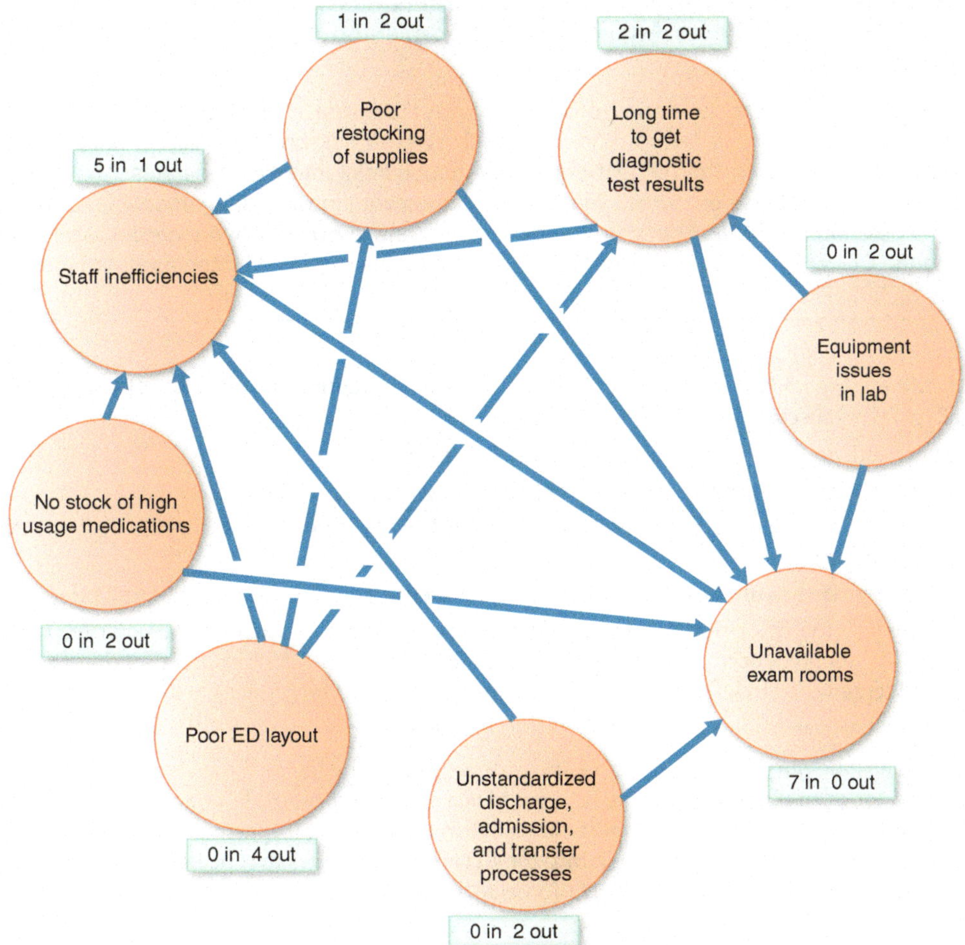

FIGURE 9.2 **Interrelationship diagram.**

FAILURE MODE AND EFFECTS ANALYSIS

The ultimate goal of FMEA is to prioritize the steps in the process that need fixing in order to prevent serious failures (e.g., adverse events) from occurring in the first place (Box 9.1). To maximize the chances of success, it is recommended that a subprocess rather than a very comprehensive process be chosen. For example, if the leaders at BAMC want to analyze the patient flow in the ED, tackling one subprocess at a time (e.g., imaging) would guarantee a more detailed description of the process steps and simplify the task of identifying failure points. Conducting FMEA requires the formation of a multidisciplinary team with all the process participants. This collaborative approach discourages the "blame game" and increases the likelihood that the proposed solutions will receive broad support. The team should accomplish the following (Institute for Healthcare Improvement, 2017):

1. Identify all steps of the process in a sequential manner. This is actually easier said than done. Even when a process is well defined and documented, there is a tendency for process participants to deviate from norms and perform steps that are unique to their way of working. For example, a nurse may call a colleague to help her with a computer problem, whereas another may call the help desk immediately.

BOX 9.1 QUALITY IN PRACTICE!

Failure Mode and Effects Analysis in ICU Admission of Potentially COVID-19 Infected Patients

A multidisciplinary team developed a flowchart of the admission process into the ICU. They identified all the potential failure modes at each step. A risk priority analysis helped them identify the modes with the highest impact on nosocomial infections: careless inquiries of epidemiological histories by nurses, inadequate implementation of management standards by nursing assistants, and exposure of attending physicians to potentially dangerous work environments. Corrective measures were proposed to improve clinical practice and management (Ye et al., 2024).

2. Identify all (big and small; likely and unlikely) potential failures at each step of the process as well as their causes: What could go wrong and why?
3. For each failure, rate the following on a scale of 1 to 10:
   a. Likelihood of occurrence (1: very unlikely to occur; 10: very likely to occur)
   b. Likelihood of detection (1: very unlikely it will NOT be detected; 10: very likely it will NOT be detected)
   c. Severity (1: very unlikely the harm will be severe; 10: very likely the harm will be severe)

   Compute the risk priority number (RPN) by multiplying all three ratings. For example, if the likelihood of occurrence for a failure point was rated at 5, its likelihood of detection at 6, and its severity at 4, the RPN for the failure mode would be $5 \times 6 \times 4 = 120$.
4. Select the best candidates for improvement. These are usually the ones with the highest RPNs.

Ultimately, the purpose is to improve the process so that the incidence of important failures is minimized, or even eliminated. Table 9.1 provides a simplified example of an FMEA. In this example, you can see that the unavailability of rooms in the Imaging Department, the need to retake images, and the exit and entrance back into the ED are major issues that need to be addressed.

A real-life use of FMEA in an organization is featured in Box 9.1.

ON THE JOB! INTERVIEW VIDEO 9.1

Stuart Carson
Performance Improvement Specialist

Prioritizing Areas Needing Improvement
Focus on quality metrics
Organizing projects across facilities
Pareto
FMEA: Reducing falls
Reconciling subjective and objective data

1. Stuart outlines one of the challenges in process improvement: a tremendous amount of data. Is having too much data detrimental? What are the downsides of having so much information?
2. How does Stuart's team use tools to determine where to focus their time and energy?
3. The third example shared during this interview was FMEA on falls. Subjectivity can skew the scoring on FMEA. Discuss the various ways that an employee's subject view or bias can alter the final RPN score.

The interview is available online by visiting www.springerpub.com/courseconnect. See inside front cover and tear-out card for CourseConnect details.

TABLE 9.1 FMEA FOR TRANSPORT OF PATIENT TO AND FROM IMAGING DEPARTMENT

Process Steps	Failure Modes	Proximate Causes	Effects	Severity (1–10)	Likelihood of Occurrence (1–10)	Likelihood of Detection (1–10)	Risk Priority Number
1. Request for transport is made	a. Request is not received	1. Request not sent 2. Request sent to wrong department 3. New staff did not know how to use the system	Patient's test and treatment are delayed	2	5	8	80
	b. Transport given wrong location of patient bed	1. Error in request 2. Confusion with another request	Transport goes back to Imaging without patient	2	3	7	42
	c. Patient is getting blood drawn	1. Requests for blood and imaging tests sent at the same time 2. Phlebotomist was delayed	Transport is delayed and falls behind on other requests	1	8	1	8
2. Patient is transported to Imaging Department	a. Exit from ED is challenging	1. Access blocked by arrival of patient in ambulance 2. Delay due to traffic to and from cardiac catheterization lab	Chaotic transport for injured patients	8	7	2	112
	b. Patient is dropped during transfer	1. Inexperienced staff 2. Patient becomes unstable and moves	Injury to patient	10	4	1	40

(continued)

TABLE 9.1 FMEA FOR TRANSPORT OF PATIENT TO AND FROM IMAGING DEPARTMENT (*CONTINUED*)

Process Steps	Failure Modes	Proximate Causes	Effects	Severity (1–10)	Likelihood of Occurrence (1–10)	Likelihood of Detection (1–10)	Risk Priority Number
3. Patient arrives at Imaging Department	a. No room available	1. Elective patients are scheduled for tests	Delay of test and treatment Prolonged pain	9	8	2	144
4. Images are obtained	a. Machine malfunctions	1. Maintenance issues 2. Inexperienced technician	Test is not performed	10	3	2	60
	b. Images have to be retaken because patient moved	1. Poor instructions given to patient 2. Patient unstable	Delayed treatment Condition worsens	9	6	3	162
5. Patient is transferred back to ED	a. Patient is dropped	1. Inexperienced staff 2. Patient becomes unstable and moves	Injury to patient	10	4	1	40
	b. Entrance into ED is challenging	1. Access blocked by arrival of patient in ambulance 2. Delay due to traffic to and from cardiac catheterization lab	Chaotic transport for injured patients	8	7	2	112
	c. Exam room occupied by another patient	1. Mistake by ED staff 2. No communication to ED staff that patient was coming back	Delayed treatment Transport falls behind on schedule	7	5	3	105
Total							905

VERIFYING ASSOCIATION BETWEEN POTENTIAL CAUSE AND EFFECT

SCATTER DIAGRAM

Scatter diagrams display the type, strength, and direction of the relationship between two variables. The independent variable is on the horizontal or x-axis, and the dependent variable is on the vertical or y-axis. Figure 9.3A displays the lack of relationship between the number of maintenance people available and the lab turnaround times, as indicated by the scattered points. The more scattered they are, the weaker the relationship. Figure 9.3B shows a negative, linear relationship between the number of stockouts and the bed turnover rate. The higher the number of stockouts in exam rooms, the lower the bed turnover rate. In Figure 9.3C, there is a positive, linear relationship between the door-to-doc time and the LWBS percentage. As the time elapsed before seeing the doctor increases, so does the LWBS. Figure 9.3D depicts a curvilinear relationship between the hourly visit rate and the ED LOS. As the number of visits per hour increases, the LOS grows at an increasing rate.

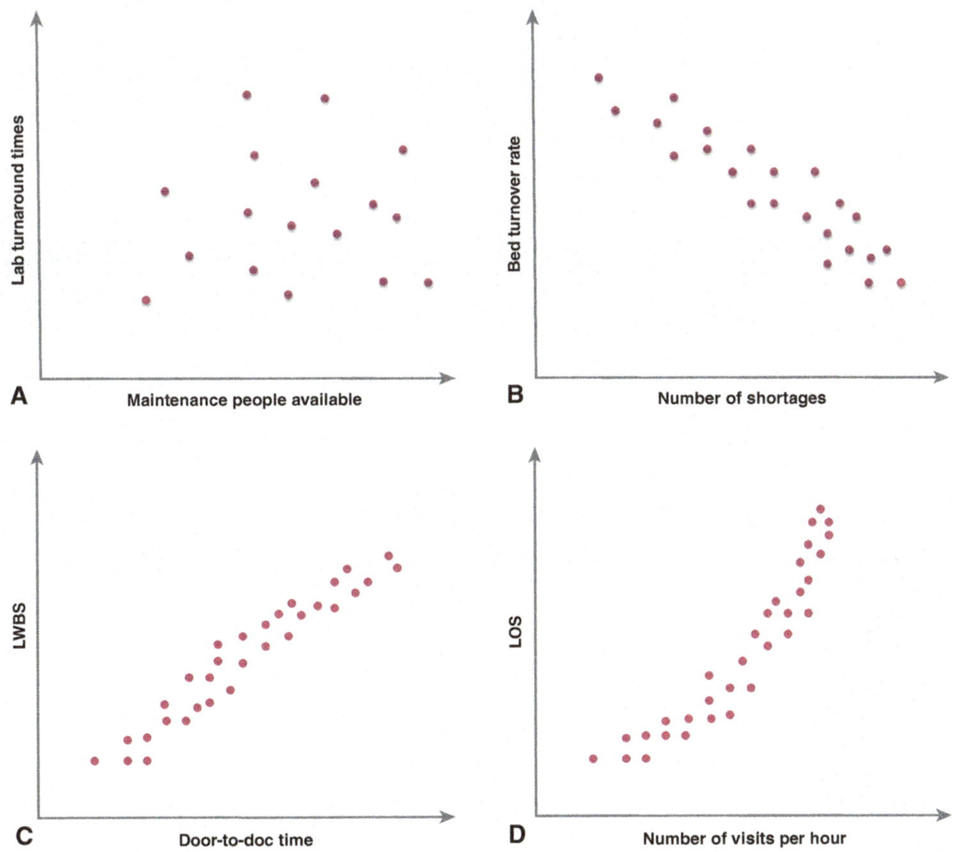

FIGURE 9.3 Scatter diagrams (see also Excel Video 9.1)

Note: (A) No relationship. (B) Negative, linear relationship. (C) Positive, linear relationship. (D) Positive curvilinear relationship.

Abbreviations: LOS, length of stay; LWBS, left without being seen.

EXCEL VIDEO 9.1

Scatter Diagram

Access the Excel video online by visiting www.springerpub.com/courseconnect. See inside front cover and tear-out card for CourseConnect details.

CORRELATION ANALYSIS

Scatter plots show whether a correlation exists. In statistics, a **correlation** is the degree to which two variables are linearly related. The **correlation coefficient**, r, expresses the strength and direction of the linear relationship between two variables, x and y, irrespective of their units of measurement. Its value is between –1 and 1, where –1 indicates a perfect negative relationship, and +1 indicates a perfect positive relationship. When r is equal to 0, there is no relationship between the two variables. For a sample,

$$r = \frac{\sum_{i=1}^{n}(x_i - \bar{x})(y_i - \bar{y})}{\sqrt{\sum_{i=1}^{n}(x_i - \bar{x})^2 \sum_{i=1}^{n}(y_i - \bar{y})^2}} \qquad [9.1]$$

where: x_i is the ith x data point,
y_i is the ith y data point,
n is the sample size,
$\bar{x}$ is the mean of the x values in the sample, and
$\bar{y}$ is the mean of the y values in the sample.

Using the door-to-doc time and LWBS percentage from the tactical dashboard (Table 4.7), the calculations to find the correlation coefficient measuring the relationship between the two variables are shown in Figure 9.4 (see also Excel Video 9.2):

B16 =CORREL(B2:B12,C2:C12)

Month	Door-to-doc time (min)	% LWBS	$x_i - \bar{x}$	$y_i - \bar{y}$	$(x_i - \bar{x})(y_i - \bar{y})$
Jan	75	2.2	-27.73	-1.95	54.07
Feb	80	2.3	-22.73	-1.85	42.05
Mar	81	2.6	-21.73	-1.55	33.68
Apr	94	3	-8.73	-1.15	10.04
May	95	3.6	-7.73	-0.55	4.25
Jun	100	3.7	-2.73	-0.45	1.23
Jul	112	4.1	9.27	-0.05	-0.46
Aug	110	6	7.27	1.85	13.45
Sep	120	5.5	17.27	1.35	23.31
Oct	128	6.2	25.27	2.05	51.80
Nov	135	6.4	32.27	2.25	72.61
Sum	1130	45.6			306.04
Mean	102.73	4.15			
r	0.947425504				

FIGURE 9.4 Calculations to find the correlation coefficient, *r*.

Abbreviation: LWBS, left without being seen.

EXCEL VIDEO 9.2

Correlation Coefficient

Access the Excel video online by visiting www.springerpub.com/courseconnect. See inside front cover and tear-out card for CourseConnect details.

$r = \frac{(306.04)}{\sqrt{(4018.18 \times 25.97)}} = 0.947$, which indicates a strong, positive relationship. The longer the door-to-doc time, the larger the percentage of patients who left without being seen at BAMC.

Of course, you can use Excel to compute the correlation coefficient. Just make sure that the two variables for which you want to compute a correlation coefficient are in adjacent columns and enter: = CORREL(array1, array2) where array1 is the column or row of x values and array2 is the column or row of y values. An important note: Correlation merely shows whether there is an association between two variables; it does not prove cause and effect.

BRIGHT ANGEL MEDICAL CENTER 9.3

It had been another long, but fruitful day. Dr. Aoki, Olina, and Adeleke were eating pizza in the staff lounge. Adeleke started, "We have some clarity now. The layout is problematic and even dangerous for patients transported to Imaging. Once they reach the Imaging Department, there is often no room available for them. I'm not sure why they have to redo the tests on a regular basis either. We need to follow up on that. And frankly, they should let us know when they are bringing a patient back. Who is running that place?"

Olina smiled. "Let's not blame them ... they will be quick to tell us that our own deficiencies delay the transports and put them behind schedule. Talking about deficiencies, I noticed that running out of stock in the exam rooms contributes to congestion as well. That's our responsibility. What about lab turnaround times?"

Adeleke sighed, "Strangely enough, there is no clear association between them and LOS. The complete blood count (CBC) test turnaround times are as erratic as can be. My hunch is that they have equipment issues at random times, but the high variability complicates our analyses. I'll check with the lab."

Dr. Aoki said, "In a nutshell, what contributes to the long LOS? Layout in general, stockouts, transport time of patients to Imaging and no room available there. And of course, the larger the number of visits, the more patients we send to Imaging! Let's order another pizza. I need some comfort food."

Besides asking the staff to work faster, what can be done to improve the efficiency of the process? Is it a good idea to assume that the problem is a lack of motivated people?

PREDICTING THE EFFECT OF THE CAUSE ON THE PROBLEM

REGRESSION ANALYSIS

Let's go back to the association between door-to-doc times and LWBS identified in the previous section. According to the scatterplot, the linear association was strong and positive. This was confirmed by a correlation coefficient equal to 0.947. **Linear regression analysis** builds on this concept, but rather than simply expressing the strength of the relationship between two variables, it shows the effect that the **independent variable** has over the **dependent variable**. The independent variable is the predictor, whereas the dependent variable is the outcome. Specifically, regression analysis produces an equation that indicates the effect that a one-unit change in the independent variable has on the dependent variable.

Regression models are very popular predictive techniques. Their use may be motivated by a desire to identify the strongest predictors of an outcome, to test hypotheses about the relationships between the predictors and the outcome, or to predict an outcome value based on specific predictor values.

SIMPLE LINEAR REGRESSION

Simple linear regression is a statistical technique that helps us study the linear relationship between *one* predictor and one outcome variable. When a one-unit change in the predictor variable is assumed to produce the same change in the outcome variable, the relationship is linear, and the model is called simple linear regression. The simple linear regression model is expressed as follows:

$$y = \beta_0 + \beta_1 x + \varepsilon \qquad [9.2]$$

where y = value of the dependent variable;

β_0 = population parameter referred to as ***y*-intercept** or value of y when $x = 0$;

β_1 = population parameter referred to as **regression coefficient (slope)**, or change in the value of y for a one-unit change in x;

x = value of the independent variable; and

ε = error term or variation in y that cannot be explained by the linear regression model. (For each value of x, the expected value of y is $\beta_0 + \beta_1 x$. The difference between that expected value and the actual y is ε.)

In reality, we do not know the population parameters and have to estimate them using sample data. The estimated regression equation is:

$$\hat{y} = a + b_1 x \qquad [9.3]$$

where $\hat{y}$ is the estimated value of the dependent variable, a is the estimated y-intercept, and b_1 is the estimated regression coefficient.

a and b can be computed using the following formulas:

$$a = \bar{y} - b\bar{x} \qquad [9.4]$$

$$b = \frac{\sum xy - n\bar{x}\bar{y}}{\sum x^2 - n\bar{x}^2} \qquad [9.5]$$

where $\bar{y}$ is the average of the y values,

$\bar{x}$ is the average of the x values, and

n is the number of data points used to compute b.

Let's reuse the data from Figure 9.4 to illustrate (Figure 9.5; see also Excel Video 9.3).

EXCEL VIDEO 9.3

Simple Linear Regression

Access the Excel video online by visiting www.springerpub.com/courseconnect. See inside front cover and tear-out card for CourseConnect details.

$b = \dfrac{4{,}990.4 - (11 \times 4.15 \times 102.73)}{120{,}100 - \left(11 \times 102.73^2\right)} = 0.076$ – For each extra minute of door-to-doc time, the % LWBS goes up by 0.076.

$a = 4.15 - (0.076 \times 102.73) = -3.66$ (rounding)—The line crosses the y-axis at -3.66.

	Month	Door-to-doc time (min)	% LWBS	xy	x^2
2	Jan	75	2.2	165.00	5625
3	Feb	80	2.3	184.00	6400
4	Mar	81	2.6	210.60	6561
5	Apr	94	3	282.00	8836
6	May	95	3.6	342.00	9025
7	Jun	100	3.7	370.00	10000
8	Jul	112	4.1	459.20	12544
9	Aug	110	6	660.00	12100
10	Sep	120	5.5	660.00	14400
11	Oct	128	6.2	793.60	16384
12	Nov	135	6.4	864.00	18225
13					
14	Sum	1130	45.6	4990.4	120100
15	Mean	102.73	4.15		

FIGURE 9.5 Calculations to find the regression equation.

Abbreviation: LWBS, left without being seen.

The equation of the line fitting the data is $\hat{y} = -3.66 + 0.076x$.

If the door-to-doc time, x, is 90 min, we predict that the % LWBS is $-3.66 + (0.076 \times 90) = 3.18\%$.

Because the relationship is linear, it can be represented by a line. Like correlation, simple regression quantifies a relationship between two metric variables. Here, the relationship is expressed by an equation which estimates the line that best fits the data. What do we mean by "best fit"? We mean the line that minimizes all the squared deviations (or errors) between the actual values of y and those estimated by the regression equation. For example, if the door-to-doc time is 94 min, the error is $e_{94} = y_{94} - \hat{y}_{94} = -0.46$ (Figure 9.6). This is why the approach used to find the regression equation from sample data is called the **least squares method**. In Figure 9.6, we used the Excel Trendline tool to find the regression equation. R^2, the **coefficient of determination**, is 0.8976. It expresses the proportion of variance in the dependent variable explained by the regression model. In our case, 89.76% of the variation in % LWBS is explained by door-to-doc time. This is a high number, thereby indicating a good fit. Remember that r, the correlation coefficient, was 0.947. As you may have guessed, $(0.947)^2 = 0.8976$. The Excel regression output is displayed in Figure 9.7.

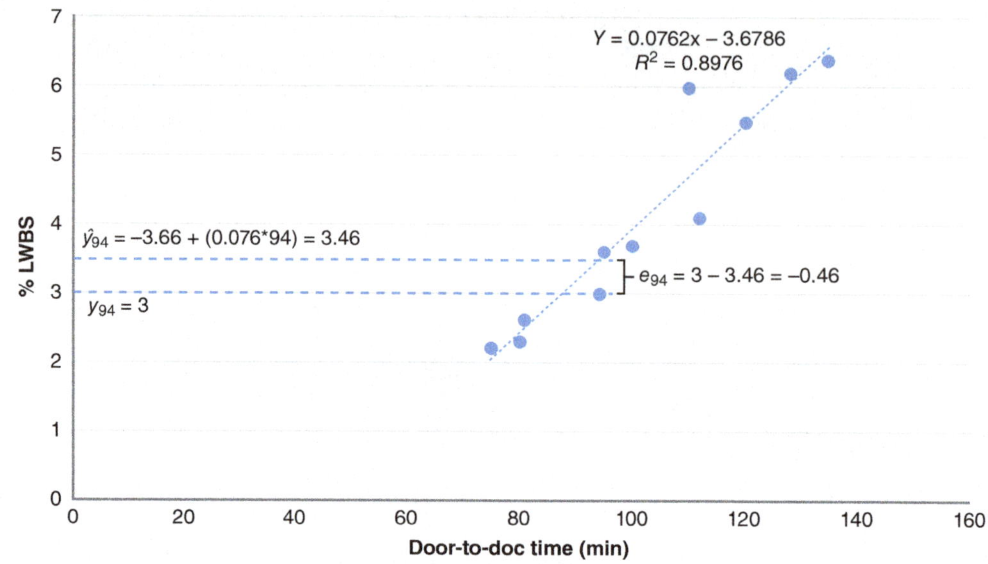

FIGURE 9.6 Regression of LWBS percentage on door-to-doc time.

Abbreviation: LWBS, left without being seen.

SUMMARY OUTPUT

Regression Statistics	
Multiple R	0.9474255
R Square	0.8976151
Adjusted R Square	0.886239
Standard Error	0.543513
Observations	11

ANOVA

	df	*SS*	*MS*	*F*	*Significance F*
Regression	1	23.30861571	23.30862	78.90357	9.50353E-06
Residual	9	2.658657014	0.295406		
Total	10	25.96727273			

	Coefficients	*Standard Error*	*t Stat*	*P-value*	*Lower 95%*	*Upper 95%*	*Lower 95.0%*	*Upper 95.0%*
Intercept	-3.678552	0.895922145	-4.10588	0.002653	-5.705268733	-1.6518353	-5.70526873	-1.65183534
Door-to-doc time (min)	0.0761629	0.00857423	8.882768	9.5E-06	0.056766641	0.0955592	0.05676664	0.095559151

FIGURE 9.7 Excel output of simple regression of LWBS percentage on door-to-doc time.

Abbreviation: LWBS, left without being seen.

Another way to assess the predictive power of our independent variable is to test the hypothesis that the regression coefficient is equal to 0:

H_0: $\beta_1 = 0$

H_A: $\beta_1 \neq 0$

Rejecting the null hypothesis would indicate that the regression coefficient is statistically significant and that, by extension, the predictor variable explains the variation in the outcome variable. To test this hypothesis, we conduct a *t* test.

The *t* statistic is computed as follows:

$$t = \frac{b_1 - 0}{SE} \quad [9.6]$$

$$= \frac{0.076 - 0}{0.0086} = 8.84 \text{ (rounding)}$$

In the output, the *t* statistic value is 8.88 (smaller rounding error), and the *p* value is 0.0000095, which is well below the usual threshold of 0.05 for significance. The ***p* value** is the probability that the null hypothesis, H_0, would be true given our data set. It is essentially the level of statistical significance for a given hypothesis test. Our *p* value indicates that this likelihood is extremely low. Therefore, we conclude that the slope, β_1, is significantly different from 0, and we reject the null hypothesis.

Analysis of variance (ANOVA) is a statistical procedure that tests the overall fit of a linear model using an *F*-ratio (Field, 2013). In simple regression, the test involves determining whether the regression coefficient is significantly different from 0. However, the *F* rather than the *t* statistic is used. The *F*-statistic value is 78.90 with a significance level of 0.0000095, which is exactly the same as for the *t* test (Figure 9.7).

MULTIPLE REGRESSION

Multiple linear regression is an extension of simple linear regression, but as its name indicates, the relationship is between multiple independent variables and the dependent variable. The multiple regression model is expressed as:

$$y = \beta_0 + \beta_1 x_1 + \beta_2 x_2 + \cdots + \beta_n x_n + \varepsilon \quad [9.7]$$

where y = dependent variable,

β_0 = intercept in regression equation,

β_1 through β_n = regression coefficients for the independent variables,

x_1 through x_n = independent variables, and

ε = error term.

The regression equation estimated from sample data is:

$$\hat{y} = b_0 + b_1 x_1 + b_2 x_2 + \cdots + b_n x_n \quad [9.8]$$

Based on the data shown in Figure 9.8 (see also Excel Video 9.4), a potential two-predictor regression model would be:

Average length of stay (ALOS) for discharged patients = $b_0 + b_1$ number of patients sent to Imaging (x_1) + b_2 average lab turnaround times (x_2).

EXCEL VIDEO 9.4

Multiple Regression

Access the Excel video online by visiting www.springerpub.com/courseconnect. See inside front cover and tear-out card for CourseConnect details.

Figure 9.9 shows the Excel output of the multiple regression analysis. The overall model fit is determined by R^2, the multiple *R*, and the ANOVA test. R^2 still indicates the percentage of variation in the dependent variable explained by the whole regression model. The **adjusted R^2** corrects the R^2 value for the number of predictors in the model and is always lower than R^2. Whereas R^2 will always increase when you add new independent variables to the model, whether or not they are significant predictors, the adjusted R^2 only increases if a new independent variable improves

	A	B	C	D
1	Month	Number of patients sent to imaging	Avge lab turnaround time for CBC (min)	ALOS for discharged patients (min)
2	Jan	823	20.2	155
3	Feb	853	25.3	185
4	Mar	928	19.7	257
5	Apr	875	18.3	265
6	May	942	10.2	285
7	Jun	925	24.6	275
8	Jul	920	23.1	285
9	Aug	997	16.5	330
10	Sep	990	20.3	325
11	Oct	1050	12.1	345
12	Nov	1152	29.8	385
13				

FIGURE 9.8 Data for multiple regression model.

Abbreviations: ALOS, average length of stay; CBC, complete blood count.

SUMMARY OUTPUT

Regression Statistics	
Multiple R	0.938451964
R Square	0.880692089
Adjusted R Square	0.850865111
Standard Error	25.97498401
Observations	11

ANOVA

	df	*SS*	*MS*	*F*	*Significance F*
Regression	2	39843.31074	19921.65537	29.52669549	0.000202618
Residual	8	5397.598353	674.6997941		
Total	10	45240.90909			

	Coefficients	*Standard Error*	*t Stat*	*P-value*	*Lower 95%*	*Upper 95%*
Intercept	-328.112335	86.25281559	-3.804076804	0.005206346	-527.0116845	-129.213
Number of patients sent to imaging	0.67540311	0.088023026	7.673027616	5.88942E-05	0.472421648	0.878385
Avge lab turnaround time for CBC (min)	-1.636091935	1.43897494	-1.136984314	0.288451861	-4.954374098	1.68219

FIGURE 9.9 Excel output of regression of ALOS on number of patients sent to radiology and lab turnaround times for CBC test results.

Abbreviations: ALOS, average length of stay; CBC, complete blood count.

the model fit more than expected by chance alone. The **multiple *R*** is the correlation coefficient between the dependent variable and the set of independent variables.

The R^2 value of 0.88 indicates that the number of patients sent to Imaging and the average lab turnaround times explain 88% of the variance in ALOS for discharged patients.

The hypothesis test for the significance of the overall regression model is:

H_0: $\beta_1 = \beta_2 = 0$

H_A: at least one of the β_i is not equal to 0.

The appropriate test statistic is the *F* test, as shown in the ANOVA output. The *F*-statistic is equal to 29.53, and its significance level is 0.0002, indicating that the model is highly significant.

However, if we look at the individual regression coefficients, we can see that for b_2, which is equal to −1.64, the *t* statistic is equal to −1.14 and is not significant given a *p* value of 0.29, well above the 0.05 threshold (Box 9.2). Why is the *F*-statistic still significant? Because the alternative hypothesis simply stated that *at least one* of the regression coefficients had to be different from 0. Let's use the model now! If 900 patients are sent to Imaging and the turnaround time for their CBC test is 20 minutes, what is the ALOS? The answer is:

$$\text{ALOS} = -328.11 + (0.68 \times 900) + (-1.64 \times 20) = 251.09 \text{ min.}$$

BOX 9.2 FAQs

Why is there a 0.05 threshold for significance? What is so particular about this number?

Because Sir Ronald Fisher, the father of modern statistics, liked it! He said: "If 1 in 20 does not seem high enough odds, we may, if we prefer it, draw the line at one in fifty (the 2% point), or one in a hundred (the 1% point). Personally, the writer prefers to set a low standard of significance at the 5% point, and ignore entirely all results which fail to reach this level. A scientific fact should be regarded as experimentally established only if a properly designed experiment rarely fails to give this level of significance" (Fisher, 1926, p. 85).

PRIORITIZING CAUSES

The list of causes for long ED LOS (Exhibit 9.1) is rather long. Verifying the association between causes and effects is a good way to cull irrelevant causes. Yet, the remaining list may still be long. Because of limited time and resources, it is imperative to uncover the few factors that have the strongest influence on the problem. This is accomplished with the development of a Pareto chart.

PARETO CHART

Pareto charts get their name from Vilfredo Pareto, the Italian engineer and economist who observed that 20% of the population owned 80% of the wealth in Italy at the end of the 19th century. This 80/20 rule was later extended to quality management. It means that 80% of the effects come from 20% of the causes. In other words, there are very few (≈20%) causes that account for the majority (≈80%) of a problem's occurrences. The Pareto chart is used to identify these "vital few" causes and, therefore, facilitate prioritization. It can also be used to uncover the most pressing problem areas. In order to construct a Pareto chart, the following steps need to be followed:

1. Determine the problem's frequency of occurrence (Table 9.2; see also Excel Video 9.5) resulting from the most influential causes. This is similar to the check sheet discussed in Chapter 6.

EXCEL VIDEO 9.5

Pareto Chart

Access the Excel video online by visiting www.springerpub.com/courseconnect. See inside front cover and tear-out card for CourseConnect details.

2. Sort the causes so that their contributions to the problem's frequency of occurrence are in descending order (Table 9.3).
3. Compute the relative importance (percentages) of each cause as a contributing factor to the problem (Table 9.3).
4. Compute the cumulative percentages (Table 9.3).
5. Develop the Pareto chart. It is a bar graph that displays the absolute or relative frequencies of occurrence and a line graph that represents the cumulative percentage. The line/curve usually has a steep incline reflecting that there are usually only a few strong influences on the problem,

TABLE 9.2 OCCURRENCES OF THE VARIOUS CAUSES OF LONG ED LOS

Cause	Number of Occurrences
Patients sent to Imaging	215
Supply shortages	37
Poor ED layout	132
Inefficient discharge process	33
Staff shortage	12
Medications unavailable	6
Total	435

Abbreviation: LOS, length of stay.

TABLE 9.3 RELATIVE IMPORTANCE OF THE VARIOUS CAUSES OF LONG ED LOS

Cause	Number of Occurrences	Percentage	Cumulative Percentage
Patients sent to Imaging	215	49.42%	49.42%
Poor ED layout	132	30.34%	79.76%
Supply shortages	37	8.51%	88.27%
Inefficient discharge process	33	7.59%	95.86%
Staff shortage	12	2.76%	98.62%
Medications unavailable	6	1.38%	100.00%
TOTAL	435	100%	

Abbreviation: LOS, length of stay.

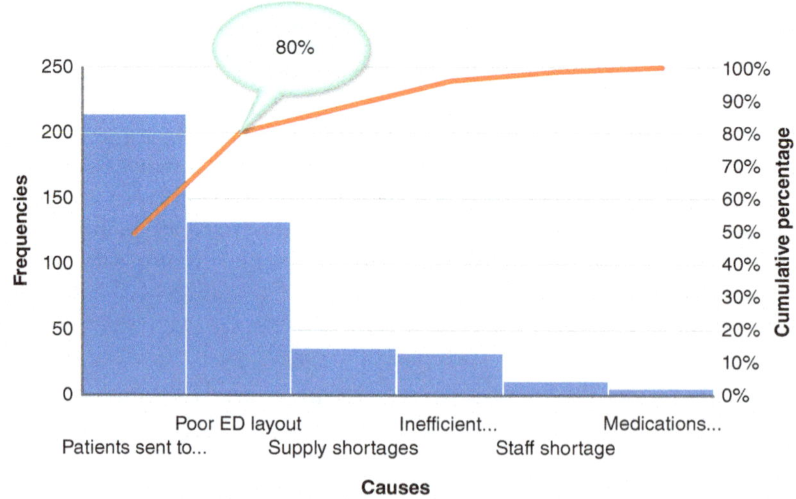

FIGURE 9.10 Pareto chart of causes of long ED LOS.

Abbreviation: LOS, length of stay.

followed by a plateau, suggesting the diminished importance of the other factors. Figure 9.10 underscores the importance of "patients sent to Imaging" and "poor ED layout" as the primary causes for long ED LOS.

BUILDING THE A3 REPORT

The *Analyze* section can now be documented on the A3 report (Figure 9.11).

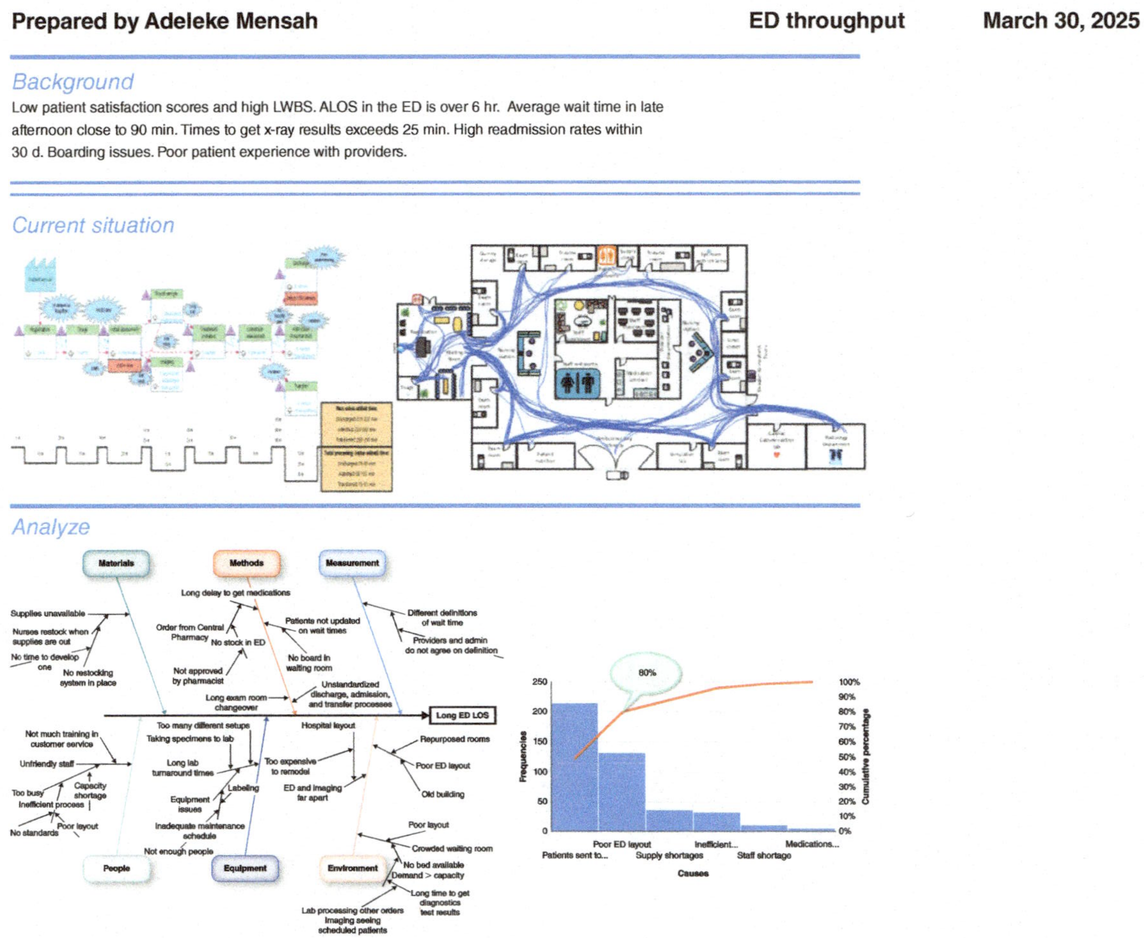

FIGURE 9.11 A3 report including the *Analyze* phase.

Abbreviations: ALOS, average length of stay; LOS, length of stay; LWBS, left without being seen.

ETHICAL SCENARIO 9.1

Relying on Evidence or Experience?

A long-standing conflict has existed between the autonomy of caregivers to deliver customized care and following evidence-based guidelines for certain disease treatments. Sometimes referred to as "cookbook" medicine, the literature is often utilized to create algorithms and protocols to guide patient treatment. Some physicians feel that these guidelines infringe on their expert training and limit their ability to effectively prescribe the treatment they feel is right for a certain patient.

Who is right in these scenarios? Should physicians follow evidence-based guidelines or have the ability to customize therapy based on their years of experience?

What are the possible ramifications of physicians being criminally prosecuted for providing care to a patient based on their best judgment rather than evidence-based medicine?

SUMMARY

Once you have measured the process rigorously, you can proceed to analyzing why waste is generated. In this chapter, you were introduced to the seven basic tools. Cause-and-effect diagrams, interrelationship diagrams, and failure mode and effects analysis are especially useful to structure the team's thoughts and assumptions about the causes of a particular problem. Scatter diagrams and correlation analysis help verify these assumptions. The effect of causes on problems can be predicted with regression techniques. So many causes need to be tackled, but which ones should be prioritized? Pareto diagrams help you identify the vital few causes that contribute the most to the problem occurrence. All these tools and techniques are widely used in organizations that have adopted total quality management in their endless search for perfect quality because they help people identify the root causes of a problem, distinguish hunches from reality, and trigger precise improvement initiatives.

CERTIFICATION TIPS

The *Analyze* portion of the certification exam contains a lot of material that could not be covered in a quality course alone.

- In addition to this chapter material, you will need to develop confidence intervals (CIs) for means and proportions and perform hypothesis tests for means, variances, and proportions. This material is provided in the book online resources (eChapter 16) for students seeking certification.
- You will also need to construct CIs for the regression coefficients. We recommend the following link: https://study.com/skill/learn/how-to-create-a-confidence-interval-for-the-slope-of-a-regression-line-explanation.html.
- Multi-vari studies and charts are not presented here because their use in healthcare would be really limited. However, they would be highly relevant in the pharmaceutical and medical device industries where positional (within-part; within-batch), cyclical (part-to-part; batch-to-batch), and temporal (over time) variation is likely and should be investigated. Good references for this material include:
    - Cavusoglu, I., & Durakbasa, M. N. (2014). The quality improvement process through application of multi-vari chart in an automotive supplier. *2014 International Conference on Production Research*, 78–81, Retrieved April 30, 2019 from https://www.researchgate.net/publication/344747263_THE_QUALITY_IMPROVEMENT_PROCESS_THROUGH_APPLICATION_OF_MULTIVARI_CHART_IN_AN_AUTOMOTIVE_SUPPLIER QualityGurus. QualityGurus. (2019, May 1). *Multi-vari study, multi-vari charts | ASQ CSSGB*. [Video] YouTube. https://www.youtube.com/watch?v=YhUTVCTZDDU
    - Zaciewski, R. D., & N'meth, L. (1995). The multi-vari chart: An underutilized quality tool. *Quality Progress*, *28*(10), 81–83.
- We have also talked about the importance of larger samples. This is related to the concept of statistical power. Check this link on sample size, power, and effect size: https://www.ncbi.nlm.nih.gov/pmc/articles/PMC7745163

KEY TERMS

Gap analysis
Failure mode and effects analysis (FMEA)
Cause-and-effect diagram
Root cause analysis (RCA)
Interrelationship diagram (or diagraph or digraph)
Scatter diagram
Correlation
Correlation coefficient
Linear regression analysis
Independent variable
Dependent variable
Simple linear regression
***y*-intercept**
Regression coefficient (slope)
Least squares method
Coefficient of determination
***p* value**
Analysis of variance (ANOVA)
Multiple linear regression
Adjusted R^2
Multiple *R*
Pareto chart

REVIEW QUESTIONS

1. What are the definition and purpose of each one of the following tools?
   a. FMEA
   b. Cause-and-effect diagram
   c. Correlation analysis
   d. Pareto chart
   e. Scatter diagram
   f. Interrelationship diagram
2. What are the four phases of analysis presented in this chapter? Briefly describe each one.

SOLVE BRIGHT ANGEL MEDICAL CENTER'S PROBLEMS

All chapter-specific data from the following problems are provided as Excel files which may be accessed via the show supplementary tab (Student Material) available online by visiting www.springerpub.com/courseconnect. See inside front cover and tear-out card for CourseConnect details.

1. Identify causes of a steady increase of supply shortages in the exam room. Classify these causes into the categories of people, methods, measurement, environment, equipment, and materials, and develop:
   a. a cause-and-effect diagram
   b. a digraph
2. Identify causes of patient falls at the elevator of a nursing home. Classify these causes into the categories of people, methods, equipment, and environment, and develop:
   a. a cause-and-effect diagram
   b. a digraph
3. Looking at a cause-and-effect diagram, the head of the Imaging Department identified reasons for long wait times (see table that follows). She wants to prioritize the factors that contribute to the problem. Her staff collected data on the frequency with which these causes contribute to long wait times over a period of a month. Based on these data, develop a Pareto chart and identify the cause(s) that require(s) immediate intervention.

Cause	Frequency of Occurrence
Patients scheduled too close together	574
Procedures that take too long	98
Patients not released on time from floor	374
Retakes on x-rays too frequent	112
Equipment inadequate for complex cases	96

4. The following are the frequencies of late lab turnaround times for various order volume levels. Develop a histogram. What can you say about the shape of the distribution? Can you make sense of it?

Daily Order Volume	Number of Late Turnaround Times
0–20	18
21–40	3
41–60	2
61–80	2
81–100	16
More than 100	22

5. At the hospital cafeteria, typical complaints about the food are that it is too salty, too mushy, too bland, too greasy, and too starchy. The manager of the cafeteria has compiled the following complaint data during the past month. Develop a Pareto chart and help him decide which problem(s) deserve(s) his immediate attention.

Complaint Type	Frequency
Too salty	184
Too mushy	60
Too bland	221
Too greasy	52
Too starchy	280
Too dry	62
Overcooked	51

6. Develop a check sheet and Pareto diagram for the following complaints regarding patients' bills. Which problems need to be prioritized?

No.	Problem	No.	Problem	No.	Problem
1	Patient never received it	12	Patient charged for services not provided	23	Total amount is inaccurate
2	Patient charged for services not provided	13	Filed late with insurer	24	Patient never received it
3	Total amount is inaccurate	14	Filed late with insurer	25	Patient charged for services not provided
4	Patient charged for services not provided	15	Total amount is inaccurate	26	Received late
5	Patient never received it	16	Patient charged for services not provided	27	Patient charged for services not provided
6	Received late	17	Filed late with insurer	28	Total amount is inaccurate
7	Filed late with insurer	18	Total amount is inaccurate	29	Patient charged for services not provided
8	Filed late with insurer	19	Patient charged for services not provided	30	Filed late with insurer
9	Patient charged for services not provided	20	Filed late with insurer	31	Received late
10	Filed late with insurer	21	Received late	32	Patient charged for services not provided
11	Received late	22	Filed late with insurer	33	Filed late with insurer

7. The table here presents failure modes, causes, and effects for each process step involved in scheduling appointments at BAMC's pediatrics clinic. Estimate the likelihood of occurrence of each failure mode, its likelihood of detection, and its severity. Compute the RPN for each step and for the entire process. Which step should be prioritized for improvement?

8. Regarding problem 7, identify actions to improve each step and reduce the occurrence of failure.
9. Use the supplemental Medical Tourism data set available in the online resources. The coding for each variable is explained in the first worksheet. Copy the data that you need and paste them on a new worksheet.
   a. Develop a scatterplot to determine whether there is a relationship between *Income* and *Likelihood to get care abroad*.
   b. Use Excel to find *r*, the correlation coefficient. Does this number confirm your findings in (a)?

Steps	Failure Mode	Failure Causes	Failure Effects	Likelihood of Occurrence (1–10)	Likelihood of Detection (1–10)	Severity (1–10)	RPN
Patient calls pediatrics clinic	Talks to someone in pharmacy who transfers patient to pediatrics	Almost identical phone numbers	Staff at pharmacy gets annoyed				
Patient listens to automatic recording and chooses appropriate option	Patient often selects wrong option or hangs up	There are nine options to select from; patient stops paying attention or gets impatient	Poor satisfaction scores and/or possible loss of revenue				
Patient is transferred to central scheduling and is put on hold	Patient hangs up	Long wait times	Poor satisfaction scores and/or possible loss of revenue				
Scheduler finds patient's name and insurance information in system	Wrong patient is found	Some names are misspelled; there are sometimes duplicate Social Security numbers	Long time to "sort things out," find the right patient, and correct the patient info				
Scheduler asks for physician's name and reason for appointment and then selects visit type	Wrong visit type is selected	Discrepancy between patient's description of reason and scheduler's interpretation	Patient's condition may require a longer visit than the one scheduled; physician has to play "catch up" with other patients				
Scheduler reviews scheduling instructions for selected visit type and physician	Scheduler skips that step	The descriptions of visit types differ from one physician to the next, which makes the review a lengthy process	Wrong type of visit is scheduled; physician is dissatisfied; billing issues				
Appointment is scheduled	Patient does not show up	No reminder is sent	Loss of revenue				

Abbreviation: RPN, risk priority number.

10. Use the supplemental Medical Tourism data set available in the online resources. The coding for each variable is explained in the first worksheet. Copy the data that you need and paste them on a new worksheet.
    a. Develop a scatterplot to determine whether there is a relationship between *Perceived Quality* and *Perceived Value*.
    b. Use Excel to find r, the correlation coefficient. Does this number confirm your findings in (a)?
    c. Add a trendline with regression equation and R^2 to the scatterplot developed in part (a). What does the R^2 value mean?
11. Use the supplemental Medical Tourism data set available in the online resources. The coding for each variable is explained in the first worksheet. Copy the data that you need and paste them on a new worksheet.

    Use Excel to find the regression equation with *Likelihood to get care abroad* as the dependent variable and *Cosmopolitanism*, *Knowledge*, and *Perceived Quality* as the independent variables.
    a. Explain the multiple R and R^2 values. Why is the adjusted R^2 value lower than the R^2 value?
    b. Explain the results of the ANOVA test.
    c. Which predictors are significant? Justify your answer.

LEARNING ACTIVITIES

1. Compare BAMC's goals in the project charter with some of the data produced in the value stream map (VSM) and the control charts. Develop a gap analysis report to show your findings.
2. Develop a fishbone diagram categorizing all the possible causes for people leaving the ED without being seen.
3. Use ChatGPT to identify all the possible causes for physicians to refuse using evidence-based treatment guidelines. Can you think of others? Explain.
4. Discussion with role-playing (three participants: CEO, CFO, and ED director). At BAMC, one of the causes for long ALOS is a poor layout. However, changing the layout is costly. The participants meet to discuss the pros and cons of changing the layout. This is a heated exchange, but hopefully, they will reach a consensus at the end of the discussion.
5. In the following article, what was the purpose of the FMEA? What problems did they discover? What were the solutions?

   Ullah, E., Baig, M. M., GholamHosseini, H., & Lu, J. (2022). Failure mode and effect analysis (FMEA) to identify and mitigate failures in a hospital rapid response system (RRS). *Heliyon*, *8*(2), e08944. https://doi.org/10.1016/j.heliyon.2022.e08944. https://www.ncbi.nlm.nih.gov/pmc/articles/PMC8857483
6. Explain why correlation does not imply causation.

REFERENCES

American Society for Quality. (2024). *What is an interrelationship diagram?* https://asq.org/quality-resources/relations-diagram?srsltid=AfmBOorSh1XBsKeYYuavj6tC1M_GfKTH85PJBjkWsR-5yy08mg5OaqPp

Field, A. (2013). *Discovering statistics using IBM SPSS statistics* (4th ed.). Sage.

Fisher, R. A. (1926). The arrangement of field experiments. *Journal of the Ministry of Agriculture of Great Britain*, *33*, 503–513. https://doi.org/10.23637/rothamsted.8v61q

Institute for Healthcare Improvement. (2017). *Failure modes and effects analysis (FMEA)*. https://www.ihi.org/resources/tools/failure-modes-and-effects-analysis-fmea-tool

Ye, M., Tang, F., Chien, C.-W., Chuang, Y.-C., Liou, J. J. H., & Qu, X. (2024). Application of failure mode and effect analysis in ICU admission of potentially COVID-19 infected patients. *American Journal of Infection Control, 52*(5), 552–562. https://doi.org/10.1016/j.ajic.2023.12.012

FOR MORE ADVANCED CONTENT ON CONFIDENCE INTERVALS AND HYPOTHESIS TESTS, SEE ECHAPTER 16: ESTIMATION AND HYPOTHESIS TESTING

eChapter 16 is available online by visiting www.springerpub.com/courseconnect. See inside front cover and tear-out card for CourseConnect details.

PART V

IMPROVE—How to Eliminate Waste?

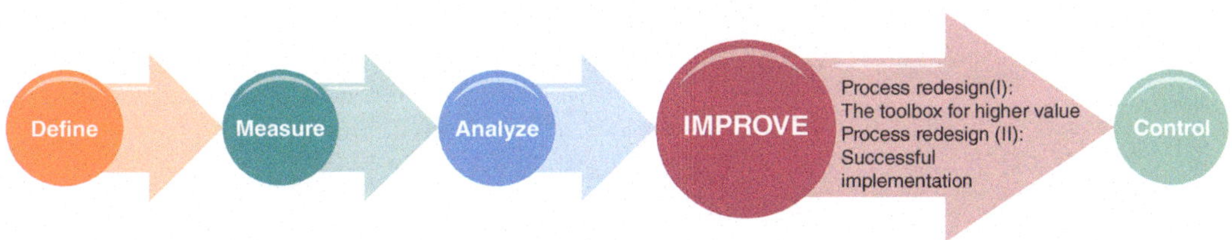

CHAPTER 10

PROCESS REDESIGN (I): THE TOOLBOX FOR HIGHER VALUE

> **BRIGHT ANGEL MEDICAL CENTER 10.1**
>
> *Barbara and everyone who had been involved in the ED throughput improvement project up to this point met in one of the large classrooms. She seemed more relaxed today than she had been for a long time. She flashed a big smile and said, "The leadership is fully on board! Your hard work and thorough analysis convinced them that we should continue to pursue the remodel of the ED. Friends, we are ready to start the most exciting phase. We are finally going to improve this place!" The room erupted in applause. "Wait, wait, I'm not finished," Barbara continued. "I want to thank all of you for helping us get this far. Now, feel free to contact Adeleke any time you have suggestions. Your insights will help the project team design effective and workable solutions. But today, let's just enjoy our progress. Lunch will be served shortly. Take a seat."*
>
> **What could go wrong during the improvement phase? How can those problems be avoided?**

LEARNING OBJECTIVES

After reading this chapter, you will be able to:

- Identify useful sources in the literature.
- Use Lean tools to implement important design principles that increase value for the customer of the process.
- Design product, functional, and hybrid layouts based on process characteristics.
- Identify and manage bottlenecks.

INTRODUCTION

After a thorough analysis of the root causes and their effects on problems, it is time to eliminate them and design robust processes. That is the most exciting phase of the project. You want to make sure the process will make it nearly impossible for waste to come back and settle in. How does the team get started? It should not waste time reinventing the wheel. The literature abounds with proven process improvement solutions. Some of these solutions will be directly applicable to the project at hand. In addition, various design principles will also prove useful to generate new, customized solutions to increase value. One of these principles is to link process and layout. A layout should support the workflow, not impede it. Finally, the theory of constraints (TOC) will help identify bottlenecks in the process and manage them to increase throughput.

WHY IS THIS MATERIAL USEFUL?

The improvement phase involves the generation of potential solutions to specific problems. This chapter offers a wide variety of improvement options designed to eradicate waste and create flow. These options will have to be customized, but they are useful starting points to unleash the team's creativity.

ON THE JOB! INTERVIEW VIDEO 10.1

Summer Johnson
Ambulatory Quality and Patient Safety Director

Every Vital Every Time Initiative
Aligning metrics with mission values
Environmental cleanliness for safety
Filling gaps in standardization
Building a sense of community
DMAIC (Define-Measure-Analyze-Improve-Control) process for sustained compliance and outcomes

1. Summer shares details about a project she led to improve the vital sign capture rate for ambulatory encounters. What does she list as some of the keys to success for process improvement projects?
2. During the implementation of this project, the quality team noted that there were some skill gaps in obtaining vital signs with various instruments used in the ambulatory environment. What potential negative outcomes can occur if the team members do not have the appropriate skills or training to use this equipment?
3. Summer highlights the DMAIC process and states that it is ingrained in her department. Did it impact the results?

The interview is available online by visiting www.springerpub.com/courseconnect. See inside front cover and tear-out card for CourseConnect details.

SECONDARY SOURCES OF INFORMATION

Formulating solutions can be both a stimulating and daunting process. What is out there? Does it work? Fortunately, many resources are readily available in the literature. Searches in Google Scholar and PubMed will yield multiple case studies of the same process problems you are facing in your organization and will explain the deployment and impact of various solutions. Furthermore, many entities have a wealth of resources available on their website (Table 10.1). For example, the Agency for Healthcare Research and Quality (AHRQ) has the RED toolkit mentioned in Box 10.1.

TABLE 10.1 ORGANIZATIONS AND QUALITY IMPROVEMENT RESOURCES

Organization	Purpose and Selected Products
AHRQ	Improving safety and quality of healthcare • Research • Teaching and training materials • Development of measures
TJC	Evaluating healthcare organizations • Educational materials and events • Sentinel event alerts • Standards

(continued)

TABLE 10.1 ORGANIZATIONS AND QUALITY IMPROVEMENT RESOURCES (*CONTINUED*)

Organization	Purpose and Selected Products
NQF	Improving outcomes, safety, equity, and affordability • Performance measurement (person- and family-centered care; prevention and treatment of leading causes of mortality; effective communication and care coordination, etc.)
IHI	Advancing and sustaining better health outcomes • Model for improvement • Tools • Systems thinking • Psychology of change • Publications
CMS	Providing health coverage and partnering with healthcare community to improve quality • Innovation models • Medicare Learning Network • Training catalog
ISMP	Preventing medication errors and promoting safe practices • Best practices • Worksheets • Experts' insights (videos)

Abbreviations: AHRQ, Agency for Healthcare Research and Quality; CMS, Centers for Medicare & Medicaid Services; IHI, Institute for Healthcare Improvement; ISMP, Institute for Safe Medication Practices; NQF, National Quality Forum; TJC, The Joint Commission.

BOX 10.1 QUALITY IN PRACTICE!

Reengineering the Hospital Discharge Process

The hospital discharge process is usually nonstandardized, leading to high variation in quality and excess costs. The Re-Engineered Discharge (RED) program was developed to address these shortcomings. This program was developed over a long period of time. In 2003, methodologies such as process mapping, failure mode and effects analysis (FMEA), and root cause analysis (RCA) were used to identify the primary process failures and their causes. With this information, a RED checklist with the essential elements of a standardized discharge process was developed. Later, a randomized controlled trial showed that the patients under the RED system had a better understanding of their condition and medications. They were also more likely to attend their follow-up appointments. As a result, the RED system was associated with a 30% decline in rehospitalizations. Other research efforts have confirmed the efficacy of RED. However, in practice, the program faced obstacles because it required overloaded nurses to spend more time with patients. To circumvent the problem, Louise, a computer-based agent, was designed to converse with patients and teach them their care plan. Eventually, Louise was replaced by Maya-RED, a more advanced system that converses with patients, addresses their concerns, reminds them about appointments, and so on. The redesign of the discharge process took a long time, and it will continue to evolve, but it has improved quality and lowered costs (Jack et al., 2023).

PROCESS DESIGN

Process design or redesign aims at creating a process that lowers the chances for error, minimizes waste, eases the flow, and allows for rapid modifications. How do we create such processes? As a general rule, simpler processes are more robust. Steve Jobs (1998) famously said:

"That's been one of my mantras—focus and simplicity. Simple can be harder than complex; you have to work hard to get your thinking clean to make it simple."

Let's explore this idea. A process is a sequence of steps. The reliability of each step is the probability that it will function effectively, that is, without errors, for a given period of time. As each step presents an opportunity—even a small one—to make errors, the more steps in the process,

BOX 10.2 QUALITY IN PRACTICE!

IDEO Human-Centered Design

IDEO is a design and consulting firm that practices human-centered design. Through a step-by-step approach, innovative solutions to complex problems are created. It is a simple concept: start with the people you are designing for and end with customized solutions that meet their needs. There are three phases: (1) the Inspiration phase involves getting to know your customers very well and learning exactly what they need (the 5 whys); (2) the Ideation phase during which you identify design alternatives and develop prototypes; and (3) the Implementation phase in which you see your creation serve its unique purpose (IDEO.org, 2024).

the greater the chances that the system/process will fail at one time or another. Furthermore, each time the responsibility for an activity is passed on to another person (a **handoff**), there is an opportunity for miscommunication and errors. Calculating the rolled throughput yield in Chapter 6 clearly illustrated this principle. Sound process design principles should therefore focus on simplicity and parsimony of tasks and movements (Laguna & Marklund, 2019). Their ultimate purpose should be the creation of meaningful value for the customer (Box 10.2).

DESIGN PRINCIPLES

The principles in Figure 10.1 are aligned with the Lean Six Sigma (LSS) philosophy introduced in Chapter 2. We will discuss each principle and link it to LSS tools.

PRINCIPLE #1: REDUCE FRAGMENTATION

For decades now, work with a narrow scope has been described as antiquated. Nevertheless, the concept remains popular thanks to well-entrenched ideas linking specialization to speed and efficiency. In an increasingly complex healthcare world, it is also tempting to divide up the work into narrowly defined areas of expertise as a justification to prevent errors. After all, one can only know so much. The problem with this approach is that it increases the fragmentation of the process, with handoffs and control/inspection points along the process. The result is more delays and possibly more errors. As much as possible, horizontal and/or vertical loading of activities should be pursued. Horizontal loading, also known as **job enlargement**, aims at increasing the variety of a job by having employees perform more activities that are immediately upstream or downstream. For example, a nurse may perform triage, provide discharge instructions, and schedule a patient for follow-up. Vertical loading, or **job enrichment**, extends the employee's regular activities to planning and control functions (Gkorezis & Theodorou, 2016). For example, the vertical loading of a nurse's tasks may entail the development of staffing schedules as well as checking proper medication reconciliation protocols. This "combination" of steps produces a simplified and continuous flow of activities. Both job enlargement and enrichment enhance the flexibility of the system.

Flexible System

A flexible system with cross-functional resources facilitates a smooth flow. Demand for services keeps on changing, not only in terms of volume but also in terms of mix. For example, during the COVID-19 pandemic, demand for ICU beds surged while demand for elective surgeries plummeted. To respond swiftly to the crisis with limited resources, New York-Presbyterian Weill Cornell Medical Center converted several operating rooms (ORs) and postanesthesia care units to ICUs, repurposed anesthesia machines as ICU ventilators, deployed perioperative staff to the newly reconfigured care units, and reassigned certified RN anesthetists as respiratory therapists (Peters et al., 2020).

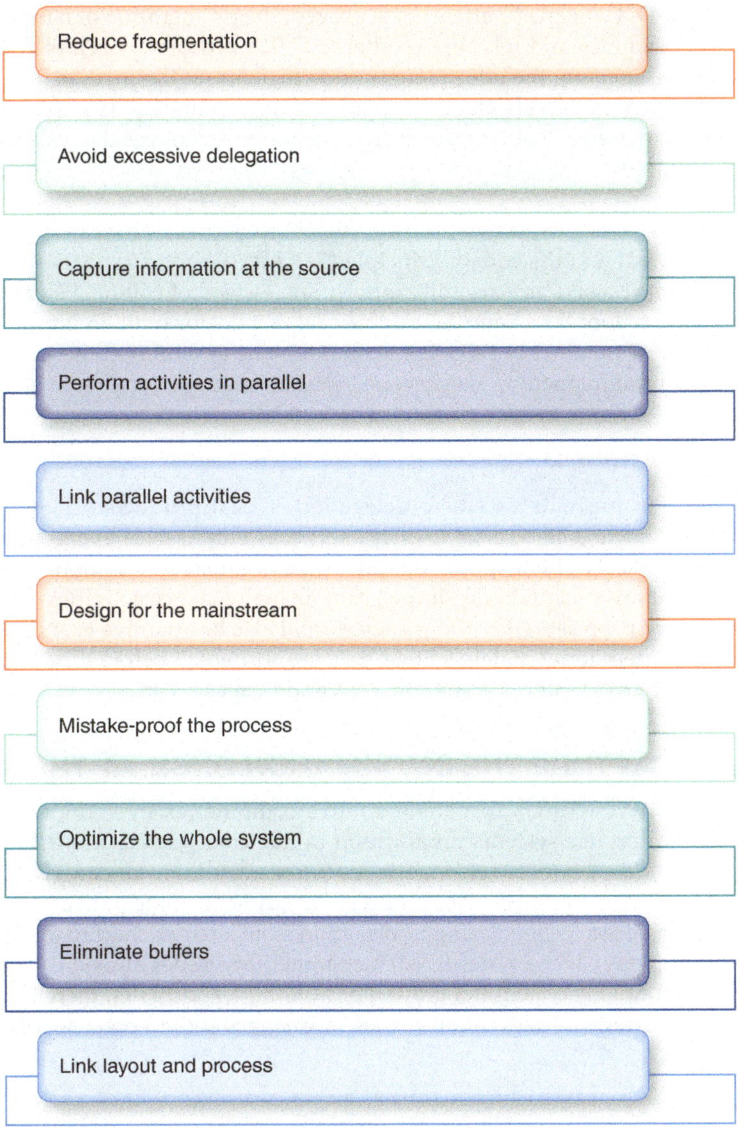

FIGURE 10.1 Design principles.

Healthcare is a multidisciplinary field in which doctors, nurses, pharmacists, technicians, dietitians, and other professionals must collaborate to provide the best possible health outcomes. This collaboration requires frequent communication and joint improvement initiatives to increase value for their patients. Yet, medicine has become increasingly specialized, somehow deepening functional silos and contributing to a disjointed flow. To be successful, process improvement team members must adopt a "whole process" or systems view. They must learn about each other's work and challenges as well as train, solve problems, and monitor performance together. Expanding one's skill repertoire and crossing over functional boundaries for the common purpose of improving patient care are truly indispensable to create a rapid and agile flow.

PRINCIPLE #2: AVOID EXCESSIVE DELEGATION

In line with Principle #1, Principle #2 attempts to prevent the proliferation of handoffs subsequent to delegating responsibilities and relying on others to "fix" problems. Lack of coordination and accountability ensues, affecting the effectiveness and efficiency of the process. In essence, Principle #2 means, "Why have somebody else do it if you can do it yourself?" Computerized physician order entry (POE) is an example of this principle in action as it reduces delays and errors associated with transcription.

Jidoka

Employee empowerment is at the core of Principle #2. *Jidoka* (Chapter 2) gives employees the authority to "stop the line" when they deem it appropriate instead of calling a supervisor to assess the problem and take action. For example, a nurse seeing a doctor omit an important step in the diagnostic evaluation or treatment of a patient can intervene and remind the doctor of that step. Preventing mistakes from happening is everyone's job, irrespective of one's level in the organizational hierarchy.

Total Productive Maintenance

Another Lean tool that prevents excessive delegation is total productive maintenance (TPM). Just like *total* quality management (TQM; Chapter 1) that emphasizes everyone's participation in quality improvements, TPM engages everyone in the organization to monitor the equipment when using it. All employees should do simple, routine maintenance activities on the equipment they use if and when appropriate (Box 10.3). They should also be attentive to small problems they cannot fix and report them immediately so that they are addressed before they become big problems that will produce errors, hinder a smooth flow, and increase costs.

PRINCIPLE #3: CAPTURE THE INFORMATION ONCE, AT THE SOURCE

It is commonplace to have written data entered into a computer, or even digital information reentered in multiple computer systems. In addition to the time wasted on performing these redundant functions, human errors are also made during reentry. Point-of-care (POC) technologies enable healthcare providers to collect electronic test data directly at the patient's bedside. As a result, they eliminate the need for reentering information from a paper chart to an electronic health record (EHR). Nevertheless, when unresolved, incompatibility issues among different technological platforms may hamper seamless integration of POC data and EHRs, thereby defeating their purpose. Therefore, a careful consideration of these challenges should precede a successful application of Principle #3.

Quality at the Source

An extension of Principle #3 is **quality at the source**. It implies that everyone is responsible for checking one's own work to avoid passing on defects to the next step or "customer" according to the next process concept, which is viewing the customer as the next step in the process (Chapter 3). Quality is built into the process at each step. This is consistent with Deming's Point #14

> **BOX 10.3 QUALITY IN PRACTICE!**
>
> **Total Productive Maintenance at Kadlec Regional Medical Center**
>
> At Kadlec Regional Medical Center in Richland, Washington, a team of clinical engineers, nurses, anesthesiologists, and one OR physician created a TPM program for the OR. They developed checklists to ensure proper start-ups of the equipment and a visual scheduled maintenance matrix to provide clinicians and engineers with a high-level view of the maintenance schedule. Clinicians also learned to perform minor repairs and replace some equipment components (Ahuja et al., 2016).

insisting on everyone's role to ensure quality. In Figure 10.2A, you see how a traditional system of quality inspection works. Only at the end of the process does the nurse check that the food to be served to a patient is hot. If it is cold—as is often the case—it is difficult to determine where the problem occurred and who is accountable. Did the food leave the kitchen cold? Did it stay on the cart too long? It is difficult to say. In Figure 10.2B, on the other hand, each participant in the process checks that the food is still at the right temperature before passing it on to the next step. This prevents the use of further resources downstream for a tray that will end up being rejected. When there is a deviation from the requirement, it is easier to track the problem to its source and find its root cause.

PRINCIPLE #4: PERFORM ACTIVITIES IN PARALLEL WHENEVER POSSIBLE

Processes can often be depicted by perfectly linear sequences of activities. When a surgery is scheduled, a patient typically waits for the medical assistant to prepare the consent form, signs it, and then goes to the scheduler's office. The patient could go to the scheduler's office *while* the medical assistant prepares the form and then sign it in the scheduler's office. Performing these activities in parallel would decrease the amount of non–value-added time for the patient and speed up the entire process, thereby easing the flow.

PRINCIPLE #5: LINK PARALLEL ACTIVITIES INSTEAD OF MERELY INTEGRATING THEIR OUTPUT

A poor implementation of Principle #4 would feature several activities being performed simultaneously and independently, without much coordination. For instance, when working on a team project, you and your teammates might divide up the tasks. Assuming each individual knows exactly what their responsibilities entail, you may all work independently. When it is time to "assemble" all the parts of the project, you realize that some of the topics may have been covered

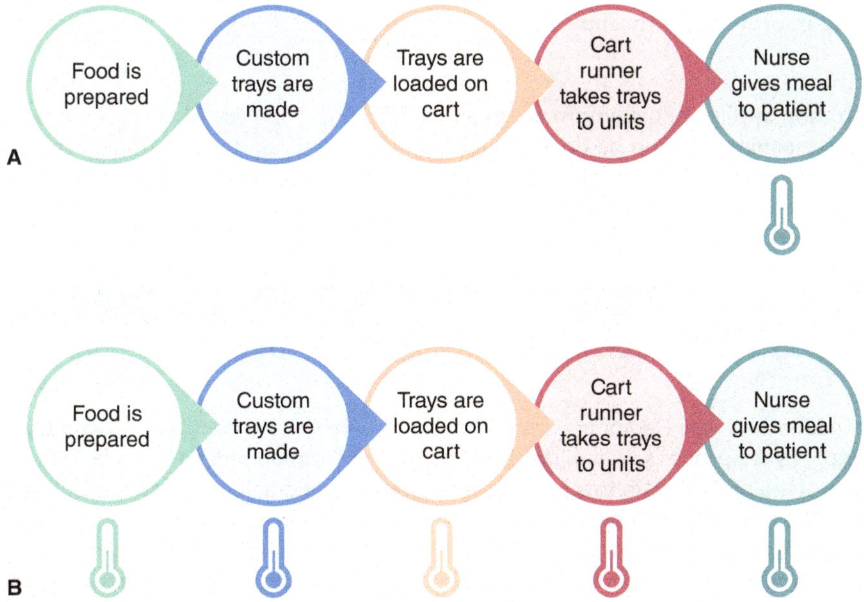

FIGURE 10.2 Approaches to quality inspection.

Note: (A) Quality inspection at the end. (B) Quality at the source.

by two or more of your teammates (redundancies), that some key parts of the project are missing (omissions/errors), and that the final output is essentially a very disjointed project report. If all of you had coordinated your activities frequently and had used a collaboration tool like Microsoft Teams to chat, videoconference, and share and edit files, chances are that the finished report might have required only a few, minor revisions, if any.

PRINCIPLE #6: DESIGN FOR THE MAINSTREAM, NOT THE EXCEPTIONS

Inefficiencies are not part of the initial process design. Often, they emerge as new services are added, the patient mix changes, modern equipment is installed, new regulations are implemented, and so on. With these changes come ad hoc process "fixes" or add-ons. Over time, they become a web of paths with complicated and jumbled flows that make it hard to track the movements of flow units. When going to your dentist for your regular checkup, you may be asked to produce your insurance card so that the staff can make a photocopy even though the information is in their electronic dental record system. A simple check on their system would indicate whether the insurance information needs to be updated, but they continue to keep paper records because "they have always done it that way." Similarly, if supplies purchased from new vendors need to be inspected, it is not necessary to create a process with inspections for all purchases, including those from well-established, certified vendors. A design for the mainstream minimizes the number of paths and thus provides a simplified platform with lower variability and increased visibility and predictability.

Standardization

Focusing on the mainstream and creating "sameness" lowers the chances of chaos related to complex processes and lack of adherence to guidelines that are just too numerous to be followed. The **standardization of work** is therefore a useful approach in that it establishes consistent processes and guidelines to produce consistent outputs and therefore eliminate variation for Six Sigma quality. Standardized work involves defining a task and specifying how it is done, when, and by whom (Safety Culture, 2024).

The example provided in Box 10.4 shows how standardization and reduction of surgical instrumentation reduced **cycle time**, that is, the time to complete all the steps (including waits) of a process, and improved quality and safety.

6S

Standardization applies to the environment as well. To make the use of the space more efficient, some "housecleaning" should be done to eliminate the clutter and ensure that each item is consistently placed in the correct location. **6S** is a tool that creates sustainable order and visibility to enhance the fluidity of the process flow (Table 10.2; Figure 10.3).

BOX 10.4 QUALITY IN PRACTICE!

Using the Six Sigma Methodology to Improve the Surgical Instruments Sterilization Process

The Bellinzona and Valli Regional Hospital in Bellinzona, Switzerland, launched a Lean initiative to improve the process of sterilization of surgical instrumentation in five ORs. The primary objectives of the project were to standardize the process and achieve a more predictable level of quality. They found that the processing of used surgical instruments involved 58 different, subsequent steps to deliver clean instruments ready for the next procedure. Using the DMAIC process, the project team focused on reducing process variation, standardizing the process to improve reliability and capability, and eliminating waste. After 18 months, the project team was able to demonstrate an improvement in the efficiency of instrument cleaning, a 0.25 increase in the sigma level, a reduction in overall cost, and a higher rate of satisfaction for the OR personnel and surgeons (Saporito et al., 2023).

TABLE 10.2 6S

S	Description
Sort out	Organize and eliminate what is unnecessary.
Systematize	Arrange items in their correct places so that they can be accessed when needed.
Scrub	Keep the environment clean.
Standardize	Do the same thing every time.
Sustain	Stick to the rules, build the previous 4Ss into the culture, and constantly improve when possible.
Safety	Always be on the lookout for safety risks and establish preventative mechanisms to reduce or eliminate them.

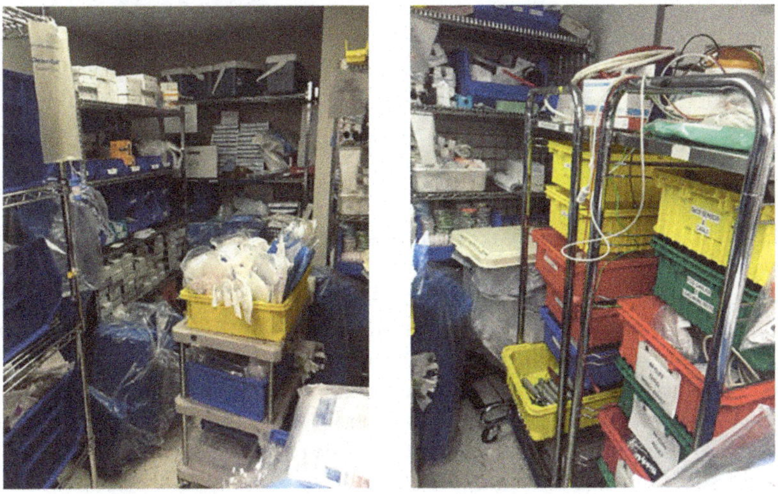

BEFORE

Anesthesia supplies need organization. An abundance of cluttered supplies leads to increased risk of expired inventory and duplication.

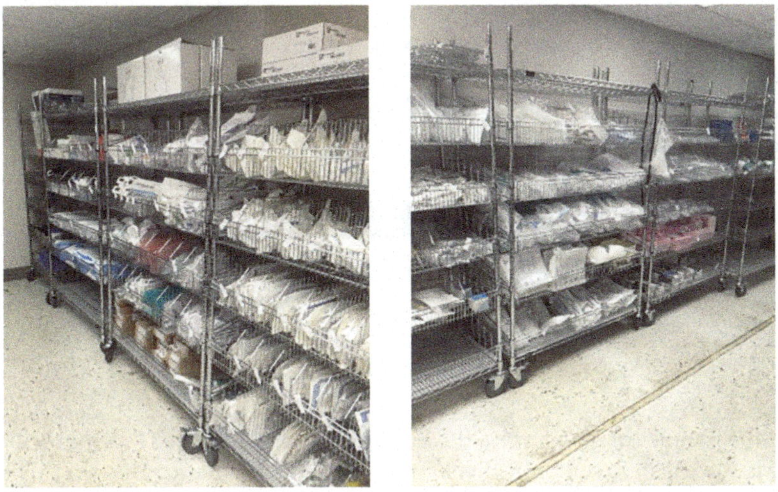

AFTER

An organized supply room increases visibility of what is missing and what needs to be replaced.

FIGURE 10.3 Anesthesiology supplies before and after using the 6s methodology.

In the case of repetitive processes such as claims processing, Lasik surgery, or orthodontics, another way of designing work for the mainstream is to level the workload.

Workload Leveling (*heijunka*)

A rapid flow through the system requires that the work keep pace with the demand rate. The "pulse" of the Lean system is referred to as **takt time**, which is the pace of work (time per unit) necessary to meet demand. To illustrate the concept, let us assume that during the flu season, Bright Angel Medical Center (BAMC) opens a flu shot clinic. The clinic is open 9 hours a day, and 50 patients are scheduled per day. The nurse giving the shots works 9 hours and takes a 1-hour lunch break as well as two 15-minute rest breaks. In order to meet the demand smoothly, the time per flu shot cannot exceed 9 minutes, as shown in the following equation:

$$\text{Takt time} = \frac{\textit{Time available for work}}{\textit{Demand}} \qquad [10.1]$$

$$= \frac{\left[9 \text{ hours} \times 60 \text{ minutes}\right] - \left[60 \text{ minutes} + \left(2 \times 15 \text{ minutes}\right)\right]}{50 \text{ patients}}$$

$$= \frac{450 \text{ minutes}}{50} = 9 \text{ minutes}$$

A flu shot should not take longer than 9 minutes to administer and document into the system in order to keep up with the demand. Ideally, this schedule would be repeated throughout the month. This is consistent with another popular Lean concept, ***heijunka***, which is **leveling the workload** in terms of volume and mix to produce a smooth and steady flow. In our previous example, let us assume that the year before, 1,000 patients received flu shots during the month of October. Demand fluctuated each day, which caused backlogs when it was high and downtime when it was low. This year, demand is expected to be about the same. However, to avoid the chaos and waste from the year before, the scheduling staff has leveled the load and has established 50 time slots for flu shots in its daily schedule: 50 flu shots × 5 days a week × 4 weeks = 1,000 flu shots. This is an example of workload leveling in terms of volume. Now, let us combine volume *and* mix. Let's assume that the past year's demand for vaccines at the BAMC clinic included 500 influenza, 400 COVID, and 100 respiratory syncytial virus (RSV) shots throughout the month of October. This year, should the staff schedule 500 influenza, followed by 400 COVID, and then 100 RSV shots? No, because the demand does not occur in that order! The demand is spread throughout the month. Therefore, the staff should establish a mixed schedule based on the demand by following these steps:

STEP 1: If not readily available, find the daily demand. Dividing the monthly demand quantities by 20 (5 days × 4 weeks), we obtain the following daily quantities:

Vaccine	Daily Demand
Influenza (I)	25
COVID (C)	20
RSV (R)	5

RSV, respiratory syncytial virus.

STEP 2: Find the number of daily cycles during which the sequence of vaccines will be repeated. This is the greatest common divisor of each shot's daily quantity. In this example, the greatest common divisor is 5. There will therefore be five cycles with the same sequence throughout the day.

STEP 3: Find the number of each type of vaccine in each cycle by dividing each daily demand quantity by the number of cycles.

Vaccine	Daily Demand	Units per Cycle
Influenza (I)	25	25/5 = 5
COVID (C)	20	20/5 = 4
RSV (R)	5	5/5 = 1

RSV, respiratory syncytial virus.

There will therefore be five cycles of 10 units, that is, 5 influenza, 4 COVID, and 1 RSV. Each cycle would repeat every 10 × 9 minutes = 90 minutes. Over a 1-day period, there will be five cycles of 90 minutes, for a total of 450 minutes, which is the time available for work.

STEP 4: Determine the daily sequence.

If the setup between the types of vaccines is minimal, we will mix the types of vaccines in such a way that we get as close as possible to a "batch" size of 1, as shown in the following.

Cycle	1	2	3	4	5
Sequence	ICICICICIR	ICICICICIR	ICICICICIR	ICICICICIR	ICICICICIR

If the setup for a particular type of vaccine is more involved, then they can be scheduled consecutively. In that case, a sequence such as IIIIICCCCR would be preferred, and if the setups were really complex, then it would be acceptable to administer 25 influenza shots, followed by 20 COVID shots, followed by 5 RSV shots. This daily sequence would be repeated each day of the month. However, efforts should be expended to reduce the **setup time**—the time required to reconfigure supplies and equipment for a different item or patient (waste in Lean)—so that a sequence producing the demand mix throughout the day (table in Step 4) could be achieved, even though it may sometimes have to be altered to accommodate patients' scheduling preferences.

You may already question the practicality of a strict adherence to this approach. If administering and documenting a vaccine takes longer than 9 minutes, patients will have to wait or the nurse will have to take shorter breaks, or another nurse may help absorb the load when the system backs up. Additionally, scheduling every 9 minutes is most unusual, and 10-minute intervals are much more likely. With 10-minute intervals, the demand would not be met unless work hours are extended or a floating nurse is assigned to the system as needed. In a nutshell, leveling the workload is difficult. It should serve as a guiding principle to enhance predictability and flow, but enough flexibility should be injected into the system to compensate for unavoidable deviations.

PRINCIPLE #7: MISTAKE-PROOF THE PROCESS

LSS aims to achieve zero defects. One of the Lean tools that facilitates this endeavor is the *poka-yoke* system (Chapter 2). This system is consistent with Deming's Point #3—"Eliminate the need for inspection by building quality into the [process] in the first place" (Chapter 1). It also supports the concept of quality at the source to avoid passing on defects. A pharmacy system that signals drug interactions for a patient is an example of a *poka-yoke* system preventing medication error. A smart pump programmed to prevent infusion of an unsafe dose of a particular drug is another example.

Checklists

Checklists are lists of actions that must be performed to achieve a successful outcome. They are formulated according to best practices in evidence-based medicine. Their use ensures that all steps of a process are followed consistently, with no omission to prevent adverse events from occurring. They are thus consistent with the standardization of methods for consistent outcomes. For example, the checklist for central line insertion at Johns Hopkins (Box 10.5) enumerates all the sequential steps to be followed to prevent infections. If a step is omitted, the reason for the omission must be documented.

BOX 10.5 QUALITY IN PRACTICE!

Central Line Insertion Checklist at Johns Hopkins (Johns Hopkins Medicine, 2024)

Date ____________________ Time ____________________

TYPE OF LINE PLACED ________________ REWIRE ☐ LOCATION OF LINE ________________

OF LUMENS ________________

Critical Steps Directions: The assistant completes this checklist by indicating with a check mark in the appropriate column when the task is performed. If the task is not performed, a comment must be added. The supervisor may also function as the assistant who completes this form.	Yes	Yes With Reminder **(If no, add a comment)**
1. Perform a time-out using the informed consent form.		
2. Clean hands.		
3. Wear a cap, mask, sterile gown/gloves, and eye protection if in contact with or crossing the sterile field *at any time during the procedure. a. All others entering the room during the procedure must wear a cap and mask.		
4. Prep site with chlorhexidine and let air dry. (*See instructions)		
5. Drape patient from head to toe using sterile technique.		
6. Prepare catheter by preflushing and clamping all lumens not in use during the procedure.		
7. Place the patient in the Trendelenburg position unless contraindicated (e.g., increased intracranial pressure [ICP]) or if femoral/peripherally inserted central catheter (PICC; place supine and flat).		
8. Maintain sterile field.		
9. Ensure grasp on guide wire is maintained throughout procedure and removed postprocedure.		
10. Aspirate blood from all lumens, flush, and apply sterile caps.		
11. Ensure venous placement. (*See instructions)		
12. Clean site with chlorhexidine, apply sterile dressing, and apply sterile caps on all hubs.		

*Checklist instructions located on back of form

Operator ________________ Supervisor ________________ Assistant ________________

Comments:

Source: Johns Hopkins Medicine. (2024). *Central Line Insertion Care Team Checklist*. https://www.hopkinsmedicine.org/-/media/heic/cl-insertion-checklist.pd

PRINCIPLE #8: OPTIMIZE THE WHOLE SYSTEM AND STOP FOCUSING ON LOCAL OPTIMIZATION

Very often, ingenious and motivated employees will work on ways to improve "their" system or process. Although their effort may improve their own operations, it may create a myriad of problems for upstream and/or downstream activities. For example, if a hospital has an integrated health information system and the Surgery Department decides to have a surgery module sold by another vendor, the surgery staff may be happy with the results. However, in the best-case scenario, it may generate excess costs to interface the surgery system with other system modules, such as lab and billing. In the worst-case scenario, information may have to be reentered, with potential for errors and additional clerical costs.

The same applies to LSS efforts. As stated in Chapter 2, these efforts will have limited impact if they are cherry-picked for implementation. Their combination is referred to as Lean bundles (Chapter 2), sets of best professional practices that are consistent with Lean. In healthcare, there are four reported Lean bundles: (a) the TQM bundle focuses on reliable and safe care; (b) the **just-in-time (JIT)** bundle targets the delivery of materials, information, and services to the patient on time; (c) the TPM bundle underscores the creation of value through efficiency and reliability of medical equipment; and (d) the Human Resources Management bundle seeks to unleash workforce participation, decentralization of authority, workload management, communication, and leadership for success.

PRINCIPLE #9: ELIMINATE BUFFERS

What is a buffer? A **buffer** is a group of flow units that have been temporarily held until capacity is freed to let them move through the process. A buffer can be an inventory of goods/supplies waiting to be used or a line of patients waiting to be seen by a provider. Buffers are often seen as an insurance policy against uncertainty in vendor lead times and demand. They also arise from variable arrivals of these flow units or variable activity times at any of the process steps the flow units go through. They are produced as well by batch processing systems that delay the movement of a flow unit from one activity to the next until a batch has been completed; hence, the goal of achieving a one-unit lot size! In any case, buffers are visual process encumbrances that halt a smooth and rapid flow. Eliminating buffers exposes weaknesses and forces redesign.

One of the Lean principles, *establish pull*, is designed to eliminate buffers. A pull system (Chapter 2) is demand-driven. It works best when there is a relatively stable demand and the process is repetitive and standardized. This is more common for administrative support services than for clinical services. However, there are some medical procedures for which a pull system works very well. For example, cataract surgeries are high-volume, relatively standardized procedures. The sequential steps are (a) patients go from the waiting room to a prep/recovery area; (b) they are then taken to the OR for their surgery; (c) next, they are taken back to the recovery area; (d) when patients have recovered and received discharge instructions, they leave. With a pull system, as soon as a bed in the recovery area becomes vacant after a patient leaves, a patient is pulled from the waiting room to be prepped. As soon as the OR is vacated by a patient and set up for the next one, a prepped patient from the prep/recovery area is pulled and placed in the OR (Figure 10.4). Because all surgery times are fairly consistent, the appointment times are set so that patients will not have to wait too long in the waiting room. The interdependence between processes requires frequent communication among the labor resources involved.

Just-In-Time

The pull system is consistent with the tightly coordinated processing system called JIT. Under that system, materials, supplies, or patients move through the system exactly when they are needed, not early and not late. For example, Toyota ordered automobile parts in small quantities based on

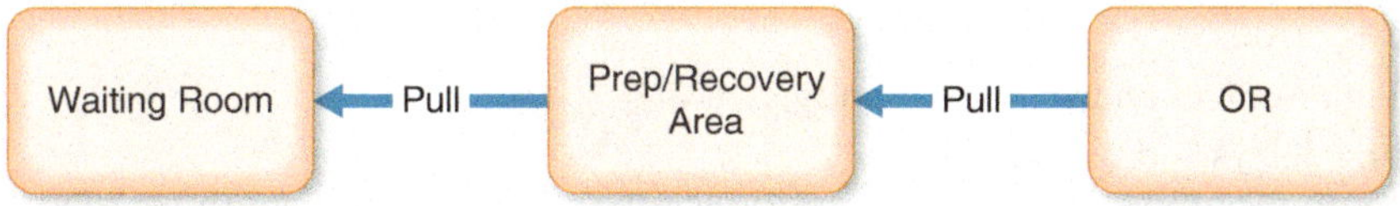

FIGURE 10.4 Pull system for cataract surgery.

Abbreviation: OR, operating room.

their short-term needs. The process was designed to ensure that a part would arrive just in time to be used, eliminating the need to keep it in inventory. Today, many healthcare organizations use a JIT system to eliminate the need to store excess supplies (Paige, 2019).

Central to the concept of JIT is *kanban*. The **kanban system** is a visual control method for JIT. It involves *kanbans*, that is, "cards" or "signals," authorizing the movement of or processing of units flowing through the system. For example, a prescription for medication is a *kanban*. It indicates the type, quantity, and dosage of medication to be dispensed. It is a signal for the pharmacist to retrieve the medication from inventory and deliver it to the patient. Similarly, a *kanban* placed with supplies in the exam room will trigger when replenishment is necessary. At a minimum, the *kanban* will display information on the item, its location in the supply room, the quantity to be ordered or moved to replenish supplies, and the safety stock. *Kanbans* are some of the visual tools used in Lean implementations. Good visual aids provide easy-to-understand information at a glance. As such, they help reduce miscommunication, a typical source of defects, delays, and other forms of waste.

Undercapacity Scheduling

You must have heard the expression "matching demand and capacity." Well, it is a bad idea! A **bottleneck** is defined as a point in the system where capacity is less than or *equal* to demand. Yes, you read correctly. When demand is equal to capacity, waiting lines or inventory build up. In fact, they build up to infinity if the system is not altered to have capacity exceed demand. This is referred to as **undercapacity scheduling**, the situation where capacity strictly *exceeds* demand. Is it inefficient? No, it is not. In Lean, employees are never idle. They are supposed to always look for ways to improve the process. Having reasonable time to do so enables them to propose ways to improve the system. Furthermore, flexible employees are routinely reassigned to areas where demand suddenly peaks in order to rebalance the workload (Principle #1).

PRINCIPLE #10: LINK LAYOUT AND PROCESS

Many of the non–value-added steps in a process consist of avoidable movements and travel. Ideally, the layout of the work environment should be designed to optimize the workflow and prevent wasteful traffic. Nursing staff spends a lot of time walking. This time would be better spent on patient care activities as well as interactions with patients' family members. Recent nursing unit designs feature decentralized nurses' stations that permit the distribution of staff members closer to the POC. The placement of medication and supply storage areas near (or in) patients' rooms also decreases time spent walking, thereby boosting productivity (Thurston, 2017). To support the continuum of care, cancer centers design facilities that optimize the patient's journey through the system with a minimum number of steps. They also create staff spaces that encourage communication and collaboration among the members of the care team (Vaughan, 2023).

THE RELATIONSHIP BETWEEN PROCESS AND LAYOUT

Ideally, the layout of the physical environment should facilitate the effective and efficient movement of flow units (patients, employees, materials, information, etc.) through the system. Common objectives include (Stevenson & Kull, 2024):

1. reducing errors;
2. utilizing resources and space efficiently;
3. avoiding delays and bottlenecks;
4. minimizing handoffs;
5. minimizing movements and transfers; and
6. ensuring safety.

TABLE 10.3 DIFFERENTIATING BETWEEN PRODUCT AND FUNCTIONAL LAYOUTS

	Product Layout	Functional Layout
1. Description	Sequential arrangement of activities dedicated to a specific service	Functional arrangement of activities accommodating a variety of services/patients
2. Process type	Standard and repetitive (with a few options)	Customized and variable
3. Demand	Stable	Fluctuating
4. Volume	High	Low
5. Resources	Specialized	Flexible
6. Flow	Fixed	Variable
7. Objective of design	Balance the workload at each step of the process	Minimize wasted movements/transfers
8. Layout design techniques	Line balancing	Block diagramming; relationship diagramming
9. Advantages	Faster processing, fewer delays, less transportation, fewer hand-offs, clear and streamlined flow	Flexibility, opportunity for high performance quality
10. Disadvantages	Low flexibility	High cost and time Jumbled flow

Source: Adapted from Russell, R. S., & Taylor, B. W. (2023). *Operations and supply chain management* (11th ed.). Wiley.

There are two basic layouts: a product layout and a functional layout. The main characteristics of each one are listed in Table 10.3 (Russell & Taylor, 2023). A product layout would be suitable for a lab: high and stable volume; a functional layout, in contrast, is the norm in hospitals where the various specialties (surgery, radiology, ophthalmology, etc.) are organized in separate departments, with each one experiencing variable demand.

DESIGNING PRODUCT LAYOUTS FOR REPETITIVE PROCESSES

In healthcare, repetitive processes are more common in high-volume support services (e.g., registration, scheduling, billing, and claims processing) than in clinical areas. However, keep in mind that blood sample processing and certain clinical procedures are high-volume, repetitive operations, similar to an assembly line in manufacturing (Box 10.6). The high volume requires a rapid flow through the process with as few hurdles and handoffs as possible. The best way to meet this requirement is to organize the resources (equipment and people) around the service and standardize procedures for consistent quality, that is, to adopt a **product layout**. This layout involves a sequential arrangement of activities dedicated to a standard product or service.

BOX 10.6 QUALITY IN PRACTICE!

Assembly Lines for Cardiac Surgeries

At Narayana Health in India, surgeons perform highly complicated cardiac procedures at a very low cost. U.K.-trained Dr. Devi Shetty, a world-renowned cardiac surgeon, founded Narayana Health in 2001 to provide high-quality cardiac care to all people, irrespective of their ability to pay. To accomplish this feat, he relied on Lean principles to eradicate waste and achieved economies of scale with high-volume surgeries in efficient operating theaters. An assembly-line approach to surgery with low setup times, surgeons practicing at the top of their license, and few unnecessary motions drives the efficiency and low error rate. A daily examination of key performance indicators (KPIs) contributes to the constant pursuit of excellence (Altstedter, 2019).

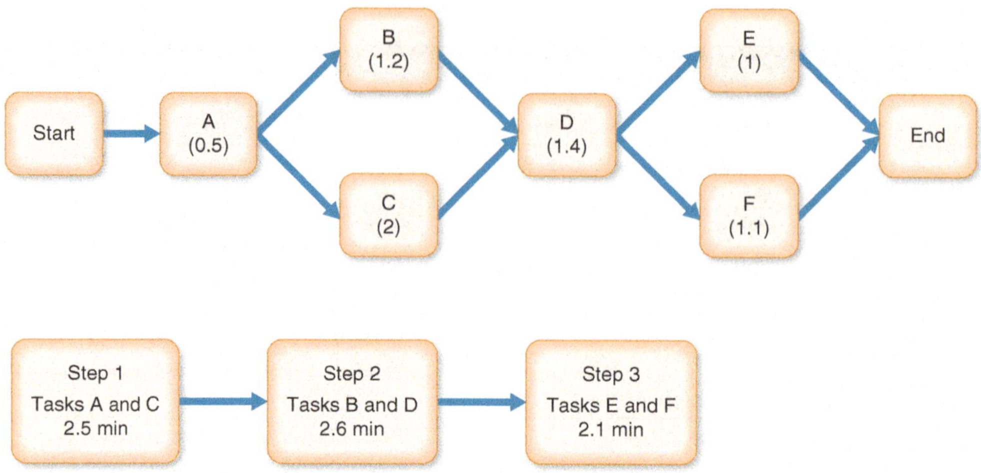

The total time to complete the 3 steps is 2.5 + 2.6 + 2.1 min. However, the resources at Step 1 start processing the second flow unit as soon as they are done with the first one, and so on. Most of the time, there will be 3 flow units in the system. Consecutive units will exit the system every 2.6 min (takt time).

FIGURE 10.5 Balanced process based on a set of tasks and their precedence relationships.

If each process task was performed sequentially by a different employee, people performing short tasks would often be idle, whereas people completing long tasks would see their backlog—buffer—increase. The stop-and-go process would be extremely inefficient and frustrating. It is thus imperative to group tasks into process steps with approximately equal workloads. **Line balancing** is a trial-and-error technique that equalizes workload requirements subject to cycle time and precedence relationship constraints. Its objective is to develop an efficient layout with the *lowest* possible number of process steps, which ensures few handoffs. Line balancing seeks to align the cycle time with the takt time. Note that a process can *never* go faster than its *slowest* step (Figure 10.5; see section on theory of constraints). Accordingly, the takt time is also viewed as the longest time allowed at a process step in order to meet output requirements. A balanced line is one of the prerequisites for a pull system.

A balanced process is shown in Figure 10.5. At the top, the network shows the various tasks to complete, their respective durations, and the order in which they have to be performed. At the bottom, the balanced process illustrates some important design features: it includes three steps, which results in only two handoffs. Moreover, the times to execute each group of tasks are relatively constant, ensuring minimal buffers between steps and steady productivity at each step. The longest step time is 2.6 minutes. It dictates the pace of the process. Every 2.6 minutes, a flow unit will exit the system.

DESIGNING FUNCTIONAL LAYOUTS FOR NONREPETITIVE PROCESSES

Functional layouts are suitable for customized, lower-volume, high-variety processes, which require flexible resources to perform diverse activities on diverse flow units. Dedicating resources assigned to fixed tasks, such as in the product layout, would result in low-capacity utilization and excess cost. Instead, a **functional layout** organizes resources into departments or areas of expertise and supports variable paths among these areas. Although less efficient than product layouts, functional layouts should also be designed with the objective of reducing waste by eliminating excess movements and transfers along the paths. A popular and intuitive method used to create functional layouts is relationship diagramming.

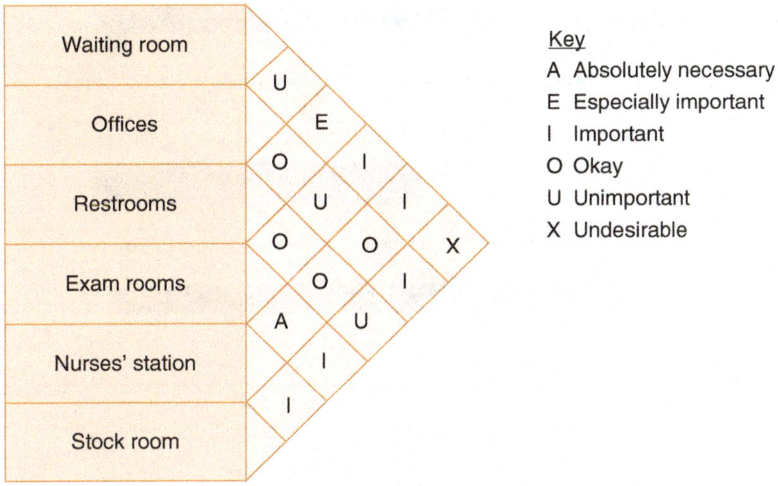

FIGURE 10.6 Muther's grid.

Relationship Diagramming

Relationship diagramming utilizes qualitative information provided by analysts, managers, and workers to establish relationship preferences between pairs of departments, workstations, or offices. It is common to use Muther's (1961) grid to reflect preferences coded as A, E, I, O, U, or X. Although X denotes an undesirable proximity between two rooms or departments, the vowels refer to various degrees of preferred proximity between such pairs. Figure 10.6 is a simple illustration of Muther's grid for a clinic. Although the waiting room should not (X) be next to the storage and supply room to prevent theft, it is absolutely necessary (A) to locate the nurses' station close to the exam rooms for easy access; it is especially important (E) to have the restrooms located close to the waiting room; it is important (I) to have the storage and supply room near the exam rooms to access medical supplies; it is okay (O) to have the nurses' station close to the offices, but it is unimportant (U) to have those offices located near the exam rooms.

Muther's grid is then used to develop a relationship diagram and evaluate the appropriateness of current or proposed layouts. The thickness of the lines indicates the extent to which close proximity is desirable. Ideally, thick lines (I, E, and A) should be short and have few, if any, angles or zigzags, whereas thin lines (U and O) can be of any length and can even be omitted from the diagram to enhance clarity. Dashed lines indicate undesirable proximity. As shown in Figure 10.7A, the storage and supply room is in very close proximity to the waiting room when it should not be; the nurses' station is too far from the exam rooms, resulting in a lot of extra traffic every day; the restrooms are not conveniently located for patients in the waiting room; and the exam rooms are too far from the stockroom to facilitate restocking. The layout in Figure 10.7B is much improved in that it fulfills most of the requirements expressed in Muther's grid. Perhaps, the building could also be remodeled to create a straight path between the nurses' station and the storage and supply room.

CELLULAR LAYOUTS

By now, you must have grasped that the main benefits of the product layout are its simplicity and efficiency, whereas the main benefit of the functional layout is its versatility in accommodating a variety of flow units. A long-held view in healthcare is that all patients are different. Manufacturers faced the same issues decades ago when the relatively low volumes of some products made it too costly for them to dedicate resources to the production of these items. The solution involved the formation of "families" of products or services with similar processing requirements

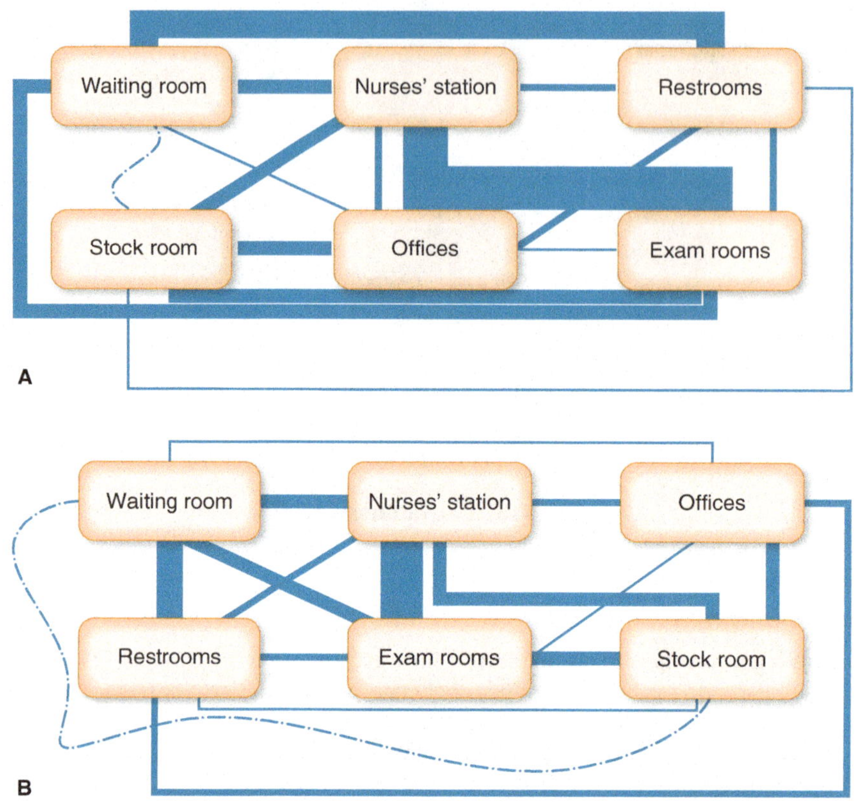

FIGURE 10.7 **(A) Relationship diagram for existing layout; (B) relationship diagram for revised layout.**

(e.g., motorcycles and jet skis). These natural groupings created a volume substantial enough to dedicate resources to their production. As the products within a family shared common process characteristics, the benefits of standardization could be reaped, and the cost penalties of switching from one product to the other were minimal.

The hybrid system that enables the coexistence of efficiency and diversity is the **cellular layout.** It does so by combining certain attributes of the product layout and certain attributes of the functional layout. It is essentially a mini-plant within a plant. In healthcare, this concept is becoming increasingly popular (Box 10.7). Let us take the example of a patient with prostate cancer. In a traditional system organized by functions, one patient may visit a urologist in one facility and then go to two separate locations for an ultrasound and lab tests. After another visit to the urology clinic, the patient may undergo surgery at the main hospital, followed by chemotherapy in yet another facility. One argument in favor of this functional layout is that it can accommodate an extremely diverse patient population with different ailments and treatment needs. The drawbacks are obvious: waste of time, waste of movements, handoffs, opportunities for communication breakdowns, patient's frustration, and fluctuations in providers' utilization. The solution is to create a urology center or wing that will diagnose and treat all urology patients. These patients are diverse, but they do share similar medical conditions. Grouping them as a "patient family" may generate the volume necessary to operate a facility dedicated to providing a comprehensive range of treatment services for these patients. The benefits are reduced movement, fewer care delays, easier tracking of patient's progress, more consistent utilization of resources, and increased standardization of care based on best practices (Figure 10.8).

BOX 10.7 QUALITY IN PRACTICE!

The Patient Hub Concept

Traditional hospitals were designed to optimize the expertise of the care team in each area and to focus on the efficient delivery of care in the most economical fashion. This resulted in siloed and segmented specialized clinics and departments, with an intent to minimize cost and maximize the use of dedicated infrastructure. Along the way, the best interest of the patient got lost. Amato et al. (2022) explored 3D software to optimize workflows that create what the authors term a patient hub. This is a patient-centric model in which all critical functions occur in the same building and on the same floor. This eliminates the non–value-added steps such as wait and transfer times, simplifies wayfinding, and reduces elevator travel. Most importantly, this allows for the delivery of multidisciplinary care and the interaction of multiple specialists who can confer and agree on the ideal treatment plan for a given patient. This proof-of-concept model still needs to be vetted in an actual clinical delivery location.

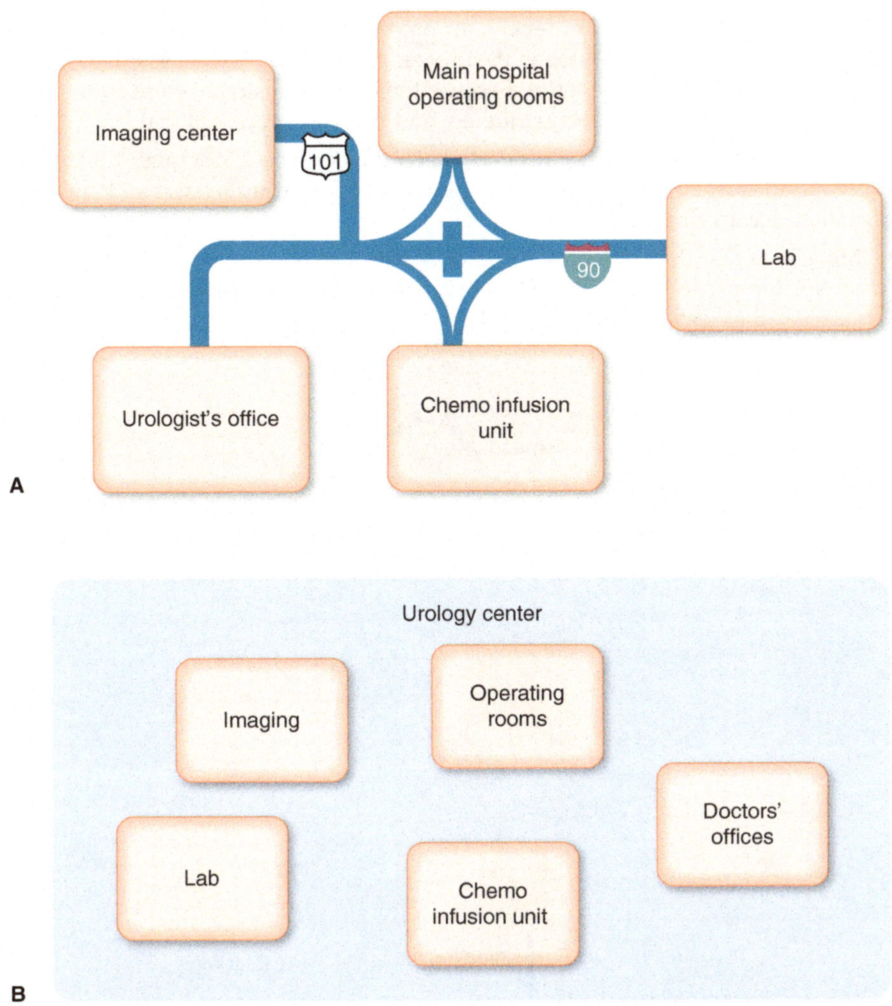

FIGURE 10.8 **Functional layout (A) versus cellular layout (B) for urology.**

THEORY OF CONSTRAINTS

As you already know, buffers cause congestion in the system. This type of congestion is called a bottleneck. As explained in Principle #9, a bottleneck involves a situation in which demand is greater than or equal to capacity (Figure 10.9). The bottleneck places a constraint on the system and restricts the flow. The constraint is the weakest link. The **theory of constraints (TOC)** is a popular methodology to identify and improve a constraint until it no longer burdens the system. "The entire bottleneck concept is not geared to decrease operating expense, it's focused on increasing throughput" (Goldratt, 2004, p. 298.).

The bottleneck is the slowest step in the process. As you know from the section on line balancing and will see in Figure 10.10, it determines the speed of the process. This is why the TOC calls for releasing flow units into the system at the pace of the bottleneck server/resource. To demonstrate the viability of this concept to business organizations, Goldratt (2004) wrote a novel, *The Goal*, which covers the troubles and eventual success of a plant manager in a fictitious manufacturing organization. The plant is plagued by late deliveries to customers and huge amounts of work-in-process (or queues) inventory inside the plant. While on a hike with a troop of Boy Scouts, the plant manager notices the similarity between the flow of goods in his plant and the flow of Boy Scouts on the trail. What happens is illustrated in Figures 10.10A to 10.10C.

TOC comprises five steps:

STEP 1: Identify the constraint or bottleneck. In process management, this would involve the identification of the slowest step in the process, that is, the one whose utilization is highest and cannot fulfill the demand. Because the pace of upstream steps in the process is faster, you will see a lot of delays, queues, and work-in-process at that step.

STEP 2: Exploit the constraint. It is important to keep the bottleneck resources utilized because every minute lost at the bottleneck is a minute lost for the entire system. Ways to accomplish this objective include:

- Make sure that the bottleneck resource always has work to do. A reasonable amount of work-in-process in front of the bottleneck is desirable because we do not want to "starve" that resource and further delay the work that it needs to perform.

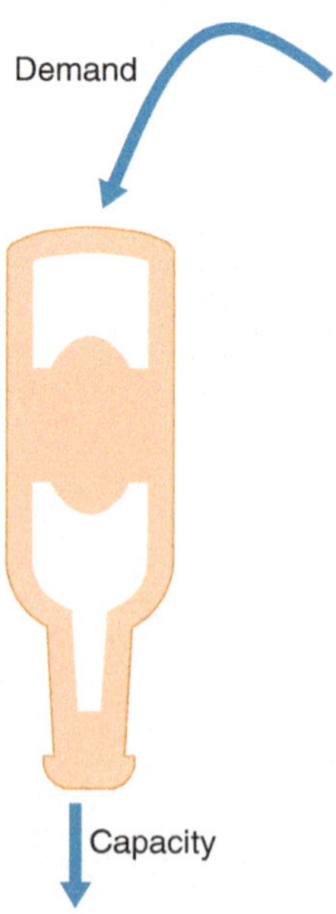

FIGURE 10.9 Bottleneck = neck of a bottle.

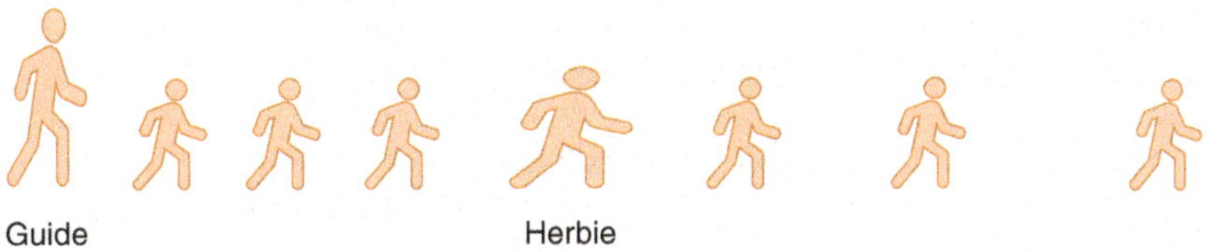

A The Boy Scouts walk in file, with the guide at the end of the file to make sure that no one stays behind. Each Boy Scout walks at his own pace, unconcerned about what is happening behind him. Soon, gaps appear between the Boy Scouts.

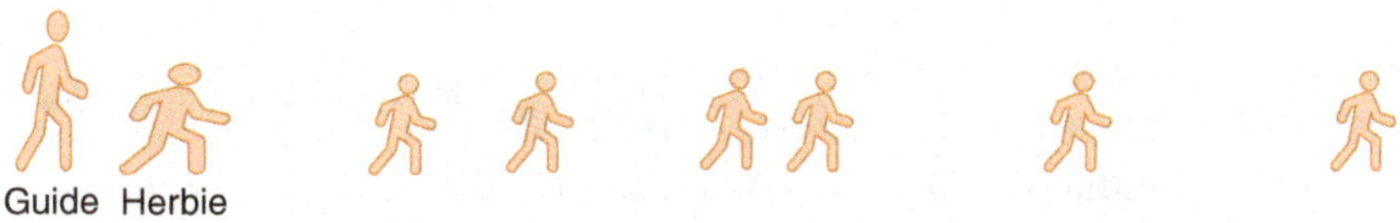

B One of the Boy Scouts, Herbie, is not very athletic and carries a heavy backpack. As time passes, his slower pace pushes him further and further behind, and the gaps between the Boy Scouts keep widening. These gaps worry the guide as he senses a loss of control over the hike.

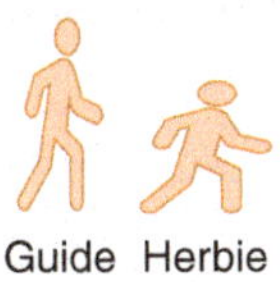

C When the first Boy Scout arrives at the camp site, can the fun begin? No, the entire troop and the guide must be at the camp site to start the fire and set up the tents. As you can see above, this only happens when Herbie, the slowest Boy Scout, arrives.

Moral of the story: *The pace of the bottleneck sets the pace for the entire system.*

The plant manager realizes that the same happens at his plant. Every work center works at its own pace, and the volume of goods each one generates exceeds the capacity of the most constrained resource, that is, the bottleneck. The result is a growing amount of work-in-process inventory in front of the bottleneck. In the end, the product cannot be sold (The GOAL) until all processing steps, including the bottleneck step, have been completed.

FIGURE 10.10 The hike as narrated in *The Goal*.

Note: (A) Boy Scouts walking in file. (B) Gaps widen; Herbie is behind. (C) Entire troop's arrival at camp site.

- Make sure that resources are always available at the bottleneck, for example, by staggering lunch breaks.
- Always perform quality control before the bottleneck. The precious time at the bottleneck cannot be wasted on defective items that might be discarded anyway.
- If equipment is used, ensure that maintenance occurs during off hours. Again, we do not want to risk a loss of productive time because of a breakdown.

STEP 3: Subordinate everything else to the constraint. Make the speed of the bottleneck the speed at which work is released (i.e., arrivals) into the process and the speed at which all other process resources work. In other words, make Herbie lead the troop to the camp site. But that will be so slow! How do we make Herbie go faster?

STEP 4: Elevate the constraint. Find ways to increase the capacity of the bottleneck by pulling unutilized resources from some other areas, or, if necessary, by subcontracting. Influence the demand placed on the bottleneck by making process changes that render the bottleneck step unnecessary for at least some flow units, and by eliminating as much non–value-added time at the bottleneck as possible. It is critical that the bottleneck resource work only on what is needed! Let's check Herbie's backpack and remove the iron skillet, the six-pack of soda, and so forth. You get the idea.

STEP 5: If the constraint is broken, do not rest on your laurels. Go back to step 1 and find a new constraint.

BRIGHT ANGEL MEDICAL CENTER 10.2

Adeleke and Olina were sitting in Barbara's office. Barbara leaned back in her chair and asked, "So, it's been less than 2 weeks since we met. Do you have a few ideas to sort out this mess?" Olina and Adeleke exchanged a smile.

"A few ideas? Just look at the first page of this report to see the list of proposed improvements," Adeleke said. Barbara sat straight up and opened the report. The first thing she saw was a bunch of bullet points. She read:

1. ***Reduce unnecessary movements***
   - *Portable x-ray machine*
   - *Medications stored in ED (kanban system for replenishment)*
   - *Improve layout (see Muther's grid; Exhibit 10.1)*
2. ***Standardize***
   - *Checklist for discharge*
   - *6S in supply and exam rooms*
3. ***Mistake-proof the system***
   - *Poka-yoke for ensuring transport gets the correct room number*
4. ***Improve predictability***
   - *Supplier certification (no need for inspection)*
   - *TPM in lab*
   - *Dedicated machine for the complete blood count (CBC) in lab*
   - *Kanban system for replenishment of supplies in each exam room*
5. ***Increase the agility of the system***
   - *Decrease turnover time in exam rooms*
   - *Training for flexibility*
   - *Staff the vaccination clinic in October with a nurse from a department other than the ED (ED is already a bottleneck)*
   - *Mixed-level scheduling at vaccination clinic*
6. ***Improve customer service***
   - *Signs in ED with expected wait*
   - *Vending machines*
7. ***Adopt a holistic approach***
   - *Lean bundles*

EXHIBIT 10.1 MUTHER'S GRID TO DESIGN NEW LAYOUT (REDUCED TRAVEL + HIGHER SAFETY)

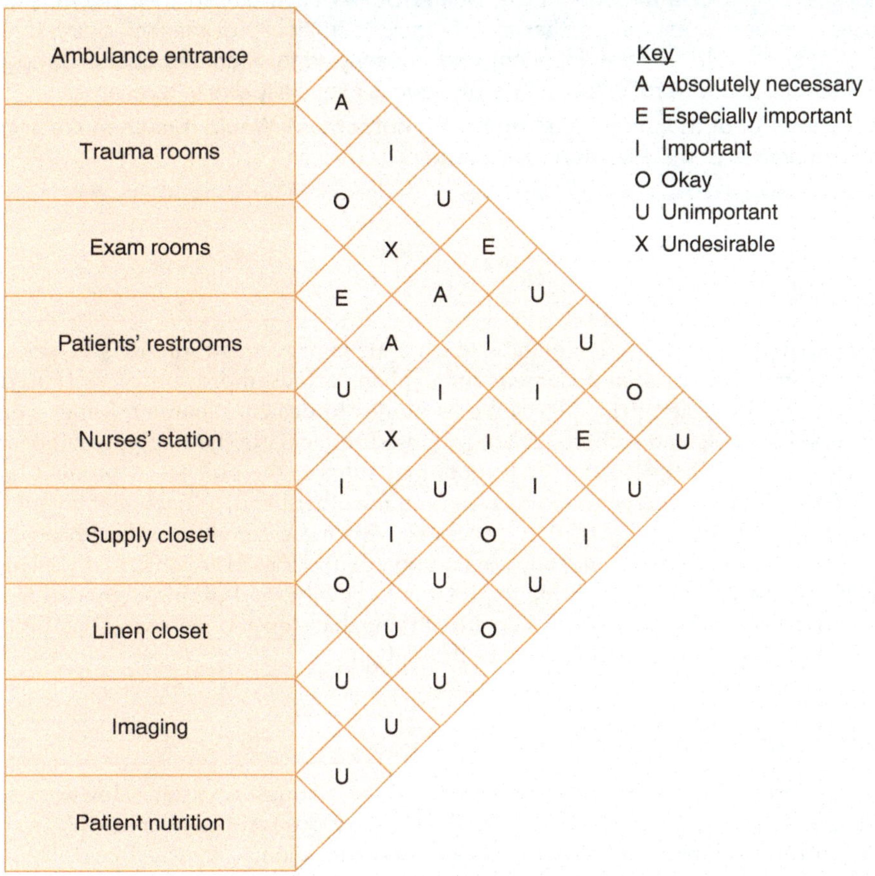

Barbara looked up, "I'm amazed. AMAZED! The team did that in just a few days?"

Olina replied, "That's the reward for being patient and doing a thorough analysis. We knew exactly what was wrong, and it made it so much easier to make suggestions for improvement."

Barbara stood up. "I'm taking this to our COO right now. Mira'd better be impressed."

Adeleke ventured, "The rumor is she is looking for a new job . . . she never got over being passed over for the CEO position."

Barbara replied, "If that is the case, this project will be a plus on her resume. I'm sure she'll be delighted."

Can you add to the list of improvements in the report? Justify your additions.

ETHICAL SCENARIO 10.1

ED or no ED? That's the Question!

Many hospital-based EDs throughout the United States have closed their doors. Some of the closures are due to mergers. Other factors include: difficulty of managing an increasing number of patients with a stable inpatient bed capacity, high operating costs, competition, safety-net status, and for-profit status. The situation is especially dire in rural areas.

What is the impact of those closures on health outcomes? Would it even make sense to redesign processes in the EDs that lose money?

SUMMARY

This chapter started the conversation on how to generate improvement solutions. A series of secondary sources are proposed that document and explain various improvement tools used in the healthcare sector. Ten design principles serve as guides to design a simpler, leaner, and more robust process. LSS tools and techniques are proposed to facilitate the implementation of each principle. One of the principles calls for layouts that support the process. A product layout is well suited for high-volume, repetitive processes. On the other hand, a functional layout is more appropriate for low-volume, high-variety processes, which are common in healthcare. Hybrid layouts are becoming more common. They accommodate situations in which a relatively high volume of flow units have similar processing requirements. Finally, the TOC highlights the fact that a process cannot go faster than its slowest step. Identifying that step and managing it appropriately help remove a process constraint and improve throughput.

CERTIFICATION TIPS

Process design principles and layouts are *not* part of the certification exam. However, all Lean tools and the TOC are included. Know each tool and its purpose and be able to *apply* it. Also, do learning activities 3, 4, 5, and 7 to prepare yourself for certification.

KEY TERMS

Process design
Handoff
Job enlargement
Job enrichment
Quality at the source
Standardization of work
Cycle time
6S
Takt time
Leveling the workload (*heijunka*)
Setup time
Just-in-time (JIT)
Buffer
Kanban system
Bottleneck
Undercapacity scheduling
Product layout
Line balancing
Functional layout
Relationship diagramming
Cellular layout
Theory of constraints (TOC)

REVIEW QUESTIONS

1. List five design principles and explain them.
2. What is *heijunka*?
3. What is *jidoka*?
4. What are the 6S? Describe each one briefly.
5. What is TPM? Should clinicians get involved in that program? Explain.

6. What is *poka-yoke*? Name three examples of its use in healthcare.
7. What are common objectives of layouts?
8. Differentiate between functional and product layouts in terms of process type, demand, volume, and resources.
9. What are the steps of the theory of constraints?
10. What is the purpose of line balancing?
11. Is a cellular layout appropriate for healthcare? Justify your answer.

SOLVE BRIGHT ANGEL MEDICAL CENTER'S PROBLEMS

1. One hundred and eighty routine complaints need to be processed by Patient Services staff in a given week. The process includes five steps, each staffed by a different employee. The staff works 8 hours a day, 5 days a week.
   a. Assuming no rest break, what is the takt time? What does it mean?
   b. If the employees take daily breaks totaling 45 minutes at the same time, what is the takt time? Compared to your answer in part (a), what do you conclude?
2. Ninety bills have to be processed by the billing office staff in a given day. The process includes four steps, each staffed by a different employee. The staff works 9 hours a day.
   a. Assuming the employees' daily breaks total 1 hour, what is the takt time? What does it mean?
   b. The longest step takes 6 minutes. How many bills can be processed in 1 day (assuming the staff takes the rest breaks mentioned in part [a])?
3. The routine complaints mentioned in problem 1 fall into three categories: quality of care, billing, and wait time. Last week (5 work days), the number of complaints in each category was as follows:

Complaint	Number
Quality of care (Q)	30
Billing (B)	90
Wait time (W)	60

   The manager of Patient Services has decided to level the workload.
   a. Find the number of daily cycles during which the complaint processing sequence will be repeated.
   b. Find the number of each type of complaint in each cycle.
   c. Determine the daily sequence if: (i) the setup between complaints is minimal, and (ii) it is not negligible, but not overly complex.
4. Jan has just finished her LSS training. Her work involves a four-step process as shown in the following graphic.

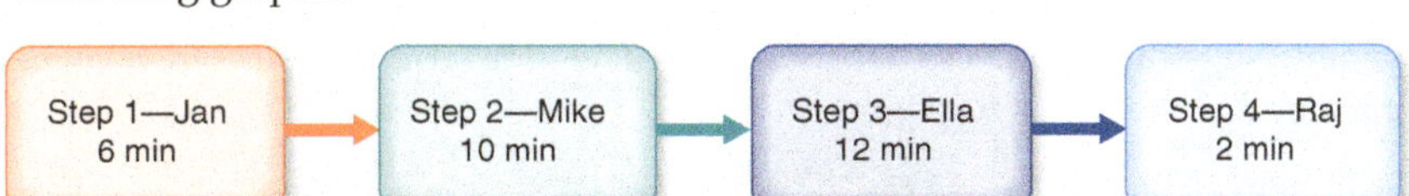

   She told her manager that she and her colleagues could each do all four steps. In other words, she would perform steps 1 to 4 and so would Mike, Ella, and Raj. Assuming that each one is equally qualified to do all steps,
   a. What is the throughput (jobs/hr) with the current process design?
   b. What is the throughput (jobs/hr) for the proposed process design?
   c. Which principles of process design did Jan use for her proposed improvement?

5. A very satisfied patient has made a sizeable donation to the plastic surgery clinic at BAMC. The funds will be used to remodel the outdated facility so that the new layout will support the workflow. After talking with the staff and making observations on her own, the office manager developed Muther's grid and then came up with the following relationship diagram. Redesign the layout according to the relationship diagram's requirements. The only constraint is that room E cannot be located anywhere else.

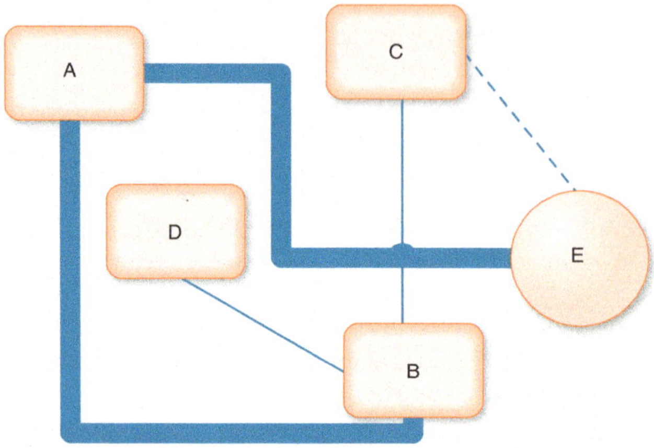

6. The Imaging Department wants to move the locations of its five clerks' offices to better improve the workflow. A team has developed Muther's grid and the following diagram. Redesign the layout according to the relationship diagram's requirements. The walls cannot be moved; each clerk's office (A, B, C, D, and E) can be placed in another location.

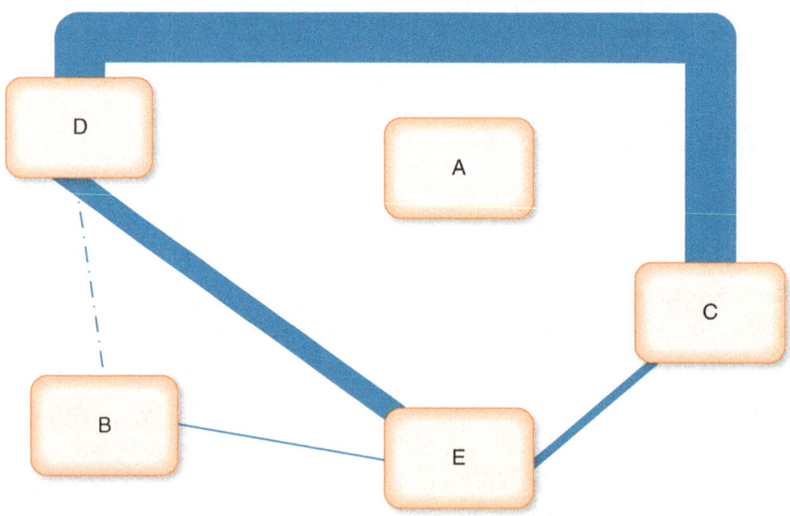

7. The following patient registration process has four steps. The time required to perform all tasks at each step is indicated in the following figure.

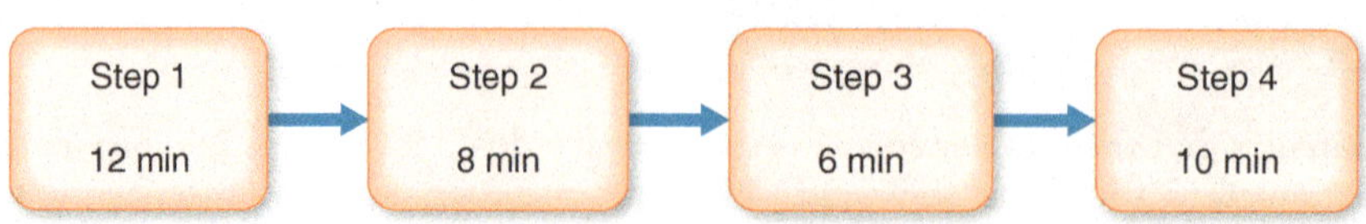

a. The demand rate is five patients per hour. Is there a bottleneck? Explain why or why not.
b. The demand rate is four patients per hour. Is there a bottleneck? Explain why or why not.
c. Which step is the constraint and limits throughput?

8. The following discharge process has five steps. The time required to perform all tasks at each step is indicated in the following figure.

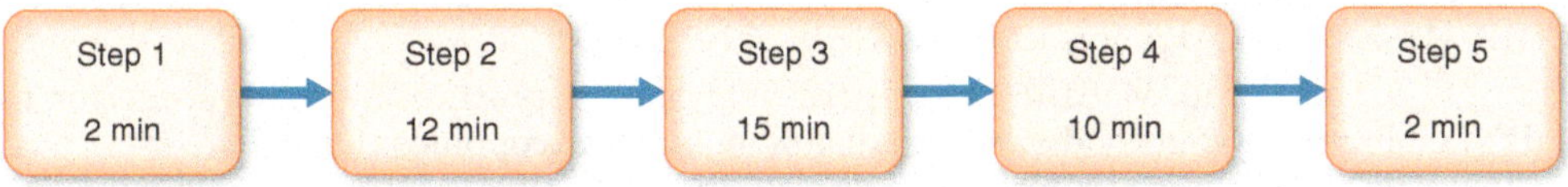

   a. Six patients need to be discharged every hour. Is there a bottleneck? Explain why or why not.
   b. Four patients need to be discharged every hour. Is there a bottleneck? Explain why or why not.

LEARNING ACTIVITIES

1. Go to one of the sources listed in Table 10.1. What valuable information did you find to improve processes?
2. Provide examples of human-centered design in healthcare.
3. Mock interview. The interviewer questions the interviewee, Dr. Devi Shetty, on cardiac surgery and layout, specifically on how to streamline the flow for lower costs and better quality. Hint: Research the biography and work of Dr. Devi Shetty before conducting the interview.
4. In the BAMC example, the imaging step is a bottleneck. List all possible ways to elevate the constraint.
5. How can you reduce setup time in the OR? What is the difference between an internal and an external setup?
6. Find an article that describes the standardization of surgical instrument trays. How did they do it? What were the benefits? Example: https://www.arthroplastyjournal.org/article/S0883-5403(21)00081-4/abstract (download the article).
7. How can you apply the 6S methodology in your own immediate work environment? In your own house?
8. You are making a presentation and must explain why capacity must always exceed demand to avoid bottlenecks. This is actually a queuing problem. Under many circumstances, the following queuing formula applies:

$$\text{Size of queue} = \frac{(\textit{Demand rate})^2}{(\textit{Capacity rate}) \times (\textit{Capacity rate} - \textit{demand rate})}$$

Use an example where capacity matches demand: demand rate = 5 patients/hr; capacity rate = 5 patients/hr. See what happens?

REFERENCES

Ahuja, D., Gullekson, R., & Kim, A. (2016). *Total productive maintenance in the OR—a case study at Kadlec Regional Medical Center Society for Health Systems*. https://www.iise.org/uploadedfiles/SHSNew/Tools_and_Resources/TPM%20Paper.doc

Altstedter, A. (2019, March 25). *The world's cheapest hospital has to get even cheaper*. Bloomberg Businessweek. https://www.bloomberg.com/news/features/2019-03-26/the-world-s-cheapest-hospital-has-to-get-even-cheaper

Amato, C., McCanne, L., Yang, C., Ostler, D., Ratib, O., Wilhelm, D., & Bernhard, L. (2022). The hospital of the future: Rethinking architectural design to enable new patient-centered treatment concepts. *International Journal of Computer-Assisted Radiology and Surgery, 17*, 1177–1187. https://doi.org/10.1007/s11548-021-02540-9

Gkorezis, P., & Theodorou, M. (2016). High-performance work practices in healthcare sector. In P. Manolitzas, E. Grigoroudis, N. Matsatsinis, & D. Yannacopoulos (Eds.), *Effective methods for modern healthcare service quality and evaluation* (pp. 16–44). Medical Information Science Reference (IGI Global).

Goldratt, E. M. (2004). *The goal: A process of ongoing improvement* (3rd ed.). Gower.

IDEO.org. (2024). *Design kit: Methods*. https://www.designkit.org/methods.html

Jack, B. W., Austad, K., Renfro, D. R., & Mitchell, S. (2023). Re-engineering the hospital discharge to improve the transition from hospital to home: Overview and a look to the future. *Journal of Healthcare Management Standards, 3*(1), 1–17. https://doi.org/10.4018/JHMS.328775

Johns Hopkins Medicine. (2024). *Central line insertion care team checklist*. https://www.hopkinsmedicine.org/-/media/heic/cl-insertion-checklist.pdf

Laguna, M., & Marklund, J. (2019). *Business process, modeling, simulation, and design* (3rd ed.). Routledge.

Muther, R. (1961). *Systematic layout planning*. Industrial Education Institute.

Paige, M. (2019). *Just-in-time inventory: Sustainability with the direct primary care*. Healthcare Business Today. https://www.healthcarebusinesstoday.com/just-in-time-inventory

Peters, A. W., Chawla, K. S., & Turnbull, Z. A. (2020). Transforming ORs into ICUs. *New England Journal of Medicine, 382*, e52. https://doi.org/10.1056/NEJMc2010853

Russell, R. S., & Taylor, B. W. (2023). *Operations and supply chain management* (11th ed.). Wiley.

Safety Culture. (2024, June 13). *What is standardized work?* https://safetyculture.com/topics/standardized-work

Saporito, A., Tassone, C., Di Iorio, A., Barbieri Saraceno, M., Bressan, A., Pini, R., Mongelli, F., & La Regina, D. (2023). Six Sigma can significantly reduce costs of poor quality of the surgical instruments sterilization process and improve surgeon and operating room personnel satisfaction. *Scientific Reports, 13*, 14116. https://doi.org/10.1038/s41598-023-41393-x

Steve Jobs. (1998). Steve Jobs: 'There's Sanity Returning'. *Business Week*.

Stevenson, W. J., & Kull, T. J. (2024). *Operations and supply chain management*. McGraw-Hill.

Thurston, T. (2017). *Top 6 design practices for patient care units*. Medical Construction Design. https://mcdmag.com/2017/12/top-6-design-practices-for-patient-care-units/

Vaughan, M. W. (2023, October 27). *A tailored approach to cancer center design*. Healthcare Design. https://healthcaredesignmagazine.com/trends/a-tailored-approach-to-cancer-center-design

CHAPTER 11

PROCESS REDESIGN (II): ENSURING SUCCESS

BRIGHT ANGEL MEDICAL CENTER 11.1

Adeleke had convened all the permanent members of the improvement team. He seemed more relaxed than usual. He started the meeting by thanking each one of them for the work accomplished thus far. He beamed, "The leadership team is impressed with our recommendations for improvement. What got us this far is our methodical approach. Let's not lose sight of that. We should create a vision for what the new process will be . . . and make sure it works before we proceed with the full implementation. What do you think?"

They all nodded.

Why is a vision of the future state of the process important? Does it delay urgent improvements?

LEARNING OBJECTIVES

After reading this chapter, you will be able to:

- Visualize the future state from different angles.
- Appreciate the role of simulation in approximating the value contributed by the new process.
- Perform a cost–benefit analysis.
- Evaluate the success of the project in general, and of the improvements in particular.

INTRODUCTION

As you all know, a picture is worth a thousand words. In Chapter 6, you visualized the "old" process and identified its shortcomings. Now, it is time to visualize the "new process" and evaluate its viability. It is important to remain focused on customers' needs and wants. How much value does the improved process add? Fortunately, you do not always have to implement the process "for real" to find out. Simulation enables you to approximate the impact of the improvements and decide whether some solutions need to be tweaked, discarded, or implemented as they are. You will also remember that one of the project constraints is cost (Chapter 5). Cost–benefit analyses should be conducted to determine whether the improvements can be implemented within budget and have a positive financial impact. Once these precautionary measures have been taken, the implementation can proceed. Again, measurement will be key to determine whether success has been achieved.

WHY IS THIS MATERIAL USEFUL?

Depicting the future state of the process is an effective way to communicate what the revised process should "look like." Process improvements can be very expensive. Making sure that their chances of success are maximized before implementation is a wise, disciplined approach. A serious project team should not let emotions and enthusiasm take precedence over caution, even at this exciting stage of the project. Once improvements deemed worthy are implemented, process metrics will help confirm their success in creating value.

ON THE JOB! INTERVIEW VIDEO 11.1

Brian Dotter
Senior Director of Pharmacy

Cross-Functional Collaboration to Ensure Success
Pharmacy supply chain
Detecting and deterring substance abuse and theft of controlled substances
Barcode medication administration
Setting up COVID vaccine clinics
Project progress reports

1. What are some of the keys to successful project management that Brian found helpful?
2. Is leading a systemwide project more complex than one involving only one department or facility? What do project leaders need to keep top-of-mind when engaging in work that includes departments or facilities in other communities?
3. Brian shares a Project Progress Report (PPR) for the barcode medication administration. What are the benefits to using this tool for the project team?

The interview is available online by visiting www.springerpub.com/courseconnect. See inside front cover and tear-out card for CourseConnect details.

THE FUTURE STATE

The **future state** of the process is essentially what it should be after improvement. Depicting the future state enables all stakeholders to visualize the opportunities for a smoother flow, higher efficiency, better outcomes, and improved customer satisfaction. In other words, it shows how waste has been minimized. The future state can be represented with a value stream map (VSM), a process activity chart, and a spaghetti diagram.

VALUE STREAM MAP

In Chapter 6, the VSM of the current process exposed the waste in the process. Remember that waste is anything that does not create value. The future state VSM does not mean that the process is completely free of waste, but it should demonstrate that the improvements will eradicate a substantial amount. The VSM developed by the Bright Angel Medical Center (BAMC) team follows. Notice the following improvements (Dalton-Norman, 2024; DeSai et al., 2021; Health Catalyst, 2024; Imhoff et al., 2022):

- **Registration**: The VSM reduced the number of questions from 17 to 3: name, date of birth, and primary complaint. The other questions are asked at the patient's bedside (performing activities in parallel). Results: Registration time is slashed by 7 minutes, and waiting time before that step decreases by 4 minutes.

- **Triage**: Vital signs are taken while patient is waiting (performing actions in parallel). Limit questions to those necessary to determine Emergency Severity Index (ESI) level. Results: Triage time is reduced from 10 to 5 minutes, and waiting time before that step decreases by 10 minutes.
- **Exam rooms**: All of them are placed close to waiting room and nurses' station. There is a straight path from the waiting room, and no obstruction from arrival of trauma patients. The changeover (setup) is divided into **internal** and **external setup**. The internal setup is the part of the changeover that must be done when the process at the relevant step is inactive (e.g., change the bedding when there is no patient in the room). The external setup can take place when the process is still ongoing (e.g., restock supply cabinet for the next patient when the exam room is still occupied). Results: Transport time is cut by 2 minutes, and changeover time is down to 6 minutes.
- **Exam by provider**: All required supplies are available in exam rooms. Result: Exam time is reduced from 20 to 17 minutes.
- **Phlebotomist**: During peak times, one floating phlebotomist is added in addition to the dedicated one. Pneumatic tube installed to send blood samples to lab. Result: Wait for phlebotomist is slashed from 10 to 3 minutes.
- **Lab**: Total productive maintenance, in addition to regularly scheduled maintenance, is implemented. There is a dedicated machine for complete blood count (CBC) tests. Results: Hardly any downtime is noted, speeding availability of test results from 35 to 15 minutes.
- **Imaging**: Most cases require a simple x-ray (Principle: design for the mainstream). A portable x-ray machine is available at the ED. For cases requiring more complex imaging, *poka-yoke* is used to ensure the transport gets the correct room number. Results: No more transport time to and from the Imaging Department in most cases; no wait at the Imaging Department in most cases; wait time for diagnostic test results is slashed from 20 to 10 minutes.
- **Medication**: High usage drugs are available in the ED with less reliance on a central pharmacy. Result: Treatment initiation is cut from 18 to 12 minutes.
- **Storage of linen and supplies**: 6S is implemented to ensure that only necessary supplies are kept and always placed in dedicated locations in the supply rooms. Result: There is easy retrieval of needed items.
- **Discharge**: A checklist helps the travel nurse perform this step properly (Principle: standardization). Discharge instructions are simplified. There is one printer at each nursing station. Patients wait in a monitored discharge lounge. Results: Discharge time is reduced by 3 minutes, and waiting time before discharge goes down to 16 minutes; reduced variation; beds in exam rooms are freed up faster; better instructions, fewer callbacks, and lower readmission rates.
- **Admission**: Training of ED providers is conducted to speed up bed request, standardization of bed request order, and communication protocol with admitting providers. Results: Admission process goes down to 15 minutes, and wait time before admission is reduced from 60 to 35 minutes, with less variation.
- **Transfer**: The VSM will centralize patient transfer so that only one number has to be called; checklist with streamlined transfer process; better collaboration with different health systems to increase provider capacity. Result: The wait for transfer goes from 90 to 30 minutes, with less variation.

PROCESS ACTIVITY CHART

In Chapter 6, you used process activity charts to determine which steps were value-added and which ones were not. Consistent with the VSM in Figure 11.1, the future state process activity chart for an admitted patient in Table 11.1 shows that when non–value-added activities could not be eliminated, their duration was reduced drastically.

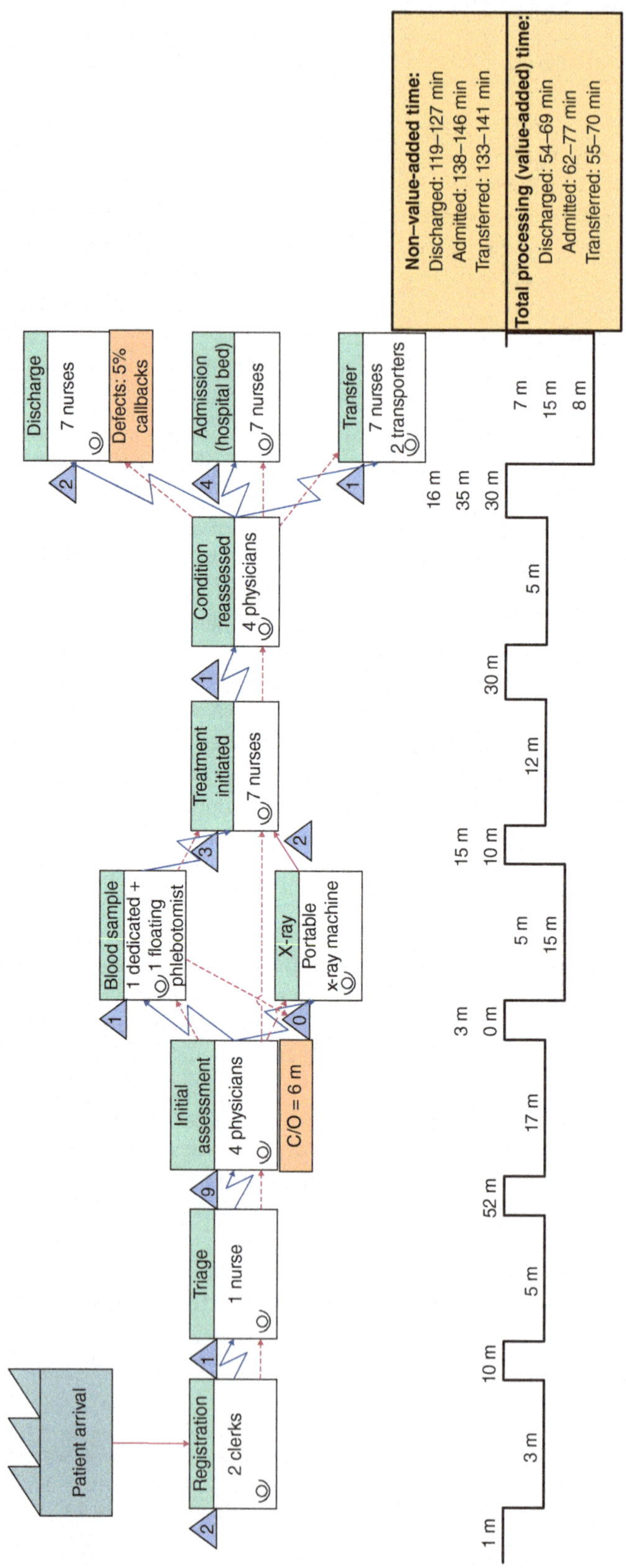

FIGURE 11.1 Future state value stream map (VSM) of patient flow in the ED.

TABLE 11.1 FUTURE STATE PROCESS ACTIVITY CHART FOR AN ED PATIENT WITH BOTH DIAGNOSTIC TESTS AND BEING ADMITTED

No.	Description	Time (min)	Distance	Value Code (V/N/B)	Symbol
1	Patient arrives.	1	100 ft	V	
2	Patient waits.	1		N	
3	Patient is registered.	3		B	
4	Patient waits.	10		N	
5	Patient is triaged.	5		B	
6	Patient waits.	51		N	
7	Patient goes to exam room.	1	100 ft	N	
8	Patient is examined by physician.	17		V	
9	Patient waits for phlebotomist.	3		N	
10	Patient's blood is drawn.	5		V	
11	Patient's images are taken.	15		V	
12	Patient waits.	10		N	
13	Treatment is initiated.	12		V	
14	Patient waits.	30		N	
15	Patient's condition is reassessed.	5		V	
16	Patient waits.	35		N	
17	Patient is admitted.	15		V	

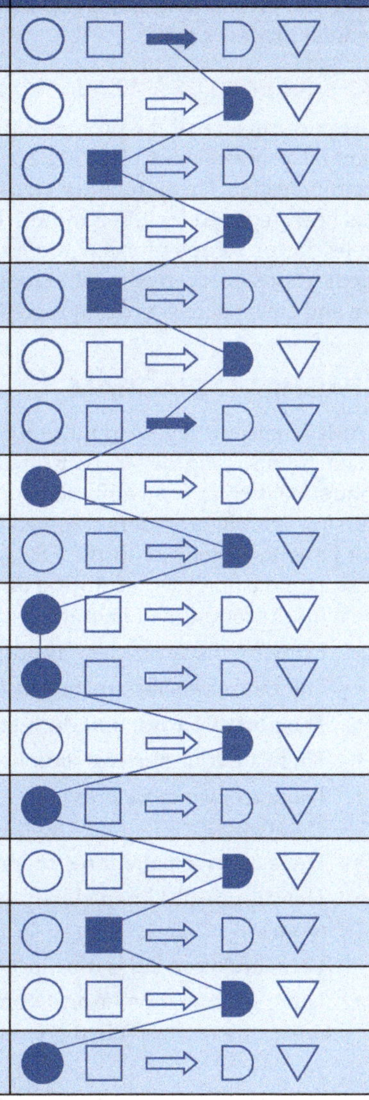

Note: B, business-value-added; N, non-value-added activities; V, value-added.

The efficiency of this process is now:

$$\text{Efficiency} = \left(\frac{\textit{Sum of the times of value-added steps in the process}}{\textit{Sum of times of all steps in the process}}\right) \times 100$$

$$= \frac{70}{219} \times 100$$

$$= 32\%$$

After the proposed redesign, the efficiency of the process would increase by 10%. Although it may still seem low, some of the non–value-added time such as Step 14 cannot be eliminated at all because it is necessary to wait 30 minutes to determine whether the treatment that was initiated is working as intended. Furthermore, the times to perform value-added steps such as triage and discharge have also been reduced, leading to a lower numerator in the efficiency ratio. In a nutshell, the future, redesigned process is much more efficient than the current one, as shown in the general process chart.

General Process Chart

The performance of the proposed process can be compared to that of the original (Table 6.6) in a **general process chart** (Table 11.2), which summarizes the extent of the improvements expected from redesign. The number of steps has been reduced by three, and the total time of the process has been reduced by 155 minutes! This is mainly the result of simplified registration and triage steps, faster setups of exam rooms, imaging available on site, proper stocking of supplies and medications, work in parallel, standardization of admission and discharge, simplification of transfer, and easier access to exam rooms.

SPAGHETTI DIAGRAM

BAMC's current layout (Figure 6.5) is problematic: long distances between waiting room and exam rooms, long distances to Imaging Department; traffic in front of trauma rooms; trauma rooms located far from ambulance entrance; patient restrooms close to supply closet and far from nursing station; providers confined in one area; only two nursing stations; the simulation lab does not have to be located in the ED; and the slit lamp is portable and can be located in any room. Based on the analysis, a future state layout was designed (Figure 11.2):

With the redesigned layout,

- Exam rooms are as close as possible to the waiting room and reached through a straight path.
- The trauma rooms are next to the ambulance entrance.
- The portable x-ray unit decreases the number of trips to the Imaging Department.
- There are four nursing stations, each with a printer.
- There are two more provider documentation stations for reduced traffic and closer proximity to patients.
- There are two patient restrooms for better customer service and limited traffic.
- The supply and linen closets are combined and enable easier access from exam and trauma rooms.
- The simulation lab is now located outside the ED.
- There are two more exam rooms but only one additional nurse during the busiest times because of a more efficient layout and streamlined process.

TABLE 11.2 GENERAL PROCESS CHART

Activities	Current Process			Redesigned Process			Difference	
	No.	Time (min)	%	No.	Time	%	No.	Time
Operations	5	78	20.86	5	64	29.22	0	–14
Inspections	3	25	6.68	3	13	5.94	0	–12
Transportation	4	14	3.74	2	2	0.91	–2	–12
Storage	0	0	0	0	0	0	0	0
Delays	8	257	68.72	7	140	63.93	–1	–117
Total	20	374	100	17	219	100.00	–3	–155

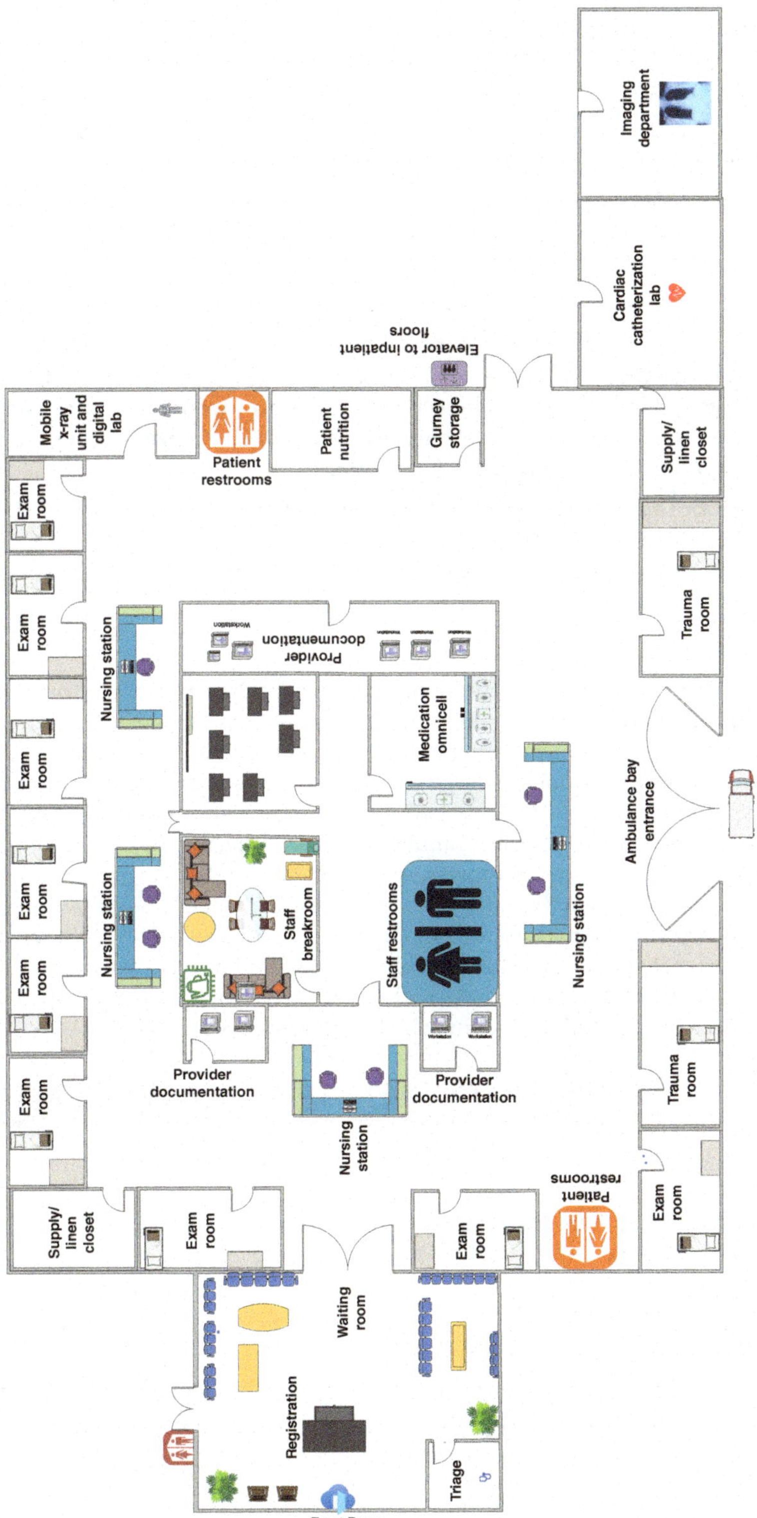

FIGURE 11.2 Future state ED layout.

BRIGHT ANGEL MEDICAL CENTER 11.2

The leadership team had gathered to review the proposed layout and other supporting documentation. Dr. Tibbets, the chief medical officer, was especially enthusiastic. "On paper, this seems to be a major improvement with no major expenses."

Michael Chen, the chief nursing officer, agreed. "I am really impressed at how the project team was able to improve both the patient and the staff experience."

Mira Martinez, the COO, added, "Based on what I computed, the length of stay (LOS) will be reduced by about 40% for discharged and admitted patients. The time reduction is even higher for transferred patients. That is a substantial improvement."

Joe García, the CFO, was pensive. "I like what I see, but it would be nice to see actual dollars and cents. How much is this really going to cost us?"

Kimberly Mitchell, the CEO, finally spoke. "Thank you for your thoughts on this matter. Like Joe, I am looking at our precarious financial situation, and I would like to know how much bang we are going to get for our buck. We approved the budget several months ago, but I'm afraid of cost overruns. I'll talk to Barbara later today."

Based on the proposed changes you have seen in the future state section of this chapter, do you think that the benefits will outweigh the costs?

SIMULATION

When evaluating the effectiveness of a new medical or behavioral intervention, experiments are usually involved. With **experiments**, investigators manipulate at least one independent variable and have direct control over the selection of participants and their exposure to the manipulated variable(s). Similarly, new process designs should undergo rigorous testing before implementation. How can we test new process designs before implementation? By simulating various design changes in isolation and simultaneously. As its name indicates, **simulation** involves the imitation or replication of a process. It is an abstraction of a real-world process. A simulation model of the patient flow through the ED is depicted in Figure 11.3. It is a simplified version of the actual patient flow because ESI levels and left-without-being-seen (LWBS) patients are not included in this model. However, the model could be modified to incorporate these and other variables. ExtendSim Pro 10.1.1 was used to develop this model. It involves a series of activities (shapes with clocks) preceded by queues (bucket-like shapes). It mimics the steps, resources, and paths shown in the future state VSM (Figure 11.1).

ON THE JOB! INTERVIEW VIDEO 11.2

Laura J. Tivis
Director of Nursing Research

Human Subjects Versus Process Improvement Research

Randomized experiments
Treatment and control
Pre- and postexperiment scores
Delphi methodology and building consensus

1. What is the difference between human subject research and quality improvement?
2. Dr. Tivis shared a study her team completed on the impact of foot reflexology on cancer patients. In what area did the study demonstrate a statically significant improvement?

The interview is available online by visiting www.springerpub.com/courseconnect. See inside front cover and tear-out card for CourseConnect details.

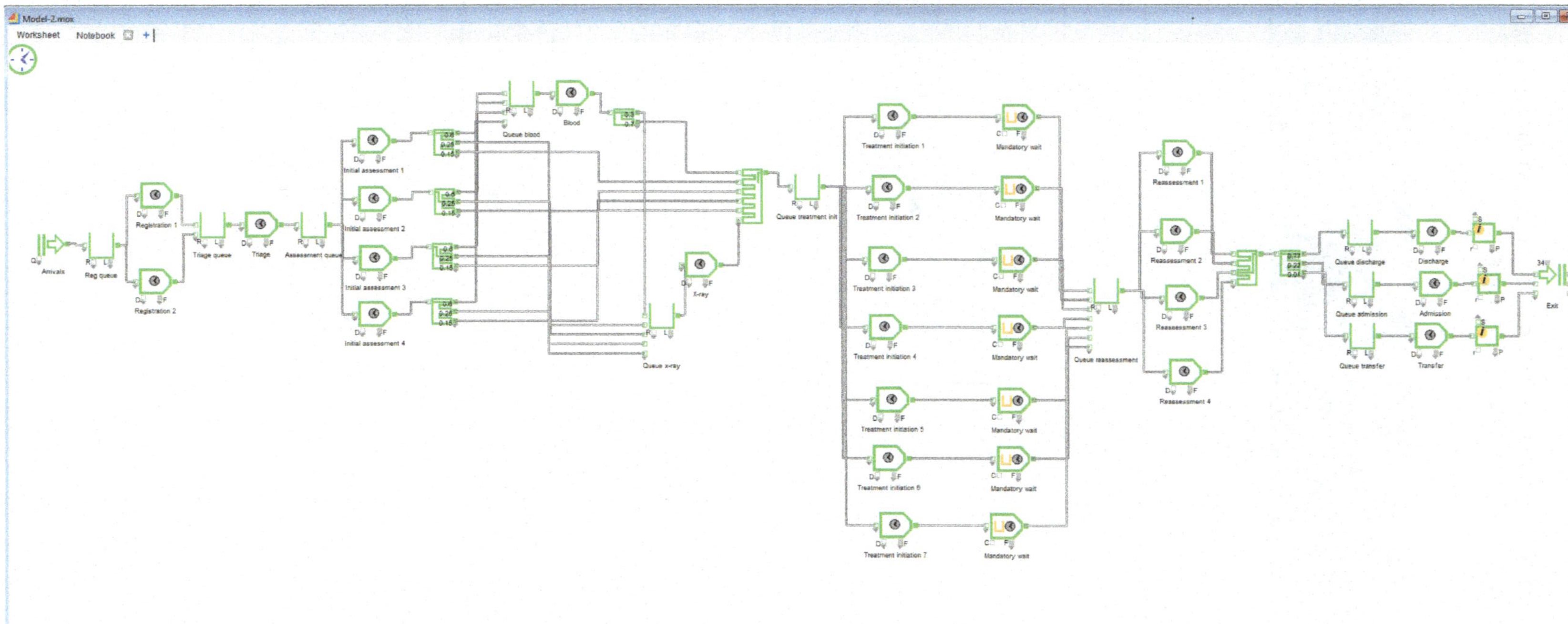

FIGURE 11.3 Simulation model using ExtendSim Pro 10.1.1.

TABLE 11.3 PERFORMANCE OF SIMULATED SYSTEM WITH ONE TRIAGE NURSE AND ONE PORTABLE X-RAY MACHINE

LOS

Random Seed		Arrivals	Average Time in Queue Triage (min)	Utilization Triage	Average Time in Queue X-Ray (min)	Utilization X-Ray	Cycle Time (min)	Exits From System
11	Overall	92	49.5	99.2%	35.9	91.1%	182.49	41
	Discharges						180.9	33
	Admissions						175.3	7
	Transfers						285.14	1
9999	Overall	110	29	81%	47.2	93%	155.12	38
	Discharges						148.4	27
	Admissions						171.6	11
	Transfers						–	0
119999	Overall	105	71.6	94%	50.6	96%	163.46	35
	Discharges						158.9	28
	Admissions						181.7	7
	Transfers						–	0

Simulation is data-intensive and requires the collection of historical data on any random variable. At a minimum, data will be collected on two variables: the arrival of flow units into the process and the processing time for each activity. Once simulation models are "run," they yield important performance statistics such as minimum, maximum, and average wait time before each activity; number of flow units held in the queue; utilization of resources, and so on. This is part of process measurement. One of the main advantages of simulation is that the process configurations can be changed easily, and the performance statistics are regenerated automatically, thereby allowing you to test different potential solutions—improvements—before selecting and implementing one. For this simulation, the distribution of arrivals to the ED from 5 to 11 p.m. (highest volume during the day) was used.

The model in Figure 11.3 was run with three different **random number seeds**, numbers that initialize a pseudorandom number generator. Each run covered a duration of 7 hours to lower the initialization effect when the simulation starts on an artificially empty system: no patient, no queue. After running the simulation, two bottlenecks emerged: triage with one nurse and taking x-rays with one portable machine. Partial results are shown in Table 11.3.

COST–BENEFIT ANALYSIS

When evaluating proposed changes, you will have to think through their effects, including the unintentional consequences of making these changes. Cost–benefit analyses are often conducted at this point to help select the most promising, yet achievable, improvement solution or bundle. Conceptually, a **cost–benefit analysis** is simple: You quantify all the projected costs and benefits of an intervention in monetary terms and select it if the benefits outweigh the costs. Of course, in practice, it is not that simple. It is difficult to predict all the costs and benefits of a proposed alternative, especially when accurate and complete data are not readily

BRIGHT ANGEL MEDICAL CENTER 11.3

Adeleke was presenting the simulation results to Barbara, Dr. Aoki, and Olina. "We collected data on the probability distributions of patient arrivals at the busiest times of the day. To duplicate the VSM, we made changes such as asking one retired nurse to fill the extra nursing position temporarily, reducing the number of questions at triage, and so on. We had to estimate distances for the new layout, but that was relatively easy. As you can see from the model and summary results (Table 11.3), the simulation of the future state VSM essentially yielded the same average lengths of stay (ALOS). This is a strong confirmation that our proposed solutions will increase throughput substantially. As for . . ."

"Stop it right there!" Barbara interjected. "What are these ridiculous waits at triage? Also, the portable x-ray machine was supposed to solve our problems with imaging. In fact, the team had estimated no wait time in both the VSM and the process activity chart. That does not appear to be the case. Your results show that the average wait for the machine can be as long as 50.6 minutes!"

Adeleke conceded, "Yes, these are the bottlenecks of the proposed system. But Loretta Romero, the ED nurse manager, had a good idea. She argued that the seventh nurse assigned to treating patients would be idle a lot if there were delays at triage. This was confirmed by the simulation results which showed low utilization of resources for treatment initiation, typically done by nurses according to physicians' orders, and practically no wait before that process step. The idle nurse could thus be floated to triage as needed. We also added a second portable x-ray machine. It is small, easy to store, and relatively inexpensive. We reran the simulation model. See the results on the screen" (Exhibit 11.1).

EXHIBIT 11.1 PERFORMANCE OF SIMULATED SYSTEM WITH TWO TRIAGE NURSES AND TWO PORTABLE X-RAY MACHINES

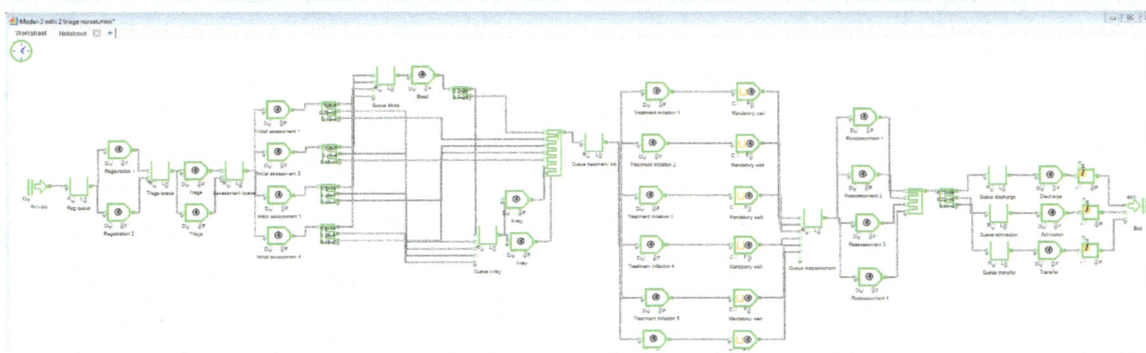

(continued)

EXHIBIT 11.1 PERFORMANCE OF SIMULATED SYSTEM WITH TWO TRIAGE NURSES AND TWO PORTABLE X-RAY MACHINES (*CONTINUED*)

Random Seed		Arrivals	Average Time in Queue Triage (min)	Average Utilization Triage	Average Time in Queue X-Ray (min)	Average Utilization X-Ray	Cycle Time (min)	Exits From System
11	Overall	92	0.9	53.7%	3.2	61.4%	156.4	48
	Discharges						180.9	38
	Admissions						175.3	9
	Transfers						285.14	1
9999	Overall	110	1.1	64.6%	4.3	60.8%	140.0	46
	Discharges						142.4	34
	Admissions						133.4	12
	Transfers						–	0
119999	Overall	105	1.4	62.5%	5.4	79.5%	155.0	48
	Discharges						152.7	38
	Admissions						164.0	10
	Transfers						–	0

Adeleke flashed a triumphant smile. "Simple reconfiguration and what do we have? Higher throughput with even lower LOS!"

Everyone clapped. Barbara questioned, "I have to say I'm impressed. Just to play the devil's advocate. . . . Did those changes create delays for treatment initiation?"

Adeleke replied, "Absolutely not! With an extra physician, we would get an even faster throughput, but that might be a tough sell."

Dr. Aoki burst out laughing. "I've been asking for one more physician for 3 years. I'm not holding my breath on this one."

"OK," Barbara concluded. "Adeleke, superb job. Now meet with the financial analyst, and hopefully our stingy CFO will like what he sees."

available. Let us demonstrate how a cost–benefit analysis is conducted with the BAMC example. BAMC is contemplating a small expansion of the ED capacity with two more exam rooms, one more nurse, and two portable x-ray machines. It is also considering a layout change with a rearrangement of existing rooms, one more patient restroom, and additional nurses' stations and provider documentation areas. To determine whether this project is worthwhile, these steps were followed:

STEP 1: Estimate all costs of improvement:

• Direct costs (building, labor, equipment, etc.)	
○ Building: remodeling	$650,000
○ Labor: one additional nurse	$180,000
○ Equipment: two portable x-ray machines, two new beds, monitors, desks, etc.	$410,000
○ Supplies: syringes, gauze, splints, suture trays, etc.	$10,000
• Indirect costs (Fixed expenses)	$0
• Contractor	$75,000
• Extra utilities during remodeling	$2,000
• Intangible costs (decrease in revenue and productivity during remodel)	$70,000
TOTAL:	$1,397,000

STEP 2: Estimate all benefits (first year in this example):

• Direct benefits	
○ Increased revenue	$1,200,000
○ Lower turnover/reduced travel nurses	$200,000
• Indirect benefits	
○ Increased payer reimbursements and interest in hospital	$600,000
• Intangible benefits	
○ Improved employee engagement	$100,000
TOTAL:	$2,100,000

The benefits definitely outweigh the costs, but BAMC's financial analyst might want to look at the cashflow projections for the next 3 years with a benefit–cost ratio. The **benefit–cost ratio** is a financial indicator used in cost–benefit analysis to determine the viability of a proposed project. It compares the **present value (PV)** of expected benefits to the PV of expected costs (Eq. 11.1). The PV assumes that the value of money received in the future is worth less today because that money could be invested now and yield a return based on a rate known as the discount rate (Corporate Finance Institute, 2024).

$$\text{Benefit–cost ratio} = \frac{PV\ of\ expected\ benefits}{PV\ of\ expected\ costs} = \frac{\sum_{t=0}^{n} \frac{Benefit_t}{(1+i)^t}}{\sum_{t=0}^{n} \frac{Cost_t}{(1+i)^t}} \qquad [11.1]$$

Where: t = period in which money is received or spent,
n = number of periods, and
i = discount rate.

Let's go back to the BAMC remodeling project. We will assume that the discount rate is 4% and that the costs for the extra nurse (during the busiest time) and supplies in the two new exam rooms ($180,000 + $10,000) will still be incurred in years 1, 2, and 3 (Table 11.4):

The benefit–cost ratio is $6,190,401.68/$1,924,267.30 = 3.22 (Table 11.5). The ratio must be greater than 1 for the project to be considered as viable. The higher the value, the more attractive the proposed project is.

If Adeleke at BAMC contemplated two other projects, let's say a 5,000 square foot (≈465 m^2) expansion or a brand-new wing, the benefit–cost ratios of all three alternatives would be compared (Table 11.6).

Once the potential success of a project has been scrutinized and validated, the project can be launched. Whenever possible, it is a good idea to pilot it on a small scale. For example, all proposed solutions (6S, *poka-yoke*, checklists, simplification of steps, etc.) could be implemented and tweaked before the layout change is completed. Then, the project implementation phase can begin. Gantt charts and PERT/CPM analysis (Chapter 5) will help keep track of activities and timelines for improvement. Following the progress of the process improvement with performance metrics and tools can demonstrate that the changes made are actually producing positive results. By the end of the *Improve* step, you should be able to document that the process was actually enhanced by your actions. Let's do that!

TABLE 11.4 EXPECTED COSTS AND BENEFITS OF ED REMODEL FOR THE NEXT 3 YEARS

Time	*t* = 0	*t* = 1	*t* = 2	*t* = 3
Costs	–$1,397,000	–$190,000	–$190,000	–$190,000
Benefits		$2,100,000	$2,300,000	$2,300,000

TABLE 11.5 COMPUTATIONS FOR BENEFIT–COST RATIO OF ED REMODEL FOR THE NEXT 3 YEARS

Time (Year)	Discounted Costs	Discounted Benefits
t = 0	$1,397,000	–
t = 1	$190,000/(1+0.04)^1 = $182,692.31	$2,100,000/(1+0.04)^1 = $2,019,230.77
t = 2	$190,000/(1+0.04)^2 = $175,665.68	$2,300,000/(1+0.04)^2 = $2,126,479.29
t = 3	$190,000/(1+0.04)^3 = $168,909.31	$2,300,000/(1+0.04)^3 = $2,044,691.62
Total	$1,924,267.30	$6,190,401.68

TABLE 11.6 BENEFIT–COST RATIOS OF THREE DIFFERENT PROJECT ALTERNATIVES

Alternative	Total Discounted Costs	Total Discounted Benefits	Benefit–Cost Ratio
Alternative A: remodeling	$1,924,267.30	$6,190,401.68	3.22[a]
Alternative B: expansion	$5,700,000.00	$8,900,000.00	1.56
Alternative C: new wing	$15,200,000.00	$16,000,000.00	1.05

[a]Best alternative.

BRIGHT ANGEL MEDICAL CENTER 11.4

It had been a few chaotic weeks at the ED while construction was going on. Now, with two extra exam rooms, conveniently placed trauma rooms, and easier access all around, the staff was in a good mood. "This is a completely different place!" one of the nurses told Loretta Romero.

"I'm finally starting to do the job I'm supposed to do . . . no more of this running around and dealing with angry patients," chimed another.

Olina walked toward the group and said, "Hey there. You look happy. Anything special going on?" "Yes," Loretta said. "The transition to the new process took some adjustments, but we like it better now. We are glad that the leadership gave us more resources when we needed them. Also, we got lucky that the new hires took some of our loads off while completing their training."

Olina nodded, "There are many reasons to be happy. The remodeling project took a little longer than expected, but by only 2 weeks. And we were slightly below budget. There's more. I've been working with Adeleke's team on documenting our progress. Wait till you see it!"

DOCUMENTING THE IMPROVEMENT

PROCESS ACTIVITY CHART

When conceived carefully, the future state should provide a close rendition of what the improved process will bring to the organization. Naturally, there will be some differences once the project is implemented. For example, you may remember that the future state VSM and process activity chart had assumed no wait for imaging with the portable x-ray machine. The simulation demonstrated that this was inaccurate and that, in fact, a second machine was needed. The simulation had also justified a second nurse in triage during peak times. As capacity changes, so do the buffers. Based on *actual* data after improvement, the revised process activity chart is now displayed in Table 11.7. Compared to the future state process activity chart (Table 11.1), the overall non–value-added time has decreased from 141 to 83.5 minutes, bringing the process efficiency to 70/161.5 = 43%! However, one more step (delay) was added before imaging. In a nutshell, the actual implementation of the process changes may bring some good surprises and some disappointments, but in the BAMC case, the new process produces much more value to the patient. Yet, it also points to the fact that more improvement is possible and should be pursued.

STATISTICAL PROCESS CONTROL CHARTS

Despite the word "control", statistical process control charts are not used exclusively in the *Control* phase of the DMAIC (Define-Measure-Analyze-Improve-Control) process. As you saw in Chapter 8, they continuously *Measure* the process to determine whether it is behaving consistently. They can also show the change that occurs after a process change. In this *Improve* phase, they should not show that a process is in control (i.e., stable and predictable). Rather, they should reveal that a major shift has occurred. Let's demonstrate this principle with an example. In Chapter 8, the *IX*- and *MR*-charts displaying the ALOS for discharged patients indicated an out-of-control situation, with ALOS averaging 276 minutes over the past 24 months and an upward trend at the end of that period (Figure 8.9). Once the project improvement was implemented, the following data were collected (Table 11.8).

The centerline value of the *IX* chart, $\overline{IX}$, is 173.8 minutes. The average moving range value, $\overline{MR}$, is 9.6 minutes. Therefore, the control limits (lower control limit [LCL] and upper control limit [UCL]) are:

$LCL_{IX} = 173.8 - (2.66 \times 9.6) = 148.3$ minutes

$UCL_{IX} = 173.8 + (2.66 \times 9.6) = 199.4$ minutes

TABLE 11.7 AFTER-IMPROVEMENT PROCESS ACTIVITY CHART FOR AN ED PATIENT WITH BOTH DIAGNOSTIC TESTS AND BEING ADMITTED

No.	Description	Time (min)	Distance	Value Code (V/N/B)	Symbol
1	Patient arrives.	1	100 ft	V	
2	Patient waits.	1		N	
3	Patient is registered.	3		B	
4	Patient waits.	1		N	
5	Patient is triaged.	5		B	
6	Patient waits.	20		N	
7	Patient goes to exam room.	1	100 ft	N	
8	Patient is examined by physician.	17		V	
9	Patient waits for phlebotomist.	1.5		N	
10	Patient's blood is drawn.	5		V	
11	Patient waits.	4		N	
12	Patient's images are taken.	15		V	
13	Patient waits.	7		N	
14	Treatment is initiated.	12		V	
15	Patient waits.	30		N	
16	Patient's condition is reassessed.	5		V	
17	Patient waits.	18		N	
18	Patient is admitted.	15		V	

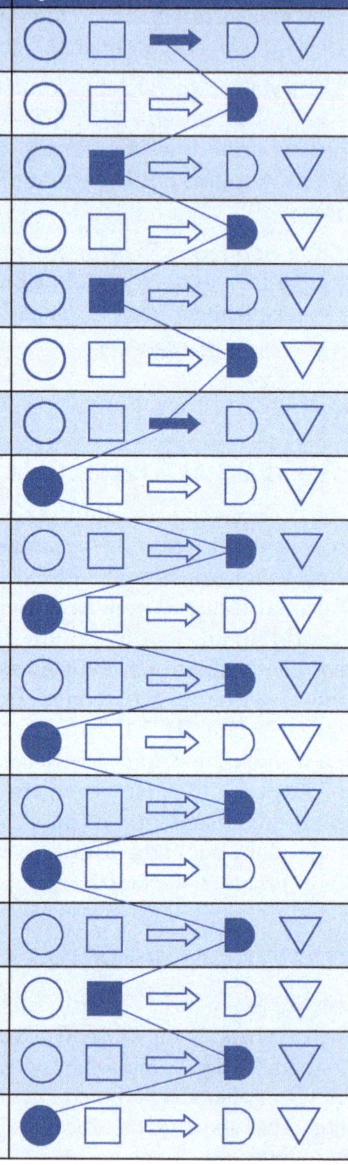

Note: B, business-value-added; N, non–value-added activities; V, value-added.

The combination of the "Before Improvement" and "After Improvement" control charts is depicted in Figure 11.4.

Quite a change! Not only has the average shifted downward from 276 to 173.8 minutes, but the variation has been substantially reduced, as shown by the spreads between the *LCL* and *UCL*. There are not enough points yet to determine whether the new process is in control or not, but 6 months after the process changes, the ALOS values are quite consistent and much more predictable.

TABLE 11.8 AVERAGE LENGTHS OF STAY (ALOS) AND MOVING RANGES (MR) AFTER IMPROVEMENT

Month	ALOS (min)	MR
1	189	-
2	178	11
3	174	4
4	158	16
5	173	15
6	171	2
Mean	173.8	9.6

SIX SIGMA METRICS

Other indicators used to document the improvement are the traditional Six Sigma metrics: yield, throughput (first pass) yield (FPY), rolled throughput yield (RTY), and sigma level.

Yield and Throughput Yield

Let' s revisit BAMC's FPY (same as throughput yield) and RTY before the improvement of ED flow for discharged patients (Chapter 6; Table 11.9).
With all the improvements made, including better training, the errors in the new process are shown in the text that follows (Figure 11.5).

The yield is now 993/1,000 = 99.3%, which is essentially a 0.3% decrease in fatalities after redesign. The computations for FPY and RTY are as follows:

$$FPY_1 = \frac{1{,}000\ \textit{units} - 8\ \textit{reworked units}}{1{,}000\ \textit{units}} \times 100\% = 99.20\%$$

$$FPY_2 = \frac{1{,}000\ \textit{units} - 11\ \textit{reworked units} - 2\ \textit{scrapped}}{1{,}000\ \textit{units}} \times 100\% = 98.70\%$$

$$FPY_3 = \frac{998\ \textit{units} - 15\ \textit{reworked units} - 2\ \textit{scrapped}}{998\ \textit{units}} \times 100\% = 98.30\%$$

$$FPY_4 = \frac{996\ \textit{units} - 21\ \textit{reworked units}}{996\ \textit{units}} \times 100\% = 97.89\%$$

TABLE 11.9 SUMMARY YIELD METRICS FOR DISCHARGED PATIENTS' FLOW THROUGH THE ED

Step	Units in	Units Reworked	Units Scrapped	Units Out	FPY (%)
1	1,000	10	0	1,000	99.00
2	1,000	22	4	996	97.40
3	996	30	2	994	96.79
4	994	29	0	994	97.08
5	994	25	3	991	97.18
6	991	10	1	990	98.89
7	990	82	0	990	91.72
					RTY 79.86%

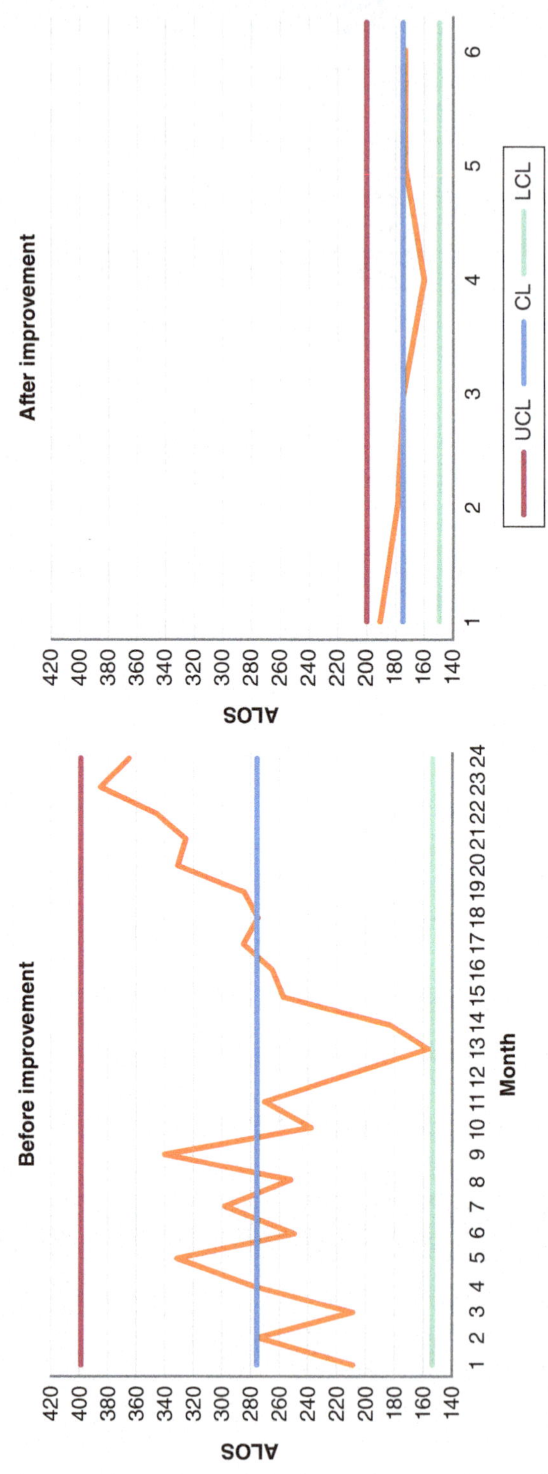

FIGURE 11.4 *IX*-charts of ALOS for discharged patients before and after improvement.

Abbreviations: ALOS, average length of stay; CL, centerline; LCL, lower control limit; UCL, upper control limit.

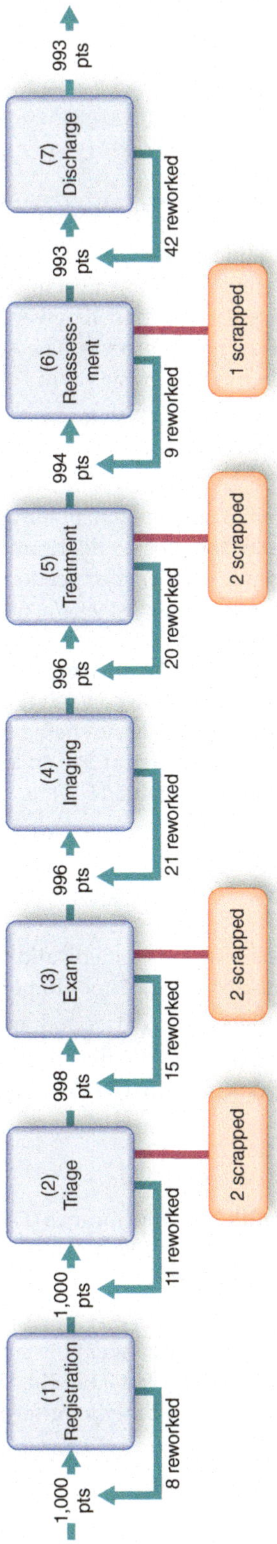

FIGURE 11.5 Errors made at each process step for discharged patients (Pts = patients) after improvement.

$$\text{FPY}_5 = \frac{996\ \textit{units} - 20\ \textit{reworked units} - 2\ \textit{scrapped}}{996\ \textit{units}} \times 100\% = 97.79\%$$

$$\text{FPY}_6 = \frac{994\ \textit{units} - 9\ \textit{reworked units} - 1\ \textit{scrapped}}{994\ \textit{units}} \times 100\% = 98.99\%$$

$$\text{FPY}_7 = \frac{993\ \textit{units} - 42\ \textit{reworked units}}{993\ \textit{units}} \times 100\% = 95.77\%$$

$$\text{RTY} = (0.992 * 0.987 * 0.983 * 0.9789 * 0.9779 * 0.9899 * 0.9577) \times 100\% = 87.34\%$$

Quality improvements occurred at almost every step. The reduction in fatalities is, of course, the most important achievement. The simplification and standardization of the discharge process has been very successful as well because it resulted in 40 fewer "reworked" units, which could be readmissions involving a repetition of the entire process. The RTY is now 87.34%, which is 7.48% higher than before improvement. This increase means that 7.48% more patients will now flow through an error-free process.

Sigma Level

The term Six Sigma refers to six *SD*s from a target value. In terms of process capability (Chapter 8), a **Six Sigma level** means that the mean of the process distribution is six *SD*s away from the lower specification limit and six *SD*s away from the upper specification limit. In other words, the C_p value is at least 2. This implies that you meet your target 99.99966% of the time (Table 11.10). This is close to zero defects! The core tenet of Six Sigma is that by removing variation from a process, you decrease the chances of introducing errors in a statistically measurable and controllable way. In fact, you will recall that a Six Sigma process is even allowed to shift 1.5σ on either side of the mean and is not generating defects. This was similar to the car not being centered when entering the garage (Figure 8.22). Today, most healthcare sectors perform at 3 to 4σ levels (Box 11.1), with a few, notable exceptions and a lot of variation within a sector (Table 11.11).

To compute the sigma level,

1. Determine the **O**pportunities for errors per unit. For example, the number of opportunities for medication administration errors is 5: wrong patient, wrong drug, wrong dose, wrong route, and wrong time.
2. Determine the number of units **(Product)**. In our medication administration example, assume that 4,000 medications were administered over a 1-month period.
3. Find the number of **D**efects during the assessment period. In our case, let us assume that there were 200 medication administration errors during the 1-month period.
4. Compute the number of defects per opportunity **(DPO)** = Defect/(Product × opportunities). In our example,

$$\text{DPO} = 200/(4{,}000 \times 5) = 0.01.$$

5. Compute the number of defects per million opportunities (**DPMO**) = DPO × one million. In our example,

$$\text{DPMO} = 0.01 \times 10^6 = 10{,}000.$$

6. Determine process sigma using a Six Sigma conversion table (www.six-sigma-material.com/Tables.html). Look for the number closest to 10,000 in the DPMO column; it is 10,724. In our case, when allowing for a 1.5σ deviation over time (long-term), the corresponding sigma level is approximately 2.3.

BRIGHT ANGEL MEDICAL CENTER 11.5

"Ch-ch-ch-ch-changes . . ." Adeleke was humming as David Bowie's song was playing in the background. The door was ajar, and Olina peered in.

"You seem very cheerful today!" she said.

"Indeed, I am. Come on in," he replied. "I've got something to show you." Olina approached the desk. Adeleke continued, "I'm especially satisfied with the discharge process. We identified 10 types of patient discharge negligence. For 1,000 discharged patients, we had 42 errors after implementing the process improvements. See our computations here. Are they correct?"

Olina looked at the following formulas and figures:

DPO = 42 errors/(1,000 patients × 10 opportunities) = 0.0042

DPMO = (0.0042) × 10^6 = 4200

Sigma level ≈ 4.10

Olina nodded. "This is good, but look at the table (https://www.six-sigma-material.com/Tables.html). This is the short-term sigma level. In the long run, the process will shift. If it shifts by 1.5 SD, the level will be 2.6."

Adeleke's smile faded. "Very discouraging," he said. "I thought we were close to Six Sigma."

Olina quickly reacted. "Look at the improvement that has been made! Getting a Six Sigma level is hard. It doesn't happen overnight."

What can BAMC do to further improve the sigma level at discharge?

TABLE 11.10 SIGMA LEVELS FOR ITEMS WITHOUT DEFECTS (YIELD)

Percentage of Items Without Defect (Yield, %)	DPMO	Sigma Level
30.85	691,462	1.0
69.15	308,538	2.0
93.32	66,807	3.0
99.38	6,210	4.0
99.98	233	5.0
99.99966	3.4	6.0

Abbreviation: DPMO, defects per million opportunities.

TABLE 11.11 SIGMA LEVELS IN THE HEALTHCARE INDUSTRY

Healthcare Sector	Metric	Incidents per Million	Sigma Level
Anesthesia (Kaira & Kopargaonkar, 2016)	Deaths	5	5.9
Laboratory (Nevalainen et al., 2000)	Sample label errors Missing information on requests (cytology, Pap smears)	5,227 100,259	4.1 2.8
Surgery (Suliburk et al., 2019)	Adverse events at three hospitals	35,042	3.3
Infectious diseases (CDC, 2020a, 2020b)	COVID-19 death rate of infected healthcare personnel Overuse of antibiotics	6,304 300,000	4.0 2.0
All (Johns Hopkins Medicine, 2016; IOM, 2007)	Deaths due to medical errors Medication errors in hospital care	100,000 15,000–99,000	2.8 3.7–2.8

Abbreviations: CDC, Centers for Disease Control and Prevention; IOM, Institute of Medicine.

BOX 11.1 QUALITY IN PRACTICE!

Performance and Service Quality Improvement in Endodontics

The Endodontics Department in a dental college adopted Lean Six Sigma methodologies to reduce waste and decrease variation. The college is funded by a charitable trust, and the walk-in patients are charged minimal amounts, if any. With high quality and low costs, the college kept attracting larger volumes of patients. Processing time averaged 115 minutes, and numerous errors were made. The sigma level for the process was 0.06. The improvement team identified poor student engagement in learning and mastering the subject as one of the root causes. In fact, the students limited themselves to rote learning the topics listed in the syllabus. Other causes included the location of the teeth where the root canals had to be performed as well as the lack of communication with patients using a different language. The implemented solutions were: (a) training of instructors in active learning strategies; (b) interns had to first be proficient at performing root canals on dummies before being assigned to actual patients; (c) only experienced interns were assigned to molar cavity cases, which take more time; (d) new, ergonomic chairs were purchased for the interns; and (e) a tracking system was installed to make sure that the patients would be treated on a first-come, first-served basis. The average processing time decreased to 84 minutes, and the sigma level increased to 4.17 (Noronha et al., 2023).

DASHBOARDS

Dashboards are also good indicators of the extent of an improvement. In Chapter 4, the tactical and operational dashboards for the ED were dismal. Consistently, the targets were not met, resulting in a lot of red on the dashboard. After the improvement, the dashboards in Tables 11.12 and 11.13 and Figure 11.6 paint a much brighter (greener!) picture.

TABLE 11.12 TACTICAL QUALITY DASHBOARD AT BAMC'S EMERGENCY DEPARTMENT AFTER IMPROVEMENT

Measures	FYTD Actual	FY Target	Jul	Aug	Sep	Oct	Nov	Dec
Process								
t-PA infusion rate for stroke, when indicated (%)	93	>95	90	92	91	93	96	96
Door-to-doc time (min)	44.3	<45	47	48	45	44	42	40
Door-to-balloon time for STEMI (min)	87.7	<90	91	90	88	86	86	85
Time between discharge order and actual discharge (min)	7.3	<10	9	8	8	6	7	6
CT scan use for pediatric patients with abdominal pain (%)	46.7	<30	52	49	48	50	42	39
Hand hygiene compliance rate (%)	97	>95	97	96	97	98	97	97
Chart closure (% in 24 hrs)	96.8	>95	96	96	96	98	97	98
Travel nurses FTEs	17.8	<20	18.3	18.9	18.1	17.9	17.2	16.5
Outcomes								
Mortality ratio—All cause (O/E)	0.8	<1	0.9	0.8	0.8	0.7	0.9	0.8
All-cause, 72-hrs return to ED (%)	4.2	<5	5	5	4	4	4	3
Average time from ED arrival to ED departure for discharged patients (min)	173.8	<150	189	178	174	158	173	171

(continued)

TABLE 11.12 TACTICAL QUALITY DASHBOARD AT BAMC'S EMERGENCY DEPARTMENT AFTER IMPROVEMENT (*CONTINUED*)

Measures	FYTD Actual	FY Target	Jul	Aug	Sep	Oct	Nov	Dec
Average time from ED arrival to ED departure for admitted patients (min)	195.8	<200	212	213	189	183	192	186
LWBS (% of arrivals)	1.8	<2	2.4	2.1	1.9	1.9	1.4	1.3
Patient Experience								
Overall (% top box)	84.1	>80	80.1	82.7	83.3	85.3	85.1	87.9
Doctors listening carefully (% top box)	61.8	>60	59	58	61	64	65	64
Courtesy and respect from doctors (% top box)	66.2	>60	62	65	67	68	66	69
Nurses listening carefully (% top box)	73	>60	67	71	72	71	79	78
Courtesy and respect from nurses (% top box)	73.3	>60	71	72	73	75	74	75
Understanding care when leaving hospital (% top box)	86.7	>85	86	86	84	87	89	88

Abbreviations: BAMC, Bright Angel Medical Center; CT, computed tomography; FTE, full-time equivalent; FY, fiscal year; FYTD, fiscal year to date; LWBS, left-without-being-seen; STEMI, ST elevation myocardial infarction.

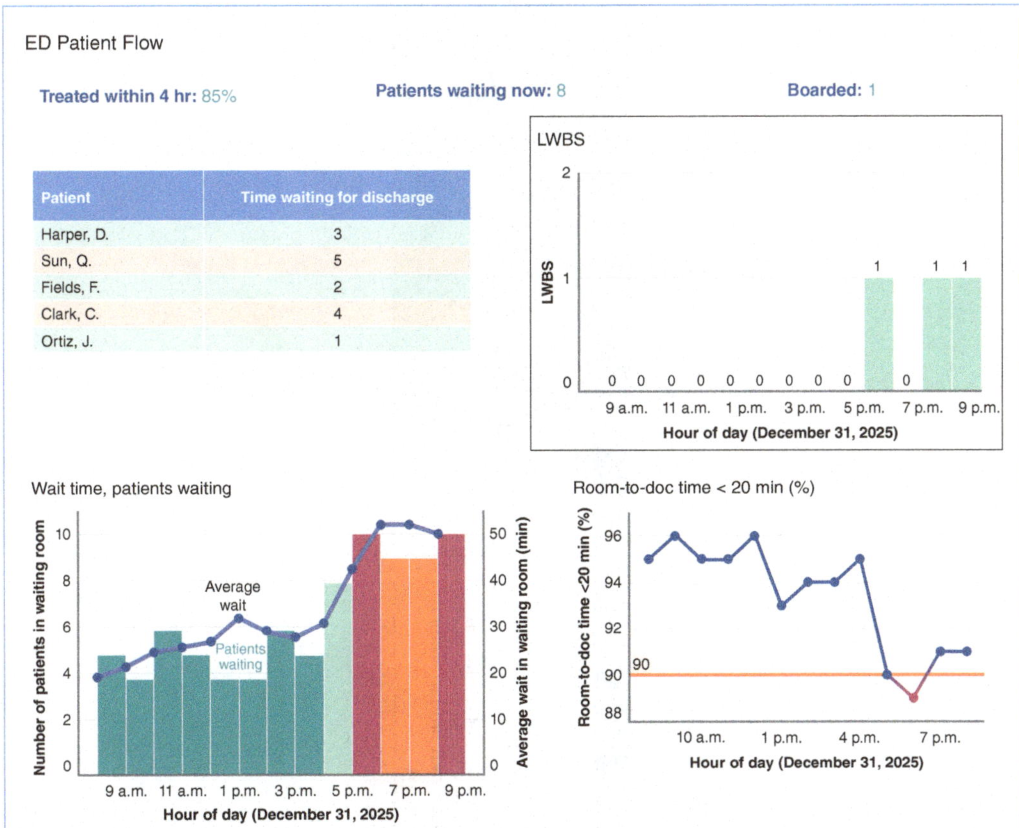

FIGURE 11.6 Wall board ED—December 31, 2025.

Abbreviation: LWBS, left without being seen.

TABLE 11.13 OPERATIONAL QUALITY DASHBOARD FOR EMERGENCY DEPARTMENT AFTER IMPROVEMENT—DECEMBER 31, 2025

Measures	Target	8:00	9:00	10:00	11:00	12:00	13:00	14:00	15:00	16:00	17:00	18:00	19:00	20:00
Number of patients waiting in waiting room	<10	5	4	6	5	4	4	6	5	8	10	9	9	10
ED LOS (min)	<180	105	115	110	125	132	151	147	158	149	162	181	179	174
Room-to-doc time <20 min (%)	>90	95	96	95	95	96	93	94	94	95	90	89	91	91
Average wait time in waiting room (min)	<50	20	22	25	26	27	32	29	28	31	42	51	51	49

Abbreviation: LOS, length of stay.

BRIGHT ANGEL MEDICAL CENTER 11.6

The executive team was gathered at the conference table. Mira Martinez's absence was noted. First on the agenda was the ED project.

Kimberly Mitchell started the meeting. "We have a lot to celebrate. Last month, the ED throughput was 31% higher than it was before the improvement. It took us a few weeks to get there, but the numbers speak for themselves: Our goal was met! For my first year as CEO of Bright Angel, I got to witness a remarkable transformation of a department known for its misfortunes and challenges. Paul, thank you for championing the effort and making sure the whole project team stayed on track, especially when they seemed discouraged."

All faces turned toward Dr. Tibbets, who sat a little straighter on his chair. "Kim, thank you for the compliment, but I had help. As chief nursing officer, Michael [Chen] was instrumental in getting the nurses engaged in the project. They provided a lot of the ideas for improvement. Also, Sam [Enapay] achieved the impossible: She oversaw the hiring and training of new nurses and made sure that everyone working in the ED got further training in customer service and service recovery. Look at our patient surveys now . . . something to be proud of. Adeleke and his team managed to make a broad range of improvements for less money than expected. We really got a lot of bang for our buck, here. Don't you think, Joe?"

Joe [Garcia] chuckled. "I agree. This was money well spent. I wish all the other projects were like that."

Kimberly spoke again. "We need to have a party for the ED staff. They deserve it. Especially Barbara. She was a true leader who inspired her staff. In fact, I heard that several are now Six Sigma Green Belts. With all the extra work they had to do during this project, that's impressive."

Dr. Tibbets nodded, "There has been a positive culture change in the organization. And it is spreading. Yesterday, C.P Rao, the director of the BAMC surgery center, reached out and asked whether he could get help to improve their throughput and get the operative cases done in a timely fashion. I put him in touch with Olina."

Kimberly beamed. "My wish is that we will have an entire system dedicated to improvement. The ED was essentially our pilot case, and it's a big success. Let's capitalize on what we have learned and expand our repertoire of best practices."

Did BAMC follow the plan-do-study-act (PDSA) cycle? Explain.

BUILDING THE A3 REPORT

At the end of the *Improve* phase, the A3 report documenting all phases should be complete. In Figure 11.7, we have added the future state, the recommendations, an implementation schedule, and the improved ALOS. Because nothing is perfect, a follow-up section with further actions to take is also included.

ETHICAL SCENARIO 11.1

Disparities in Orders of Diagnostic Tests

Physicians and providers have a large amount of discretion when ordering diagnostic laboratory and imaging tests to help substantiate or disprove a medical diagnosis. There is a lot of variability in the amount of testing ordered from one physician to another. Some physicians order an entire battery of tests on every patient to ensure they don't miss anything, however trivial.

What impact on cost and resource utilization does "blanket" ordering have?

From a quality standpoint, are patients better off if they undergo more tests?

As a manager, how would you improve the ordering process?

Prepared by Adeleke Mensah **ED Throughput** **December 30, 2025**

Background

Low patient satisfaction scores and high LWBS. ALOS in the ED is over 6 hr. Average wait time in early evening exceeds 2 hr. Delays to get x-rays and lab results. High readmission rates within 72 hr. Boarding issues. Poor patient experience with providers.

Current situation

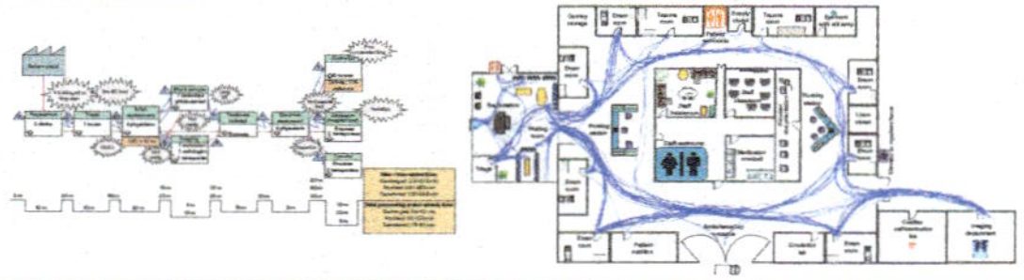

Analyze

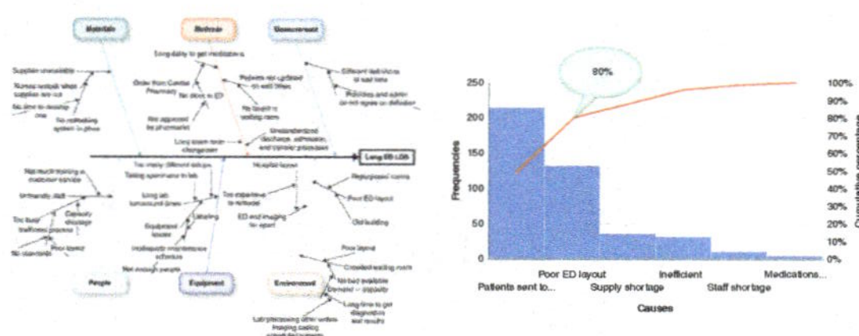

Target

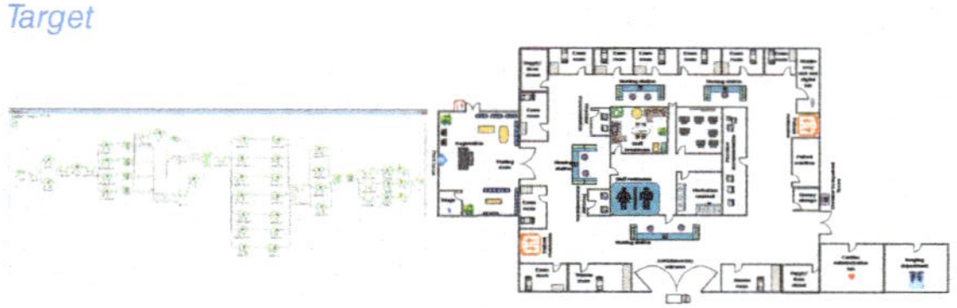

Recommendations

- Simplify registration and triage; send ED nurse to triage at busy times.
- Change layout for easy access to trauma rooms, exam rooms, nurse stations.
- Inventory control and 6S in exam rooms and supply room.
- Have 2 portable x-ray machines in ED.
- Store high-usage medications in ED.
- Standardization of discharge and admission (checklists); centralization for transfer.

Implementation schedule

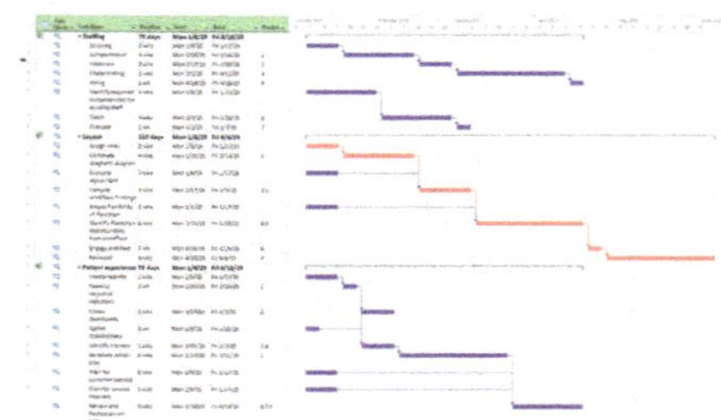

Improvement

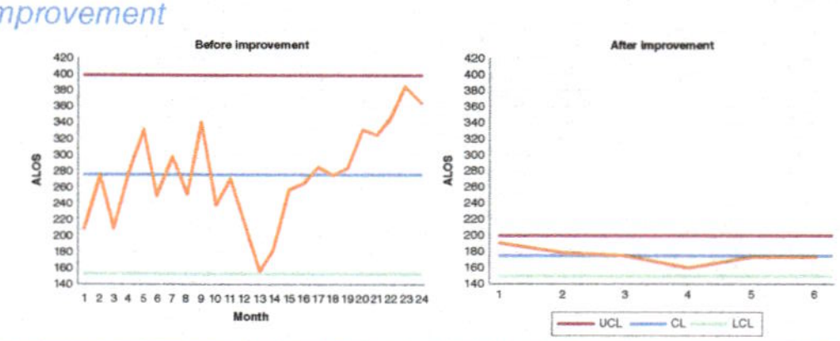

Follow-up

Evaluate LSS training program
Update targets

FIGURE 11.7 Complete A3 report.

Abbreviation: ALOS, average length of stay; LSS, Lean Six Sigma; LWBS, left without being seen.

SUMMARY

Before implementing a process improvement, it is necessary to visualize its future state. VSMs, process activity charts, and planned layouts can depict the improved process envisioned by the team. Simulating the improved process will generate performance metrics that will support the improvement as is or suggest revisions. The performance metrics may even lead to the generation of multiple alternatives for improvement. Cost–benefit analysis will help determine which one of these alternatives delivers the most value. During the implementation, project managers document progress in terms of time, cost, and quality. After implementation, general process charts, side-by-side control charts, Six Sigma metrics, and dashboards will reveal the actual extent of the improvement. Some "kinks" might need to be addressed shortly after implementation, but over time, the merits of the revised process will become more obvious. The *Improve* phase is documented in the A3 report with the future state graphics, the proposed solutions, the schedule for implementation, the results, and follow-up.

CERTIFICATION TIPS

The two chapters on process improvement offer a good overview of the principles and techniques to generate and scrutinize improvements. Yet, they do not cover all items that might be expected on the certification exam. Those of you seeking certification should review the following topics:

- Design of experiments (DoE): https://asq.org/quality-resources/design-of-experiments (The DoE template is especially useful)
- Trystorming, a combination of brainstorming and rapid prototyping: https://www.leansixsigmadefinition.com/glossary/trystorming/#:~:text=Trystorming%20is%20a%20combination%20of,will%20work%20quickly%20or%20not
- Setup reduction—single-minute exchange of die: https://www.lean.org/lexicon-terms/single-minute-exchange-of-die
- One-piece flow (ideal lot size = 1): https://safetyculture.com/topics/one-piece-flow

KEY TERMS

Future state
Internal setup
External setup
General process chart
Experiment
Simulation
Random number seed
Cost–benefit analysis
Benefit–cost ratio
Present value (PV)
Six Sigma level

REVIEW QUESTIONS

1. What is referred to as "the future state"?
2. List and describe two tools that can be used to depict the future state.
3. What is the difference between the internal and external parts of the setup? How can you decrease the setup time?
4. What is a general process chart?
5. What are the advantages of using simulation in process redesign?
6. What is a cost–benefit analysis?
7. Why is the PV of money used when computing the benefit–cost ratio?
8. Why should we use before and after intervention control charts?
9. What is the Sigma level?
10. What does a Sigma level of 6 indicate?

SOLVE BRIGHT ANGEL MEDICAL CENTER'S PROBLEMS

1. In a small dental clinic, placing a crown involves the steps shown in the following graphic. The dentist had 300 cases for which installing a crown was necessary. Determine the yield and RTY. State the meaning of these performance metrics.

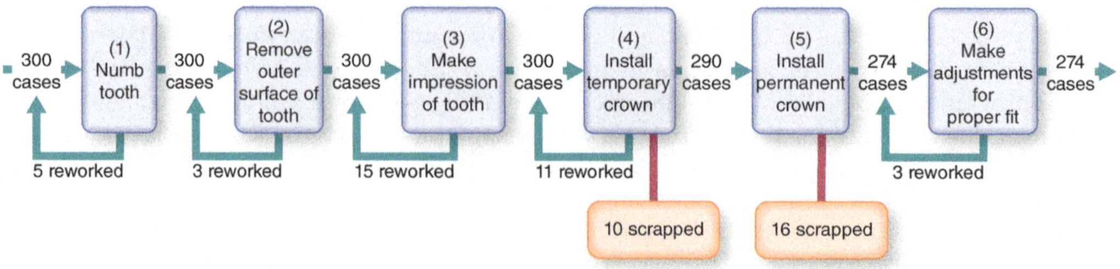

2. Processing blood samples is done in 7 steps. Five hundred blood samples were recently processed at BAMC, and the number of reworked and scrapped units is shown in the following table. Compute the yield and the RTY. State the meaning of these performance metrics.

Step	Number Reworked	Number Scrapped
1. Collection	3	1
2. Labeling	4	0
3. Documentation	5	0
4. Handling	1	2
5. Centrifugation	0	1
6. Testing	4	0
7. Transport	1	2

3. Determine the short- and long-term sigma levels (1.5σ deviation) for the following process scenarios. Use a Six Sigma conversion table (e.g., www.six-sigma-material.com/Tables.html).
   a. A total of 100,000 blood transfusions took place the past year. Five of those resulted in a fatality. There are three opportunities for defect (preanalytical, analytical, and postanalytical).
   b. In the past year, 5,000 patients were discharged. Of those, 111 had their personal items misplaced. There are four opportunities for defect (identification, placement in storage, recordkeeping, and retrieval from storage).
   c. In the past quarter, 1,694 heart attacks were treated. Out of those, 91% of the cases resulted in defect-free care. There are six components of care.
   d. Five hundred blood samples were drawn last week. The nurses who observed the phlebotomists identified 10 mistakes. Errors typically fall into seven domains.
   e. The primary types of errors that can be made in the registration process are wrong patient name, Social Security number, address, birth date, and insurance information. In all, 1,000 patients were registered, and 47 mistakes were made.
4. The following table shows three alternatives for a redesign of the ED. Compute the benefit–cost ratios for each alternative and decide which one appears to be the most attractive.

Alternative	Costs	Benefits
Alternative A: full expansion	$4,270,000	$5,000,000
Alternative B: medium expansion	$3,100,000	$4,500,000
Alternative C: small expansion	$1,900,000	$2,300,000

5. The following chart shows the projected costs and benefits for a process improvement in the Surgery Department over the next 4 years. The discount rate is 3%. Organize them into costs and benefits and perform a cost–benefit analysis.

Time	t = 0	t = 1	t = 2	t = 3	t = 4
Costs	–$600,000	–$220,000	–$220,000	–$180,000	–$160,000
Benefits		$1,200,000	$1,300,000	$1,500,000	$1,500,000

6. The following table shows the projected costs and benefits for a process improvement in the Imaging Department over the next 3 years. The discount rate is 5%. Organize them into costs and benefits and perform a cost–benefit analysis.

Time	t = 0	t = 1	t = 2	t = 3
Costs	–$1,600,000	$0	$0	$0
Benefits		$900,000	$900,000	$900,000

7. The process for ordering and delivering food to inpatients was redesigned. The following table shows the before and after improvement steps and their durations.

	Current Process			Redesigned Process		
Activities	No.	Time (min)	% of Total	No.	Time (min)	% of Total
Operations	12	65	?	10	57	?
Inspections	4	8	?	2	6	?
Transportation	3	12	?	1	4	?
Storage	0	0	?	0	0	?
Delays	5	26	?	2	20	?

a. Determine the percentage that each type of activity contributes to total time.
b. Develop the general process chart and discuss the magnitude of the improvements.
c. If operations are the only value-added activities, how much more/less efficient is the new process?

8. The process for scheduling elective surgeries was redesigned. The following table shows the before and after improvement steps and their durations.

	Current Process			Redesigned Process		
Activities	No.	Time (min)	% of Total	No.	Time (min)	% of Total
Operations	7	24	?	4	18	?
Inspections	2	12	?	2	10	?
Transportation	2	4	?	2	3	?
Storage	0	0	?	0	0	?
Delays	3	15	?	3	12	?

a. Determine the percentage that each type of activity contributes to total time.
b. Develop the general process chart and discuss the magnitude of the improvements.
c. If operations are the only value-added activities, how much more/less efficient is the new process?

9. In BAMC 11.2, Mira Martinez says that, based on her computations, the projected decrease in LOS time for discharged and admitted patients is 40% or more. Use the VSM in Chapter 6 (Figure 6.2) and the future state VSM (Figure 11.1) in this chapter to verify or dispute her findings. If a range of values is provided in the VSM, take the midpoint to represent the LOS.

LEARNING ACTIVITIES

1. Role-playing with two discussants: Dr. C.P. Rao, Director of Surgery, and Olina Petrenko, Director of Quality. Start a discussion between C.P. and Olina on the inability to get cases started on time, resulting in staff staying late and patients complaining about the delays. Discuss potential causes and solutions.
2. When there are no best practices for a specific condition, what should the provider do?
3. What happens when improvements suggest that there are redundant positions in the organization? Discuss the pros and cons of firing people whose positions are obsolete. What would you do if you had to fire these people who are the "victims" of a process improvement?
4. Ask ChatGPT (https://chatgpt.com): "What are the elements of the best layout for an ED?" Follow up with "Where should these areas be located?"

   How does the proposed solution differ from the layout in Figure 11.2? Are there constraints that prevent "ideal" layouts to be implemented? Explain.
5. Mock interview. You and a fellow student conduct a 10-minute interview on the standardization of procedures for better safety, with one of you being Dr. Atul Gawande, and the other the interviewer. Hint: Review information on Dr. Gawande's professional accomplishments and writings before the interview.

SPRINGER PUBLISHING CONNECT™ A robust set of instructor resources designed to supplement this text is located at **http://connect.springerpub.com/content/book/978-0-8261-7976-0.** Qualifying instructors may request access by emailing **textbook@springerpub.com.**

REFERENCES

Corporate Finance Institute. (2024). *Benefit–cost ratio (BCR)*. https://corporatefinanceinstitute.com/resources/accounting/benefit-cost-ratio-bcr

Dalton-Norman, C. (2024). *Optimize transfer center practices to improve patient acquisition whitepaper*. Conduit Health Partners. https://www.conduithp.com/news/optimize-transfer-center-practices-to-improve-patient-acquisition

DeSai, C., Janowiak, K., Secheli, B., Phelps, E., McDonald, S., Reed, G., & Blomkalns, A. (2021). Empowering patients: Simplifying discharge instructions. *BMJ Open Quality*, *10*(3), e001419. https://www.ncbi.nlm.nih.gov/pmc/articles/PMC8442096

Health Catalyst. (2024). *Quick registration dramatically reduces delays in ED patient care*. https://www.healthcatalyst.com/success_stories/emergency-department-registration-process-mission-health

Imhoff, B., Marshall, K., Nazir, N., Pal, A., & Parkhurst, M. (2022). Reducing time to admission in emergency department patients: A crossfunctional quality improvement project. *BMJ Open Quality*, *11*, e001987. https://doi.org/10.1136/bmjoq-2022-001987

Institute of Medicine. (2007). *Preventing medication errors*. Washington, DC: The National Academies Press. https://doi.org/10.17226/11623

Johns Hopkins Medicine. (2016). *Study suggests medical errors now third leading cause of death in the U.S.* https://hub.jhu.edu/2016/05/03/medical-errors-third-leading-cause-of-death/#:~:text=Analyzing%20medical%20death%20rate%20data,Prevention's%20third%20leading%20cause%20of

Kaira, J., Kopargaonkar, A. (2016). Quality improvement in clinical laboratories: A Six Sigma concept. *Pathology and Laboratory Medicine*, *1*(1), 11–20. https://www.researchgate.net/publication/304580459_Quality_Improvement_In_Clinical_Laboratories_A_Six_Sigma_Concept

Nevalainen, D., Berte, L., Kraft, C., Leigh, E. Picaso, & Morgan, T. (2000). Evaluating laboratory performance on quality indicators with the Six Sigma scale. *Archives of Pathology & Laboratory Medicine*, *124*, 516–519. https://doi.org/10.5858/2000-124-0516-ELPOQI

Noronha, A., Bhat, S., Gijo, E. V., Antony, J., Laureani, A., & Laux, C. (2023). Performance and service quality enhancement in a healthcare setting through Lean Six Sigma strategy. *International Journal of Quality & Reliability Management*, *40*(2), 365–390. https://doi.org/10.1108/IJQRM-07-2021-0226

Suliburk, J. W., Buck, Q. M., Pirko, C. J., Massarweh, N. M., Barshes, N. R. et al. (2019). Analysis of human performance deficiencies with surgical adverse events. *JAMA Network Open*, *2*(7), e198067. https://doi.org/10.1001/jamanetworkopen.2019.8067

PART VI

CONTROL—How to Keep Waste at Bay?

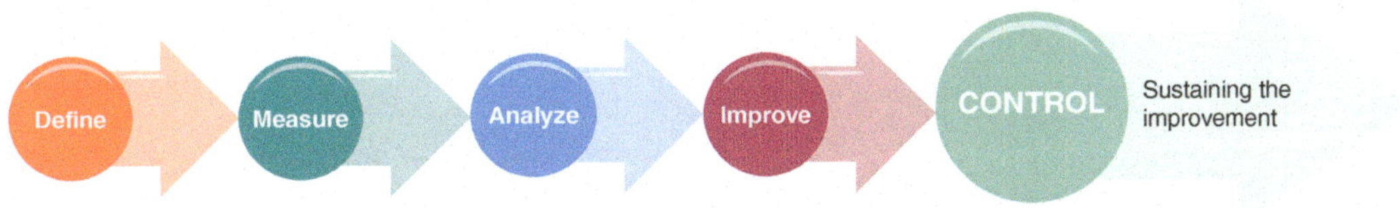

CHAPTER 12

SUSTAINING THE IMPROVEMENT

BRIGHT ANGEL MEDICAL CENTER 12.1

Barbara Waters had just come back from a week at the beach. She was relaxed and ready to get back to business. She turned on her computer and started reading her emails. The routine: meetings, reports, inquiries from staff, and upcoming conference announcements. Someone knocked on her door. "Come in," she said cheerfully. Adeleke and Olina entered the office. "Welcome back, stranger," Adeleke said.

"Nice tan," Olina complimented. They all laughed and chatted for a couple of minutes. Olina sighed. "I hate to bring this up on your first day back," she said, "but we have had a few issues—nothing serious—with some of the older care providers. Not only are they reluctant to use checklists, but even when they do, the methods they use to perform some of the tasks are also antiquated."

Adeleke added, "There is an ego issue, and it runs counter to our desire to standardize best practices. Also, it irritates the providers who stick to the rules."

"For example?" Barbara inquired.

"For example, one of the physicians still orders too many CT scans for pediatric patients, often violating the pediatric CT protocols. Also, for transfers, some providers still bypass the central office."

"Time for a Gemba walk," Barbara said as she stood up.

How can older providers be persuaded to adopt new protocols?

LEARNING OBJECTIVES

After reading this chapter, you will be able to:

- Develop a control plan.
- Differentiate standard operating procedures (SOPs) from checklists.
- Establish a system to safeguard document integrity and ensure appropriate storage.
- See how internal audits can be proactive agents of compliance and change.
- Understand the importance of statistical process control (SPC), routine, simplicity, and visual aids in sustaining the improvement.
- Recognize the collaborative effort in taking the improvement to the next level.

INTRODUCTION

Once the improvement is implemented and deemed successful, we must ensure that it stays that way. It is easy to go back to our "old" ways of doing things, thus jeopardizing the improvement. This chapter focuses on retaining the benefits of the process redesign. This effort will start with proper documentation of the improvement, including a control plan, SOPs, document control, and regular audits. The documents can be consulted whenever uncertainty occurs or "bad" habits reemerge. Then, mechanisms and tools to monitor the process are established: SPC, 6S, total productive maintenance (TPM), visual management (VM), and huddles; they contribute to systematizing and routinizing the improvements. As you know, there is no such thing as perfection, and there is always room for further improvement. Participative structures such as quality circles (QCs) and kaizen blitzes help us reach the next frontier in excellence and disseminate the lessons learned. This material is presented in three sections:

- Documenting the New Process
- Systematizing the Improvement
- Institutionalizing the Improvement

WHY IS THIS MATERIAL USEFUL?

After expending so much effort and so many resources to improve a process, it would be a pity to let time and apathy chip away at achievements benefiting patients and staff. Learning how to sustain the improved process and staying focused on further progress are therefore critical components of quality management.

DOCUMENTING THE NEW PROCESS

CONTROL PLAN

Sustaining the gains over time starts with the development of a **control plan**. This document outlines the improved process steps and characteristics and specifies the actions needed to maintain performance (Croft, 2024). A control plan typically includes the following items (Croft, 2024; Usifo, 2024).

1. **The process steps**. All process steps must be listed. A flowchart is a useful tool for this purpose because it also depicts the process flow. The failure mode and effects analysis (FMEA) is also valuable because it specifies all possible failure points in the process; these points need to be monitored closely.
2. **The performance metrics of interest and their specifications**. The critical-to-quality characteristics (CTQs) that are relevant to control the process should be clearly defined. In Bright Angel Medical Center (BAMC)'s case, they will include: average lengths of stay (ALOS), left-without-being-seen (LWBS), door-to-doc time, number of stock shortages in exam rooms, time from decision to discharge to actual discharge, return visits within 72 hours, and so on. The specifications are expressed as a target value and a tolerance range (e.g., 120 minutes ± 15 minutes). Throughput yield and sigma level are other important metrics to track performance.
3. **The measurement methods**. How will you measure the CTQs? The methods should spell out:
   a. The tools, instruments, and recording methods used to measure the CTQs. These may be electronic health records, sampling method and size, patient experience survey results, observations, and so on.
   b. Frequency of data collection and reporting. How often will the data be collected and their results reported? For example, length of stay (LOS) may be recorded continuously and reported in real time, whereas hand hygiene compliance may be observed through daily samples and reported monthly.
   c. The measurement units: These might include minutes or hours, percentages or rates per 1,000 patient-days, and so on.

4. **The control methods**. How will you ensure that the process does not deviate from its specifications? Statistical process control (SPC), checklists, *poka-yoke*, visual aids such as wall boards, dashboards, and **standard operating procedures (SOPs)** help detect deviations from expected performance and trigger prompt, corrective action. For SPC, the centerline and control limit values should be stated.
5. **The response plan**. If the process metrics fall outside the control limits or specifications, the actions necessary to identify the root causes, eliminate them, and bring the process back into control should be stipulated. These actions should be documented as well for future reference.
6. **Roles and responsibilities**. To ensure accountability, the people who will be responsible for taking the measurements, analyzing the data, reporting the results, and taking corrective action should be named in the plan.
7. **Review and revision**. In a dynamic environment, conditions change. The control plan should therefore be evaluated regularly; it is a living document. When revisions are made, the date when the plan was updated and its version number should be clearly indicated.

The following is an example of a control plan for BAMC (Figure 12.1). To save space, the flowchart is omitted.

STANDARD OPERATING PROCEDURES

SOPs are detailed sets of written instructions to perform routine operations correctly and consistently (Gaskin, 2022). These instructions should always be followed in the same way to guarantee regulatory compliance and adherence to best practices. Their purpose is threefold: (1) improve performance (quality, efficiency, and reliability); (2) establish a standard for quality control; and (3) protect against knowledge loss. To develop an SOP, perform the following steps (Hashemi-Pour & Brush, 2024; Oragui, 2024).

1. **Define the objectives of the SOP.** Is it meant to increase efficiency, improve communication between providers, prevent adverse events, or something else? A group of stakeholders should brainstorm and identify the SOP's specific goals.
2. **Identify the end user(s).** The SOP must focus on the specific activities carried out by the end users. As a result, it should be written in a way that they can easily understand and use terms which are common in their work environment.
3. **Determine the scope.** In this step, one has to decide which elements will be included in the SOP. These may be: What specific tasks should be addressed, by whom (see previous step), when, where, and how (tools, instruments, system, etc.; Box 12.1).
4. **Select the format.** This step depends on the audience for which the SOP is created. The format can be:
   - a step-by-step list for short and straightforward instructions,
   - a hierarchical list for a longer and more complex series of steps and substeps,
   - a flowchart for procedures that involve decision points with alternate paths and outcomes, or
   - a video that demonstrates how certain tasks need to be performed (e.g., on a computer system).
5. **Collect all information and draft the SOP**. Research all aspects of the operation that need to be documented, observe the tasks involved, talk to subject matter experts, and so on. Then develop an outline and start writing the SOP.
6. **Pretest and revise**. Solicit feedback from a group of targeted end users and revise the SOP accordingly.
7. **Train the end users and implement the process**. Once the SOP is finalized, employees must be trained or retrained to perform and practice the operation as specified in the SOP.
8. **Review periodically and revise**. In the quest for continuous improvement, process changes will occur on a regular basis. The SOP must be updated accordingly, and the users should be trained or made aware of the new version.

	A	B	C	D	E	F	G	H	I	J	K	L	M	N	O
4		Customer:	Patients, Staff, Payers, Community, TJC				Email:	amensah@bamc.net						Revision date:	9/4/2025
5							Phone:	111-111-1111						Version	1.1
6															
7–8	Step	CTQ/Metric	Specification Target	LSL	USL	Measurement Method	Sample Size	Measure Frequency	Responsible for Measurement	Control Chart Type	CL	LCL	UCL	Corrective Action Code	Responsible for Action
9	Registration	Wait time (min)	1	0	2	Observation (sampling)	5	1X each shift	Intern	X-bar and R	0.9	0	1.8	A or B,C	Patient Registration Supervisor
10	Triage	Door-to-triage time (min)	3	1	5	EHR system	Shift subgroup	End of shift	Data analyst	X-bar and s	3.2	1.4	5	A or B,C	Nurse manager
11	Initial exam	Door-to-doc time (min)	35	25	45	EHR system	Shift subgroup	End of shift	Data analyst	X-bar and s	32	21	43	B, C, D	Nurse manager
12		LWBS (%)	1	0	2	EHR system	Shift subgroup	End of shift	Data analyst	p-chart	1.5	1.2	1.8	B, C, E	Service representative
13		Hand hygiene (%)	96	95	100	Pokayoke; Observation (sampling)	shift subgroup; 20 min	Daily	Rotating observation team	p-chart	96	92	100	F,G	Observation team
14		Exam time (min)	15	10	30	Observation (sampling)	5	1X each shift	Nurse	X-bar and R	17	5	29	A, B, G	ED Medical Director
15	Blood drawn	Wait time (min)	4	0	8	EHR system	10	1X daily	Data analyst	X-bar and s	5	2	8	A,B,C,F	Lab manager
16		Lab turnaround time (min)	15	10	20	EHR system	10	1X daily	Data analyst	X-bar and s	18	14	22	A,B,C	Lab manager
17	x-rays taken	Wait time (min)	2	0	5	EHR system	10	1X daily	Data analyst	X-bar and s	2	0	4	A, B, C	Nurse manager
18	Treatmt. Init.	Stockouts (#)	0	0	3	Pokayoke; Observation	Each occurrence	Daily	Nurse	u-chart	1	0	2	B,C,F	Nurse
19		Sigma level	5	4.5	6	EHR system	Each occurrence	Monthly	Data analyst		4.2	4	4.4	B,C,D,E,F,G	ED Medical Director
20	Cond. Reass.	Wait time (min)	25	20	30	EHR system	4	1X each shift	Data analyst	X-bar and R	25	20	30	A,B,C,F,G	ED Medical Director
21		Sigma level	5	4.5	6	EHR system	Each occurrence	Monthly	Data analyst		4.4	4.2	4.6	B,C,D,E,F,G	ED Medical Director
22	Discharge	Wait time (min)	7	4	10	EHR system	shift subgroup	1X each shift	Data analyst	X-bar and s	18	12	24	A,B,C,D,G	Nurse manager
23		ALOS (min)	120	90	150	EHR system	All occurrences	Monthly	Data analyst	IX-bar and MR	162.8	148	199	B,C,D,G	ED director
24		Teach-back (%)	95	90	100	Observation (sampling)	shift subgroup; 30 min	1X each shift	Intern	p-chart	94	91	97	B,C,D,F,G	Nurse manager
25		Return to ED < 72 hrs (%)	2.5	0	5	EHR system	Each occurrence	Monthly	Data analyst	p-chart	4	3	5	B,C,E,F,G	ED Medical Director
26	Admission	Wait time (min)	30	20	40	EHR system	shift subgroup	1X each shift	Data analyst	X-bar and s	27	21	33	A,B,C,D,G	ED Medical Director, Admissions
27		ALOS (min)	160	150	200	EHR system	All occurrences	Monthly	Data analyst	IX-bar and MR	162	135	189	B,C,D,G	ED Medical Director, Admissions
28	Transfer	Wait time (min)	25	5	60	EHR system	shift subgroup	1X each shift	Data analyst	X-bar and s	30	20	40	A,B,C,D,G	Central call center
29		ALOS (min)	200	100	240	EHR system	All occurrences	Monthly	Data analyst	IX-bar and MR	197	127	267	B,C,D,G	Central call center
30															
31															
32	A	Check capacity and demand													
33	B	Determine root cause and solve problem													
34	C	Verify corrective action is effective													
35	D	Deploy customer service protocol													
36	E	Deploy service recovery protocol													
37	F	Communicate results to accountable staff													
38	G	Post results in designated areas													
39		Candidate for improvement or reevaluation of specs.													
40															

FIGURE 12.1 Control plan for BAMC.

Abbreviation: BAMC, Bright Angel Medical Center.

BOX 12.1 FAQs

What is the difference between a checklist and an SOP?

A checklist is a simple step-by-step list of *what* tasks need to be done in sequential order.

An SOP is more detailed. Besides the *what*, it also specifies *when*, *where*, and especially *how* a task is to be done, in addition to *who* will do it. It is much more granular than a checklist.

Abbreviation: SOP, standard operating procedure.

SOPs should be distributed to users and, in some cases, posted in locations where the operation is performed. For easy reference, it is a good idea to make the SOPs available online. An example of an SOP is provided in Box 12.2.

DOCUMENT CONTROL

As mentioned earlier, control plans and documents must be aligned with a changing environment. In other words, control is dynamic. **Document control** involves the systematic management of critical documents related to process quality. It includes the creation, approval, storage, organization, review, and distribution of documents so that "the right version is available to the right people at the right time" (Accruent, 2024). This practice follows the International Organization for

BOX 12.2 QUALITY IN PRACTICE!

Standard Operating Procedure for Patient Transfer (Isakov, 2024)

The Centers for Disease Control and Prevention (CDC) provides an example of SOP for patient handoff between a healthcare facility and an ambulance. The format of the SOP is a hierarchical, bulleted list of tasks to be performed in chronological order. They include:

- mobilizing for patient transfer
- preparing for transfer of patient and patient care
  - sending facility tasks
  - transporting ambulance provider tasks
    - before transport
    - during transport
    - upon arrival
  - receiving facility tasks

The full SOP example is available online at: https://stacks.cdc.gov/view/cdc/156207/cdc_156207_DS1.pdf

Abbreviation: SOP, standard operating procedure.

Standardization (ISO)'s requirements for document control. These requirements include (Byrne, 2023; Randig, 2009):

1. **Get approval of documents before release**. New documents (e.g., process changes, SOPs) must be checked for accuracy and approved by designated individuals before they are distributed and used. To avoid long and unnecessary delays, only process owners and other stakeholders should approve the new documents.
2. **Update documents and get them reapproved.** We can be certain of one thing: work never stays the same. External conditions such as new technologies or regulations bring about change, and so does an organization's commitment to continuous improvement. Processes will change accordingly, and documents will have to be updated and reapproved.
3. **Make sure changes can be identified**. When you collaborate with others on a document, you want to be able to see the changes they make (think about the "Track Changes" option in a word processor). The same is true for document control. It would be careless to keep only the most recent version. Rather, the people approving the changes want to see the old and new versions, with dates and changes typed in red, for example. This facilitates the change audit trail.
4. **Make the documents available at points of use**. The people using the documents should have easy, but controlled, access to them. Fortunately, most documents are now stored digitally, and permissions for access can be granted or rescinded. When paper documents are involved, it becomes more difficult to control access and ensure that the correct version is in use.
5. **Identify documents of external origin and control their distribution**. Documents from external suppliers (e.g., safety instructions for equipment used in process) and customers (e.g., Centers for Medicare & Medicaid Services [CMS] requirements) may be stored with all other process documents. These do not require approval and updates by your organization, but it is imperative that the authorized users of these documents have access to the correct version.
6. **Prevent the unintended use of obsolete documents**. As mentioned in Points #3 to #5, it is important that the most recent version of a document be used. It is therefore critical to communicate version updates to all relevant users and deny access to obsolete documents stored digitally. With paper copies, instructions to destroy old documents or to stamp them as "obsolete" should be clearly communicated.

AUDITING

An **audit** is a systematic performance review based on selected criteria or standards (Jamtvedt et al., 2019). Although auditing in healthcare often emphasizes billing to detect fraud and abuse, it can also pertain to medical practices. The intent is to identify areas (structure, process, outcomes) where clinical care deviates from evidence-based guidelines or best practices and identify improvement opportunities. Audits may be external (Box 12.3) when conducted by entities such as The Joint Commission (TJC), or internal when performed by the organization's quality officers or healthcare professionals. They can be based on readily available information (e.g., readmissions within 72 hours or patient experience survey results) or on new observations and sampling. Although they are part of accreditation and certification (see Chapter 13), audits can serve a more proactive purpose in achieving excellence and getting closer to a desired benchmark. The ultimate goal is to improve compliance, safety, health outcomes, and patient experience. In a systematic review of the literature, Hut-Mossel and colleagues (2021) identified several factors that influence the impact of an audit on the quality of care:

1. External audits initially improve care, then gains taper off because of complacency.
2. A situation has to feel unsustainable for healthcare professionals to engage with internal audits.
3. Successful, internal audits require champions to be deemed worthy by healthcare professionals.
4. Bottom-up initiated audits are more likely to result in meaningful and sustainable improvements.
5. Audit findings motivate healthcare professionals to persuade high-level management of the need to improve.
6. Audits stimulate feedback across disciplines and foster collaboration.

BOX 12.3 QUALITY IN PRACTICE!

External Audit of the Emergency Medical Services (EMS) Preparedness in the Czech Republic

The preparedness of EMS depends on real experience as well as tactical and verification exercises. In the Czech Republic, there is no standardized methodology to evaluate EMS preparedness, resulting in inconsistent responses across the country. To improve the evaluation process, a group of academics and 32 EMS experts developed an auditing tool with specific metrics. The development of this tool started with an examination of the obligations of EMS units as stipulated by law. They identified three important criteria to measure: (1) collaborative preparedness with other units of the Integrated Rescue System; (2) the preparedness of EMS forces for emergency events; and (3) the means of communication during an emergency. These criteria were measured by 13 indicators, weighted based on their importance. The scores received on each indicator were multiplied by the respective weights, and the sum of these weighted values determined the level of preparedness. This tool was used successfully for external audits, but it can also serve as a self-assessment and guide for improvement (Tušer et al., 2023).

SYSTEMATIZING THE IMPROVEMENT

Sustaining the improvement goes beyond establishing the administrative safeguards covered in the previous section. It also involves making the "new" process the everyday routine. SPC is especially useful in that regard.

STATISTICAL PROCESS CONTROL (REVISITED)

In Six Sigma, SPC is a true multitasker: it *measures* the process (Chapter 8), shows whether the *improvement* has taken place (Chapter 11), and indicates whether the "new" process remains in *control*. The *IX*-chart displaying the ALOS for discharged patients (Figure 11.4) displays a major reduction in random variation for 6 months after improvement. Remember that for a process, the state of being "in control" means that the process behaves as expected with no assignable or nonrandom variation. This is why SPC systematically tracks process indicator values and signals when an out-of-control situation has already arisen or is imminent. To illustrate, let's revisit the ALOS for a year after improvement.

You may recall from Chapter 11 that the centerline value of the *IX* chart, $\overline{IX}$, was 173.8 minutes, and the average moving range value, $\overline{MR}$, was 9.6 minutes. Therefore, the control limits (lower control limit [LCL] and upper control limit [UCL]) were:

$$LCL_{IX} = 173.8 - (2.66 \times 9.6) = 148.3 \text{ minutes}$$

$$UCL_{IX} = 173.8 + (2.66 \times 9.6) = 199.4 \text{ minutes}$$

$$LCL_{MR} = 0 \times 9.6 = 0 \text{ minute}$$

$$UCL_{MR} = 3.267 \times 9.6 = 31.4 \text{ minutes}$$

ALOS was tracked every month (Table 12.1), and the next 6 months of data were plotted on the existing SPC charts for the new process (Figure 12.2).

As you can see, the MR are in control, but the ALOS are definitely not. There is a visible downward trend with the last three points below the LCL. Should the people at BAMC be worried? Find out in Bright Angel Medical Center 12.2.

TABLE 12.1 A YEAR OF AVERAGE LENGTHS OF STAY (ALOS) AND MOVING RANGES (MR) AFTER IMPROVEMENT

Month	ALOS (min)	MR
1	189	–
2	178	11
3	174	4
4	158	16
5	173	15
6	171	2
7	168	3
8	154	14
9	158	4
10	142	16
11	148	6
12	141	7
Average	162.8	8.9

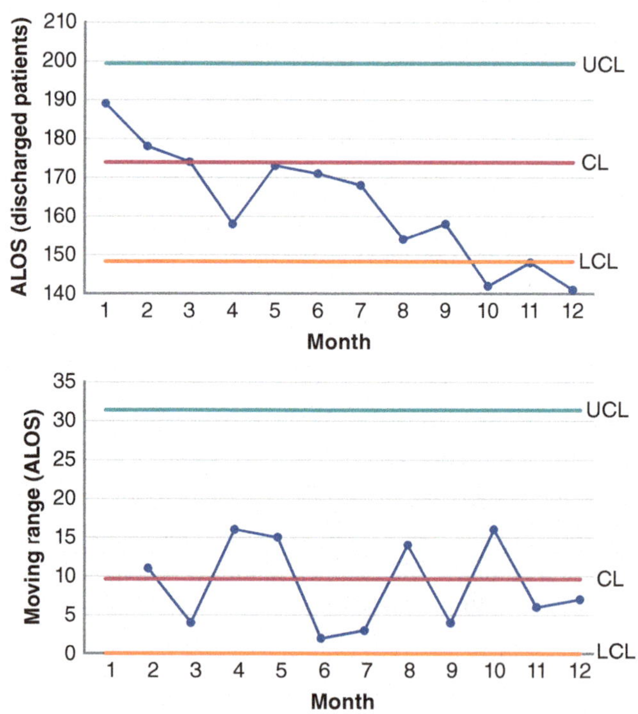

FIGURE 12.2 *IX*- and *MR*-charts for 12 months after improvement.

Abbreviations: ALOS, average lengths of stay; CL, centerline; LCL, lower control limit; MR, moving range; UCL, upper control limit.

BRIGHT ANGEL MEDICAL CENTER 12.2

Barbara stormed into Olina's office. "What is this? The new process is already out of control! What went wrong?" she exclaimed.

Olina replied: "Please calm down. Yes, the process is out of control, but think of it as the initial phase. We only had six points to establish the new control limits, which was not much to start

(continued)

BRIGHT ANGEL MEDICAL CENTER 12.2 (*CONTINUED*)

with. After the new process was implemented, we tweaked a few things, and this downward trend is looking very good to us. We may be on our way to meet our target of 2 hours for discharged patients."

Barbara's expression softened. "That makes sense, I overreacted. What shall we do now?"

Olina answered, "We know why the process is out of control, and it is a good thing. We are waiting for a few more data points and we will build a new control chart."

Barbara got up and said, "Very good. Did you share this with Adeleke?"

Olina smiled. "Of course," she said. "He had noticed too. You know he just got his Black Belt, don't you?"

Barbara smiled back. "Yes, I know. I have a little gift for him . . . a small judoka figure . . . with a black belt!" They both laughed.

If the ALOS keeps going down, what would you recommend?

6S (REVISITED)

In Chapter 10, you saw how 6S created a platform for order, standardization, and visibility to promote an unencumbered process flow and continuously improve quality. These elements are important to hold the gains achieved with the improved process. Let's see how each element of 6S can benefit the redesigned process (Rodriguez, 2024; Six Sigma Daily, 2020).

- **Sort out**: When unnecessary items are eliminated (e.g., obsolete SOPs, expired medications), efficiency and productivity increase as employees spend less time searching for the items needed, and freed up space eases access and flow.
- **Systematize**: When each item is stored in one place and stays in that place, efficiency and productivity further increase because unnecessary movements and searches are eliminated.
- **Scrub**: Cleanliness improves safety, especially in healthcare, with fewer slips and falls and a lower risk of contamination. It may also boost staff morale and patient satisfaction.
- **Standardize**: Repetitiveness (e.g., checklists, warnings, labels) is the antidote to excess variation, thereby decreasing defects. It also eases problem detection by flagging abnormalities.
- **Sustain**: Sticking to the rules is the necessary condition for control. It promotes adherence to a new and better way of doing things. It also encourages people to work together and generate new ideas.
- **Safety**: Being mindful of safety risks and finding ways to minimize or eradicate them further reinforces people's engagement in continuous process improvement.

The 6S methodology is therefore an integral part of controlling the process to maintain the improvements. It is also one of the prerequisites for total productive maintenance (TPM).

TOTAL PRODUCTIVE MAINTENANCE

The order and discipline created by 6S are critical to secure well-running equipment and spot malfunctions. In Chapter 10 (Principle #2), you saw that TPM prevents excessive delegation by engaging employees to perform small, routine maintenance activities on the equipment they use. That way, maintenance personnel is free to address maintenance problems requiring more advanced technical expertise. TPM also encourages employees to report problems they could not handle right away to avoid safety issues, defects, delays, and breakdowns later on. In that regard, TPM also plays an important role in the control phase of a Six Sigma project by safeguarding the reliability of the equipment and the integrity of the process. Why is it considered "total"? Because it includes everyone in the organization, spans the entire life cycle of the equipment, and covers all equipment in every department or office.

Types of Maintenance

There are two primary types of maintenance: preventive and corrective. **Preventive maintenance** refers to scheduled maintenance activities to prevent problems from occurring when the equipment is used for productive purposes. Think about taking your car for service so that it will not break down when you drive it. **Corrective (or breakdown) maintenance** entails the activities performed to restore the equipment to its proper working condition after a breakdown has already occurred. In this case, think about taking your car to a repairman because of a transmission fluid leak. These two types of maintenance can be further divided into more specific types, and there is no shortage of classification schemes in the literature. Generally speaking, corrective maintenance has two subcategories (Tarlengco, 2024):

- Emergency maintenance that is undertaken after a machine failure; for example, a service call is made when a computer system has crashed.
- Deferred maintenance that is postponed due to lack of resources (e.g., budget, manpower, or spare parts). An example of this type of maintenance could be delaying the repair of a ventilation system because no replacement parts are readily available.

Preventive maintenance is often subdivided into (Wu, 2024):

- Time-based maintenance, according to which maintenance activities are scheduled at regular time intervals. An example would be inspecting fire extinguishers in a hospital once a month.
- Usage-based maintenance that depends on the amount of usage of the equipment. For example, breathalyzers may be recalibrated every 100 uses.
- Predictive maintenance that depends on sensors to detect whether maintenance is needed. For example, a color printer will indicate when an ink cartridge is running low and needs to be reordered or replaced.
- Prescriptive maintenance, which is an advanced type of preventive maintenance that relies on data analytics, machine learning, and artificial intelligence (AI) to predict when maintenance will be required. For example, analysis of vibration data on certain parts could identify the extent of wear and make maintenance suggestions.
- TPM is also an advanced type of preventive maintenance in that it promotes a proactive, holistic approach to eliminating all forms of waste and improving equipment reliability.

A summary of the types of maintenance is shown in Figure 12.3.

Benefits of Total Productive Maintenance

We have already mentioned the general benefits of TPM, but here is a more comprehensive list showing the broad impact of this Lean methodology:

- **Human benefits** with employee ownership, knowledge, higher morale, teamwork, and increased autonomy.
- **Cost benefits** through lower repair costs, freed up capacity of specialized maintenance personnel, reduced unplanned downtime, and lower scrap and rework.

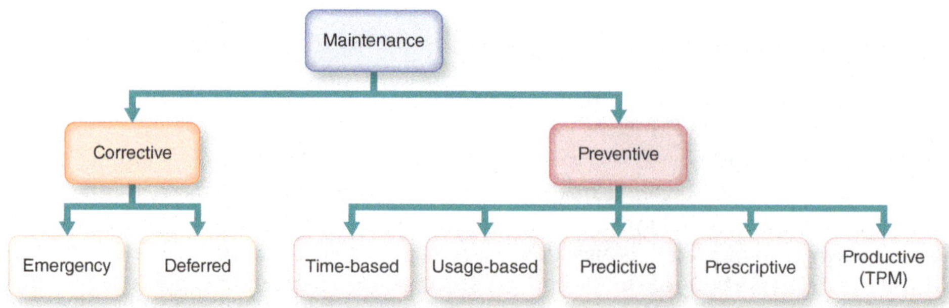

FIGURE 12.3 Types of maintenance.

- **Quality benefits** with increased system reliability, higher safety, fewer defects, lower variation, continuous improvement, and ultimately better customer satisfaction.
- **Speed benefits** with optimal productivity and fewer delays and stoppages.

In summary, TPM contributes to process performance gains and their sustainability.

VISUAL WORKPLACE

Lean wants problems to be visible, not hidden. Why? So that they can be detected easily and corrected promptly. **Visual management (VM)** is therefore one of the pillars of Lean. It is a system that uses visual cues to provide workers with process information, often in real time, and trigger swift corrective action when required.

Benefits of Visual Management

Some of the advantages of using VM include (Tezel et al., 2016):

- process transparency
- discipline in maintaining correct procedures
- continuous improvement
- job facilitation and time saving
- learning while working
- shared ownership
- management-by-facts
- simplification

In this book, we have already talked about operational dashboards or wall boards, value stream maps, kanban systems, and 6S as useful visual tools to identify problems when they occur, but a host of other tools are reported in the literature. Table 12.2 displays a few of them and their purposes.

Huddle boards and huddles obviously go hand in hand. In Chapter 2, we had briefly discussed daily huddles. Let's examine them in more detail.

TABLE 12.2 TYPES OF VISUAL TOOLS AND THEIR PURPOSES

Tool	Purpose
Color coding	Identification (e.g., good in green and bad in red) Designation of location (e.g., yellow signs for warnings; blue containers for surgical tape [Figure 12.4])
Floor markings and signage	Designation of specific zones (e.g., where special PPE is required) Directions to access specific areas (e.g., Imaging)
Shadow boards	Marking of where each piece of equipment must be placed (e.g., tool board with drawings of tools in different spots)
Andon lights	Flashing when a major problem has occurred and the process must stop (e.g., code blue)
Kanban boards with cards	Authorization to perform certain activities to ensure flow (e.g., replenishment cards for some supplies)
Huddle boards	Communication of issues and team progress in daily or weekly meetings (e.g., review of various KPIs at the beginning of a shift in the ED)
Digital signage	Real time communication of process status (e.g., patients waiting for discharge instructions; estimated wait time in ED)

Abbreviations: KPIs, key performance indicators; PPE, personal protective equipment.

Source: Adapted from McLean, T. (2024). *Types of visual management tools and visual controls*. TXM Lean Solutions. https://txm.com/5-types-of-visual-controls/; Croft, D. (2024). *Visual management*. Learn Lean Sigma. https://www.learnleansigma.com/lean-tools/visual-management

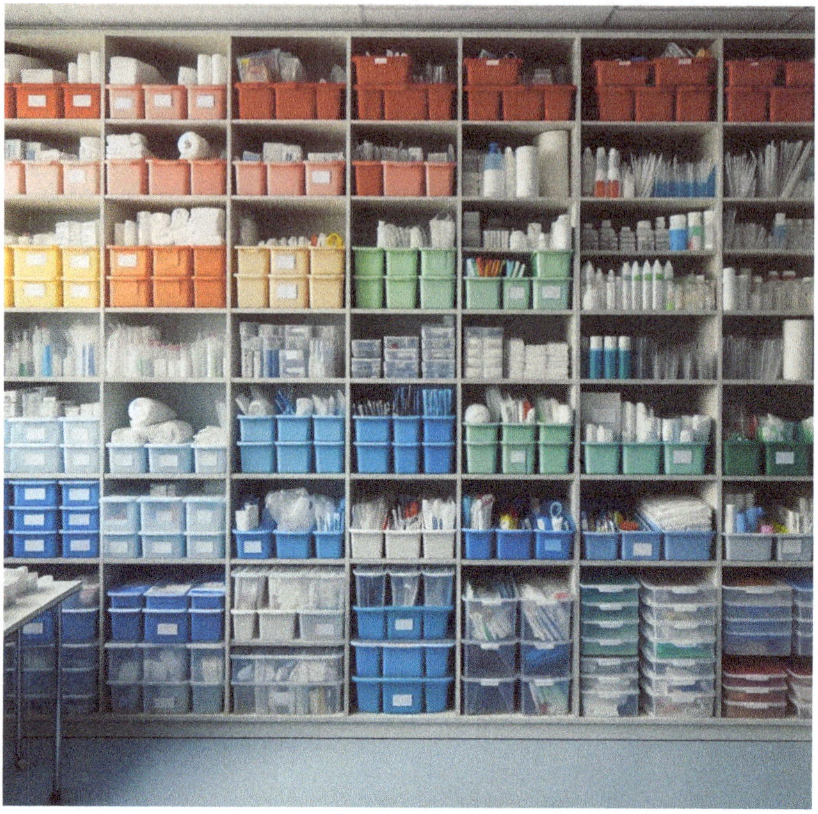

FIGURE 12.4 Color-coded containers in supply room.

Note: Created with Microsoft Copilot|Designer.

HUDDLES

Huddles are short meetings occurring at the beginning of the workday or shift. They provide the opportunity to update the team regarding new initiatives, review the progress made from the previous day, and address the day's agenda, especially in the area of safety (e.g., risks associated with today's scheduled patients). The compressed, standardized format requires that: (a) the huddle occur at the same time for consistency; (b) the members stand; (c) the agenda be posted, not read, on a board; (d) safety concerns be escalated for resolution, not solved on the spot; and (e) only unusual patients scheduled for the day be mentioned (Agency for Healthcare Research and Quality, 2017).

A typical agenda comprises (Institute for Healthcare Improvement, 2024):

1. **Yesterday's safety issues.** Wins of the day should be listed. If there are concerns, the CUS (Concern, Uncomfortable, Safety) tool may be used for this purpose as participants will (a) state their **C**oncern; (b) say why it made them **U**ncomfortable, and (c) state that there is a **S**afety issue. The link to a very good video illustrating this concept is: https://www.youtube.com/watch?v=LvO-4qM_aig&t=10s.
2. **Today's issues.** Issues about some patients scheduled for the day are discussed. A table with the patients' names and issues should be posted on the board to speed up review and serve as a reminder during the day.
3. **Tracked issues.** Updates on issues that have been monitored by the team are mentioned.
4. **Inputs.** Team members are asked one more time if they have any special concern.
5. **Announcements.** New initiatives and other changes/updates are communicated.

Benefits of Huddles

Huddles have multiple benefits (Shaikh, 2020):

- continuous safety improvement
- quick and sharp focus on daily safety issues
- face-to-face communication
- empowerment of frontline staff
- increased accountability
- proactive control of quality

As problem detection is prioritized and promptly communicated, huddles not only help monitor process performance, but they also fulfill the quest for continuous improvement (see ON THE JOB! video).

ON THE JOB! INTERVIEW VIDEO 12.1

Jennifer Gartner
Internal Medicine Practice Manager

Daily Huddles to Drive and Sustain Change
Organizing daily huddles
Remote nurse support for in-basket management
Managing challenges with COVID
Accountability through huddle participation

1. Jennifer discusses her role as a practice manager and shares some tips about daily huddles. What are some of the tactics used in her daily huddles?
2. The remote in-basket support is a project that the clinic implemented and discussed at the daily huddle. What are the benefits of this format when new projects are launched?
3. How can daily huddles contribute to accountability? How does psychological safety impact the effectiveness of the huddles?

The interview is available online by visiting www.springerpub.com/courseconnect. See inside front cover and tear-out card for CourseConnect details.

INSTITUTIONALIZING THE IMPROVEMENT

In the previous sections of this chapter, we have mentioned continuous improvement several times. Consistent with the "Act" stage in the Deming Wheel (Chapter 1), you want to expand the knowledge to a wider domain and even push the envelope further. This philosophy of continuous improvement is *kaizen* (Chapter 2). All process stakeholders should be continuously engaged in improving the process.

QUALITY CIRCLES

Quality circles (QCs) are groups of three to 12 frontline employees who meet regularly to find ways to solve problems in their work area. Participation is voluntary, and workers meet during work hours (International Society of Six Sigma Professionals, 2024). They play an important part in controlling a process as they continuously identify problems that will inevitably surface over time. They are trained in Lean concepts and quality improvement tools such as SPC, Pareto charts, and cause-and-effect diagrams. They formulate suggestions for improvements, present them to their supervisors or middle management, and, if lucky, they get to implement them.

Because they are continuously involved in the process, they are ideal candidates to spot problems, fix them, and prevent later occurrences. Therefore, they can be guardians of process improvements. QCs encourage a culture of quality control awareness among employees. However, over time, they tend to yield diminishing returns. Rejected suggestions by management, fewer meetings, apathy, cynicism, and burnout creep up over time and halt the momentum that this participative structure once had (Lawler & Mohrman, 1985). Once popular, they have now been replaced by groups tasked to meet a precise objective over a short time frame. One example is teams in rapid process improvement workshops.

RAPID PROCESS IMPROVEMENT WORKSHOPS

Also known as a **kaizen event or kaizen blitz**, a **rapid process improvement workshop (RPIW)** is a short-term event that targets a specific problem area or process to deliver a significant improvement. Teams involving process owners and key stakeholders gather with a facilitator for 3 to 5 days (Reyes, 2023). The DMAIC (Define-Measure-Analyze-Improve-Control) methodology is applied, but the five steps are collapsed into three phases: preparation, event, and follow-up (Box 12.4). A typical schedule is shown in Table 12.3 (ad-esse.com, 2025; Feldman, 2023; Reyes, 2023).

Benefits

RPIWs or kaizen blitzes are not meant for major projects involving a large number of participants and requiring intensive data analysis. Rather, they are meant for narrow-focused problems which can be solved promptly. Their main advantages include:

- compressed time frame
- intense collaboration
- sense of urgency
- use of simple tools and techniques
- quick implementation of workable solutions
- impressive results

CLOSURE: LESSONS FROM THE PROJECT AND MOVING ON

As projects do come to a close, several lessons have been learned. Did the project achieve the aim of delivering a quality output within its scope, time, and budget constraints? Going back to the project charter is a good way to establish whether the project delivered on its promises (Table 12.4).

BOX 12.4 QUALITY IN PRACTICE!

A Lean Six Sigma Rapid Process Improvement Workshop to Implement eScreening at the Veterans Health Administration

The evidence on electronic self-report screening for patients prompted the Veterans Health Administration (VHA) to develop a comprehensive mobile screening technology (eScreening) for veterans to self-report mental and physical screenings on a tablet. A team of researchers collaborated with the National VHA Office of Patient Care Services to facilitate the eScreening implementation in VHA clinics. In the first phase of their project, they conducted an RPIW to write the eScreening Playbook, a process guide for implementation. In the second phase, they combined the Playbook with training and facilitation components to obtain a comprehensive implementation strategy for eScreening. An interdisciplinary group comprised of 12 members with a Lean Six Sigma Black Belt facilitator met during 3 days to: finalize current value stream maps, define roles, examine the eScreening process, visualize the target state, perform a gap analysis, evaluate propositions, and develop implementation, staffing, and communication plans. These outputs helped create the Playbook. Eventually, eScreening was found to be aligned with clinical practice at the VHA, and the implementation guide was deemed to provide a clear plan for usage (Pittman et al., 2021).

Abbreviation: RPIW, rapid process improvement workshop.

TABLE 12.3 THE THREE PHASES OF A KAIZEN EVENT

Phase	Activities	Time
PREPARATION (Define)	• Identify sponsor. • Define scope and objectives. • Select team members and leader. • Provide necessary training. • Collect data on current performance.	1–4 wk before workshop
EVENT Day 1 (Measure)	• Do a Gemba walk, observe, and record. • Identify key issues (more specific than objectives). • Develop a VSM. • Check relevant metrics.	1 work wk
Day 2 (Analyze/ Improve)	• Identify root causes and validate them. • Envision the future state.	
Days 3 and 4 (Improve)	• Generate high-impact solutions and make sure they are workable. • Create a list of actions for implementation. • Implement the majority of the solutions. • Ensure process is capable.	
Day 5 (Control)	• Develop SOPs. • Develop plan to monitor results. • Present recommendations and findings to upper management and get approval for full implementation.	
FOLLOW-UP	• Continue implementation. • Monitor process. • Measure performance. • Present achievements to upper management and celebrate.	0–60 d

Abbreviations: SOP, standard operating procedure; VSM, value stream map.

TABLE 12.4 ASSESSMENT OF PROJECT PERFORMANCE

Project Charter		
Improving Throughput in the ED for Better Health Outcomes and Greater Patient Satisfaction		**Achievements**
Goal Statement	Improve ED throughput by 30% by the end of the calendar year.	40%
Outcome Measures	Hand hygiene compliance rate >95%	97%
	LWBS rate <2% of arrivals	1.3%
	ED LOS (discharged) <150 min	171 min (141 now)
	ED LOS (admitted) <200 min	186 min
	Door-to-doc time <45 min	40 min
	Room-to-provider time <20 min, >90% time	93.25%
	Return to ED in <72 hrs <5%	3%
	Patient satisfaction scores in top box >80%	87.9%
	Travel nurses FTEs <20	16.5
	Lean training >85%	82%

(continued)

TABLE 12.4 ASSESSMENT OF PROJECT PERFORMANCE (*CONTINUED*)

Project Charter			
Improving Throughput in the ED for Better Health Outcomes and Greater Patient Satisfaction			**Achievements**
Milestones and Deliverables	• Staffing	4/18/25	4/18/25
	• Layout	6/6/25	6/20/25
	• Patient experience	4/18/25	4/11/25
Budget	• Staffing	$600,000	$659,000
	• Layout	$1,500,000	$1,397,000
	• Patient experience	$100,000	$98,500

Abbreviations: FTE, full-time equivalent; LOS, length of stay; LWBS, left-without-being-seen.

Some mistakes will be acknowledged. For example, the team may have realized that some metrics did not provide a precise measure of process performance, or that some activities required more levels of approval and took longer to complete. All-important observations will need to be documented. In an organization committed to continuous quality improvement, failures must be recognized, successes must be celebrated, new standards must be set, and knowledge transfer must take place. Some of these concepts are illustrated in Bright Angel Medical Center 12.3.

BRIGHT ANGEL MEDICAL CENTER 12.3

Dr. Aoki had asked Barbara to meet her for lunch at a nearby restaurant. They talked briefly about a possible visit by TJC, but it was obvious that Dr. Aoki was distracted.

"Everything OK, Hana?" Barbara inquired.

Dr. Aoki let out a deep sigh. "Frankly, no. After the changes we made, throughput has soared, and LOS has decreased by more than we could hope for. Unfortunately, some people have started to slack off a little. Some say they no longer need the checklists, others miss the huddles once in a while. Get the picture?"

Barbara hesitated for a moment and asked, "Have you talked to them?"

Dr. Aoki replied, "Of course, I did. They don't see a problem as long as we meet the target. I reminded them it was all about the patient, not just a mere target."

"I'll talk to Adeleke and Olina," Barbara promised.

A few days later . . .

Olina and Adeleke were briefed in Barbara's office. Olina started, "This is not unusual. Not everyone likes the discipline that the new system requires. Perhaps we could move the target from 150 to 145 minutes to get their attention?"

Adeleke scratched his head, "Hold on for a sec. It may be a good idea to get them to strive for even better, but it should not be perceived as the stick rather than the carrot. Perhaps Dr. Aoki and you, Barbara, should seek the staff's input about how to reach the next level of excellence. It's their process, and it's up to them to audit it and find ways to make it better. Something like that. In stressing process ownership, you might also remind them about accountability and the need to document failures when they occur. We have been a little lax

(continued)

BRIGHT ANGEL MEDICAL CENTER 12.3 (*CONTINUED*)

on that. Also, we need to get back to the habit of celebrating small wins. We all appreciate a little pat on the back."

Barbara nodded, "Very wise, Adeleke. We can't blame them for becoming complacent if we do the same thing. I'll talk to Hana."

Olina added, "Talking about wins, we have a new one at the Surgery Center. Remember that Dr. Rao was having problems with operating cases not starting on time? These problems are now fixed, and the staff and patients are much happier."

Barbara smiled, "The ED is now a model for the rest of Bright Angel! How about that? Kimberly Mitchell should thank us."

Adeleke whispered, "The rumor is that she plans to do just that!"

How do you motivate employees to strive for the next level?

ETHICAL SCENARIO 12.1

Artificial Intelligence in Healthcare

AI can offer comprehensive clinical decision support which, in turn, can lead to a better quality of care and health outcomes. Ideally, it is used as an aid, not a replacement, for decision-making. For example, it can augment human proficiency in diagnosing certain ailments. As AI capabilities continue to improve at warp speed, adoption of AI-health is likely to increase, and overreliance on the tool could occur. Could AI become a primary agent in healthcare decision-making rather than a mere control check? Several questions need to be answered.

If a misdiagnosis occurs, who is responsible for the mistake? The clinician or the tool?

What evidence is needed to prove the effectiveness and safety of the AI-health solution?

Should patients be informed of the use of AI in their healthcare?

SUMMARY

Once process improvement gains have been secured, it is crucial to sustain them as time passes. This chapter stressed the importance of documentation to track potential deviations from progress and record methods and procedures for future use. Continuous monitoring of the process, simple and disciplined organization of the work environment, and VM routinize the improvement into employees' daily tasks and ensure success through repetition. Finally, as new problems arise, it is important to prevent inertia and complacency. The team should not rest on its laurels. Rather it should aim to raise the bar higher through structured, collaborative, problem-solving efforts.

CERTIFICATION TIPS

- The American Society for Quality certification materials include all SPC charts in the *Control* section of the exam. We covered them in Chapter 8. You should be able to *apply* (select appropriate charts, do computations, and solve problems) the materials on SPC charts.
- The format of control plans varies from one source to the other. They are indeed adaptable to every situation. As you can see from Figure 12.1, they provide instructions to collect data and build control charts. They also indicate what action needs to be taken when deviations from the plan occur. You should be able to *apply* your knowledge of control plans (i.e., develop a control plan easily if you understand sampling, SPC, and improvement options).

- Simply *understand* the nature and purpose of SOPs and document control. Also *remember* what audits involve and why they are conducted.
- The material on training plans (not covered in this chapter) should be *applied*. Sources to develop training plans include: https://www.coursera.org/enterprise/articles/power-of-effective-employee-training-plan and https://www.indeed.com/hire/c/info/training-plan-templates.
- *Apply* your knowledge of 6S to create and sustain order in a particular situation.
- *Understand* how the various types of maintenance can be used to control the improvement.
- *Understand* how VM tools can improve control.
- Review the Plan-Do-Study-Act cycle (Chapter 1) and be able to determine (*Apply*) what is being done at each stage.

KEY TERMS

Control plan
Standard operating procedure (SOP)
Document control
Audit
Preventive maintenance
Corrective (or breakdown) maintenance
Visual management (VM)
Quality circle (QC)
Rapid process improvement workshop (or kaizen event or kaizen blitz)

REVIEW QUESTIONS

1. What is a control plan? List and explain three elements that are included in the plan.
2. What are SOPs?
3. What is the difference between an SOP and a checklist?
4. List the ISO's requirements for document control.
5. What is an audit?
6. Is a process always in control after an improvement? Explain.
7. How can the 6S help control the new process?
8. What are the various types of maintenance?
9. Explain how TPM can help control the redesigned process.
10. List three visual management (VM) tools and explain their purpose.
11. What is typically covered during a daily huddle?
12. What is a kaizen event? How does it follow the DMAIC process?

LEARNING ACTIVITIES

1. Develop a Pecha Kucha (presentation with 20 slides, 20 seconds each) about the importance of VM in controlling a process.
2. Create a video of your workspace (or your garage) as it undergoes a 6S transformation.
3. Discussion with role-play. A nurse manager has noticed that a nurse is not following SOPs for clinical documentation. The manager addresses the issue with the nurse, who feels that she is doing a great job. How does the nurse manager address the situation in a productive way? Show the back-and-forth between the two individuals.
4. Modify the control plan in Figure 12.1 as you see fit: add process steps, change the performance metrics and specifications, modify the measurement methods and control charts, and identify different courses of action.

REFERENCES

Accruent. (2024). *What is document control? Why is it important?* https://www.accruent.com/resources/blog-posts/document-control

ad-esse. (2025). *Rapid Improvement Workshops (RIW)*. https://www.ad-esse.com/rapid-improvement-workshop-riw

Agency for Healthcare Research and Quality. (2017). *Daily huddle component kit*. Author. https://www.ahrq.gov/hai/tools/ambulatory-surgery/sections/sustainability/management/huddles-comp-kit.html

Byrne, J. (2023, February 21). *Understanding document control in ISO 9001:2015*. Cognidox. https://www.cognidox.com/blog/document-control-iso-90012015

Croft, D. (2024). *Guide: Control plan*. Learn Lean Sigma. https://www.learnleansigma.com/guides/control-plan

Feldman, K. (2023, July 29). *Kaizen blitz explained: An intensive approach to solving problems*. iSixSigma. https://www.isixsigma.com/dictionary/kaizen-blitz

Gaskin, J. (2022, September 15). *Standard operating procedures: Definition, purposes, examples, and templates*. Venngage. https://venngage.com/blog/standard-operating-procedure

Hashemi-Pour, C., & Brush, K. (2024, June). *Standard operating procedure (SOP)*. TechTarget | Business Analytics. https://www.techtarget.com/searchbusinessanalytics/definition/standard-operating-procedure-SOP

Hut-Mossel, L., Ahaus, K., Welker, G., & Gans, R. (2021). Understanding how and why audits work in improving the quality of hospital care: A systematic realist review. *PLoS One*, *16*(3), e0248677. https://10.1371/journal.pone.0248677

Institute for Healthcare Improvement. (2024). *Patient safety essentials toolkit: Huddles*. Author. https://www.ihi.org/resources/tools/huddles#downloads

International Society of Six Sigma Professionals. (2024). *Quality circles: Overview, advantages, and disadvantages*. https://isssp.org/quality-circles-overview-advantages-and-disadvantages/

Isakov, A. (2024, May 15). *Example: Standard operating procedure (SOP) for patient handoff between a healthcare facility and a transporting ambulance*. CDC Stacks. https://stacks.cdc.gov/view/cdc/156207/cdc_156207_DS1.pdf

Jamtvedt, G., Flottorp, S., & Ivers, N. (2019). Audit and feedback as a quality strategy. In R. Busse, N. Klazinga, D. Panteli, & W. Quentin (Eds.), *Improving healthcare quality in Europe: Characteristics, effectiveness and implementation of different strategies*. European Observatory on Health Systems and Policies. https://www.ncbi.nlm.nih.gov/books/NBK549284/

Lawler, E. E. I., & Mohrman, S. A. (1985, January). Quality circles after the fad. *Harvard Business Review*. https://hbr.org/1985/01/quality-circles-after-the-fad

Oragui, D. (2024, June 20). *How to create a standard operating procedure*. Helpjuice. https://helpjuice.com/blog/standard-operating-procedure

Pittman, J. O. E., Rabin, B., Almklov, E., Afari, N., Floto, E., Rodriguez, E., & Lindamer, L. (2021). Adaptation of a quality improvement approach to implement eScreening in VHA healthcare settings: Innovative use of the Lean Six Sigma rapid process improvement workshop. *Implementation Science Communications*, *2*, 37. https://doi.org/10.1186/s43058-021-00132-x

Randig, M. A. (2009). *ISO 9001—Document control (4.2.3)*. MAS Solutions. https://www.masquality.com/uploads/7/2/3/4/72345885/iso_9001_-_document_control__4.2.3.pdf

Reyes, J. (2023, December 13). *Understanding the kaizen blitz method*. https://safetyculture.com/topics/kaizen-blitz

Rodriguez, D. (2024, August 2). *5s method in Six Sigma: Definition, importance, and implementation*. Invensis. https://www.invensislearning.com/blog/5s-method-in-six-sigma

Shaikh, U. (2020, January 29). *Improving patient safety and team communication through daily huddles*. Agency for Healthcare Research and Quality. https://psnet.ahrq.gov/primer/improving-patient-safety-and-team-communication-through-daily-huddles

Six Sigma Daily. (2020, November 9). *Getting organized with 5S: Sort, set, shine, standardize, sustain*. https://www.sixsigmadaily.com/5s-sort-set-shine-standardize-sustain

Tarlengco, J. (2024, August 24). *Corrective maintenance*. SafetyCulture. https://safetyculture.com/topics/corrective-maintenance

Tezel, A., Koskela, L., & Tzortzopoulos, P. (2016). Visual management in production management: A literature synthesis. *Journal of Manufacturing Technology Management*, *27*(6), 766–799. https://doi.org/10.1108/JMTM-08-2015-0071

Tušer, I., Bekešiene, S., & Navrátil, J. (2023). Emergency management and internal audit of emergency preparedness of pre-hospital emergency care. *Quality & Quantity*, *57*, S293–S305. https://doi.org/10.1007/s11135-020-01039-w

Usifo, D. (2024, March 19). *Using a control plan in Six Sigma*. Deeprojectmanager. https://deeprojectmanager.com/six-sigma-control-plan

Wu, W. (2024, March 25). *What is preventive maintenance? Types, benefits, cost, and examples*. Coast. https://coastapp.com/blog/preventive-maintenance

PART VII

Reaping the Rewards and Building Resilience

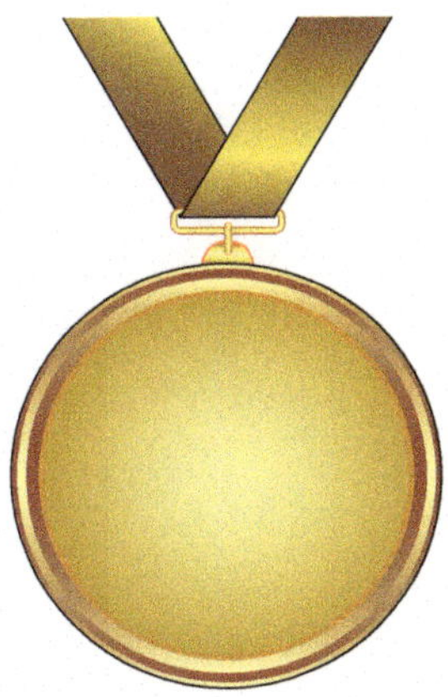

CHAPTER 13

ACCREDITATION, AWARDS, AND THE HIGHLY RELIABLE ORGANIZATION

BRIGHT ANGEL MEDICAL CENTER 13.1

Kimberly Mitchell and several members of the executive team had invited Barbara Waters, Dr. Aoki, and the ED improvement project team to give them a final update on the progress they had made in the ED.

"We are so impressed by all that you've done. Could you share with our team the key learnings throughout this journey?"

"Well," Barbara started, "this project did not really involve radical change. In other words, it was not disruptive like ***kaikaku****. Yet, it required considerable effort and coordination, and we are happy that it was very successful. But we haven't arrived at the finish line yet. While our throughput is improved, we are still seeing patients in the waiting room get frustrated and leave on busy days. We'll keep working on it. And we can always do better on our quality metrics. Our focus now is kaizen or small, incremental improvements. That said, I think the keys to our success so far have been to follow the data and include frontline employees in the process. Probably the biggest mistake we avoided was trying to solve all the problems on our own. We continue to believe that those doing the work are in the best position to determine how it should be done."*

Dr. Tibbets joined in, "I am just amazed at how much you were able to accomplish in so little time." Barbara blushed. "It really was a team effort," she said, gesturing to Olina, Adeleke, and the rest of the team. "We all brought our own set of skills and together, we were really able to make things happen."

Michael Chen, the chief nursing officer, approved. "The ED story has inspired several departments and clinics. They now have some quality improvement projects under way. And that's the type of enthusiasm we need before The Joint Commission (TJC)'s visit. You should give input into the planning process, all three of you."

Why was it important for the leaders to bring the team back to recognize them and celebrate their success?

Does it make sense to have a process improvement team participate in the accreditation process?

LEARNING OBJECTIVES

After reading this chapter, you will be able to:

- Describe why institutions undergo accreditation.
- Explain the difference between accreditation and certification.
- Articulate why the Malcolm Baldrige National Quality Award (MBNQA) holds such prestige.
- Describe the criteria for the MBNQA.
- Recognize the characteristics of leaders of institutions that achieve high performance in quality and safety.
- Learn the principles that make an organization highly reliable.
- Explain the importance of anticipation and containment for highly reliable organizations (HROs).

INTRODUCTION

In this book, everything has always been about the patient! Indeed, the overarching theme has been to deliver value to the patient. Yet, as discussed in Chapter 3, healthcare organizations have multiple customers, including payers, accreditation agencies, certification organizations, and the community.

Healthcare organizations must undergo accreditation and/or certification on a regular basis. Accreditation and certification validate an institution and may bring distinction for high standards. In this chapter, we review the ways healthcare organizations and provider groups achieve accreditation, and we describe the most notable healthcare award in the United States. We also discuss how organizations can become more consistent and reliable.

WHY IS THIS MATERIAL USEFUL?

Accreditation ensures that healthcare organizations have the systems and processes in place to achieve high-quality care. It is a stamp of approval that strengthens patient confidence when using the services provided by the institution. As a healthcare professional, you will be asked to participate in your organization's accreditation process. This chapter familiarizes you with the process. It also shows you how to go beyond accreditation to achieve excellence in patient care while building a **highly reliable organization (HRO)**.

ACCREDITATION

Accreditation is a rigorous and comprehensive validation process that examines the systems, processes, and performance of healthcare organizations. It is performed by impartial outside groups to ensure that business is being conducted in a way that meets national quality standards (Table 13.1). In order for an organization to receive federal payment from Medicare or Medicaid, it must have a certification called Conditions of Participation (CoPs) or Conditions for Coverage (CfCs) that complies with the government's health and safety requirements. Accrediting bodies must have quality standards and a survey process that meets or exceeds Medicare and Medicaid requirements. The process that the Centers for Medicare & Medicaid Services (CMS) uses to recognize an accreditation body that can evaluate a healthcare organization is called "deeming." CMS monitors and validates the surveys of these entities with "deeming authority." In this section, we will look more closely at three accrediting bodies: The Joint Commission (TJC), **Det Norske Veritas (DNV)**, and the **National Committee for Quality Assurance (NCQA)**.

TABLE 13.1 SELECTED LIST OF ORGANIZATIONS WITH DEEMING AUTHORITY AND THEIR PRIMARY SCOPE

Organization	Scope of Accreditation
The Joint Commission (TJC)	• Ambulatory surgical centers • Clinical laboratories • Critical access hospitals • Home health agencies • Hospice agencies • Hospitals • Psychiatric hospitals
Det Norske Veritas (DNV)	• Hospitals • Critical access hospitals
Accreditation Commission for Health Care (ACHC)	• Hospitals • Ambulatory surgical centers • Clinical laboratories • Critical access hospitals • Home health agencies • Hospice agencies
Community Health Accreditation Program (CHAP)	• Home health agencies • Hospice agencies
Accreditation Association for Ambulatory Healthcare (AAAH)	• Surgical centers • Primary care providers • Health plans
National Committee for Quality Assurance (NCQA)	• Health plans • Behavioral health clinics

THE JOINT COMMISSION

In 1951, the American College of Physicians, the American Hospital Association, the American Medical Association, and the Canadian Medical Association joined the American College of Surgeons to create the Joint Commission on Accreditation of Hospitals (JCAH), whose main purpose was to provide voluntary accreditation. The Social Security Amendment of 1965 created two major healthcare programs in the United States: Medicare and Medicaid. At the time, only hospitals accredited by the JCAH were "deemed" to be in compliance with the Medicare CoPs and could participate in the Medicare and Medicaid programs. In 1987, JCAH was renamed the Joint Commission on Accreditation of Healthcare Organizations, and in 2007, the name was shortened to TJC. Currently, this agency accredits and certifies more than 22,000 healthcare organizations in the United States. TJC accreditation or certification is recognized as symbolizing quality and an organizational commitment to meeting certain performance standards (TJC, 2024c). A basic tenet of TJC is that healthcare organizations can go beyond accreditation and achieve exemplary safety records. Their program called "Leading the Way to Zero™" helps healthcare organizations change the way they work to prevent patient harm. Zero harm does not mean that mistakes never happen. It means that systems and processes are put in place to catch errors before they cause harm (TJC, 2024d). TJC has expanded its survey process to non–hospital-based services. Many payers now require accreditation as a condition for reimbursement.

How Is Accreditation Achieved?

TJC standards form the basis of an objective survey process that uses the **tracer methodology** to evaluate healthcare organizations (Box 13.1). The survey process is data-driven and focused on the evaluation of the actual care processes that affect patients. Trained surveyors perform an onsite assessment every 3 years for hospitals and health systems (every 2 years for lab accreditation), checking for compliance with standards founded on the most current evidence-based practices.

BOX 13.1 QUALITY IN PRACTICE!

Tracer Methodology

The tracer methodology involves following patients through the entire care delivery process to evaluate the care provided by an organization as well as the effectiveness of its systems. Surveyors can then identify quality problems at any step of a process or at transition points between processes. TJC utilizes three types of tracers:

1. Individual tracer activity to assess patient care experience, treatment, and services and evaluate standards compliance. High-risk services are usually selected.
2. System tracer activity to evaluate system integration, care coordination, data management, infection control, and medication management.
3. Accreditation program-specific tracers to identify risk and safety issues relevant to the organization being surveyed (TJC, 2024e).

The surveys are unannounced. Following the path of care throughout a hospital stay, the team can randomly select patient records to evaluate the quality of care provided against TJC-established criteria. After the survey, the "findings" or areas of noncompliance with national standards are shared with the organization. The organization is required to develop a "plan of correction" to ensure they can meet the standard. Depending on the severity of the finding, TJC can return to repeat parts of the survey and verify compliance.

Priorities

The standards aim to help organizations improve their progress toward safe, reliable, sustainable, and patient-centered care (TJC, 2024b). Their primary areas of focus are briefly described in Table 13.2.

Performance Measurement

TJC works with CMS and other experts to identify and implement standardized performance measures. TJC distinguishes between accountability and nonaccountability measures and places a greater emphasis on the former (TJC, 2024a). Accountability measures are the best indicators of improvement on patient outcomes and must meet the criteria for process indicators outlined in Chapter 4: evidence-based, reflecting the quality of the process itself, directly related to outcomes, proven safe, systematic and timely, stable, and valid.

TABLE 13.2 THE JOINT COMMISSION'S PRIORITIES AND THEIR PURPOSES

Priority	Purposes
Quality and safety	• Infection prevention • Suicide prevention • Emergency management
Healthcare equity	• Equal rights and access to quality care for minorities, women, people of color, those with disabilities, and people living in rural communities or in poverty
Environmental sustainability	• Greener healthcare practices to reduce the negative impact on the environment and the resulting effects on chronic conditions and the ability to provide undisrupted care
Workforce safety and well-being	• Decrease healthcare workers' burnout which threatens safety and quality care

Benefits of Accreditation

There is consistent evidence that ensuring standards compliance improves healthcare organizations' care processes (Jha, 2018). But, in addition, there are benefits to the organizations themselves:

- helping to organize and strengthen patient safety efforts
- strengthening community's confidence in care provided by the institution
- providing education to enhance staff performance
- building a framework for organizations to structure safety and quality efforts
- providing a thorough and in-depth review of care processes

ON THE JOB! INTERVIEW VIDEO 13.1

Danika Severe
Senior Director for Quality and Patient Safety
Continual Readiness

High reliability: Safety together
Safety and accreditation
Patient, medication, and workforce safety
Accreditation programming
Establishing minimum standards
Creating high reliability
Preparing for TJC survey
SMART program cards: Checklists
Survey preparation schedule
Senior leader training
Planning boards

1. What suggestions does Danika make to help organizations prepare for TJC surveys?
2. How can a hospital or health system know if it is adequately prepared for a survey?
3. Within a hospital or health system, who contributes to completing a successful TJC survey?

The interview is available online by visiting www.springerpub.com/courseconnect. See inside front cover and tear-out card for CourseConnect details.

Another accrediting agency that has been gaining traction worldwide is DNV.

DET NORSKE VERITAS

DNV is an international accrediting certification body headquartered in Norway. It provides a variety of services across multiple sectors, including healthcare. It has been accrediting hospitals since 2008. Like TJC, its accreditation standards, the National Integrated Accreditation for Healthcare Organizations (NIAHO®), follow closely the Medicare CoPs and cover the following (DNV, 2024):

- **Quality management system and governance**: These standards guarantee that the governing body establish and sustain a robust quality management system. The system must be data-driven and focus on quality improvement with measurement (outcomes, process, and patient perception), assessment, corrective and preventive actions, and monitoring. The system should conform to the ISO 9001 standard (see later section in this chapter) within 3 years after the initial accreditation.
- **Proactive risk management**: These standards call for the identification and management of risks threatening patient safety. They include medical errors and adverse patient events. Once detected, these risks should be reported and their sources investigated. Preventive and corrective actions should ensue, and the effectiveness of these actions should be continuously monitored.

- **Higher risk services**: Services such as anesthesia, obstetrics, nuclear medicine, and ED present higher levels of risk. Special procedures must be in place in these areas to ensure utmost proficiency and safety.
- **Medication management**: The organization seeking accreditation should have pharmacy services with written policies and procedures based on best practices for patient care. The policies cover ordering, storage, handling, dispensing, and administration.
- **Patient rights**: The organization should abide by the nondiscrimination provisions of the Affordable Care Act (ACA), inform patients and/or representatives of patients' rights before providing or discontinuing care, tell them about their visitation rights, and allow them to develop advanced directives. These rights should be communicated in the patient's chosen language.
- **Physical environment**: Construction, layout, equipment, and maintenance of the facility should promote patient safety. Multiple maintenance strategies (e.g., preventive vs. corrective) can be implemented, but their use should be justified based on equipment type and safety risk.

TJC and DNV have very similar standards, leading to similar health outcomes and patient experience (Box 13.2).

The NCQA accreditation scope is different from TJC's and DNV's. It targets insurance plans and provider groups.

NATIONAL COMMITTEE FOR QUALITY ASSURANCE

Founded in 1990, the NCQA is a private, not-for-profit organization dedicated to improving healthcare quality (NCQA, 2024b). NCQA accredits health plans, provider groups, and health insurance organizations. The accreditation process is an onsite, rigorous review of more than 60 standards performed every 3 years. Every year, health plans must report on their performance. These performance reviews are tracked, and assessment scores, based on a set of clinical measures and consumer experience, are reported to the public.

When NCQA reviews a health plan, provider group, or health insurance company, it looks at structure, organization, and results in these areas (NCQA, 2024a):

- Quality management and improvement using:
  - **healthcare effectiveness data and information set** with measures comprising five domains: effectiveness of care, access/availability of care, utilization and risk-adjusted utilization, health plan descriptive information, and measures reported using electronic clinical data systems
  - Consumer Assessment of Healthcare Providers and Systems performance measures

BOX 13.2 QUALITY IN PRACTICE!

It's the Standards That Count!

A study compared the differences in six disease-specific 30-day mortality and six hospital-acquired infection rates among U.S. hospitals accredited by TJC, DNV, the Center for Improvement in Healthcare Quality, and the Healthcare Facilities Accreditation Program (HFAP). The data were obtained from the American Hospital Association and CMS's Hospital Compare databases. Statistically significant differences between hospitals were observed only for the 30-day mortality rates related to chronic obstructive pulmonary disease and heart failure, with TJC-accredited hospitals performing better than DNV- and HFAP-accredited hospitals, respectively. The authors concluded that overall, the accreditation agencies do not have a significant impact on hospital outcomes and patient experience. As a result, they recommend considering membership and other costs when selecting an accreditation agency (Kato & Zikos, 2022).

TABLE 13.3 DIFFERENCES BETWEEN ACCREDITATION, CERTIFICATION, AND LICENSURE

Designation	Who or What?	Voluntary	Agency
Accreditation	Organization	Yes	Nongovernmental
Certification	Program or Service	Yes	Nongovernmental
Licensure	Individual	No	Governmental

- Utilization management
- Population health management
- Network management
- Credentialing and re-credentialing of providers
- Members' rights and responsibilities
- Member connections
- Medicaid benefits and services

Any health plan sold on the health insurance exchanges as outlined by the ACA requires accreditation through NCQA, but many unaccredited plans are still sold through employers or in the private market. NCQA scores are posted, and consumers can compare plans according to these parameters.

Accreditation is an acknowledgment that a whole organization (e.g., a hospital) is complying with recognized standards of practice. In contrast, **certification** focuses on programs or functions (e.g., heart disease care; Table 13.3). A highly regarded certification agency is the **International Organization for Standardization (ISO)**.

CERTIFICATION

THE INTERNATIONAL ORGANIZATION FOR STANDARDIZATION

The ISO, a nongovernmental agency counting over 160 member countries, established ISO 9000 certification in 1987, with the latest version of the 9001 standard released in 2015. The ISO provides standards to organizations wanting to ensure that their products and/or services consistently meet consumers' requirements and that the quality continuously improves. It is thus consistent with DNV's requirement that ISO 9001 certification be required for reaccreditation.

ISO 9001:2015 builds on the Plan-Do-Study-Act cycle (Chapter 1) and centers on the documentation and review of effective quality management practices in leadership, process interactions, human resources management, service continuum, sustainability, and measurement-analysis-improvement activities (American Society for Quality [ASQ], 2024a).

In healthcare, ISO certification covers various sectors: patient safety, streamlined supply chains, and innovations in digital health and sustainability. It is based on seven principles that help build a quality management system for healthcare organizations (ASQ, 2024a; Table 13.4).

TABLE 13.4 ISO'S SEVEN PRINCIPLES

Principle	Objective
1. Customer focus	Meeting and trying to exceed customers' needs
2. Leadership	Create unity of purpose, good communication, and strategy alignment
3. Engagement of people	Build a culture of motivated, committed workers at all levels through open discussion and sharing of knowledge
4. Process approach	Coordinate work processes and reduce variation to provide the most value to customers

(continued)

TABLE 13.4 ISO'S SEVEN PRINCIPLES (*CONTINUED*)

Principle	Objective
5. Continuous improvement	Continuously examine and improve processes to lead to faster, more efficient, and higher quality operations
6. Evidence-based decision-making	Analyze and evaluate data to make informed decisions based on facts
7. Relationship management	Create a mutually beneficial relationship with suppliers to optimize resources and cost

ISO, International Organization for Standardization.

Source: Adapted from American Society for Quality. (2024a). *What is ISO 9001:2015—Quality management systems?* https://asq.org/quality-resources/iso-9001#Revision

BRIGHT ANGEL MEDICAL CENTER 13.2

The board members and executive team had gathered. Stewart Baldrige, the board chair, opened the meeting by welcoming everyone, showed the agenda items on the screen, and said, "Kimberly, you're first! Is today a good day?"

Kimberly smiled and replied, "It certainly is! You all trusted me with turning this hospital around 2 years ago. There were more challenges than any of us could have imagined, but this place is experiencing a transformation we can be proud of. What started as a long-shot project to increase the throughput in the ED became a source of inspiration. The results motivated Dr. Rao to revamp the elective surgery schedule and decrease downtime. Soon after that, the pharmacy standardized its ordering process and improved its inventory control system, lowering costs while decreasing out-of-stock situations. As this transformative culture started taking hold, we were able to get reaccredited by TJC. The visiting team highlighted a few areas where we need to work harder, but they recognized our tremendous change for the better. The Bright Angel team has delivered!"

Everyone in the room clapped.

Emily Bates, the new board member, asked "So, what's next?"

Kimberly did not hesitate, "How about the Malcolm Baldrige National Quality Award (MBNQA)?"

Stewart Baldrige smiled, "I like the sound of it." The room erupted in laughter. "Also, we need to fill Mira's position . . . Kimberly, what do you think of asking Barbara if she's interested?"

Is it premature for Bright Angel Medical Center (BAMC) to think about the MBNQA at this stage?

MALCOLM BALDRIGE NATIONAL QUALITY AWARD

Unlike accreditation or certification, which indicates that specified standards are being met, a growing number of healthcare organizations are trying to differentiate themselves by seeking awards. Awards suggest that an institution is not just meeting the standards but exceeding them in certain ways. Achievement of this type adds luster to an institution's image, sets it apart from the competition, and is a focal point for employee pride.

There are numerous national, regional, and state awards in healthcare, but the **Malcolm Baldrige National Quality Award (MBNQA)** is especially coveted. The U.S. Congress established this award in 1987 to recognize all types of companies that have implemented successful quality management systems (ASQ, 2024b). The MBNQA is the only presidential award for performance excellence in the United States. The National Institute of Standards and Technology manages the award, and the president of the United States presents it annually. There are now seven categories of awards representing different segments of the economy, and an independent board judges the competition:

1. manufacturing
2. service

3. small business
4. education
5. healthcare
6. nonprofit
7. community

The Baldrige Excellence Framework provides a comprehensive performance management approach that focuses on results, learning, and sharing of information (National Institute of Standards and Technology, 2021). It does not tell leaders how to run their organizations but instead helps guide the assessment of systems and outcomes. Similar to the balanced scorecard (Chapter 4), the framework stresses an integrated approach to deliver ever-improving value to customers, develop organizational capabilities, and promote personal learning. This framework encompasses excellence criteria covering seven areas of organizational management and performance (Figure 13.1):

1. **Leadership**: The leaders do not just need to lead the organization well. The MBNQA goes beyond that and is interested in how the organization leads within the community.
2. **Strategy**: The organization must have a planning process that defines its direction and delineates how the strategy will be implemented. Strategic planning should lead to positive action, and the strategic plans should not just sit on the shelf.
3. **Customers**: The organization must show that it values its customers and builds strong and lasting relationships. These relationships are put in the context of the market as a whole. In healthcare, this means putting the patient at the center of its focus, but customers of various processes, such as physicians and other staff, are also valued.
4. **Measurement, analysis, and knowledge management**: The organization must be able to collect and use data to support its decisions, improve key processes, and manage performance. The organization must turn data into information that can be used to drive its business.

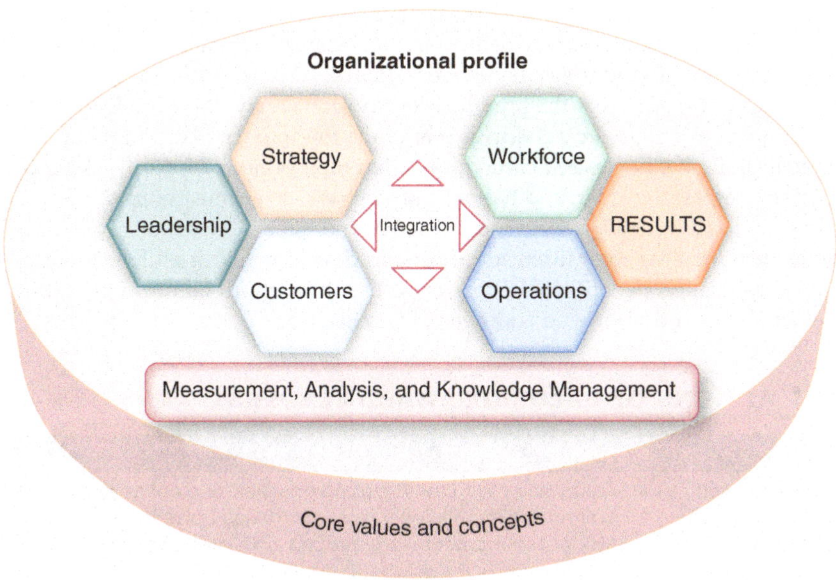

FIGURE 13.1 MBNQA framework overview.

Abbreviation: MBNQA, Malcolm Baldrige National Quality Award.

Source: National Institute of Standards and Technology. (2021). *How Baldrige works*. https://www.nist.gov/baldrige/how-baldrige-works

5. **Workforce**: Organizations that value their human resources, train them, and empower them to do their jobs are more resilient and flexible. Workforce morale spills over into taking care of customers and organizational excellence. Organizations taking care of their people tend to perform better and maintain higher efficiency.
6. **Operations**: Operations management determines how well the organization is run. Excellent organizations are interested in identifying the processes that matter, designing them well, managing the variables, and continuously improving so that the outcomes are enhanced.
7. **Business/organizational performance results**: Organizations that focus on results have a broad portfolio of performance indicators: customer satisfaction, finance, human resources, supplier and partner performance, operations, governance and social responsibility, and competitiveness. Healthy organizations learn from comparing themselves to others and strive to adopt best practices.

LEADERSHIP

The first criterion of the MBNQA, and possibly the most important, is an evaluation of leadership. Let us explore this concept a bit further. Although there is no specific leadership style that defines Baldrige leaders, the Baldrige Foundation Institute for Performance Excellence (Strahan, 2019) found some common behaviors that leaders of high-performing organizations display. These leaders: (a) create and maintain a focused vision for their organization, and (b) ensure the effective execution of that vision (Table 13.5). Achieving a focused vision involves clarifying and aligning strategic priorities and defining performance criteria. For these leaders, the organization's mission, vision, and values are more than words on paper; they are the compasses that guide the organization's actions. This happens through effective communication and consistency of action at all levels.

Exceptional leaders encourage innovation to address difficult problems. They provide a safe environment to share new ideas and challenge the workforce to think creatively. Lean Six Sigma (LSS) methodology can be used to foster innovation since the most effective way to improve a process is to eliminate areas of little value, augment existing value, and produce areas of new value (Hansen, 2018). Enhancing quality while decreasing costs requires innovation.

Leaders of exceptional organizations must model desired behaviors. They must be consistent with their actions and words. They model the organization's mission and courageously stand up in tough situations. These leaders truly believe in the mission of their organizations and use continuous improvement to realize their vision of excellence.

Ensuring effective execution of the organization's vision is how Baldrige leaders achieve their goals. A clear theme articulated by Baldrige leaders is the importance of data and using objective metrics to incentivize the desired behaviors within their organizations. Tracking performance measures, using comparative data, and having a structure to select meaningful metrics are vital to operating an organization while improving efficiency and effectiveness.

Baldrige leaders are also committed to leadership development at all levels within the organization. The organization benefits by having expertise throughout its ranks and allows for both personal development and improved competencies of staff.

TABLE 13.5 ACTIONS OF BALDRIGE AWARD LEADERS

Behaviors	Methods
1. Create and maintain a focused vision for their organization.	a. Clarify and align strategies and priorities, and define performance criteria. b. Encourage innovation to address difficult problems. c. Model desired behaviors through consistency in words, actions, and values.
2. Ensure effective execution of the vision.	a. Align and manage the organization through measurement and data. b. Develop leaders at all levels.

Source: Data from Strahan, J. (2019). *Strategy execution and sustainability: Using the Baldrige leadership model to overcome evasive organizational challenges.* https://www.ache.org/-/media/ache/about-ache/baldrige-foundation-institute-for-performance-excellence-white-paper-201901.pdf

Leaders must understand their organizations and how the different components work together. Indeed, healthcare organizations must be appreciated as a system, the components of which work together to provide high-quality care. The many leaders within the organization (the governing body, the chief executive and other senior leaders, and the leaders of the licensed independent practitioners) should also work well together.

As institutions evolve, leaders must grow and change. Leaders do not have to know the answers to all the questions; instead, they need to create an environment where the right questions are asked (Box 13.3). At times, it may be uncomfortable to ask or respond to hard questions, but it is important to take all questions seriously and try to answer them honestly (Figure 13.2). Greater institutional tolerance and diversity of thought lead to higher performing organizations. The best leaders view every situation, no matter how challenging, as an opportunity to learn. If leaders are not willing to take a hard look inward and are willing to assess their own strengths and weaknesses, they will find it difficult to create an organizational culture where assessment is the norm.

BOX 13.3 QUALITY IN PRACTICE!

Wellstar Paulding Hospital Earned the Malcolm Baldridge National Quality Award

In 2020, Wellstar Paulding Hospital (WPH), part of the Wellstar health system, was recognized for outstanding quality outcomes with the MBNQA. Culture for an organization is set at the top and the senior leadership at WPH were credited for creating an environment focused on patient safety and high-quality care. Senior leaders actively participated in daily safety and voice of the customer (VOC) huddles and performed frequent leadership rounds. They also drove the "Neighbors Caring for Neighbors" initiative, personally reviewing safety concerns that were escalated and compliance audit findings. Senior leaders recognized and celebrated team members who had the courage to bring forward safety concerns. This hands-on approach set the tone for the remainder of the organization and positioned WPH to excel in several areas, including performing in the top 10% for mortality index and inpatient complication index as reported by IBM Watson. The team at WPH also sustained a pressure ulcer rate of zero for several years. The senior leadership team created the conditions for the caregivers to excel in their work and put in place systems and processes to optimize safe care (https://www.nist.gov/baldrige/wellstar-paulding-hospital).

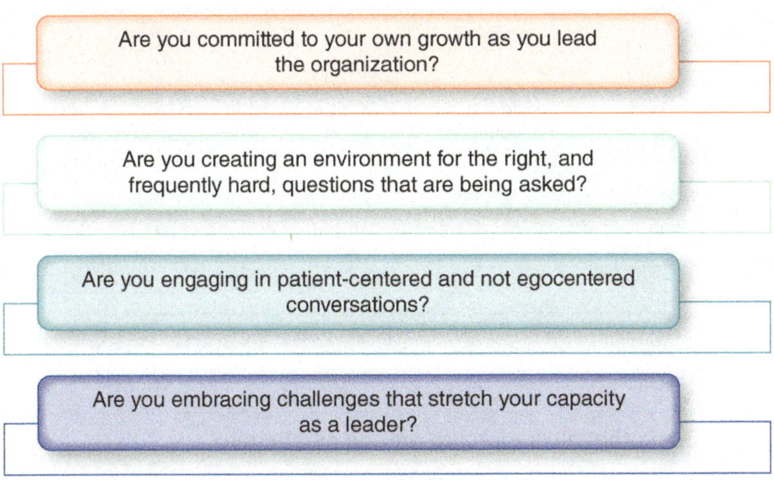

FIGURE 13.2 Questions for leaders to ask themselves.

Source: Modified from Hines, S., Luna, K., Lofthus, J., Marquardt, M., & Stelmokas, D. (2008). *Becoming a high-reliability organization: Operational advice for hospital leaders*. https://archive.ahrq.gov/professionals/quality-patient-safety/quality-resources/tools/hroadvice/hroadviceref.html

Different leadership groups that may be found within an organization are listed in the following sections. Although each of the leadership groups must work together as a team, each has a distinct role as it relates to quality. In small organizations, these groups may overlap, and a single individual may assume several roles.

The Governing Body

In Chapter 1, you may remember that when Kimberly Mitchell took over as BAMC's CEO, one of her first actions was to discuss her plans with the board of directors. The commitment to patient safety and quality must start with the governing body or board of directors. A component of Baldrige's leadership development is the education and monitoring of board performance. A strong and capable board helps the organization maintain a constant focus on excellence and motivates leaders to achieve their vision. Delivering quality healthcare is increasingly recognized as a corporate responsibility, and the healthcare organization's board must be fully engaged. In order to hold senior management accountable for the performance of the institution, the board must be involved in identifying the quality and safety goals. Boards must prioritize quality and safety agendas and commit sufficient resources for the implementation of continuous improvement programs.

The CEO and Other Senior Leaders

The CEO and senior leaders of an organization must take strong steps to create the expectation of quality. In Chapter 1, Kimberly Mitchell and the executive leadership team of BAMC analyzed the hospital's operations and developed a strategic plan. The senior leadership team is responsible for the development and implementation of the strategic plan of the organization. This group must prioritize projects, adopt quality measures to track, and set goals to accomplish (Figure 13.3).

STRATEGY

By now, you probably realize that the contents of this book parallel the Malcolm Baldrige performance framework. In Chapter 1, you learned how to take into account the organization's strengths, weaknesses, opportunities, and threats (SWOT). Based on the SWOT analysis, a strategic path is

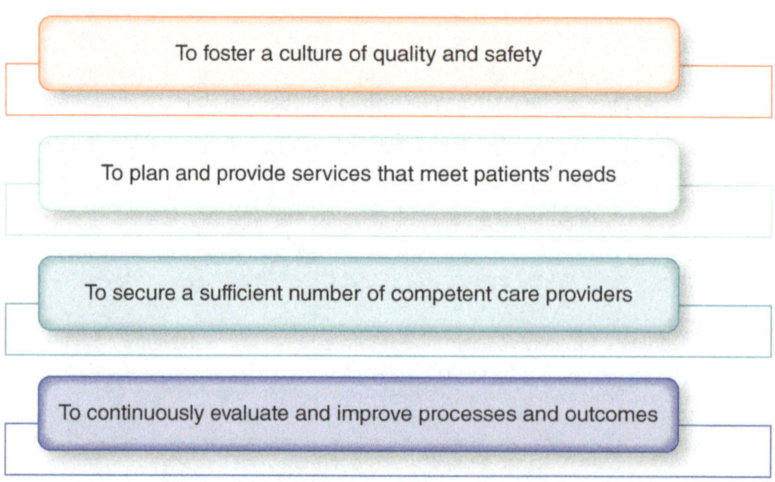

FIGURE 13.3 Goals that all leadership groups must share.

Source: Adapted from Schyve, P. M. (2009). *Leadership in healthcare organizations: A guide to Joint Commission leadership standards*. The Governance Institute. https://psnet.ahrq.gov/issue/leadership-healthcare-organizations-guide-joint-commission-leadership-standards chosen, and the primary functions within the organization—marketing, operations, finance, human resources, and information technology (IT)—must align their strategies with the business strategy. As per the cumulative model, building a strategic advantage in operations means competing on the basis of quality, cost, timeliness, and flexibility, with quality as the building block for overall excellence.

CUSTOMERS

The ultimate customers of the chain of interconnected healthcare processes are known collectively as the "market." They define the meaning of quality. In Chapter 4, you learned how to capture the VOC. The VOC reflects the customers' opinions and perceptions regarding the service provided by the organization. In healthcare, the VOC often captures the following service characteristics: responsiveness, reliability, communication with providers, empathy, courtesy, ease of making an appointment, and tangible aspects of the service such as lighting, noise, cleanliness, and so on. The house of quality framework helps ensure that the VOC is translated into the voice of the process (VOP) and is measured through quality indicators along the three stages of the healthcare delivery system: structure (or input), process, and outcomes (or output). Many of the tools described in this text are designed to measure, analyze, and improve a process so that the customer's needs and wants are met.

MEASUREMENT, ANALYSIS, AND KNOWLEDGE MANAGEMENT

Throughout the chapters, you were introduced to tools and methodologies that can be used to diagnose and improve workflows and processes. These tools and methodologies are summarized in Appendix B. LSS tools help signal problems, identify opportunities for improvement, and design targeted corrective actions. They are especially useful for systematically communicating to others within the organization what is needed to align activities with performance.

WORKFORCE

LSS is much more than a collection of tools. It is based on a systemwide collaboration of individuals in all functions of an organization—marketing, finance, IT, operations, and human resources—working together to support the overall organizational goals. Total quality management (TQM) and LSS (Chapters 1 and 2) stress employee respect and empowerment. Similarly, some of the process design principles in Chapter 10 emphasized employee autonomy and collaboration, increased flexibility through job enlargement, cross-training, and job enrichment. Supervisors and leaders must learn from those actually doing the job and allow them to solve problems and improve processes when they see fit. Respect is a fundamental value in a continuously learning organization.

OPERATIONS

Process management is the core of operations. Processes must be designed to support the organizational strategy. At the beginning of this text, you learned about the Institute of Medicine (IOM)'s call to design a system that makes it harder to do something wrong and easier to do something right. This idea paralleled Deming's Point #3, which advocated productive systems geared toward prevention of errors rather than correction. Chapter 10 presented several process design principles, which were built upon this concept as well as TQM and LSS paradigms. The principles urge organizations to emphasize mistake-proofing, simplification, integration, collaboration, and reduction of variability to achieve world class performance.

In the dynamic healthcare environment, processes cannot be static. Rather, they must evolve to continue to support changing strategies. Change is hard! Sometimes, even the simplest process modifications are met with harsh resistance (Box 13.4).

BOX 13.4 QUALITY IN PRACTICE!

The Semmelweis Reflex

In the 1840s, a gifted physician named Ignaz Semmelweis worked in the Vienna General Hospital's first obstetrical clinic. The clinic was set up so that physicians delivered babies on some days of the week, and midwives delivered babies on the other days. Semmelweis was very observant. He noticed that patients cared for by the midwives had fewer deaths related to childbed fever compared to those cared for by the physicians. He also noted that physicians would come to the clinic from the autopsy suite and not wash their hands prior to delivery. Remember, this observation was prior to Pasteur's discovery in 1865 that germs caused disease. Semmelweis came up with the idea that doctors should wash their hands prior to delivering babies.

One would think that this would be considered a rational idea that was based on observation, right? Well, Semmelweis's suggestion was met with anger and dismissed by all his colleagues. In fact, Semmelweis was ridiculed by all for his suggestion. Why could the physicians not embrace this new concept? Was it because they did not want to appear "dirty" or thought Semmelweis was critical of the way they took care of their patients? No one really knows, but this response to new information is very common among all people. It is called the Semmelweis reflex, the rejection of the results of research and observable facts because it conflicts with established beliefs. It is not a person's personality or intelligence that causes this response but rather the result of the deeply held beliefs of the person.

The Semmelweis reflex is a common occurrence during organizational change. Each of us is susceptible to this reflex. We need to recognize it and be sure that we are responding to change in a positive way.

BUSINESS/ORGANIZATIONAL PERFORMANCE RESULTS

In Chapter 11, the BAMC dashboards showed marked improvements in several performance metrics. The lower door-to-doc time leads to a lower left-without-being-seen rate and increased revenue. The average lengths of stay was drastically shortened, boosting throughput and revenue. The lower number of travel nurses full-time equivalents (FTEs) slashed labor costs. The higher top box percentages in patient experience and the better health outcomes increase Medicare reimbursements and enhance the organization's image, ultimately leading to increased revenue and lower costs of poor quality. Furthermore, the enhanced working conditions for staff with less waste and higher skill utilization are likely to lower turnover costs. Therefore, over time, the added value to processes and their outputs triggers financial benefits. This is one of the requirements of the MBNQA: to translate quality improvements into significant business outcomes. This is another reminder that a systems approach to quality yields an end result greater than the sum of its parts. This was illustrated in our balanced scorecard (Figure 4.11). Listening to the VOC and developing the human capital of an organization improve processes, which in turn enhance the financial health of the organization. When quality is the driving force of an organization, and the Malcolm Baldrige framework for performance excellence is achieved, business success follows (Box 13.5). Deming taught that strong, visionary leadership is needed to drive organizational learning and cooperation (Chapter 1). But leadership alone cannot lead to a quality organization. It takes a culture of quality and continuous improvement throughout the organization to achieve excellence in healthcare.

BOX 13.5 QUALITY IN PRACTICE!

GBMC Healthcare, 2020 Malcolm Baldrige Award Winner

The GBMC Healthcare system includes a vast network of healthcare facilities including an acute care hospital, primary and specialty care practices, and hospice care in the greater Baltimore area. All senior leaders take regular Gemba walks through all medical units to have face-to-face discussions with frontline workers about achievement of GBMC's Four Aims of better health,

(continued)

BOX 13.5 QUALITY IN PRACTICE! (*CONTINUED*)

better care, least waste, and more joy. The use of visual displays facilitates these discussions and helps gauge performance toward goal achievement. Furthermore, the CEO participates in all employee orientations to reinforce the organization' s purpose, vision, and values.

The relentless pursuit of excellence has resulted in:

- a 5-star rating from CMS
- industry-leading performance in process metrics
- outstanding physician performance in communication with patients
- excellent nurse residency program
- enterprise-wide medical record system with 10 Gold Star Status

These achievements led to financial rewards with an increased cash flow even during the pandemic, a healthy cash-to-total debt ratio, a larger market share, and a higher ED volume. Outstanding performance on all criteria of the MBNQA Framework helped GBMC earn the prestigious award in 2020. https://www.nist.gov/baldrige/gbmc-healthcare-system

NEW BALDRIGE AWARD CRITERIA FOR 2024

In 2024, the Baldrige Award program updated its award criteria. The program still builds on the framework shown in Figure 13.1, but the *Measurement, Analysis, and Knowledge Management* criterion is now subsumed in all other criteria. Besides leadership, strategy, customers, operations, workforce, and financial performance, the criteria also include organization description, community relationships, and organizational learning. There is a renewed emphasis on resilience, the topic of the next section (National Institute of Standards and Technology, 2024).

THE HIGHLY RELIABLE ORGANIZATION

Healthcare is a complex world with constant change and high risk. Doctors, nurses, and technicians work hard to deliver the best possible care. But in an environment of frequent and routine interruptions, patient variability, and occasionally emergent situations, it is difficult to consistently provide quality care or the "right care for the right patient at the right time—every time" (Hubing, 2013). As healthcare providers focus on improving quality and safety, they have turned to other industries that share characteristics of complexity and risk to learn how to avoid accidents. Industries such as aviation, nuclear power, and the military have studied past disasters to develop practices leading to improved safety. Weick and Sutcliffe (2007) demonstrated how the concepts of high reliability apply to healthcare and help prevent errors and avoid crises.

HROs work to decrease or eliminate errors that can lead to patient harm despite operating in complex and risky domains. The only way that organizations can become highly reliable is by putting time and resources into what they value. For example, the airline industry values airplanes not crashing. Consequently, 2023 was a record-breaking year for safety with a fatality risk rate dropping from 0.03 per million flight sectors to 0.03 fatalities per million flights (Flight Safety Foundation, 2024). However, airlines still occasionally lose a traveler's bag. This doesn't mean that the individuals in baggage claim are not good at their jobs; it likely suggests that out of all of the airline's competing priorities, traveler safety ranks higher than baggage handling. Organizations must decide where they want to excel and put time and resources into the effort. Determining an organization's strategy and priorities defines the areas where resources are targeted. In an organization that has quality as a core strategy, resources can be allocated to designing thoughtful processes to help employees reduce error, building a culture that is collaborative and information-sharing, and developing surveillance systems to identify mistakes early.

In Chapter 6 (*rolled throughput yield*), we looked at the concept of **reliability**, or the probability that each step will function effectively, without error, for a determined period of time. We will now explore how health systems can become HROs.

COMMON PRINCIPLES OF HIGHLY RELIABLE ORGANIZATIONS

Weick and Sutcliffe (2007) studied complex, high-risk organizations that coped well with sudden disasters and adapted in ways that prevented future catastrophes. They found that the culture of these organizations was constantly organizing and planning to handle the known, expected events, but they were always alert to the fact that unexpected things could happen. They were prepared to manage the unexpected. It was based on strong principles that were embraced at all levels of the organization and went beyond the process improvement concepts explained in Chapters 10 and 11 when we talked about the *Improve* stage in the DMAIC (Define-Measure-Analyze-Improve-Control) process. The principles were as follows (Figure 13.4):

1. **Sensitivity to operations**: Leaders in HROs need to be aware of how processes and systems affect the organization. They appreciate that employees involved in direct patient care understand best the state of the equipment and the adequacy of the processes to care for patients. HROs ensure that leaders and staff at all levels become aware of the risks to patients and work collectively to correct problems to improve the quality and safety of the care provided.

   Being sensitive to operations means being aware of how messy reality is in most processes and identifying abnormalities around them. When individuals are involved in a complex activity, they often lose sight of what is going on around them. However, in an HRO, everyone must learn how to notice. For example, a laboratory manager saw data that several environmental services workers had sustained needlestick injuries while cleaning her department. She went to the blood drawing area and observed the venipuncture technicians depositing the used needles in the sharps container. A few of the needles fell out of the sharps container into the trashcan that was positioned below. The manager moved the trashcan location away from the sharps container, and the needlestick injuries stopped occurring.

   In HROs, clear focus on problematic processes leads to important observations that can result in improvement. Employees must be able to ask questions and challenge assumptions. If everyone is clearly observing what is actually happening, problems can be identified sooner.

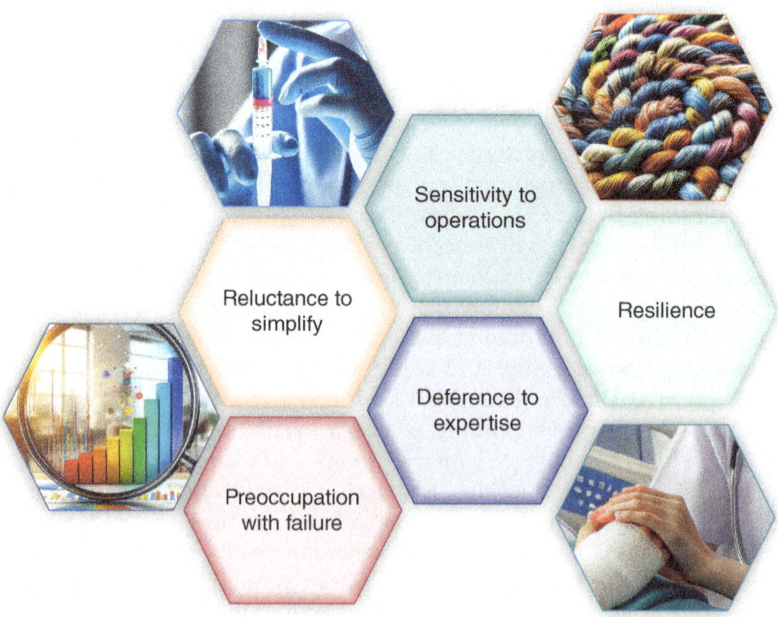
Sensitivity to operations
Reluctance to simplify
Resilience
Deference to expertise
Preoccupation with failure

FIGURE 13.4 Principles of HROs.

Abbreviation: HRO, highly reliable organizations.

2. **Reluctance to simplify**: LSS taught us that simplifying processes leads to improved quality and decreased variability. Then, why should we be reluctant to simplify? When analyzing a problem (not a process), it is important to understand the complexity of issues surrounding failures and not link the solution to a simple cause. Broad, rational excuses are often used when something is not working well. Assigning blame to a single staff member, faulting inadequate training, citing poor communication, and so on, may be easy, but the true reason for the failure will not be found and corrected unless (a) all possible causes, including the seemingly insignificant ones, have been identified and evaluated; and (b) the underlying causes of symptoms have been unearthed. People often jump into simple explanations for problems, but it does not get them closer to solving them. For example, attributing low patient satisfaction scores to an increase in ED admissions that had delays in transfers to a bed seems logical. But examination of data can suggest alternative reasons for the problem. Groups must be resistant to accepting the first possible answer and should dig deeper to uncover other potential causes. Brainstorming sessions must have a diversity of perspectives, and there must be trust within the group so people feel free to question and speak up.
3. **Preoccupation with failure**: Every organization has failures. In HRO organizations, employees are encouraged to look at their work processes and ask themselves, "What could possibly go wrong?" This shared attentiveness is constant. When issues are identified, employees are encouraged to come forward, and the focus is then placed on how to safeguard the process (Box 13.6).

   HROs destigmatize failures and consider the identification of failure points as a success. When issues are identified, they are communicated across the organization to help other areas correct a failure point or stimulate ideas to improve more processes. For example, during the early days of the COVID-19 pandemic, hospitals were fearful of not having enough personal protective equipment (PPE) to keep their employees safe. Multidisciplinary groups brainstormed about what to do if N95 facemasks ran low. Other health systems were called, and potential solutions were compiled. One health system decided to stave off the risk of running out of N95 facemasks by assigning labeled facemasks to individuals and resterilizing them as needed. This prevented a shortage that could have resulted in staff exposure to the virus.

BOX 13.6 QUALITY IN PRACTICE!

O-Rings and the *Challenger* Accident

On January 28, 1986, the space shuttle *Challenger*, in its 10th flight, exploded 73 seconds after takeoff, killing the seven crew members inside. The entire event, captured on television, was horrifying to watch. What happened? Everyone wanted to know.

A Presidential Commission was convened and tasked with solving this mystery. And what was uncovered was no mystery at all. The point of failure should have been identified prior to the mission and corrected, but the complex situation was simplified to a point where the danger was ignored.

The failure that caused the *Challenger* explosion was an O-ring whose seal was breached, allowing pressurized burning gas from the solid rocket motor to reach the external fuel tank. Several factors, including the wear and tear of the aircraft after nine previous flights, the material used to make the O-rings, and the reaction of the joints as the shuttle launched, complicated the National Aeronautics and Space Administration (NASA) engineers' jobs. However, one factor, the temperature of the day, played a large role. The ambient temperature at Cape Canaveral, Florida, was 36° Fahrenheit. This was much colder than for any of the previous flights of the *Challenger*. Engineers had been concerned about the O-ring sealant at low temperatures, but this concern was not thought to be important enough to fix. Also, on that cold morning, the temperature or a possible O-ring failure was not factored into the calculations as the *Challenger* team was preparing for takeoff. The result of not considering all possible failure points resulted in disaster (Presidential Commission on the Space Shuttle *Challenger* Accident, 1986).

HROs also focus their attention on the little problems in order to prevent bigger mistakes. These small issues are viewed as symptomatic of underlying problems that need more attention. The failure mode and effects analysis tool (Chapter 9) is especially well suited to engage teams in identifying all points of *possible* failure and mistake-proof the system accordingly.

4. **Deference to expertise**: In every organization, some people are technical experts on processes or technology. The experts know how things work and the risks that patients face. Leaders of HROs must understand that these are the individuals who must be drawn into the conversations if they want to build a culture of high reliability. Leaders (without the expertise) should not call the shots when circumstances call for those with specific expertise to direct the way. Often, these experts do not have the most seniority and need to be encouraged to speak out. The worst thing that a leader can say is, "I know that." This will shut down communication, and people will stop voicing their concerns and ideas. In order to build an HRO, leaders and supervisors must listen to staff and create a culture of openness.
5. **Resilience**. There are always unexpected events. Leaders and staff in HROs are trained and prepared to respond when system failures occur. The capacity to recover quickly from unexpected events is called **resilience**. Resilient leaders design redundancy into their systems so that there will not be a single point of failure. Emergency situations are discussed, and the organization learns from errors. Planning efforts are organized so that all employees know their roles and have personalized plans of action so that they are not crippled when errors occur (Box 13.7).

With the rapid changes occurring in healthcare, such as delivery redesign, increased data reporting, and more rigid payment models, physicians and other providers are experiencing increased stress. In order to achieve high-quality care, a resilient and well-supported clinical team is paramount. The National Academies of Sciences, Engineering, and Medicine (2019) recognized the importance of preventing clinician burnout and improving well-being and resilience. The result was a collaborative platform entitled "Action Collaborative on Clinician Well-Being and Resilience," which focused on individual approaches to increase personal resilience and organizational approaches to reduce stressors.

For example, in the context of the COVID-19 pandemic, health system administrators and clinicians needed to quickly and significantly change their workflow throughout the organization. Universal virus testing, masking, closing of patient care units, acquisition of increased numbers of ventilators and PPE devices, transition from in-person clinic visits to telehealth, modifying infection control strategies, and so on, stressed all personnel. The organizations that had incorporated high-reliability methods into their cultures were able to adapt and continue to provide quality care.

BOX 13.7 QUALITY IN PRACTICE!

Mercy Hospital Defying the Odds After EF-5 Tornado

On May 22, 2011, Mercy Hospital Joplin was struck by an EF-5 tornado resulting in devastating damage to the facility and other surrounding homes and buildings. The hospital itself was almost completely destroyed. Despite the chaotic environment, power outages, and debris littered everywhere, the physicians and staff performed heroically to save as many patients as they could from injury. Leadership's first priority was to ensure that all 2,000 coworkers were accounted for and safe. The hospital then focused on safely transferring inpatients to other facilities for their continued care and getting the hospital back online. Many employees stayed through the night to help triage, treat, and support those doing their very best in a challenging situation. Dozens of community members were injured from the tornado and presented to the damaged facility seeking care. The U.S. Secretary of Homeland Security, Janet Napolitano, praised Mercy physicians and coworkers for their quick response and resilience in the face of such devastation. This was an incredible example of grit and determination. The health system continued to support all 2,000 coworkers financially during the subsequent years, and a new hospital opened its doors almost 4 years later, showing the resilience of the medical teams and the community at large to come back from a traumatic event (Mercy, 2024).

THE IMPORTANCE OF MINDFULNESS IN HIGHLY RELIABLE ORGANIZATIONS

The aforementioned five principles are interrelated and must be understood by everyone in the organization in order to have a collective "mindfulness." **Mindfulness** is a rich awareness of detail that allows one to discover and correct errors that could escalate into a crisis. Performance can be improved by paying attention to one's surroundings and actively working to eliminate distractions. Inattention to detail caused by stress and fatigue creates conditions that lead to errors. In HROs, everyone is engaged in the mission and strives to identify ways to improve the workings of the organization (Box 13.8).

So, what actually happened in the incident narrated in Box 13.8? A young recruit saw a piece of paper fly onto the flight deck. He saw the paper and could anticipate that something bad could happen as a result. Anticipation encompasses three of the five concepts of HROs:

1. Preoccupation with failure: The recruit was actively looking for signs that could indicate an error.
2. Reluctance to simplify: Foreign-object debris on the flight deck is a hazard. It can be sucked into jet engines and cause failure. The recruit saw the piece of paper and did not convince himself that the paper was too minor to cause problems.
3. Sensitivity to operations: The recruit understood how jet engines are able to draw foreign objects into them and how damage to engines and personnel can result.

Anticipation can also make healthcare safer. Imagine that instead of a young recruit on an aircraft carrier, you see a young nurse in the medical ICU. She is helping a physician insert a central venous catheter, a catheter that is placed in a large vein and is at high risk for infection. The nurse, using the sterile technique, has set up all of the equipment needed for the catheter insertion. The doctor comes into the room and puts on sterile gloves. However, the nurse notices that he has not washed his hands. Her mind is racing. She can anticipate that the error of not washing hands can result in a potentially life-threatening infection. In an HRO, she must speak up and stop the catheter from being placed. Anticipation is more than sensing early events that will lead to a problem; it also includes acting on observations to prevent future events from occurring. That is related to the Lean concept of *jidoka*.

Anticipation is important, but errors do happen. Unexpected events or mistakes, no matter how carefully one tries to avoid them, occur. HROs are able to respond appropriately when errors occur to contain the damage. The last two principles of HROs are related to containment:

4. Deference to expertise: In the last example, the physician must defer to the expertise of the nurse and respect her ability to see errors that will lead to infection. Even though the nurse did not have the same number of years of training, she did have the knowledge and experience to call out the error.

BOX 13.8 QUALITY IN PRACTICE!

Lessons From an Aircraft Carrier

The Navy has significantly reduced risk in their operations over the years by adopting the mindset of highly reliable organizations. In his post, Dr. Muething described one example of how a culture of mindfulness improves safety. He was touring a naval aircraft carrier and watching the crew during a routine aircraft landing. A piece of paper floated up onto the deck, and a young trainee immediately responded by raising his hand. He understood how this could lead to distraction and danger. When other members of the crew saw his hand raised, they also raised their hands. The landing was aborted. The commander, when he heard of the trainee halting the landing, commended him and praised him by name. Safety is of utmost concern in HROs (Muething, 2011).

5. Resilience: The nurse and physician must regroup, absorb any strain, and preserve a professional relationship as they gather the necessary materials to restart the catheter insertion under sterile conditions. Both parties must also learn and grow from the episode.

HROs act mindfully to *manage* the unexpected. Note that we say "manage" and not "expect" the unexpected. Always expecting the unexpected is very stressful and signals that there is no expectation of stability within the organization. In managing the unexpected, HROs organize themselves to anticipate and notice aberrations to stop the development of errors. If they cannot halt mistakes, they focus on containment. If an event cannot be contained, HROs work to restore system functioning as soon as possible.

This book has been about a relentless pursuit of quality. But in the end, it is about being able to respond effectively and quickly to dramatic changes. It is the "obsession" with quality that prepares the organization to be responsive to patients' needs, and the efficient use of resources that allows it to react to the most unanticipated changes. Embracing the concepts of HROs will help you create a better healthcare organization.

BRIGHT ANGEL MEDICAL CENTER 13.3

"Who can tell me something about a highly reliable organization or HRO?" asked Dr. Tibbets. His style of teaching revolved around asking questions, dating back all the way to when he was a resident in training to be a physician.

"It's an organization that doesn't make mistakes," Dr. Aoki stated. Olina shook her head as she knew no organization was flawless.

"Nope," said Dr. Tibbets, noticing Olina's head shakes. "What do you think, Olina?" "Well," she started, "an HRO is an organization that is obsessed with safety and puts systems and processes in place to catch most errors before they reach the patient. They continue to grow and evolve to meet the needs of the ever-changing healthcare environment. And they are a learning organization, ensuring that they recover promptly from their mistakes and don't repeat them once they understand the underlying causes."

Dr. Tibbets grinned. "Exactly," he said. "Now that we better understand process improvement and the elements behind what it takes to function like an HRO, we need to engrain these in how we function day to day. Becoming an HRO doesn't happen by accident. It takes commitment and intentional effort to evolve over time to truly become highly reliable."

The group committed to continuing the journey toward becoming an HRO and ensuring they stayed that way.

—The end—

ETHICAL SCENARIO 13.1

When a Patient's Health Can No Longer Be Improved

Futile care is defined as care that will serve no useful purpose to improve the health of a patient. Patients can reach a point in their illness where there are no more options to return them to a state of health. Some examples include advanced cancer, multiorgan failure, or severe brain injury. Understandably, families often struggle when hearing the news that implementing additional therapies will not impact their loved one. Physicians occasionally encounter family members who cannot accept the reality that additional treatments will be futile. Many hospitals have an ethics committee to help provide guidance in these types of situations where families and caregivers are not on the same page regarding future care.

What are the implications of continuing to provide treatment to patients with no hope for improvement?

SUMMARY

This chapter does not really conclude our journey toward excellent quality because, as you know, it is a continuous pursuit. The chapter simply provides an overview of the rewards reaped from a commitment to excellence. Accreditation testifies to the organization's adherence to stringent, evidence-based standards of quality. Awards, whether they are granted at the community, regional, or national level, demonstrate that a healthcare organization's performance has surpassed that of all others. As such, it can be considered a role model. Becoming an HRO requires a fixation on safety and quality to prevent errors from occurring in the first place or being prepared to recover if they occur unexpectedly. The HRO essentially takes this quality journey full circle as you remember from Chapter 1 the IOM's insistence on building processes that make it difficult for errors to occur. We hope this book has given you the motivation to do just that.

KEY TERMS

Kaikaku
Highly reliable organization (HRO)
Accreditation
Det Norske Veritas (DNV)
National Committee for Quality Assurance (NCQA)
Tracer methodology
Healthcare effectiveness data and information set
Certification
International Organization for Standardization (ISO)
Malcolm Baldrige National Quality Award (MBNQA)
Reliability
Resilience
Mindfulness

REVIEW QUESTIONS

1. What does zero harm mean, and why is TJC encouraging health systems to adopt this goal?
2. What is the tracer methodology?
3. What are the main areas of focus of TJC's standards?
4. What are the benefits of accreditation?
5. Are DNV's and TJC's standards very different? Explain.
6. What is the difference between accreditation and certification?
7. What organizations are accredited by NCQA, and why would this be important for consumers?
8. What is ISO 9001, and why was it established?
9. List the seven traditional criteria of the MBNQA. Explain how they are integrated.
10. How do the 2024 MBNQA standards differ from the traditional ones?
11. What is the Semmelweis reflex? How is it related to the contents of this book?
12. What are the five principles of an HRO? Explain.
13. How can mindfulness prevent errors in the healthcare setting? Give one example.
14. The U.S. Army Medical Command is adopting the principles of a HRO. What possible barriers might there be in the military to "deferring to expertise"? Why must these be overcome?

SOLVE BRIGHT ANGEL MEDICAL CENTER'S PROBLEMS

1. BAMC is preparing for a TJC survey. TJC uses a "tracer method," which follows the patient through the healthcare organization and looks at processes at each point along the way. How would you advise BAMC to prepare for this type of survey?

2. As BAMC starts to develop systems to become an HRO, how would you begin to incorporate the five principles of an HRO into the organization? Use the example of an upper-level management meeting that is discussing pharmacy errors and near misses over the past month. Give an example of how the five principles of HROs could be demonstrated in the meeting.

LEARNING ACTIVITIES

1. Why would the CMS allow an independent organization to survey healthcare organizations to ensure that they are complying with CMS standards?
2. Mock interview with two students. One student interviews Dr. Ignaz Semmelweis about resistance to change in healthcare. Hint: Research Dr. Semmelweis's biography before the interview.
3. Find two healthcare organizations that have received the MBNQA to see whether the processes they followed prior to achieving this honor were similar or different. What is the underlying commonality that allowed the two organizations to be recognized for this award?
4. In Box 13.6, "O-Rings and the *Challenger* Accident," why were individuals hesitant to bring forward their concerns with O-ring failure? At the time, what were the potential cultural barriers at NASA that contributed to the disaster?
5. During the COVID-19 pandemic, health systems needed to adapt to rapidly changing circumstances. One challenge was to increase the testing capabilities. One organization, the University of Alabama at Birmingham Health System, was asked to dramatically increase testing (from 1,000/day to >10,000/day) so that all students at colleges around the state could be checked regularly. Using the principles of HROs, describe how this organization could address this daunting challenge.

SPRINGER PUBLISHING CONNECT™ | A robust set of instructor resources designed to supplement this text is located at **http://connect.springerpub.com/content/book/978-0-8261-7976-0.** Qualifying instructors may request access by emailing **textbook@springerpub.com.**

REFERENCES

American Society for Quality. (2024a). *What is ISO 9001:2015—Quality management systems?* https://asq.org/quality-resources/iso-9001#Revision

American Society for Quality. (2024b). *What is the Malcolm Baldrige National Quality Award (MBNQA)?* https://asq.org/quality-resources/malcolm-baldrige-national-quality-award

Det Norske Veritas. (2024). *Hospital accreditation*. https://www.dnv.com/services/hospital-accreditation-7516

Flight Safety Foundation. (2024, March 13). *Exceptionally safe*. https://flightsafety.org/asw-article/exceptionally-safe

Hansen, M. T. (2018). *Great at work: How top performers do less, work better, and achieve more*. Simon & Schuster.

Hubing, K. (2013). The Right Care at the Right Time, Every Time. The George Washington University. https://smhs.gwu.edu/news/right-care-right-time-every-time

Jha, A. K. (2018). Accreditation, quality, and making hospital care better. *JAMA, 320,* 2410–2411. https://doi.org/10.1001/jama.2018.18810

Kato, M., & Zikos, D. (2022). Association between hospital accrediting agencies and hospital outcomes of care in the United States. *Journal of Hospital Management and Health Policy, 6*(12). https://dx.doi.org/10.21037/jhmhp-21-24

Mercy. (2024). *Rebuilding after Joplin tornado*. https://www.mercy.net/about/history/joplin/joplin-tornado/

Muething, S. (2011, January 27, 2011). *Lessons from an aircraft carrier*. Cincinnati Children's. https://blog.cincinnatichildrens.org/hospital-operations/patient-safety/lessons-from-an-aircraft-carrier/

National Academies of Sciences, Engineering, and Medicine. (2019). *Taking action against clinician burnout: A systems approach to professional well-being* The National Academies Press. https://nap.nationalacademies.org/catalog/25521/taking-action-against-clinician-burnout-a-systems-approach-to-professional

National Committee for Quality Assurance. (2024a). *Health plan accreditation*. https://www.ncqa.org/programs/health-plans/health-plan-accreditation-hpa

National Committee for Quality Assurance. (2024b). *Why we're here*. https://www.ncqa.org/about-ncqa

National Institute of Standards and Technology. (2021). *How Baldrige works*. https://www.nist.gov/baldrige/how-baldrige-works

National Institute of Standards and Technology. (2024). *New Baldrige Award criteria for 2024*. https://www.nist.gov/system/files/documents/2023/12/20/New-Baldrige-Award-Criteria-for-2024_0.pdf

Presidential Commission on the Space Shuttle Challenger Accident. (1986). *An accident rooted in history*. NASA Retrieved from https://www.nasa.gov/history/rogersrep/v1ch6.htm

Strahan, J. (2019). *Strategy execution and sustainability: Using the Baldrige leadership model to overcome evasive organizational challenges*. https://www.ache.org/-/media/ache/about-ache/baldrige-foundation-institute-for-performance-excellence-white-paper-201901.pdf

The Joint Commission. (2024a). *Accountability measures fact sheet*. https://www.jointcommission.org/resources/news-and-multimedia/fact-sheets/facts-about-accountability-measures

The Joint Commission. (2024b). *Building a better tomorrow*. https://www.jointcommission.org/our-priorities

The Joint Commission. (2024c). *Facts about The Joint Commission*. Author. https://www.jointcommission.org/who-we-are/facts-about-the-joint-commission/#eb1599ff871b471d8af75e327afca50c_f89791abb8f042859d8264a6b3f31233

The Joint Commission. (2024d). *Leading the way to zero*. https://www.jointcommission.org/resources/patient-safety-topics/zero-harm

The Joint Commission. (2024e). *Tracer methodology fact sheet*. https://www.jointcommission.org/resources/news-and-multimedia/fact-sheets/facts-about-tracer-methodology/

Weick, K. E., & Sutcliffe, K. M. (2007). *Managing the unexpected: Resilient performance in an age of uncertainty* (2nd ed.). Jossey-Bass.

ECHAPTER PART VIII: ADVANCED QUALITY MANAGEMENT AND LEAN SIX SIGMA PROJECT TOOLS (ECHAPTERS 14, 15, AND 16)

eChapters 14, 15, and 16 are available online by visiting www.springerpub.com/courseconnect. See inside front cover and tear-out card for CourseConnect details.

APPENDIX A

CUMULATIVE STANDARD NORMAL DISTRIBUTION TABLE

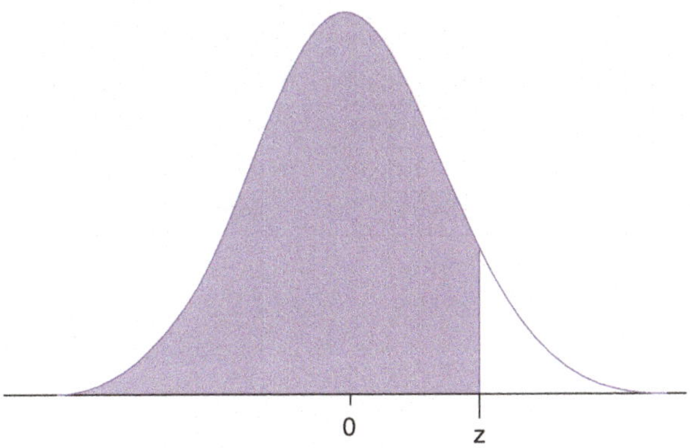

z	0.00	0.01	0.02	0.03	0.04	0.05	0.06	0.07	0.08	0.09
0.0	0.5000	0.5040	0.5080	0.5120	0.5160	0.5199	0.5239	0.5279	0.5319	0.5359
0.1	0.5398	0.5438	0.5478	0.5517	0.5557	0.5596	0.5636	0.5675	0.5714	0.5753
0.2	0.5793	0.5832	0.5871	0.5910	0.5948	0.5987	0.6026	0.6064	0.6103	0.6141
0.3	0.6179	0.6217	0.6255	0.6293	0.6331	0.6368	0.6406	0.6443	0.6480	0.6517
0.4	0.6554	0.6591	0.6628	0.6664	0.6700	0.6736	0.6772	0.6808	0.6844	0.6879
0.5	0.6915	0.6950	0.6985	0.7019	0.7054	0.7088	0.7123	0.7157	0.7190	0.7224
0.6	0.7257	0.7291	0.7324	0.7357	0.7389	0.7422	0.7454	0.7486	0.7517	0.7549
0.7	0.7580	0.7611	0.7642	0.7673	0.7704	0.7734	0.7764	0.7794	0.7823	0.7852
0.8	0.7881	0.7910	0.7939	0.7967	0.7995	0.8023	0.8051	0.8078	0.8106	0.8133
0.9	0.8159	0.8186	0.8212	0.8238	0.8264	0.8289	0.8315	0.8340	0.8365	0.8389
1.0	0.8413	0.8438	0.8461	0.8485	0.8508	0.8531	0.8554	0.8577	0.8599	0.8621
1.1	0.8643	0.8665	0.8686	0.8708	0.8729	0.8749	0.8770	0.8790	0.8810	0.8830
1.2	0.8849	0.8869	0.8888	0.8907	0.8925	0.8944	0.8962	0.8980	0.8997	0.9015
1.3	0.9032	0.9049	0.9066	0.9082	0.9099	0.9115	0.9131	0.9147	0.9162	0.9177
1.4	0.9192	0.9207	0.9222	0.9236	0.9251	0.9265	0.9279	0.9292	0.9306	0.9319
1.5	0.9332	0.9345	0.9357	0.9370	0.9382	0.9394	0.9406	0.9418	0.9429	0.9441
1.6	0.9452	0.9463	0.9474	0.9484	0.9495	0.9505	0.9515	0.9525	0.9535	0.9545
1.7	0.9554	0.9564	0.9573	0.9582	0.9591	0.9599	0.9608	0.9616	0.9625	0.9633

(continued)

z	0.00	0.01	0.02	0.03	0.04	0.05	0.06	0.07	0.08	0.09
1.8	0.9641	0.9649	0.9656	0.9664	0.9671	0.9678	0.9686	0.9693	0.9699	0.9706
1.9	0.9713	0.9719	0.9726	0.9732	0.9738	0.9744	0.9750	0.9756	0.9761	0.9767
2.0	0.9772	0.9778	0.9783	0.9788	0.9793	0.9798	0.9803	0.9808	0.9812	0.9817
2.1	0.9821	0.9826	0.9830	0.9834	0.9838	0.9842	0.9846	0.9850	0.9854	0.9857
2.2	0.9861	0.9864	0.9868	0.9871	0.9875	0.9878	0.9881	0.9884	0.9887	0.9890
2.3	0.9893	0.9896	0.9898	0.9901	0.9904	0.9906	0.9909	0.9911	0.9913	0.9916
2.4	0.9918	0.9920	0.9922	0.9925	0.9927	0.9929	0.9931	0.9932	0.9934	0.9936
2.5	0.9938	0.9940	0.9941	0.9943	0.9945	0.9946	0.9948	0.9949	0.9951	0.9952
2.6	0.9953	0.9955	0.9956	0.9957	0.9959	0.9960	0.9961	0.9962	0.9963	0.9964
2.7	0.9965	0.9966	0.9967	0.9968	0.9969	0.9970	0.9971	0.9972	0.9973	0.9974
2.8	0.9974	0.9975	0.9976	0.9977	0.9977	0.9978	0.9979	0.9979	0.9980	0.9981
2.9	0.9981	0.9982	0.9982	0.9983	0.9984	0.9984	0.9985	0.9985	0.9986	0.9986
3.0	0.9987	0.9987	0.9987	0.9988	0.9988	0.9989	0.9989	0.9989	0.9990	0.9990
3.1	0.9990	0.9991	0.9991	0.9991	0.9992	0.9992	0.9992	0.9992	0.9993	0.9993
3.2	0.9993	0.9993	0.9994	0.9994	0.9994	0.9994	0.9994	0.9995	0.9995	0.9995
3.3	0.9995	0.9995	0.9995	0.9996	0.9996	0.9996	0.9996	0.9996	0.9996	0.9997
3.4	0.9997	0.9997	0.9997	0.9997	0.9997	0.9997	0.9997	0.9997	0.9997	0.9998

APPENDIX B

TOOL KIT

Phase	Tool [Chapter #]	Purpose
DEFINE	A3 report [2, 4, 6, 9, 11, 12]	Summarizes the DMAIC (Define-Measure-Analyze-Improve-Control) activities and tracks progress of improvement project in one page.
	Gemba walk [2, 6]	Gathers facts through actual observation of the process and interaction with frontline employees.
	Case for action [3]	Makes a compelling argument for change and the resources to implement it.
	Benefits/Effort matrix [3]	Displays the values of potential projects based on an assessment of the efforts and benefits they involve in order to prioritize them.
	SIPOC (Suppliers–Inputs–Process–Outputs–Customers) diagram [3]	Summarizes the suppliers, inputs, process steps, outputs, and customers to facilitate process definition and requirements.
	Flowchart [3]	Depicts the sequential steps along the path(s) of a process in a basic way.
	Swimlane diagram [3]	Shows the various participants in the sequence of process activities.
	5w2h framework [3]	Facilitates: (a) process understanding by answering seven important questions, and (b) identification of improvement opportunities.
	House of quality (HOQ) matrix [4]	Depicts the relationship between customer and process requirements.
	Kano model [4]	Helps gain a deep understanding of customers' expectations and their relationships to satisfaction.
	Critical-to-quality (CTQ) tree [4]	Helps generate important, objective performance requirements—CTQs—from the voice of the customer (VOC).
	Affinity diagram [4]	Encourages people to think creatively about new concepts and/or to organize large amounts of language data (ideas, opinions, problems, etc.) into logical groupings.
	Consumer Assessment of Healthcare Providers and Systems (CAHPS) [4]	Captures patient experience in multiple domains.
	SERVQUAL [4]	Captures the five domains of quality of services. It can be adapted for healthcare services.
	Benchmarking [4]	Compares an organization's performance to the best in order to identify and follow best practices for improvement.
	Balanced scorecard [4]	Conveys critical information on key performance indicators in finance, marketing, operations, and human resources at a glance.

(continued)

Phase	Tool [Chapter #]	Purpose
DEFINE	Dashboard [4, 7, 11]	Tracks key performance indicators at the strategic, tactical, or operational level.
	Project charter [5]	Provides a road map for the project with justification, expected benefits, team members and their roles, and timeline for completion.
	Force field analysis [5]	Facilitates change by strengthening the favorable forces and reducing the opposing ones.
	SMART framework [5]	Helps define project goals that are Specific, Measurable, Attainable, Relevant, and Time-bound.
	Risk assessment assignment matrix [5]	Helps visualize the significance of various risks in terms of severity and probability with a color-coded “traffic light” system.
	Work breakdown structure [5]	Depicts a project’s components at various levels of detail to help the planner identify all the work requirements of a project and organize them in a logical fashion.
	Gantt chart [5]	Shows the scheduling of activities and/or resources.
	Project plan [5]	Communicates to all concerned parties what is going to happen and when and establishes performance expectations.
	Variance [5]	Shows schedule, cost, scope, or technical deviations from the project plan.
	Critical path method (CPM) [5]	Plans and schedules project activities; identifies those that are critical to timely project completion.
	Network diagram [5]	Graphically represents the project activities and their precedence relationships.
MEASURE	Value stream map [6]	Depicts a process flow from a Lean perspective, indicating areas that need improvement (kaizen).
	Process activity chart [6]	Displays all steps, categorizes them (operations, inspections, storage, delays, and transportation), and indicates whether or not they create value.
	Flow process chart [6]	Incorporates the symbols of the process activity chart into a flowchart.
	Yield [6]	Determines the percentage of units that are nondefective when they exit the process.
	First pass yield [6]	Determines the percentage of units that passed through a process step without rework.
	Rolled throughput yield [6]	Determines the percentage of units that passed through the entire process without ever requiring rework.
	Check sheet [6]	Tracks problem occurrences and organizes them by category to identify critical problem areas.
	Spaghetti diagram [6]	Depicts traffic intensity and patterns within a physical area or across areas to visualize where movements are wasted.
	Data visualization [7]	Graphically represents information and data.
	Bar chart [7]	Represents the frequency of nominal or categorical data. The variable labels can be displayed on the horizontal axis or the vertical axis. The length of the bars indicates the absolute or relative frequencies of the data.
	Pie chart [7]	Displays relative frequencies or percentages of various categories or groups.
	Doughnut chart [7]	Displays relative frequencies or percentages of various categories or groups. Variation of pie chart with a hole in the middle.
	Histogram [7]	Displays the frequencies for each value or range of numeric (ordinal, interval, or ratio) data.

(*continued*)

Phase	Tool [Chapter #]	Purpose
MEASURE	Line chart [7]	Displays interval or ratio data over time with a line connecting data points.
	Box-and-whisker plot (or boxplot) [7]	Graph that depicts the center (median) and spread (minimum, maximum, interquartile range) of a metric variable.
	Central tendency [7]	Indicates the center of the distribution of a variable.
	Variation or dispersion [7]	Reflects the spread of the data distribution.
	Probability sampling [A.7.1]	Randomly selects units from a population, with each unit having a known probability of being selected.
	Simple random sampling [A.7.1]	Randomly selects units from a population so that every sample of a certain size has a known and equal probability of being selected. The number in each stratum of sample units is proportionate to the size of the stratum in the population.
	Proportionate stratified random sampling [A.7.1]	Randomly selects units from each stratum of a population. The number of sample units from each stratum is proportionate to the size of the stratum in the population.
	Systematic sampling [A.7.1]	Selects sample units from the population according to a fixed interval.
	Cluster sampling [A.7.1]	Selects sample units in a cluster or mini-population.
	Nonprobability sampling [A.7.1]	Selects units from a population using a subjective or non-random method.
	Convenience sampling [A.7.1]	Selects sample units based on availability.
	Judgment sampling [A.7.1]	Selects sample units based on relevance to topic of interest.
	Statistical process control [8, 11, 12]	Determines whether a process is performing as expected.
	Control charts [8, 11, 12]	Depict the consistency of process performance indicators over time. They are line graphs with a centerline representing the overall process average and control limits set by the random variation of the process.
	p-chart (Attributes) [8]	Tracks the proportion defective in a sample (equal or different sample or subgroup sizes) over time.
	np-chart (Attributes) [8]	Tracks the number of defective items in a sample (equal or similar sample or subgroup sizes) over time.
	c-chart (Attributes) [8]	Tracks the number of defects per unit over time.
	u-chart (Attributes) [8]	Tracks the number of defects per unit over time when the area of opportunity fluctuates.
	IX chart (Variables) [8]	Displays individual data points collected individually or as overall averages and reported infrequently over time.
	MR chart (Variables) [8]	Depicts moving ranges or absolute difference between two consecutive, individual measures or *IX*s over time.
	$\bar{X}$ chart (Variables) [8]	Tracks sample means over time.
	R chart (Variables) [8]	Tracks sample ranges over time.
	s-chart (Variables) [8]	Tracks sample SDs over time.
	Pattern test [8]	Detects patterns in a control chart divided into zones A, B, and C.
	Cumulative sum (CUSUM) chart [8]	Detects sudden and small deviations from a target value quickly.
	Process capability ratio, C_p [8]	Determines whether a process in control has a distribution narrow enough to fit within specification limits.
	Process capability index, C_{pk} [8]	Determines whether a process in control is properly centered with respect to a specified target value.

(continued)

Phase	Tool [Chapter #]	Purpose
ANALYZE	Gap analysis [9]	Compares the actual with the desired process performance.
	Cause-and-effect diagram (fishbone diagram) [9]	Displays potential sources of quality problems.
	Root cause analysis (RCA) [9]	Systematically searches for the root cause of a problem.
	The 5 Whys [2, 9]	Identifies the root cause(s) of a problem.
	Interrelationship diagram (or diagraph or digraph) [9]	Depicts the links among different aspects of a complex situation.
	Failure mode and effects analysis [9]	Helps identify potential failure points in a process and assess the relative impact of these failures.
	Scatter diagram [9]	Displays the type, strength, and direction of the relationship between two variables.
	Correlation analysis [9]	Measures the degree to which two variables are linearly related.
	Linear regression analysis [9]	Fits a trend line to historical data points by minimizing the sum of the squared deviations between points on the line and the actual data points.
	Least squares method [9]	Estimates the equation that minimizes the sums of the squares of the deviations from the estimate (see linear regression analysis).
	Simple linear regression [9]	Examines the linear relationship between only *one* predictor and one outcome variable.
	Analysis of variance (ANOVA) [9]	Tests the overall fit of a linear model using an *F*-ratio.
	Multiple linear regression [9]	Examines the linear relationship between two or more independent variables and the dependent variable.
	Pareto chart [9]	Identifies the "vital few" issues (e.g., causes) that need to be prioritized based on the 80/20 rule.
IMPROVE	Job enlargement [10]	Increases the variety of a job by having employees perform more immediately upstream or downstream activities.
	Job enrichment [10]	Extends the employee's regular activities to planning and control functions.
	Jidoka [2, 10]	Gives employees the authority to "stop the line" when they deem it appropriate.
	Total productive maintenance (TPM) [10, 12]	Engages everyone in the organization to monitor the equipment when using it, thereby increasing equipment reliability.
	Quality at the source [10]	Makes everyone responsible for checking one's own work to avoid passing on defects to the next step or "customer."
	6S [10, 12]	Creates sustainable order and visibility to enhance the fluidity of the process flow.
	Leveling the workload (*heijunka*) [10]	Sets an even daily schedule that follows customer demand in terms of volume and mix.
	poka-yoke [10]	Mistake-proofs a task or process so that errors are identified.
	Checklist [2, 10]	Lists all the actions that must be performed to reach a successful outcome.
	Lean bundle [2, 10]	Creates efficient operations and combines best practices and concepts of Lean management.

(*continued*)

Phase	Tool [Chapter #]	Purpose
IMPROVE	Just-in-time (JIT) [10]	Makes materials, supplies, or patients move through the system exactly when they are needed, not early and not late.
	Kanban system [10, 12]	Authorizes the movement of or processing of units flowing through the system to ensure that they are available just in time. Uses a visual control system with a system of cards or signals.
	Undercapacity scheduling [10]	Schedules work so that the capacity of a process exceeds the demand placed on it in order to avoid bottlenecks.
	Line balancing [10]	Equalizes workload requirements subject to cycle time and precedence relationship constraints (high-volume, repetitive processes).
	Relationship diagramming [10]	Utilizes qualitative information provided by analysts, managers, and workers to establish relationship preferences between pairs of departments, workstations, or offices (low-volume, high-variety processes).
	Theory of constraints (TOC) [10]	Identifies and improves a constraint until it no longer burdens the system.
	General process chart [11]	Compares current and proposed process designs and displays the extent of improvement.
	Simulation [11]	Imitates or replicates a real-world process and produces performance metrics to guide redesign.
	Cost-benefit analysis [11]	Compares the expected financial costs and benefits of a project.
	Sigma level [11]	Determines the number of standard deviations between the process average and the closest specification limit.
CONTROL	Control plan [12]	Outlines the improved process steps and characteristics and specifies the actions needed to maintain performance.
	Standard operating procedure (SOP) [12]	Provides a detailed set of written instructions to perform routine operations correctly and consistently.
	Document control [12]	Manages critical documents related to process quality in a systematic fashion.
	Audit [12]	Reviews process performance based on selected criteria or standards.
	Preventive maintenance [12]	Prevents problems from occurring when the equipment is used for productive purposes.
	Visual management (VM) [12]	Uses visual cues to provide workers with process information and prompt swift corrective action when required.
	Color coding [12]	Facilitates identification of items and designation of location.
	Shadow board [12]	Marks where each piece of equipment must be placed.
	Andon light [12]	Flashes when a major problem has occurred and the process must stop.
	Daily huddle [12]	Quickly addresses progress toward performance goals and keeps team members aligned and focused.
	Huddle board [12]	Displays issues and team progress in daily or weekly meetings.
	Quality circle (QC) [12]	Meets regularly to find ways to solve problems in their work area.
	Rapid process improvement workshop (RPIW) or kaizen event or kaizen blitz [2, 12]	Targets a specific problem area or process to deliver a significant improvement in a short period of time.

(*continued*)

Phase	Tool [Chapter #]	Purpose
ACCREDITATION	Tracer methodology [13]	Follows patients through the entire care delivery process to evaluate the care provided by an organization as well as the effectiveness of its systems.
	Healthcare effectiveness data and information set (HEDIS) [13]	Measures the quality of health plans.

INDEX

A3 report, building, 50, 108–109, 171–173, 298–300, 361–362
absolute frequencies, 183
abuse, 6
ACA. *See* Affordable Care Act
accountable care organizations (ACOs), 9
accreditation, 394–399
  achieving, 395
  benefits of, 397
  Det Norske Veritas (DNV), 397–398
  The Joint Commission (TJC), 392
  higher risk services, 398
  medication management, 398
  National Committee for Quality Assurance (NCQA), 392, 396–397
  patient rights, 398
  physical environment, 398
  proactive risk management, 397
  quality management system and governance, 397
accrediting agencies, 68
ACOs. *See* accountable care organizations
act, 20
activity schedule, 140–143
addition, 82
adjusted R^2, 295
admission, 339
affinity diagrams, 46, 92–93
Affordable Care Act (ACA), 5, 82
Agency for Healthcare Research and Quality (AHRQ), 93, 310
AHRQ. *See* Agency for Healthcare Research and Quality
ALOS. *See* average length of stay
analysis of variance (ANOVA), 295
ANOVA. *See* analysis of variance
appraisal costs, 16
area of opportunity, 236
assignable/special causes of variation, 225–226
assurance, 95
attributes, 230
auditing, 376–377
average length of stay (ALOS), 244, 295, 372

backward pass, 141, 143
balanced scorecard, 103–104
BAMC. *See* Bright Angel Medical Center
bar chart, 183–184
basic flowchart symbols, 70
basic quality, 86
benchmark, 47, 103
benchmarking, 102–103
benefits/effort matrix, 64–65
  types of, 64
binomial distribution, 193–195
Black Belts, 50
bottleneck, 322
Bright Angel Medical Center (BAMC), 3, 23–24, 64, 75, 83, 228, 338
buffers, eliminating, 321–322
business case for action, 63–64
  business environment, 64
  cost of inaction, 64
  diagnosis, 64
  objectives, 64
  problem, 64
business strategy, 12

c-charts, 236–240
CAHPS. *See* Consumer Assessment of Healthcare Providers and Systems
care delivery models, 9–10
  accountable care organizations (ACOs), 9
  hospital value-based purchasing (VBP), 10
  medical homes, 9
  merit-based incentive payment system (MIPS), 10
categorical data, 182
cause-and-effect diagram, 280–284
  basic quality tools, 281–282
  environment, 281
  equipment, 281
  materials, 280
  measurement, 280
  methods, 280
  people, 280
cause on the problem, predicting the effect of, 291–297
causes of variation, 225–226
cellular layouts, 325–327
central limit theorem (CLT) in statistics, 179, 191
central tendency, 198–200
  mean, 200
  measures of, 198–200
  median, 198–200
  mode, 198
centerline, 228
certification, 399–400
  International Organization for Standardization (ISO), 399–400
CfCs. *See* Conditions for Coverage
check sheet, 170
checklists, 48, 319–320
  standardizing with, 49
clinical productive system, 18
closure conversations, 35
CLT. *See* central limit theorem
cluster sampling, 218
co-creating value, 90
coefficient of determination, 293

collecting data, 158
collection methods, 92
common causes of variation, 226–227
competitive priorities in operations strategy, 15
  cost, 15
  flexibility, 15
  quality, 15
  timeliness, 15
computerized physician order entry (POE), 314
computing slack, 143–144
Conditions for Coverage (CfCs), 394
Conditions of Participation (CoPs), 394
construct validity, 120
Consumer Assessment of Healthcare Providers and Systems (CAHPS), 93–94
consumers, 67
content validity, 120
continuous data, 195
continuous distributions, 195
control, 351
control charts, 227
  for attributes, 230–243. *See also* *c*-charts; *np*-charts; *p*-charts; *u*-charts
  decision tree, 256
  factors for, 276
  patterns, 255–257
  for variables, 243–255. *See also* *MR* charts; *IX* charts; $\bar{X}$ charts; *R* charts; *s*-charts
control limits, 228–229
control methods, 373
control phase, 351
control plan, 49, 372–373
controlled experiments, 47
convenience sampling, 219–220
convergent validity, 120
conversations, 35
  closure conversations, 35
  initiative conversations, 35
  performance conversations, 35
  understanding conversations, 35
COPIS method, 65
  for BAMC'S ED throughput improvement project, 66
CoPs. *See* Conditions of Participation
corrective (or breakdown) maintenance, 380
correlation analysis, 290–291
correlation coefficient, 290
cost–benefit analysis, 346–351
costs, 15
  appraisal costs, 16
  external failure costs, 16
  internal failure costs, 16
  prevention costs, 16
CPM. *See* critical path method
criterion validity, 120
critical activities, 139
critical path, 139
critical path method (CPM), 124, 137–144
  activity schedule, 140–143
  advantages, 145
  computing slack, 143–144
  critical path, 139–140
  disadvantages, 145
  evaluating, 145
  network diagram, 137–139
critical-to-quality (CTQ) tree, 81, 83, 87–89, 372
  partial CTQ tree for BAMC, 87
cross-sector collaboration for a healthy living environment, 127
CTQ. *See* critical to quality
culture, 22
cumulative model, 17–18
cumulative sum (CUSUM) charts, 224, 257–262
  IX chart as basis for, 258
customers, 405
customers in healthcare, 67–68
  accrediting agencies, 68
  patients' perspectives, 67
  providers' perspectives, 67–68
  third-party payers' perspectives, 68
cycle time, 160, 316

daily huddle, 40
dashboards, 104–108, 189–190, 358–361
  operational dashboards, 104
  strategic dashboards, 104
  tactical dashboards, 104
data analytics, 180
  descriptive analytics, 180
  predictive analytics, 180–181
  prescriptive analytics, 180–181
  types, 180–181
data collection methods, 91–93, 158
  affinity diagram, 92–93
  idea generation, 92
  plan and sequence, 158
data sets, 181
data visualization and description, 179–221. *See also* central tendency; dispersion
  bar chart, 183–184
  binomial distribution, 193–195
  continuous distributions, 195
  dashboards, 189–190
  discrete distributions, 193
  doughnut charts, 184–186
  empirical distributions, 191–198
  histogram, 186–187
  interval data, 182–183, 186–190
  line chart, 187–189
  measurement levels, 182–183
    examples, 183–190
  measures of dispersion, 200–203
  nominal or categorical data, 182–186
  normal distribution, 195–197
  ordinal data, 182–186
  pie charts, 184–186

Poisson distribution, 195
population, 190
probabilities, 191
ratio data, 182–183, 186–190
sample, 190
sample size, 190
sampling frame, 190
standard normal distribution, 197–198
theoretical distributions, 191–198
defects, errors, 36
defects per million opportunities (DPMO), 356
defects per opportunity (DPO), 356
deference to expertise, 410
deferred maintenance, 380
Define-Measure-Analyze-Improve-Control (DMAIC) process, 44, 351, 384, 408
degree of freedom, 202
Deming wheel, 20
Deming's 14 points, 20–22
demographics, 90
dependent variable, 292
descriptive analytics, 180
design principles, 312–322
buffers, eliminating, 321–322
capturing the information once, at the source, 314–315
checklists, 319–320
designing for the mainstream, not the exceptions, 316–319
excessive delegation, avoiding, 314
flexible system, 312–313
fragmentation, reducing, 312–313
Just-In-Time (JIT), 321–322
link layout and process, 322
linking parallel activities, 315–316
mistake-proof the process, 319–320
performing activities in parallel, 315
quality at the source, 314–315
standardization, 316–318
total productive maintenance (TPM), 314
undercapacity scheduling, 322
whole system optimization, 320–321
workload leveling (*heijunka*), 318–319
Det Norske Veritas (DNV), 394, 397–398
diagnosis-related group (DRG), 5
direct-to-employer arrangements, 11
discharge, 339
discrete data, 193
discrete distributions, 193
discriminant validity, 120
dispersion, measures of, 200–203
range, 200–201
standard deviation (*SD*), 202
standard error (*SE*), 202–203
variability or dispersion, 200
variance, 201–202
DMAIC. *See* Define-Measure-Analyze-Improve-Control
DNV. *See* Det Norske Veritas
do, 20
document control, 375–376
documenting the improvement, 351–358
process activity chart, 351
Six Sigma metrics, 353
statistical process control charts, 351–352
documenting the new process, 372–377
auditing, 376–377
control plan, 372–373
document control, 375–376
standard operating procedures (SOPs), 373–375
Donabedian triad, 97
doughnut charts, 184–186
Dow Jones Industrial Index, 200
DPMO. *See* defects per million opportunities
DPO. *See* defects per opportunity
DRG. *See* diagnosis-related group
dysfunctional processes, 62–63

EF-5 Tornado, 410
effectiveness, 9
efficiency, 9
EHR. *See* electronic health record
electronic health record (EHR), 314
emergency maintenance, 380
Emergency Severity Index (ESI) classification, 72, 164
empathy, 95
empirical distributions, 191–198
employees in functional areas, 128
endodontics, 358
equitable treatment, 9
errors, 7
ESI. *See* Emergency Severity Index
exam by provider, 339
exam rooms, 339
excellent quality, 82
excitement quality, 86
Executive sponsor or champion, 50
executives, 128
experimental probability, 191
experiments, 344
external failure costs, 16
extra processing, 36

failure mode and effects analysis (FMEA), 47, 69, 280, 285–288
for transport of patient to and from imaging department, 287–288
feasibility, 62
fee-for-service (FFS), 5
FFS. *See* fee-for-service
first pass yield (FPY), 166
fishbone (cause-and-effect or Ishikawa) diagram, 46
5 Whys, 47

5w2h framework, 72–76
cost, 75
location, 74
method, 74
people, 74
purpose, 74
sequence, 74
subject matter, 74
flexibility, 15
flexible system, 312–313
flow process chart, 166–168
flow unit, 70
flowchart, 70–72
of current patient flow, 71
FMEA. *See* failure mode and effects analysis
focus group interviews, 91
force field analysis, 130
form, 117
forward pass, 140, 143
Four Conversations, 35
FPY. *See* first pass yield
fraud, 6
frequency distribution, 183
FTEs. *See* full-time equivalents
full-time equivalents (FTEs), 236
functional layouts, 324–325
versus product layouts, 327
for nonrepetitive processes, designing, 324–325
functional strategies, 14
future state process activity chart, 341

Gantt charts, 48, 124, 133
gap analysis, 279
Gemba walk, 35
general process chart, 342
governing body, 404
Green Belts, 50
green healthcare, 11

handoffs, 15, 312
HCAHPS. *See* Hospital Consumer Assessment of Healthcare Providers and Systems
health co-creation, 11
health disparities, 8
health maintenance organization (HMO), 5
healthcare effectiveness data and information set, 398
heijunka (leveling the workload), 318–319
high-level view, of the process, 65–67
highly reliable organization (HRO), 407
common principles of, 408–410
deference to expertise, 410
mindfulness importance in, 411–412
preoccupation with failure, 409
reluctance to simplify, 409
resilience, 410
sensitivity to operations, 408
histogram, 186–187
HMO. *See* health maintenance organization
HOQ. *See* house of quality
Hospital Consumer Assessment of Healthcare Providers and Systems (HCAHPS), 93
hospital value-based purchasing (VBP) program, 10, 93, 101
house of quality (HOQ), 82–89
HRO. *See* highly reliable organization
huddles, 372, 382–383

IDEO human-centered design, 312
imaging, 339
improve phase, 351
independent variable, 292
information technology, 11
initiative conversations, 35
innovation centers, 11
institutionalizing the improvement, 383–387
quality circles (QCs), 383–384
rapid process improvement workshop (RPIW), 384
insurers' roles in care delivery, 10
internal failure costs, 16
International Organization for Standardization (ISO), 399–400
interquartile range, 201
interrelationship diagrams/diagraphs/digraphs, 284–285
interval data, 182–183, 186–190
inventory, 36
ISO. *See* International Organization for Standardization
IX charts, 243–255
all individual *X* values, plotting, 246
control limits, determining, 246
determining whether the process is in control, 246
mean of the individual *X* values, computing, 245–246

JCAH. *See* Joint Commission on Accreditation of Hospitals
jidoka (automation with a human touch), 42
JIT. *See* Just-In-Time
job enlargement, 312
job enrichment, 312
The Joint Commission (TJC), 21, 376, 394
joint commission, 395–397
performance measurement, 396
priorities, 396
Joint Commission on Accreditation of Hospitals (JCAH), 395
judgment sampling, 220
Just-In-Time (JIT), 40–41, 321–322

Kadlec Regional Medical Center, 314
Kaikaku, 393
kaizen blitz, 372, 384
kaizen event, 41, 384

kanban system, 322
Kano model, 85–86
basic quality, 86
excitement quality, 86
performance quality, 86
question and answer format in, 86
key performance indicators (KPIs), 103
KPIs. *See* key performance indicators

lab, 339
law of large numbers (LoLN), 179, 191
layout improvement project, 139
leadership, 402–404
CEO and other senior leaders, 404
governing body, 404
leadership importance in project management, 129–131
Lean, 34–42
four conversations, 35
implementations in healthcare, shortcomings, 42–43
just-in-time (JIT), 40–41
leadership and training for, importance, 35–36
Lean culture, 35–36
Lean system, 318
principles, 37–42
create flow, 39
establish pull, 39–41
identify value, 37–38
map the value stream, 38–39
seek perfection, 41–42
after the COVID-19 crisis, 43
waste elimination, 36–37
Lean bundles, 42
Lean Six Sigma (LSS) certification, 22
Lean Six Sigma (LSS) framework, 22, 32–55, 402. *See also* Six Sigma methodology
analyze, 23
benefits of, 52–53
certification tips, 53–54
control, 23
define, 23
improve, 23
measure, 23
methodologies, 32
rapid process improvement workshop, 384
Leapfrog, 101–102
least squares method, 293
length of stay (LOS), 157
line balancing, 324
line chart, 187–189
linear regression analysis, 291
LoLN. *See* law of large numbers
LOS. *See* length of stay
LSS. *See* Lean Six Sigma

maintenance, 380. *See also* total productive maintenance (TPM)
corrective (or breakdown), 380
deferred, 380
emergency, 380
predictive, 380
prescriptive, 380
preventive, 380
time-based, 380
types, 380
usage-based, 380
Malcolm Baldrige National Quality Award (MBNQA), 400–407
business/organizational performance results, 402, 406–407
customers, 401, 405
leadership, 401
measurement, analysis, and knowledge management, 401, 405
new Baldrige Award criteria for 2024, 407
operations, 402, 405–406
strategy, 401, 404–405
workforce, 402, 405
MAP. *See* Measure Applications Partnership
Master Black Belts, 50
MBNQA. *See* Malcolm Baldrige National Quality Award
mean, 200
Measure Applications Partnership (MAP), 99
measurement, analysis, and knowledge management, 405
measurement methods, 372
median, 198–200
medical errors, 7
medical homes, 9
medication, 339
mergers and acquisitions, 10
merit-based incentive payment system (MIPS), 10
mindfulness, 411–412
MIPS. *See* merit-based incentive payment system
mode, 198
motion, 36
moving ranges [*MR*] charts, 224
MR charts, 243–255
all moving ranges, plotting, 245
centerline and control limits, 245
determining whether the process is in control, 245
mean moving range, computing, 245
MR for each data point, computing, 244
multiple linear regression, 295
multiple *R*, 296
multiple regression, 295–297
Muther's grid, 325

National Committee for Quality Assurance (NCQA), 394, 398–399
National Integrated Accreditation for Healthcare Organizations (NIAHO®), 397
National Surgical Quality Improvement Program (NSQIP), 103

NCQA. *See* National Committee for Quality Assurance
network diagram, 137–139
"next process" concept, 69
NIAHO®. *See* National Integrated Accreditation for Healthcare Organizations
nominal data, 182, 183–186
nonprobability sampling, 209, 219–220
  convenience sampling, 219–220
  judgment sampling, 220
nonrandom variation, 46
nonresponse bias, 220
non–value-added time, 160
normal distribution, 195–197
np-charts, 235–236
  average number of defective items, computing, 235
  centerline, drawing, 236
  daily number of LWBS patients, plotting, 236
  determining whether the process is in control, 236
  UCL and LCL of the *np*-chart, determining, 235
NSQIP. *See* National Surgical Quality Improvement Program

O-Rings and the *Challenger* accident, 409
objective quality indicators, 83
  outcomes, 99
  process, 98
  structure, 98
occupational medicine clinic, value stream mapping in, 163
OECD. *See* Organisation for Economic Co-operation and Development
operational dashboards, 104
operations, 405–406
  competitive priorities in, 15
  strategy, 15
opioid misuse and abuse, 109
order qualifiers, 18
order winners, 18
ordinal data, 182–186
Organisation for Economic Co-operation and Development (OECD) countries, 6
  healthcare-related errors in, 7
  life expectancy at birth in, 8
  national health spending for, 6
outcome indicators, 99, 191
overall hospital quality star rating, 100–101
overproduction, 36
overuse, 6

p-charts, 230–235
  control limits, drawing, 233
  control limits or upper and lower bands of the chart, determining, 232
  determining whether the process is in control, 235
  each sample *SD* of the proportion, computing, 231
  mean proportion of LWBS patients, computing, 231
  plotting the proportion defective, 234
p value, 295
parameters, 191
Pareto chart, 297–298
path, 139
patient- and family-centered care (PFCC), 90
Patient-Centered Medical Home (PCMH), 93
Patient-Centered Outcomes Research Institute (PCORI), 9
patient-centeredness, 9
patient hub concept, 327
patients, 67
patients' perspectives, 67
pattern tests, 257
  zones and patterns, 257
PCMH. *See* Patient-Centered Medical Home
PCORI. *See* Patient-Centered Outcomes Research Institute
PDSA. *See* plan-do-study-act
performance
  conversations, 35
  measurement, 396
  quality, 86
personal protective equipment (PPE), 409
PFCC. *See* patient-and family-centered care
phlebotomist, 339
pie charts, 184–186
plan, 20
plan-do-study-act (PDSA) cycle, 20
POC. *See* point-of-care
point-of-care (POC) technologies, 314
Poisson distribution, 195
poka-yoke (mistake-proofing), 42
population, 190
  health, 11
  size, 190
  variance, 201
potential cause and effect, verifying association between, 289–291
PPE. *See* personal protective equipment
precedence relationships, 138
predictive analytics, 180–181
predictive maintenance, 380
prescriptive analytics, 181
prescriptive maintenance, 380
present value (PV), 349
prevention costs, 16
preventive maintenance, 380
priorities, 396
prioritizing causes, 297–298
probabilities, 191
  experimental, 191
  subjective, 191
  theoretical, 191

probability distribution, 191
probability sampling, 210–219
problem-solving, 279–305. *See also* scatter diagrams; simple linear regression
  A3 report, building, 298–300
  basic tools, 280
  correlation analysis, 290–291
  multiple regression, 295–297
  organizing the team's thoughts, 280–288. *See also* cause-and-effect diagram; failure mode and effects analysis (FMEA); interrelationship diagrams/diagraphs/digraphs
  Pareto chart, 297–298
  prioritizing causes, 297–298
process(es), 18–19, 97–98
  in a hospital, 19
  Deming wheel, 20
  productive system, 18
process activity chart, 164–166, 339–342, 351
  future state process activity chart, 341
  general process chart, 342
  symbols in, 164
process and layout, relationship, 322–327
process capability, 46, 262–267
  analogy, 266
  index, 265
  process centering, 265
  process distribution, 263
  ratio, 263
  specification or tolerance limits, 262
process control charts, 229–230
process design, 311–312
process efficiency, 160
process improvement candidate, 63
process indicators, 98
process measurement, 157–178. *See also* value stream map (VSM)
  A3 report, building, 171–173
  check sheet, 170
  data collection, 158
  flow process chart, 166
  spaghetti diagram, 170–171
  value-added activities and waste, 158–159
  value categorization of process activities, 159
  yield, 166–169
process modeling, 69–72
  flowchart, 70–72
  swimlane diagram, 72
process owners, 62
process redesign, ensuring success, 337–366. *See also* dashboards; spaghetti diagrams; value stream map (VSM)
  cost–benefit analysis, 346–351
  documenting the improvement, 351–358. *See also* *individual entry*
  future state, 338–344
  simulation, 344–346
process selection and description, 61–76
  benefits/effort matrix, 64–65
  business case for action, 63–64
  customers, 67–68
  describing the process, 65–69
  dysfunction, 62
  feasibility, 62
process stability and capability, 224–276. *See also* control charts: for variables; cumulative sum (CUSUM) charts
  attributes, 230
  centerline, 228
  control charts for attributes, 230–243
  control limits, 228–229
  process control charts, 229–230
  variables, 230
  variation, 225–227
process steps, 68–69, 372
  subprocesses and steps, 69
process variation, 225
product layouts for repetitive processes, designing, 323–324
productive system, 18
project champions, 128
project charter and roles, 125–128
  for BAMC, 126
project management, 123–152
  employees in functional areas, 128
  executives, 128
  leadership importance in, 129–131
  personal relationships in project teams, 147
  phases of a project, 131–137
    closure, 131, 137
    control, 131, 136–137
    execution, 131, 136
    initiation, 131–132
    planning, 131–137
  project champions, 128
  project charter and roles, 125–128
  project management office, 127
  projects failure, reasons, 145–147
  team dynamics and communication, 146–147
  triple constraint, 124
project manager, 127
project plan, 136
project team, 128
  characteristics of, 128
projects failure, reasons, 145–147
proportionate stratified random sampling, 216
providers' perspectives, 67–68
psychographics, 90
pull system, 40
Purchasing (VBP) program, 93, 101
push system, 39
PV. *See* present value

QCs. *See* quality circles
QFD. *See* Quality function deployment
qualitative research data collection methods, 91

quality, 15, 82–89. *See also* house of quality (HOQ)
  costs of, 16
  basic quality, 86
  excellent quality, 82
  excitement quality, 86
  house of quality (HOQ), 82
  performance quality, 86
quality at the source, 314–315
quality circles (QCs), 372, 383–384
quality first, 3–26. *See also* strategic importance of quality; total quality management (TQM); value-based care
  cumulative model, 17–18
  value, 3
quality function deployment (QFD), 82
quality indicators, 83
quality issues threatening value-based care, 7–8
  errors, 7
  medical errors, 7
  variation, 7–8
quality measures, use of, 100–108
  benchmarking, 102–103
  dashboards, 104–108
  hospital value-based purchasing (VBP) program, 93, 101
  Leapfrog, 101–102
  overall hospital quality star rating, 100–101
quantitative research data collection methods, 92
questionnaire design, basic concepts of, 116
questionnaire development, 116–119
  construct validity, 120
  content validity, 120
  convergent validity, 120
  criterion validity, 120
  discriminant validity, 120
  form, 117
  pretest, 119
  relevance, 117
  reliability, 119–120
  sequencing, 118
  wording, 117–118

R chart, 249–251
random causes of variation, 226–227
random number seeds, 346
random variation, 46
range, 200–201
  interquartile, 201
rapid process improvement workshop (RPIW), 384
  three phases of, 385
ratio data, 182–183, 186–190
RCA. *See* root cause analysis
RED toolkit, 310
registration, 338
regression analysis, 291–292
regression coefficient (slope), 292
relationship diagramming, 325
relative frequencies, 184
relevance, 117
reliability, 95, 119–120, 407
resilience, 410
responsiveness, 95
risk assessment assignment matrix, 132
rolled throughput yield (RTY), 166, 353
root cause analysis (RCA), 47, 69, 280
RPIW. *See* rapid process improvement workshop
RTY. *See* rolled throughput yield

s-chart, 253–254
safety, 8
sample, 190
sample size, 190
sample variance, 201
sampling distribution, 192
sampling frame, 190
Saskatchewan Health Authority (SHA), 90
scatter diagrams, 289–290
school nurses' access to children's electronic records, 72
scope creep, 125
SD. *See* standard deviation
SE. *See* standard error
secondary sources of information, 310–311
semistructured personal interviews, 91
sequencing, 118
SERVQUAL survey instrument, 95–96
setup time, 319
SHA. *See* Saskatchewan Health Authority
sigma level, 353, 356–358
simple linear regression, 292–295
  regression coefficient (slope), 292
  y-intercept, 292
simple random sampling, 210–213
  using Excel, 213–215
simulation, 344–346
SIPOC. *See* Suppliers–Inputs–Process–Outputs–Customers
6S, 316
6S (revisited), 378–380
  total productive maintenance, 380–381
  visual tools and their purposes, types, 379
six aims for quality improvement, 8–9
  effectiveness, 9
  efficiency, 9
  equitable treatment, 9
  patient-centeredness encompasses, 9
  safety, 8
  timeliness, 9
Six Sigma methodology, 43–53
  A3 report, 50
  analyze the process, 23, 46–47
    5 Whys, 48
  control the improved process, 23, 49
  define the process, 23, 45–46
  history, 44
  improve the process, 23, 47–49

learning culture in, 50–52
Black Belts, 50
Executive sponsor or champion, 50
Green Belts, 50
Master Black Belts, 50
White Belts, 50
Yellow Belts, 50
measure the process, 23, 46
principles, 44–49
Six Sigma metrics, 353–356
rolled throughput yield (RTY), 353
sigma level, 353
throughput (first pass) yield (FPY), 353
yield, 353
slack, 139
SMART framework, 132
social determinants of health, 11
SOPs. *See* standard operating procedures
spaghetti diagrams, 170–171, 342–344
SPC. *See* statistical process control
specification or tolerance limits, 262
stakeholders, 64
standard deviation (*SD*), 202
standard error (*SE*), 202
standard normal distribution, 197–198
standard operating procedures (SOPs), 49, 371, 373–375
standardization, 316–318
statistical process control (SPC), 49, 226, 351–352, 371
control phase, 351
improve phase, 351
Six Sigma metrics, 353–356
statistics, 191
storage of linen and supplies, 339
strategic dashboards, 104
strategic importance of quality, 12–18
business strategy, 12
competitive priorities, 15
functional strategies (HOW), 14
operations strategy, 15
SWOT analysis, 13–14
structural indicators, 97
study, 20
subgroup, 228
subjective probability, 191
Suppliers–Inputs–Process–Outputs–Customers (SIPOC), 45, 62, 65
customers, 65
inputs, 65
outputs, 65
process, 65
suppliers, 65
surgical instruments sterilization process, 316–317
symptoms versus root causes, 47
sustaining the improvement, 371–388. *See also* documenting the new process; institutionalizing the improvement
swimlane diagram, 72
SWOT analysis, 13–14
systematic (or periodic) sampling, 216–218
systematizing the improvement, 377–383
huddles, 382–383
statistical process control, 373, 377
6S, 379
total productive maintenance, 379, 380
visual workplace, 381
systems thinking, 12

tactical dashboards, 104
takt time, 318
tangibles, 95
target value, 265
team dynamics and communication, 146–147
Thai Public Hospital, 52
theoretical distributions, 191–198
theoretical probability, 191
theory of constraints (TOC), 309, 328–332
constraint, exploiting, 328
constraint or bottleneck, identifying, 328
elevating the constraint, 330
find the new constraint, 330
subordinating everything else to the constraint, 329
third-party payers' perspectives, 68
throughput (first pass) yield (FPY), 353
throughput yield (TPY), 46, 166
time-based maintenance, 380
timeliness, 9, 15
TJC. *See* The Joint Commission
TOC. *See* theory of constraints
toolbox for higher value, 309–336. *See also* theory of constraints (TOC)
cellular layouts, 325–327
functional layouts for nonrepetitive processes, designing, 324–325
organizations and quality improvement resources, 310–311
process and layout, relationship, 322–327
process design, 311–312. *See also* design principles
product layouts for repetitive processes, designing, 323–324
relationship diagramming, 325
secondary sources of information, 310–311
"top box" score, 93
total processing time, 160
total productive maintenance (TPM), 49, 314, 372, 380–381
benefits of, 381
cost benefits, 381
human benefits, 381
quality benefits, 381
speed benefits, 381
types of maintenance, 380

total quality management (TQM), 19–22
  in a hospital, 19
  Deming wheel, 20
  Deming's 14 points, 20–22
  process(es), 18–19
  productive system, 18
TPM. *See* total productive maintenance
TQM. *See* total quality management
tracer methodology, 395
transfer, 339
transport, 36
triage, 339
triple constraint, 124

u-charts, 240–243
undercapacity scheduling, 322
understanding conversations, 35
underutilization, 36
unstructured personal interviews, 91
U.S. healthcare system, 5–7
  national health spending, 6
usage-based maintenance, 380

value, 3
value-added activities and waste, 158–159
value-based care, 4
  care delivery models, 9–10
  current threats to, 4–8
    high costs, 4–7
    inadequate quality, 7–8. *See also* quality issues in value-based care
  direct-to-employer arrangements, 11
  green healthcare, 11
  health co-creation, 11
  increasing approaches, 8–12
  information technology, 11
  innovation centers, 11
  insurers' roles in care delivery, 10
  long pursuit of, 4
  mergers and acquisitions, 10
  new opportunities, 10–12
  population health, 11
  six aims, 8–9
value-based purchasing (VBP), 10
value categorization of process activities, 159
value stream, 157
value stream map (VSM), 38, 157, 159–164, 338–339
  admission, 339
  all areas of waste, identifying and listing, 161
    delays, 161
    errors/defects, 161
    variation, 163
  capacity at each process step, entering, 160
  delays and transports involved in the process, 160
  discharge, 339
  exam by provider, 339
  exam rooms, 339
  future state, 340
  imaging, 339
  lab, 339
  list of opportunities for improvement, developing, 163
  medication, 339
  phlebotomist, 339
  process steps, identifying, 160
  registration, 338
  relevant process data, entering, 160
  steps in, 159–160
  storage of linen and supplies, 339
  transfer, 339
  triage, 339
  value-added time or process efficiency, computing the percentage of, 160
variability or dispersion, 200
variables, 230
variance, 201–202
  population variance, 201
  sample variance, 201
variation, 46, 225–227
  assignable causes of, 225–226
  common or random causes of, 226–227
  nonrandom variation, 46
  process variation, 225
  random variation, 46
VBP. *See* value-based purchasing
visual management (VM), 372, 381
  benefits of, 381
  tools, 41
visual workplace, 381
vital few, 99–100
VM. *See* visual management
VOC. *See* voice of the customer
voice of the customer (VOC), 81–82, 90–96
  capturing, 83
  data collection methods, 91–93
  focus group interviews, 91
  perceived healthcare quality, dimensions of, 96
  qualitative research data collection methods, 91
  semistructured personal interviews, 91
  SERVQUAL survey instrument, 95–96
  translating VOC into VOP, 83, 109
  unstructured personal interviews, 91
voice of the process (VOP), 81–82, 97–99, 405
  outcome indicators, 99
  outcomes, 97
  process, 97–98
  structure, 97–98
VOP. *See* voice of the process
VSM. *See* value stream map

waiting, 36
Walmart's Centers of Excellence Program, 68
waste, 34, 36–37
  defects, errors, 36
  elimination, 36–37, 47–49
  extra processing, 36

    inventory, 36
    motion, 36
    overproduction, 36
    transport, 36
    underutilization, 36
    waiting, 36
WBS. *See* work breakdown structure
Wellstar Paulding Hospital (WPH), 403
White Belts, 50
wording, 117–118
work breakdown structure (WBS), 124, 132
    for Bright Angel's ED throughput improvement project, 134–135
workforce, 405
workload leveling (*heijunka*), 318–319
WPH. *See* Wellstar Paulding Hospital

x-axis, 187
$\overline{X}$ chart, 249–251, 253–255

y-axis, 187
y-intercept, 292
Yellow Belts, 50
yield, 166–169, 353
    first pass yield (FPY), 166
    rolled throughput yield (RTY), 166
    throughput yield (TPY), 166